Atlas of

Sexually Transmitted Diseases and AIDS

Second Edition

Atlas of
Sexually Transmitted Diseases and AIDS

Second Edition

EDITORS

Stephen A. Morse, MSPH, PhD
Associate Director for Science
Division of AIDS, Sexually Transmitted Diseases and
Tuberculosis Laboratory Research
Center for Infectious Diseases
Centers for Disease Control and Prevention
1600 Clifton Road
Atlanta, GA 30333
USA

Adele A. Moreland, MD
Olmsted Medical Group
210 Ninth Street
Rochester
Minnesota, 55903
USA

King K. Holmes, MD, PhD
Director, University of Washington Center for AIDS and STDs
1001 Broadway
Seattle,
Washington, 98122,
USA

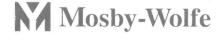 Mosby-Wolfe

London Baltimore Barcelona Bogotá Boston Buenos Aires Caracas Carlsbad, CA Chicago Madrid Mexico City Milan Naples, FL New York Philadelphia St. Louis Seoul Singapore Sydney Taipei Tokyo Toronto Wiesbaden

Published in 1996 by Mosby-Wolfe, an imprint of Times Mirror International Publishers Limited.

Printed by Grafos S.A. Arte sobre papel, Barcelona, Spain.

ISBN 0-7234-2143-9

For full details of all Mosby-Wolfe titles please write to Times Mirror International Publishers Ltd, Lynton House, 7–12 Tavistock Square, London WC1H 9LB, England.

A CIP catalogue record for this book is available from the British Library.

Library of Congress Cataloging-in-Publication data has been applied for.

This book should not be used as a prime source for prescribing and dispensing drugs. The publisher, editor, and contributors have undertaken reasonable endeavours to check dosage for accuracy. We recommend that the reader should always check the manufacturer's product information for changes in dosage or administration before administering any medication.

Project Manager:	Louise Crowe
Development Editor:	Jennifer Prast
Designer:	Lara Last
Layout Artist:	Rob Curran
Illustrations Manager:	Lynda Payne
Illustrator:	Maurice Murphy
Production:	Jane Tozer
Indexer:	Cathy Croom
Publisher:	Richard Furn

PREFACE

Even a lifetime of clinical experience does not produce an expert clinician. The expert must also sort out the wheat from the chaff in the accelerating number of changes in many clinical and laboratory disciplines. The bewildered beginner needs a practical synthesis of the essential facts, the classical and typical clinical manifestations, and the most useful techniques, tests, and therapy. We thank each of the authors of this *Atlas*, who were selected on the basis of their outstanding reputations as clinicians and teachers. It is gratifying how they have been able to combine succinct text with a wealth of photographs and helpful illustrations to distill essential, practical information into a uniquely accessible format. Specialists and generalists alike, can literally complete the book in a day, and like the editor, will learn dozens of important new findings and approaches (while relearning many old ones!). They will find this a very useful resource to return to, again and again. The student or trainee will be surprised at how easy it is to understand and assimilate new information, because it is so richly illustrated and so clearly presented. When finished with the *Atlas*, they will have acquired a broad and solid foundation from which to pass board examinations, and to go on to become expert clinicians themselves.

King K. Holmes

ACKNOWLEDGEMENTS

We would like to recognise and express deep gratitude to Sumner E. (Sam) Thompson, MD, and Sidney Olanksy, MD, for their inspiration, teaching, clinical expertise, and hard work. Dr Thompson inspired us to tackle the project and was a coeditor of the first edition of this *Atlas of Sexually Transmitted Diseases*. His contributions as author and as editor are deeply embedded within the second edition. His clinical vision inspires physicians, medical students, and clinicians at Emory and its affiliates. Dr Sidney Olanski transmitted his vast knowledge and love of dermatology and syphililogy to all those that he taught. His long associations at the Fulton County Health Department in conjunction with his teaching in the dermatology department at Emory University provided a great deal of the inspiration and interest in STDs at Emory that ultimately resulted in this book. We would also like to express special thanks to the physicians, staff, and patients at the Fulton County Health Department in Atlanta, Georgia, for their teaching patience and generosity.

Stephen A. Morse, Adele A. Moreland, and King K. Holmes

CONTENTS

CONTRIBUTORS

Miriam J. Alter PhD
Chief, Epidemiology Section
Hepatitis Branch
Division of Viral and Rickettsial Diseases
National Center for Infectious Diseases
Centers for Disease Control and Prevention
1600 Clifton Road
Atlanta, GA 30333
USA

Robert J. Arko, DVM
Assistant Chief, Gonorrhea, Chlamydia, and Chancroid Branch
Division of AIDS, Sexually Transmitted Diseases and Tuberculosis
Laboratory Research
National Center for Infectious Diseases
Centers for Disease Control and Prevention
1600 Clifton Road
Atlanta, GA 30333
USA

Ronald C. Ballard, PhD
Director, National Reference Center for Sexually Transmitted Diseases
South African Institute for Medical Research
2000 Johannesburg
South Africa

Robert C. Barnes, MD
800 Chestnut Street
Bellingham, WA 98225
USA

Consuelo Beck-Sague, MD
Assistant Chief, Treponemal Pathogenesis and Immunobiology Branch
Division of AIDS, Sexually Transmitted Diseases and Tuberculosis
Laboratory Research
National Center for Infectious Diseases
Centers for Disease Control and Prevention
1600 Clifton Road
Atlanta, GA 30333
USA

John Bryan, MD
Professor
Department of Pathology and Laboratory Medicine
Emory University School of Medicine
Director, Division of Laboratory Medicine
Emory University Hospital
Atlanta GA 30322
USA

Gail H. Cassell, MS, PhD
Professor and Chairman
Department of Microbiology
University of Alabama at Birmingham
Birmingham, AL 35294
USA

Sharon Hillier, PhD
Department of Obstetrics, Gynecology and Reproductive Sciences
University of Pittsburgh School of Medicine
Pittsburgh, PA 15261
USA

Catherine Ison, PhD
Senior Lecturer
Department of Medical Microbiology
St Mary's Medical School
Norfolk Place
Paddington
London W2 1PG
UK

Peggy Keen, MD
Grady Memorial Hospital
80 Butler Street
Atlanta, GA 30335
USA

Joan S. Knapp, PhD
Chief, Gonorrhea, Chlamydia, and Chancroid Branch
Division of AIDS, Sexually Transmitted Diseases, and Tuberculosis
Laboratory Research
National Center for Infectious Disease
Centers for Disease Control and Prevention
1600 Clifton Road
Atlanta, GA 30333
USA

Sandra A. Larsen, PhD
Chief, Treponemal Pathogenesis and Immunobiology Branch Division of
AIDS, Sexually Transmitted Diseases, and Tuberculosis Laboratory Research
National Center for Infectious Diseases
Centers for Disease Control and Prevention
1600 Clifton Road
Atlanta, GA 30333
USA

Joel S. Lewis, MS
Research Microbiologist
Treponemal Pathogenesis and Immunobiology Branch
Division of AIDS, Sexually Transmitted Diseases and Tuberculosis
Laboratory Research
National Center for Infectious Diseases
Centers for Diseases Control and Prevention
1600 Clifton Road
Atlanta, GA 30333
USA

John G. Long, MD, MPH
Consulting Physician
Division of Pediatric Infectious Diseases
Scottish Rite Children's Medical Center
Atlanta, GA
USA

Bhagirath Majmudar, MD
Professor of Pathology and Associate Professor of Obstetrics and
Gynecology
Department of Pathology
Emory University Hospital
Atlanta, Georgia 30322
USA

Marilynne McKay, MD
Professor of Dermatology and Gynecology/Obstetrics
Emory University School of Medicine
Atlanta, Georgia 30322
USA

Adele A. Moreland, MD
Olmsted Medical Group
210 Ninth Street
Rochester
Minnesota, 55903
USA

Stephen A. Morse, MSPH, PhD
Associate Director for Science
Division of AIDS, Sexually Transmitted Diseases and Tuberculosis
Laboratory Research Center for Infectious Diseases
Centers for Disease Control and Prevention
1600 Clifton Road
Atlanta, GA 30333
USA

Jorma Paavonen, MD
Department of Obstetrics and Gynecology
Naisden Clinic
Haartman Street No 2
00290 Helsinki
Finland

Philip Pellett, PhD
Chief, Molecular Genetics Section
Viral Exanthems and Herpesvirus Branch
Division of Viral and Rickettsial Diseases
National Center for Infectious Dieseases
Centers for Disease Control and Prevention
1600 Clifton Road
Atlanta, GA 30333
USA

Roselyn J. Rice, MD
Office of Minority Health
National Center for Infectious Diseases
Centers for Disease Control and Prevention
1600 Clifton Road
Atlanta, GA 30333
USA

Samuel K. Sarafian, PhD
1802 McClendon Ave.
Altanta, GA 30307
USA

Julius Schachter, PhD
Professor of Epidemiology and Laboratory Medicine
Department of Laboratory Medicine
University of California at San Francisco
San Francisco, CA 94143
USA

Stephen D. Shafran, MD, FRCPC
Division of Infectious Diseases
University of Alberta
Edmonton
Alberta
Canada T6G 2B7

Craig Shapiro, MD
Deputy Chief, Epidemiology Section
Hepatitis Branch
Division of Viral and Rickettsial Diseases
National Center for Infectious Diseases
Centers for Disease Control and Prevention
1600 Clifton Road
Atlanta, GA 30333
USA

David Spach, MD
University of Washington
Center for AIDS and STDs
1001 Broadway, Suite 206
Seattle, WA 98122
USA

David Taylor-Robinson, MD, FrcPATH
Professor of Genitourinary Microbiology and Medicine
St Mary's Hospital Medical School
Head, MRC Sexually Transmitted Diseases Research Group
St Mary's Hospital
Praed Street
London, W2 1NY
UK

Sumner E. Thompson, MD
Division of Infectious Diseases
Emory University School of Medicine
Atlanta, GA 30322
USA

Suzanne D Vernon, MD
Research Microbiologist
Viral Exanthems and Herpesvirus Branch
Division of Viral and Rickettsial Diseases
National Center for Infectious Diseases
Centers for Disease Control and Prevention
1600 Clifton Road
Atlanta, GA 30333
USA

Ken B. Waites, MD
Department of Pathology
University of Alabama at Birmingham
Birmingham, AL 35233
USA

William Whittington
University of Washington Center for AIDS and STDs
1001 Broadway
Seattle
Washington 98122
USA

CHAPTER ONE

Genital Anatomy and Dermatologic Examination

A Moreland and M McKay

INTRODUCTION

Skin changes (cutaneous disorders) of the genital skin may be assumed either by patient or physician to be of a sexually transmitted nature because of their location. This chapter will review genital anatomy and examination, and general principles of dermatologic examination. The latter will include common cutaneous disorders of the genitalia that are not sexually transmitted, but that may be seen in a sexually transmitted disease (STD) clinic or be mistaken for a STD.

GENITAL ANATOMY AND EXAMINATION

The examination of both the male and female genital region should begin below the umbilicus at the mons pubis. It is generally unsatisfactory to try to evaluate a partially clothed patient, because important ancillary findings (e.g. lymph nodes) may be missed. The patient should be undressed below the waist and gowned or draped; the gloved physician then exposes the lower abdomen and genitalia in a systematic manner. Inspect the inguinal folds, noting erythema or scaling and palpating for nodes. Exam table stirrups afford better visualization of the genitalia and perianal area in either sex, and should be used if available. Examine pubic hair for nits and look for papules of molluscum contagiosum, folliculitis, human papillomavirus (HPV), or scabies burrows. Other skin lesions such as blisters (herpesvirus, HSV) or scaly plaques (tinea, syphilis) should be noted, as well as ulcerations anywhere on the genitalia. At the inferior midline near the male penis or female clitoris, the hair becomes more sparse.

MALE GENITAL EXAMINATION

Penis and Scrotum

Male genital anatomy is shown in *Fig. 1.1*. Deep pigmentation is usual on the shaft of the penis and the hair is almost absent. A few minute yellowish papules may be seen (*Fig. 1.2*). These are pilosebaceous units (sometimes a vestigial hair and its associated oil gland). Sweat glands are also present on the base, shaft and glans of the penis

The redundant prepuce (foreskin) projects over the glans where sebaceous glands (of Tyson) secrete a keratinous material called smegma which may accumulate between the prepuce and gland in an uncircumcised male. The inner surface of the prepuce has a moist appearance, much like a mucous membrane. Scattered sebaceous glands empty directly to the surface of the glans and are not associated with hair follicles.

The ridge encircling and bordering the glans is called the corona and the sulcus below it the coronal sulcus. A varying number of smooth or slightly pebbly flesh-colored papules in one or two orderly rows may rim some or all of the corona; these are a normal variant called 'pearly penile papules'. They may be mistaken for condylomata (HPV) but histologically are angiofibromas (*Fig. 1.3*). The urethral meatus is usually located on the posterior or undersurface of the glans and should be carefully examined for discharge, ulcers, or growths such as condylomata.

The skin of the scrotum is thin and more deeply pigmented than the surrounding skin. Scrotal skin is closely adherent to the underlying dartos muscle, which gives it a rugose wrinkled appearance with contraction of the muscle (e.g. at rest in younger individuals, and in the cold at all ages). The scrotum has numerous pilosebaceous, eccrine and apocrine glands. Hair is sparse and coarse.

Fig. 1.1 Male genitals.

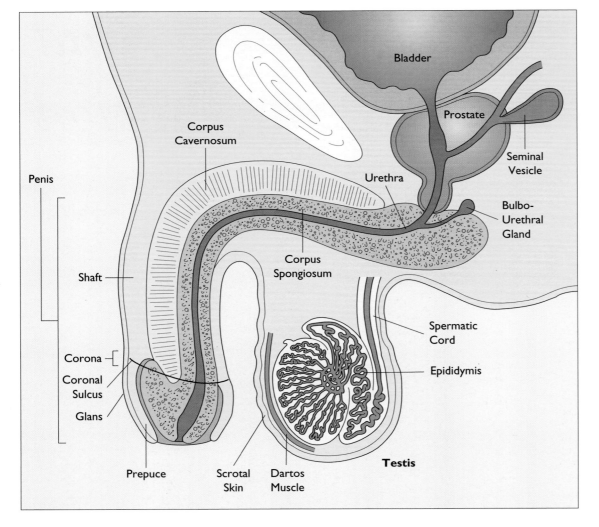

Gentle palpation of the testes, spermatic cord and epididymis within the scrotal sac will reveal any tenderness or masses which may indicate infection. Raise the scrotum to examine the perineal skin between the scrotum and the anus. Sparse, coarse hair covers the skin up to the anal mucosa and sweat and sebaceous glands are present.

Anus and Rectum

The folds of the anus are hairless and pale and should be examined for hemorrhoids, fissures, ulcers, erosions, and growths. By gentle pressure with a gloved finger the rectal mucosa can be palpated for tenderness, ulcers, discharge, or masses beyond the anal sphincter.

FEMALE GENITAL EXAMINATION

The Vulva

The female genitalia are shown in *Fig. 1.4*. The commonest diagnostic error in evaluation of the vulva is failure to systematically examine the area. Proceed from the labia majora inward, and routinely perform the examination in the same way for all genital complaints to assure recognition of the range of normal anatomic variations. During the examination, the physician can reassure the patient by verbalizing normal findings, and an office hand-mirror may help communication between patient and physician regarding specific areas of concern.

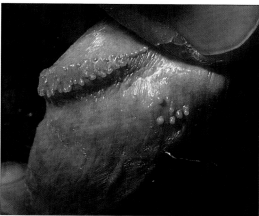

Fig. 1.3 'Pearly penile papules.' A normal variant, these tiny papules are sometimes mistaken for condylomata.

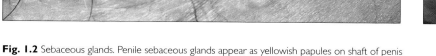

Fig. 1.2 Sebaceous glands. Penile sebaceous glands appear as yellowish papules on shaft of penis and may also be present on the scrotum. These may be quite prominent on some individuals.

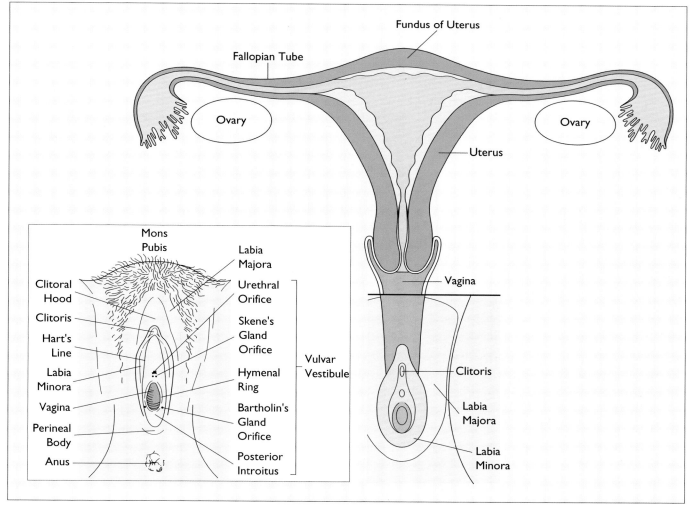

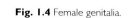

Fig. 1.4 Female genitalia.

The Labia Majora

The plump paired labia majora fuse anteriorly at the mons pubis and posteriorly merge with the perineal area. They are bounded laterally by the intertriginous folds and are covered by coarse hair. Sweat and sebaceous glands are present. Abnormal findings or signs of infection may be difficult to see because of the pubic hair.

The Labia Minora

In addition to the pigmentation of the outer labia minora, there are two other normal findings which can confuse the untrained examiner. First are the normal smooth yellowish 'pebbly' papules that are most numerous at the outer edges of the labia minora. These are sebaceous glands and normally occur along the outer minora and inner majora (*Fig. 1.5*). Under the clitoral hood, sebaceous secretions called smegma may accumulate. The sebaceous glands usually stop about halfway along the surface of the inner minora, and this line (Hart's line) demarcates mucosal from squamous epithelium (*see Fig. 1.4*). Patients sometimes mistake these papules for vesicles or pustules and become concerned. In some cases, the sebaceous glands give rise to inclusion cysts; small ones are called milia and larger ones develop into epidermoid cysts. If they are not symptomatic, they can be ignored.

The second normal variant is the presence of small, often asymptomatic, cutaneous papillae on the inner labia minora, especially at the posterior vaginal introitus (*Fig. 1.6*). Longer papillae in the posterior introitus have been described as a normal variant and a rough, papillomatous labial mucosal surface often becomes more prominent in inflammatory conditions or lichenification. The clinician should be careful not to overdiagnose benign papillomatosis as 'subclinical HPV'. Condylomatous HPV lesions in the posterior introitus are typically plaque-like and are relatively easy to differentiate from the delicate stalk-like papillae.

Some investigations of vulval mucosal papillae initially implicated HPV infection, especially when magnified inspection of papillomatous epithelium revealed an associated mosaic or punctate vascular pattern with capillaries extending into individual papillae. Since there might not have been either a history of previous infection nor obvious condylomata acuminata, it was suggested that papillomatosis represented 'subclinical' HPV infection. Subsequent studies using polymerase chain reaction (PCR) technology have made this assumption valid.

The Vulvar Vestibule

The vestibule is the inner portion of the vulva extending from Hart's line on the labia minora inward to the hymenal ring. Within the vestibule are located the urethral meatus and the openings of Skene's and Bartholin's glands (*Fig. 1.4*). Smaller minor mucous glands are found throughout the vestibule, mostly in the posterior fourchette and in the groove at the base of the hymenal ring, where they may be seen as tiny pit-like openings. Vulvar vestibulitis should be suspected by the patient's complaint of significant and persistent entry dyspareunia and discomfort at the opening of the vagina. The diagnosis is made by finding erythema and point tenderness upon palpation of the gland orifice with a cotton-tipped applicator.

Visible changes (plaques, scarring, thickening) should be biopsied, preferably in the thickest portion of a lesion. Acetowhitening (application of vinegar or 3–5% acetic acid for 1–2 minutes) can be used to highlight thickened areas if there is a history of HPV. If HPV infection is found on the vulva, colposcopy of the vagina and cervix is recommended; if on the anus, proctoscopy. Biopsies should be performed on any diagnostically questionable areas, especially if intraepithelial neoplasia is suspected, but biopsies are rarely helpful for nonspecific inflammation or vestibulitis. Findings such as koilocytosis without obvious condylomata should be considered nonspecific; many women with this histology are asymptomatic and others with vulvar burning have no evidence of HPV.

The Vagina and Cervix

Before inserting a speculum into the vagina, gentle pressure with two fingers on the posterior fourchette relaxes the muscles at the vaginal opening. To view the vagina, a warm speculum of proper size, moistened with water, should be inserted with the blades closed and positioned obliquely. The blades are then slipped horizontally and opened slowly.

The moist vaginal mucosal lining is erythematous and has a slightly irregular surface. Numerous transverse and longitudinal folds give the vaginal canal a rugose appearance. The cervix appears at the end of the vaginal vault as a firm, smooth, somewhat circular or dome-shaped mass with a central concavity, the os (*Figs 1.7–1.10*), which is the entrance to the endocervical canal. Notations of vaginal discharges, lesions, or ulcers, and cervical mucosal abnormalities, ectropion, or lacerations should be made. Before the speculum is removed, samples can be obtained for cytology, cultures, and other diagnostic tests, and direct microscopy of vaginal and cervical secretions.

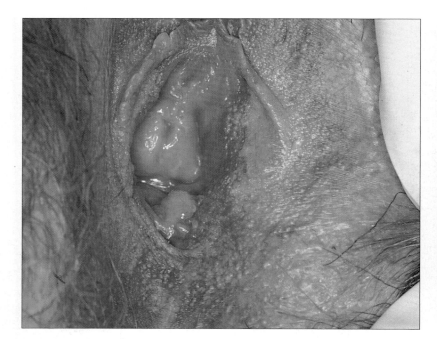

Fig. 1.5 Normal vulva with finely textured papular sebaceous glands on the inner labia majora and labia minora. In this case, glands are confluent over the outer minora, producing an almost white appearance. By contrast, the vestibular mucosa inside Hart's line appears red, although this is normal coloration. There is much individual variation in the size and distribution of genital sebaceous glands, but in general, they decrease in number with age.

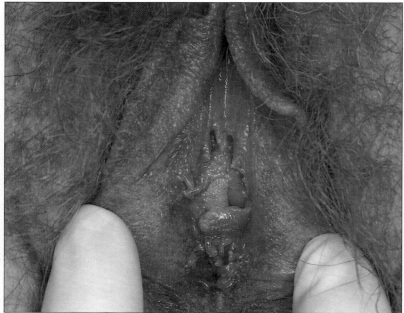

Fig. 1.6 Normal vulva with prominent vestibular papillae on the mucosa inside Hart's line and at the posterior fourchette. Although they are frequently mistaken for condylomata, biopsied papillae are typically negative for human papillomavirus (HPV). HPV lesions are usually more keratotic and less translucent than papillae; the latter are often symmetrical and/or linear on both sides of the vulva, unlike condylomata. No treatment is necessary.

Bimanual Examination

The middle and index fingers of one hand should be inserted along the posterior vaginal wall after the speculum is withdrawn. The cervix is then lifted toward the abdominal wall and the opposite hand presses down to palpate the uterus, which can be gently moved to determine presence of tenderness or tumors. The ovaries and Fallopian tubes (adnexa) are found laterally or posterolaterally to the uterus. Bimanual palpation will usually ascertain tenderness and presence of masses. A clean glove should be used for the rectovaginal examination. The examining finger is gently placed into the anal opening and when the sphincter is relaxed the examination can comfortably proceed. The index finger is placed into the vagina and the middle finger into the rectum to palpate the posterior uterine and vaginal structures. Rectal hemorrhoids, polyps, and tumors can be observed and noted.

PRINCIPLES OF DERMATOLOGIC EXAMINATION OF THE GENITALIA

Although it is traditional to classify and discuss infectious diseases and conditions with respect to etiology, this approach has significant shortcomings when applied to cutaneous disorders. A 3 mm papule, for example, can be a congenital nevus, a benign or malignant neoplasm, or the result of infection with a bacteria, a virus, or a fungus. Since the skin lesion itself is the usual starting point for the development of a differential diagnosis, the traditional dermatologic approach is to seek out a so-called 'primary lesion', one that recreates the pathophysiology of the disease process. This usually implies a search for a fresh, fully developed lesion, rather than one that has dried,

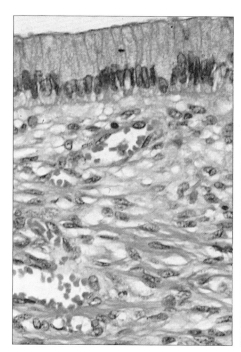

Fig. 1.7 Normal cervix. The squamocolumnar junction is seen and also the lower part of the endocervical canal.(See also **4.27**.)

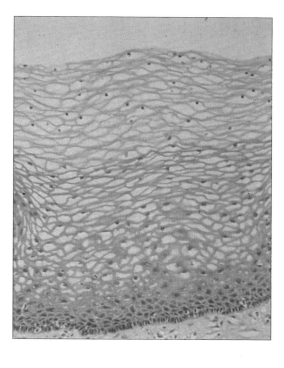

Fig. 1.8 Stratified squamous epithelium covers the ectocervix. Like those of the vagina, the cells are rich in glycogen during the period of sexual maturity.

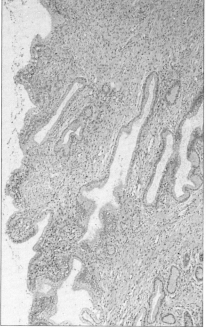

Fig. 1.9 (Left) the endocervical canal is lined by a single layer of tall columnar mucus-secreting epithelium. (Right) numerous deep invaginations of the mucus-secreting epithelium extend into the cervical stroma and greatly increase the surface for mucus production.

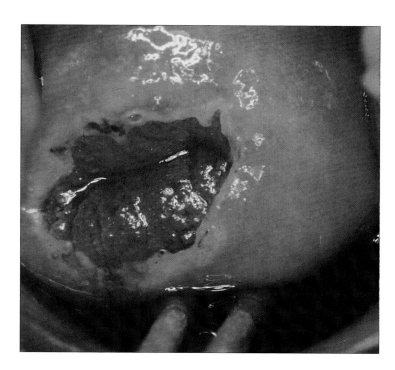

Fig. 1.10 Colposcopy. Ectopy showing early squamous metaplasia. (See also **4.28**.)

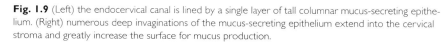

crusted, been scratched, or become secondarily infected. In addition to describing the morphology of the primary process, observation of the distribution and configuration of the lesions on the skin helps to identify the disorder, as it may be one of many dermatoses that are more easily identified by finding similar lesions on other areas of the body.

With these principles in mind and for the purpose of this discussion, the nonvenereal genital dermatoses will be grouped into seven different morphologic categories. Six of these are defined by the primary lesion, such as pustules, pigmentary disorders, and dermatitis. The seventh category, erosions and ulcers, deals with the so-called 'minus' lesions, wherein the original morphology has been altered by the loss of superficial epidermis (erosion) or of the entire skin surface itself (ulcer). This latter category may be difficult to assess, for normal morphologic clues to differential diagnosis frequently are absent.

The final category is itching, defined by the symptom. This section will discuss evaluation of pruritus ani, scrota, and vulvae.

Dermatitis/Eczema

The term dermatitis simply means inflammation of the skin. The Greek root eczema, which means 'boiling over or out', is remarkably descriptive of the oozing, wet appearance of dermatitic skin. Eczemas characteristically are pruritic. The patient complains of itching, and scratch marks (excoriations) may be seen on the skin surface. Dermatitis typically changes its appearance over time. The first sign simply may be erythema, which is followed by a pebbly appearance to the skin surface that rapidly evolves into small blisters which may ooze and crust (*Fig. 1.11*). As dermatitis evolves, the skin becomes thickened, leathery, and often

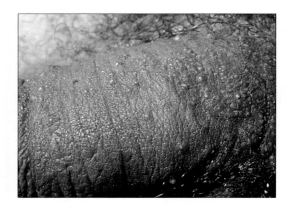

Fig. 1.11 Allergic contact dermatitis of the penis due to spermicidal jelly. Note the typical appearance of microvesicles on the glans penis. This patient complained of pruritus and rash developing approximately 2 days after use of the product.

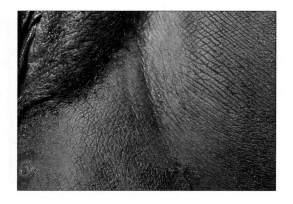

Fig. 1.12 Lichenification of intertriginous skin as a result of chronic rubbing and scratching with an ulcer due to scratching (excoriation).

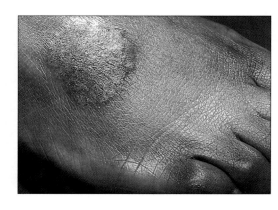

Fig. 1.13 Lichen simplex chronicus on the foot. The hallmark of this diagnosis is the leathery appearance of the skin.

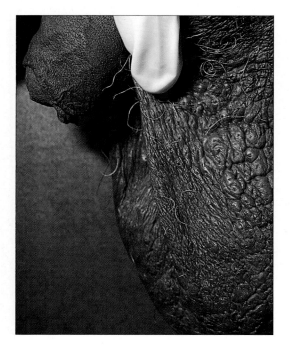

Fig. 1.14 Lichen simplex chronicus of the scrotum. The accentuation of normal skin markings is shown clearly. The inguinal area is hyperpigmented — a milder sign of continuous rubbing.

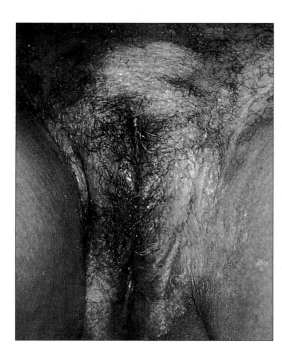

Fig. 1.15 Vulvar lichen simplex chronicus. The extensiveness of the area involved suggests that pruritus has been present for several months or more. The skin is lichenified, scaly, and in some areas hyperpigmented.

scaly, with increased skin markings. These findings are the hallmark of lichenification (*Fig. 1.12*) and are even more important than scaling in making this diagnosis. The patient's rubbing or scratching of the initial condition will increase the likelihood of lichenification, which persists long after the original insult has been removed. Acute dermatitis, then, is seen as a plaque that is erythematous, edematous, and oozing; chronic dermatitis is a plaque that may be purplish, hyperpigmented, and lichenified. In the latter case, the patient is said to have lichen simplex chronicus, a descriptive term that indicates only that the patient has a plaque of thickened skin that has been rubbed or scratched. Any area of the body may be involved (*Fig. 1.13*), but genital skin is a common area of involvement (*Figs. 1.14* and *1.15*). Some underlying skin conditions, such as atopic dermatitis, may make it more likely that the patient will develop areas of lichen simplex chronicus. In other cases, the skin reaction is due to something that has come in contact with the epidermis. The offending substance may be an irritant such as urine or a true allergen. Neomycin and benzocaine are relatively common allergens found in nonprescription topical medications. These medications may be self-prescribed by patients or prescribed by physicians to treat both pruritus and any type of irritation, abrasion, or ulcer.

Papulosquamous Disorders

The papulosquamous dermatoses, as the name implies, are characterized by papules and plaques that typically have a scaly surface. While a plaque of lichen simplex chronicus might fit this description, it should be noted that lichenification is *secondary* to rubbing and scratching of the affected skin. The papulosquamous dermatoses, on the other hand, begin with a scaly papule as the primary lesion. Of all dermatologic disorders, probably the most commonly encountered are those in the papulosquamous category, and it is important for the clinician to develop a logical approach to the differential diagnosis of these problems (*Fig. 1.16*).

The acute onset of a pruritic annular lesion anywhere on the body, especially in intertriginous areas, should raise the suspicion of a dermatophyte (*Fig. 1.17*) infection. Scraping a bit of scale from the border of a lesion and

DIFFERENTIAL DIAGNOSIS OF COMMON PAPULOSQUAMOUS DERMATOSES

CONDITION	ERYTHEMA	SKIN CHANGES THICKENING	PRURITUS	ASSOCIATED LESIONS
Psoriasis	++	+++	+/–	Red plaques with silvery scale on knees, elbows, scalp. Nail pitting. Little or no scaling on genital psoriasis.
Seborrheic dermatitis	++	+	+	Scaling/erythema on eyebrows, nasolabial folds, hairline, occasionally on axillae, inguinal folds, or genitals.
Dermatophyte (tinea cruris)	++	Raised border	++	Annular plaque with central clearing and peripheral scale. KOH shows hyphae.
Candidiasis	++	Edema	+++	Acute erythema, edema, peeling, satellite pustules. Gram stain shows budding yeast.
Lichen simplex chronicus	++	+++	+++	May be limited to vulva; other common sites are ankle, nape of neck, arm.
Chronic dermatitis (contact or irritant)	+++	++	++	Often eczematous and oozing. May involve congruent areas, eyelids. May generalize.
Lichen planus	Violaceous	++	++	Purple polygonal papules and plaques, especially on wrists and legs. Lacy white pattern on buccal mucosa.
Lichen sclerosus and mixed dystrophy	+	–	+/–	Usually limited to vulva, anus ('keyhole' pattern). White, and nonscaly. Dermis thick, epidermis atrophic.

Fig. 1.16 Differential diagnosis of common papulosquamous dermatoses.

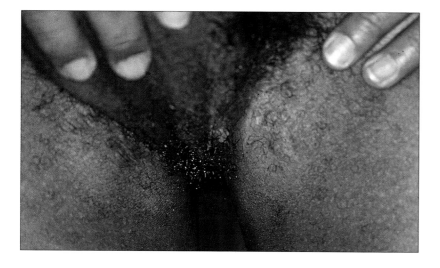

Fig. 1.17 Tinea cruris. Erythema and scaling associated with pruritus are typical features of a dermatophyte infection. Scrapings for potassium hydroxide (KOH) and fungal cultures should be taken from the leading edge of the involved skin, even though scaling there may be minimal.

examining it under 10–20% potassium hydroxide (KOH) solution will allow the visualization of fungal hyphae *(Figs. 1.18–1.21)*. Dermatophyte infections are more common in men than in women, but the latter are more likely to develop candidal infections, usually as a result of spread from the vagina (see section on pustular disorders, p. 13). Griseofulvin is effective only for dermatophytes and nystatin only for *Candida*, but the imidazole antifungals are effective treatment for both dermatophyte and candidal infections. Annular lesions also may occur in secondary syphilis, but syphilis only rarely itches, and no hyphae can be seen on KOH and, of course, the serology is positive. Psoriasis is another commonly encountered papulosquamous disorder

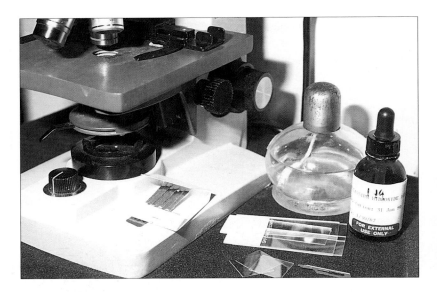

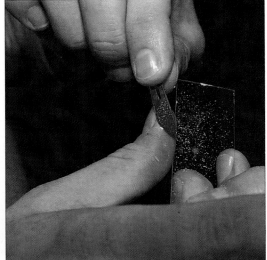

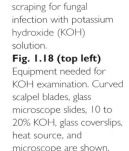

Figs. 1.18–1.21 Examination of skin scraping for fungal infection with potassium hydroxide (KOH) solution.
Fig. 1.18 (top left) Equipment needed for KOH examination. Curved scalpel blades, glass microscope slides, 10 to 20% KOH, glass coverslips, heat source, and microscope are shown.
Fig. 1.19 (top right) A curved scalpel blade allows gentle scraping of the skin with minimal trauma. The scale should be collected directly onto a glass slide and the coverslip applied.
Fig. 1.20 (lower left) KOH applied by dropper to the edge of the covered specimen allows it to penetrate under the coverslip by capillary action. The slide is gently warmed, without boiling, to allow clearing of the specimen. The alcohol lamp produces a cleaner flame than do matches.
Fig. 1.21 (lower right) Microscopic view of branched hyphae among cleared keratinocytes as they appear in a positive KOH preparation.

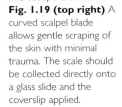

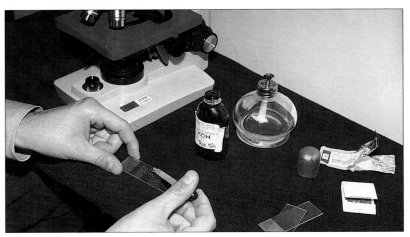

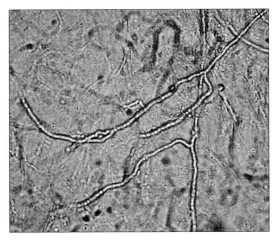

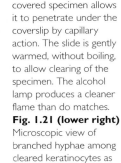

Fig. 1.22 Psoriasis. Thick reddish plaques with an adherent thick white scale are typical on nongenital skin such as the arms, elbows, knees, and scalp.

Fig. 1.23 Psoriasis of the vulva. The typical thick scale seen here is sometimes absent when psoriasis occurs on the genital skin, leaving erythematous patches and plaques with a more macerated and moist scale, or with no scale at all.

with a distinct familial association, even though many patients are unaware of family members with psoriasis. Typically seen as thick, red plaques with adherent white scales, psoriasis occurs most commonly on the arms (*Fig. 1.22*), knees, elbows, trunk, and sacrum, as well as the scalp. Genital lesions, however, are apt to have little if any scale, and may be seen simply as persistent intertriginous erythema (*Figs. 1.23* and *1.24*). Scaly plaques may be seen on the penis and scrotum as well as on the pubic area, and in some cases may closely resemble the papulosquamous form of secondary syphilis (see *Fig. 2.48*), with minimal involvement of the rest of the body. Fingernail pitting may lead one to suspect the diagnosis of psoriasis in a persistent genital papulosquamous disorder. A mild topical corticosteroid (hydrocortisone 1%) generally is effective in treating genital psoriasis. The use of strong fluorinated steroids on genital skin may lead to the development of striae, which are permanent and unsightly.

Seborrheic dermatitis usually is seen as scaling in the hairy areas of the body, with a more or less prominent erythematous and papular component. Most commonly diagnosed in the scalp as 'dandruff', seborrheic dermatitis also affects the eyebrows, nasolabial folds (*Fig. 1.25*), axillae, central chest, and

genital region. Women usually experience only mild erythema and scaling on the mons pubis (*Figs. 1.26* and *1.27*), but men may have erythematous plaques on the penis (*Fig. 1.28*) that are difficult to differentiate from psoriasis or secondary syphilis (see *Fig. 2.50*). Treatment with mild corticosteroids is effective in this condition, as well.

Lichen planus (classically described as purple, pruritic, polygonal papules and plaques) is not as scaly as are the above disorders. The typical areas of involvement are the flexor surfaces of the wrists, the trunk (*Fig. 1.29*), and the anterior shins. An examination of the tongue (*Fig. 1.30*) or buccal mucosa (*Fig. 1.31*) may show a lacy white pattern and sometimes erosions difficult to distinguish from *Candida* or thrush. This lacy white pattern also may be seen on genital mucosal surfaces, but violaceous papules with or without scale (*Figs. 1.32* and *1.33*) also may be seen. Treatment of lichen planus is symptomatic, with corticosteroids and, if necessary, antipruritic agents. Lichen sclerosus and the so-called mixed dystrophies (see below) may be responsible for thickened, scaly plaques appearing on the genitalia. Although these disorders are not always pruritic, itching may occur

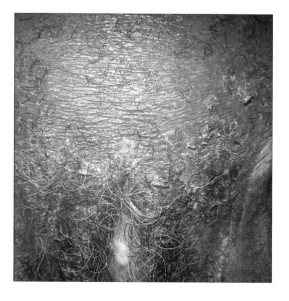

Fig. 1.24 Psoriasis of the penis. The typical intense erythema of psoriatic plaques, but with complete lack of scale, is seen in this largely intertriginous plaque of psoriasis under the foreskin.

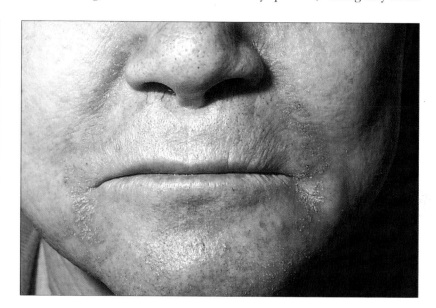

Fig. 1.25 Typical seborrheic dermatitis in the nasolabial crease. Erythema with mild scaling is seen.

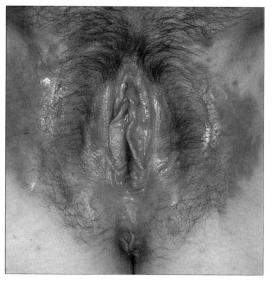

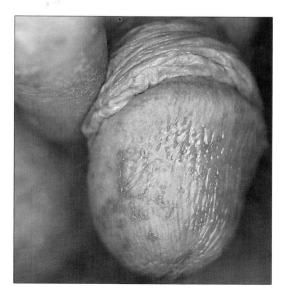

Figs. 1.26 (left) and **1.27 (right)** Seborrheic dermatitis of the vulva may present as pruritus of the vulva or mons. The skin appears red or slightly pigmented and thick 'dandruff' scales may be seen.

Fig. 1.28 Seborrheic dermatitis on the penis. Erythematous changes are sometimes difficult to differentiate from psoriasis, and may resolve with a mottled hypopigmentation.

primarily or may be secondary to medications that have been applied to the affected area. A biopsy may be necessary to differentiate lichenified dermatitis from a primarily papulosquamous disorder.

Pigmentary Disorders
Hyperpigmentation

A black macule on the genitalia is an obvious lesion of concern, for it is important to rule out *malignant melanoma* as a diagnostic possibility. Typically, however, a melanoma (*Fig. 1.34*) is a single lesion with an irregular 'notched' border with variable hyperpigmentation, which also may show areas of depigmentation within the larger macule. This malignant change should be distinguished from that of *freckle* or *lentigo* (*Fig. 1.35*) — benign macules having regular borders and smooth pigmentation. Diffuse hyperpigmentation as a result of chronic inflammation, *postinflammatory hyperpigmentation*, also can occur as multiple macules, giving a 'spotty' appearance to genital skin, especially around the vaginal introitus (*Fig. 1.36*).

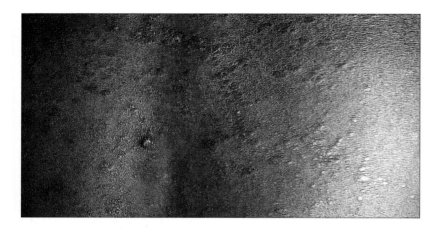

Fig. 1.29 Lichen planus on the trunk. Typical violaceous flat-topped papules are seen, some with angular borders and adherent scale in the form of Wickham's striae.

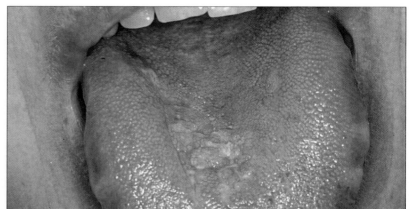

Fig. 1.30 Oral lichen planus of the tongue. Whitish plaques are seen centrally.

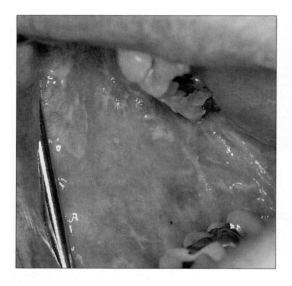

Fig. 1.31 Oral lichen planus. Thin whitish linear streaks or Wickham's striae are seen on the buccal mucosa. This is not symptomatic unless it is erosive.

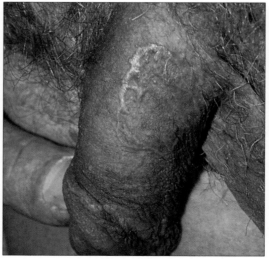

Fig. 1.32 Flesh-colored papules of lichen planus have a lacy white surface and assume an annular configuration.

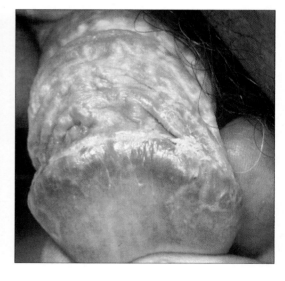

Fig. 1.33 These papules on the glans are scalier and more extensive than those in **1.32**.

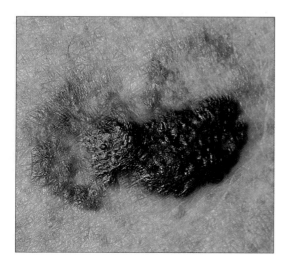

Fig. 1.34 Malignant melanoma. Note the asymmetry, irregular contours, and variable pigmentation that are the hallmarks of this malignancy.

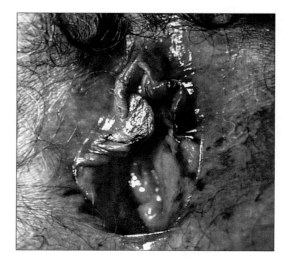

Fig. 1.35 Lentigines of the vulva. Multiple dark macules or freckles on the labia minora and vaginal introitus may appear as a result of previous inflammation, but single lesions should be evaluated carefully to rule out the possibility of malignant melanoma.

Another form of diffuse hyperpigmentation, but with a thickened velvety appearance to the skin, is that of *acanthosis nigricans*. This pigmentary change may be seen around the neck (*Fig. 1.37*), genitalia (*Fig. 1.38*), and the axillae of genetically predisposed obese individuals or in some patients with endocrine abnormalities. This 'benign' or pseudoacanthosis nigricans cannot be distinguished clinically or histologically from the form that is associated with internal malignancy, usually a gastric adenocarcinoma. Thus a thorough evaluation for malignancy should be made in patients who present with new-onset acanthosis nigricans. Unfortunately, the malignancy may be well established by the time the cutaneous changes are seen.

Hypopigmentation

By far the most common color change on the genitalia is the loss of pigment in the form of *vitiligo*. This pigment loss is quite remarkable in persons with dark complexions and may be overlooked entirely in fair-skinned people. Characteristically symmetric in distribution, it may be seen as white patches on the glans penis (*Fig. 1.39*) or as a 'keyhole' pattern around the vagina (*Fig. 1.40*) and anus. When it occurs on other areas of the body, it also is often periorificial, around the mouth, eyes (*Fig. 1.41*), and nares. Vitiligo also may develop distally over the fingers and toes, again, in a typically symmetric pattern. Asymmetric vitiligo is unusual but does occur, often in a dermatomal distribution. Some vitiligo patients have autoimmune thyroid

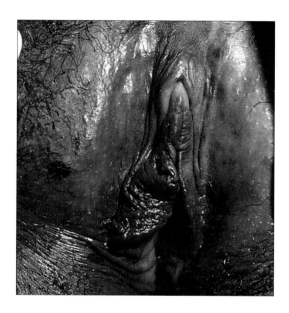

Fig. 1.36 Postinflammatory hyperpigmentation of the vulva. The spotty hyperpigmentation on the right labium majus and left labium minus seen in association with a more diffuse hypopigmentation around the clitoris and the lower introitus.

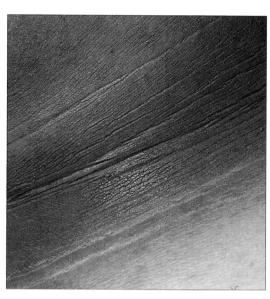

Fig. 1.37 Pseudoacanthosis nigricans of the neck. The finely papillated surface of the skin gives it a velvety appearance. This feature, in combination with hyperpigmentation, is the cardinal sign of acanthosis nigricans of any etiology.

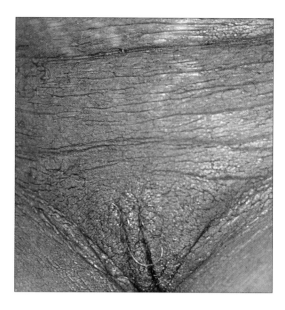

Fig. 1.38 Acanthosis nigricans of the vulva. This patient, who has extensive involvement of all intertriginous skin and of the hands and mouth, was found to have gastric adenocarcinoma — the most common cancer associated with this disorder. The acute onset of thick, velvety intertriginous plaques, hyperpigmented or not, should prompt a thorough evaluation for internal malignancy.

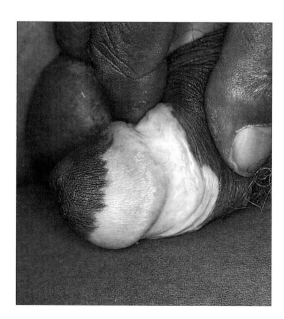

Fig. 1.39 Vitiligo of the glans penis. This is a relatively common condition, which, although asymptomatic, may be a source of great anxiety for the patient.

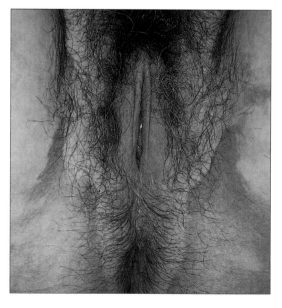

Fig. 1.40 Vitiligo of the vulva. This photograph shows the typical symmetric loss of pigmentation from the periorificial skin. Notice that the epidermis is quite normal in appearance. There is no sign of the atrophy usually associated with lichen sclerosus, which also may be hypopigmented.

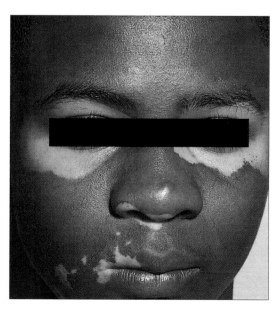

Fig. 1.41 Periorificial facial vitiligo. The patchy symmetric loss of pigmentation in vitiligo may be localized to one area of the body or it may involve many sites. In this patient, the vitiligo was confined to the face and extremities.

disorders or diabetes, but many have no systemic abnormalities. Treatment should be directed to a dermatologist, but spontaneous repigmentation has been known to occur. Post-inflammatory hypopigmentation may be seen after an episode of primary or secondary syphilis (*Fig. 1.42*), any form of genital ulcer, a dermatophyte infection, or chronic dermatitis or intertrigo (*Figs. 1.43* and *1.44*).

Atrophy

Itching or burning may be the presenting symptom in *lichen sclerosus* (*lichen sclerosus et atrophicus*). Occurring more commonly on female genitalia, this condition is seen clinically as depigmentation of the skin (*Fig. 1.45*). The atrophic epidermis shows fine 'cigarette paper' wrinkling, while the sclerotic or thickened dermis obscures normal capillary filling, giving a white appearance to the skin. Severe cases may result in complete resorption of the labia minora, and vulvar adhesions are not uncommon. The etiology of this condition is unknown, and occasionally it may be seen in young girls, in some cases resolving at puberty. Symptoms vary in such cases of lichen sclerosus, ranging from the patient's complete unawareness of the problem to severe itching and burning. The thinned epidermis is extremely friable, and petechiae or purpura may be seen as a result of scratching. When seen in the male, lichen sclerosus may cause the glans penis to have an extremely white, scarred-down appearance known as *balanitis xerotica obliterans* (*Fig. 1.46*). As with lichen sclerosus in the female, balanitis xerotica may respond to topical treatment with glucocorticoids.

In some cases, lichen sclerosus may develop discrete areas of thickened hyperkeratotic stratum corneum (*Fig. 1.47*). Several biopsies should be taken

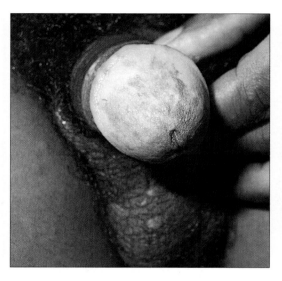

Fig. 1.42 Postinflammatory hypopigmentation and hyperpigmentation of the penis. A syphilitic chancre may have been the cause of the spotty pigmentation of the glans that appeared months prior to the development of a generalized papular eruption. This generalized eruption, visible on the penis, scrotum, and legs, proved to be a manifestation of secondary syphilis.

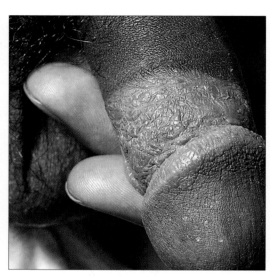

Fig. 1.43 Postinflammatory hypopigmentation of the foreskin and corona of the penis. Seborrheic dermatitis caused the pigment changes in this patient, who visited the STD clinic for this problem.

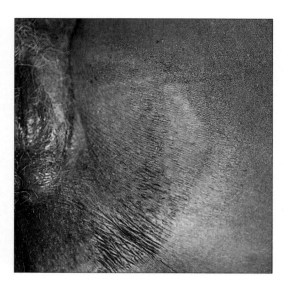

Fig. 1.44 Postinflammatory hypopigmentation and hyperpigmentation of chronic intertrigo. Pigment variations may be seen as inflammatory cutaneous conditions flare and resolve.

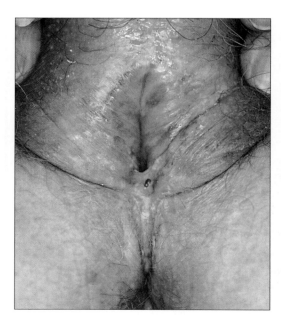

Fig. 1.45 Lichen sclerosus of the vulva. Thinning and atrophy of epidermal skin are seen with loss of architecture of the labia minora, including adhesion formation at the posterior introitus. Note the presence of erosions and petechiae secondary to mild trauma of the fragile skin.

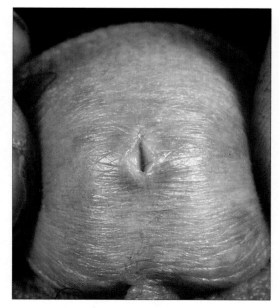

Fig. 1.46 Balanitis xerotica obliterans. Lichen sclerosus on the glans penis exhibits white atrophic patches similar to those seen on the vulva. Meatal stenosis may occur.

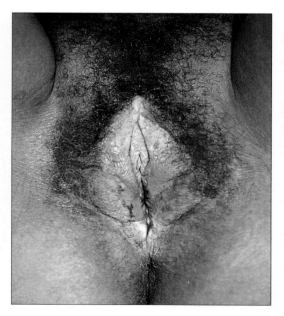

Fig. 1.47 Hypertrophic, white thickened areas of vulvar skin in association with lichen sclerosus. This patient has biopsy-proven lichen sclerosus with areas of cutaneous hyperplasia. There was no evidence of malignancy. This condition was previously called 'mixed dystrophy' of the vulva, but this terminology is no longer used.

from different areas of thickened dystrophic skin to rule out the possibility of vulvar intraepithelial neoplasia (VIN). Atrophic vaginitis may be seen in the postmenopausal woman, though cutaneous changes may consist only of mild thinning and loss of subcutaneous substance.

Pustules

Most physicians regard the presence of pustules on the skin as prima facie evidence of infection. In most cases this is true, and infection certainly should be ruled out when pus-containing papules are seen. The presence

of pus generally implies infection; however, there are certain cutaneous conditions that are characterized by the presence of aggregates of white cells that are sterile to culture for bacteria, fungi, or a virus. In the following section, we will discuss the pustular conditions of the genitalia (*Figs. 1.48* and *1.49*).

Infectious pustules

One of the most common causes of genital pustules, especially with inflammation, is cutaneous *candidiasis* or *monilia* (*Fig. 1.50*). Skin lesions generally

INFECTIOUS PUSTULAR CONDITIONS OCCURRING ON THE GENITALIA

Fig. 1.48 Infectious pustular conditions occurring on the genitalia.

CONDITION	FINDINGS	TREATMENT
Candida	Most common, itches and burns. Intense erythema; often edema, satellite lesions.	Imidazole or azole creams and suppositories. Nystatin vaginal suppositories. Oral ketoconazole or fluconazole in resistant cases — short courses.
Tinea	Serpiginous 'active' border, itchy, relatively unusual in women.	Oral griseofulvin. Topical imidazoles.
Impetigo	Usually secondary to pruritic dermatitis, excoriations, secondary bacterial colonization.	Topical antibacterial scrubs. Erythromycin or dicloxacillin.
Folliculitis	Pustules at base of hairs (rule out Gram-negative infection if patient is on antibiotics).	Erythromycin or dicloxacillin unless Gram-negative; then according to sensitivities.
Furunculosis 'boils'	Painful, deep-seated nodules may be topped by pustules; may suppurate; recurrent lesions may indicate transmission by close contact.	Early treatment with erythromycin or dicloxacillin may abort early lesions and prevent suppuration.
Herpes simplex	WBCs in old intact vesicles may cause lesions to look pustular.	Acyclovir or topical antibiotics in mild cases.
Syphilis	Scattered scaly pustules may be seen in secondary syphilis.	Penicillin: see treatment schedule in Chapter 2.

NONINFECTIOUS PUSTULAR CONDITIONS OCCURRING ON THE GENITALIA

Fig. 1.49 Noninfectious pustular conditions occurring on the genitalia.

CONDITION	FINDINGS	TREATMENT
Pseudofolliculitis	Ingrown hairs indicate mechanical trauma.	Stop shaving.
Acneiform rashes	Withdrawal of potent topical steroids; contact with oils, hydrocarbons.	Wean off with hydrocortisones. Eliminate work-related industrial exposure.
Hidradenitis suppurativa	Chronic acneiform condition with sinus tracts and scarring.	Minocin, 100 mg *po* daily. Surgical excision of affected area.
Pustular psoriasis and/or Reiter's	Often associated with arthritis; usually a previous history of disease.	Methotrexate or retinoid therapy. Refer to dermatologist.
Pemphigus	Chronic familial form (Hailey–Hailey) or acquired (pemphigus vulgaris).	Antibiotics and oral corticosteroids. Refer to dermatologist.

While the presence of pus generally implies infection, this finding is not specific. Just as there are nonpyogenic infections, there are certain pustular skin conditions not at all associated with infectious organisms. Gram stains of pustule contents should be examined for bacteria and Gram-positive budding yeast forms; KOH of the pustule roof may reveal fungal hyphae; and bacterial cultures should be done on material from cleaned, intact lesions. If lesion morphology suggests herpes, Tzanck smears and viral cultures should also be performed; dark-field examination should be done if syphilis is suspected.

are seen in conjunction with a candidal vaginitis in the female (*Fig. 1.51*). Males may also harbor the organism (*Candida albicans*) in the inguinal or gluteal folds, on the scrotum, and, especially if uncircumcised, on the penis (*Fig. 1.52*). Factors predisposing to cutaneous candidiasis include immuno-suppression, diabetes mellitus, and the administration of systemic antibi-otics. While candidal pseudohyphae sometimes may be seen on KOH examination of material from superficial intertriginous erosions, the better diagnostic tests for this organism are a Gram or PAS stain of material from a pustule. The typical budding yeast forms are Gram-positive and somewhat larger than lymphocytes (*Fig. 1.53*).

Acute inflammatory tinea infections may have a vesiculopustular scaly border (*Fig. 1.54*). KOH of blister or pustule roof will demonstrate fungal hyphae. In the presence of a chronic intertrigo, foci of dermatophyte infec-tions may remain deep in follicles, which can occasionally become nodular (Majocchi's granuloma). The diagnosis of fungal folliculitis should be con-sidered when the patient fails to respond to systemic antibiotics.

Discrete, scattered pustules in hairy areas of the body generally are caused by staphylococci and streptococci (Bockhart's impetigo). Since many cuta-neous staphylococci are penicillinase producers, treatment should be with erythromycin or with penicillinase-resistant penicillins such as dicloxacillin.

In susceptible individuals, folliculitis may develop into a larger cutaneous abscess called a *carbuncle* or a *furuncle* (*Fig. 1.55*). Typically caused by *Staphylococcus aureus*, early lesions will respond to systemic antibiotics. Most later lesions benefit from application of warm compresses until spontaneous rupture of the abscess occurs, but fully developed walled-off abscesses may require incision and drainage. Recurrent furunculosis does not necessarily imply that a patient has an immune deficiency. Phage-typing of staphylo-cocci has been used to identify cluster groups of patients who pass the infec-tion back and forth, usually in a close-living or sexually active situation. Pustules also may be seen in mixed bacterial *impetigo* (*Fig. 1.56*), an extreme-ly common skin infection that may be the result of secondary bacterial col-onization of a pre-existing dermatitis.

While the umbilicated papules of *molluscum contagiosum* (*Figs. 1.57* and *1.58*) are not actually pustules, the initial appearance of these lesions may mislead the patient and physician. Since usually they are pale or flesh-colored, they can give the appearance of pustules; however, they are actual-ly rather sturdy papules, which may persist for many weeks. The central dell or umbilication is characteristic of the viral etiology of these lesions, which

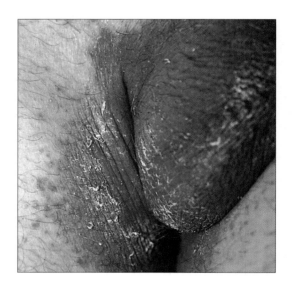

Fig. 1.50 *Candida* infection showing the intense inflammation with satellite pustules. Note that the pustules are superficial and not located at the base of hairs.

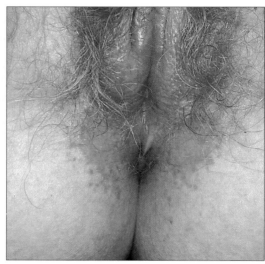

Fig. 1.51 *Candida* vulvovaginitis. Intense erythema and edema appear around the introitus, perineum, and perianal areas. The discrete erythematous macules at the active borders are resolving pustules.

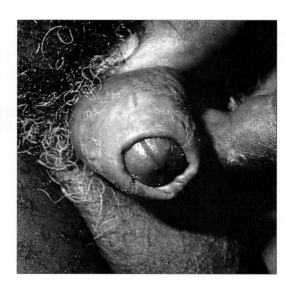

Fig. 1.52 *Candida* balanitis showing edema and erythema with satellite pustules. This is seen most commonly in uncir-cumcised males. *Candida* should be considered a sexually transmissible disease, and treatment with imidazole creams may facilitate satisfactory topical treatment of both partners.

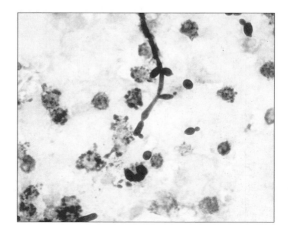

Fig. 1.53 PAS stain of budding yeast and pseudohyphae seen in *Candida albicans*.

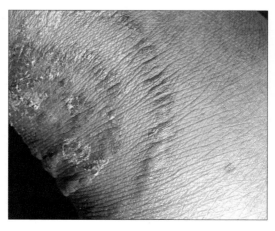

Fig. 1.54 Tinea corporis showing vesicles and pustules at the active advancing edge of a typical scaly plaque.

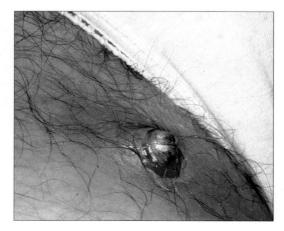

Fig. 1.55 Carbuncle on the upper thigh. A thick crust with surrounding erythema and tenderness is characteristic.

are caused by a pox virus. Therapy is directed toward destruction of the lesion, with curettage or blistering agents applied to the lesions.

Noninfectious Pustules

In most clinical situations, the presence of pus implies infection, and it is entirely appropriate to obtain bacterial, fungal, and/or viral cultures in this setting. There are certain dermatologic conditions, however, in which pustules or the accumulation of white cells in the epidermis is initiated by stimuli other than bacterial infection.

While bacterial superinfection can play an important part in *hidradenitis suppurativa* (*Figs. 1.59* and *1.60*), the mechanism of this severe acneiform eruption in the groin and/or axillae is related to occlusion of hair follicles and retention of follicular contents, resulting in an inflammatory process that includes hair follicles and sweat glands. Secondary bacterial infection is common. The presence of multiple papules, pustules, cysts, and sinus tracts is the cutaneous constellation common to cystic acne, hidradenitis, and dissecting folliculitis of the scalp, which may occur together. In some chronic cases, keloid formation may be the most prominent feature of a 'burned-

out' case of hidradenitis. Antibiotic therapy can be helpful in acute flares of this disease, and resistance to tetracycline or erythromycin should raise the suspicion of superinfection with Gram-negative organisms. Surgical excision and grafting remains the treatment of choice for recalcitrant cases, although the vitamin A analogs (e.g. isotretinoin) have shown some promise in the treatment of this distressing condition.

Pustular psoriasis (*Fig. 1.61*) may begin as groups of sterile pustules in intertriginous areas. These rapidly enlarge and spread across the trunk and extremities in waves that coalesce, forming 'lakes' of pus in the superficial epidermis. This severe form of psoriasis is associated with high fevers and malaise. It occurs primarily in patients already diagnosed with psoriasis and is seen sometimes as a result of systemic steroid therapy. Acute episodes may be difficult to manage, and generally respond best to systemic therapy with antimetabolites such as methotrexate or with the vitamin A analog etretinate.

Reiter's disease is an uncommon condition in which urethritis and arthritis may be associated with psoriasis-like lesions on the skin, including an inflammatory condition of the penis known as *circinate balanitis*. The urethritis and involvement of genital mucosa make the STD clinic a likely

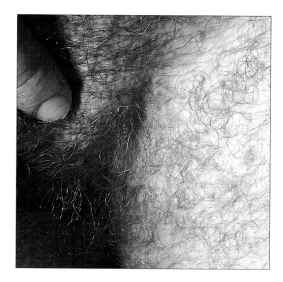

Fig. 1.56 Impetigo. Pustules, pus-filled bullae, crusts, and erosions are all present in this superficial bacterial skin infection, which may be localized to the groin in sexually active patients.

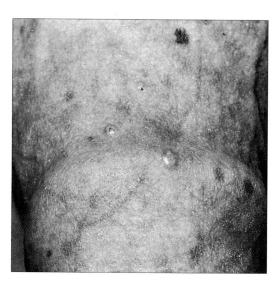

Figs. 1.57 (left) and **1.58 (right)** Molluscum contagiosum. Flesh-colored papules of molluscum may be distinguished by their umbilicated centers. The papules contain a white cheesy substance, which may be stained for the presence of viral inclusion bodies.

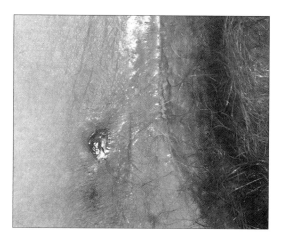

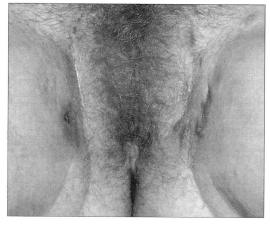

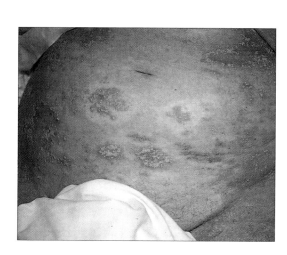

Figs. 1.59 (left) and **1.60 (right)** Hidradenitis suppurativa of the vulva. Indolent painful pustules and nodules are associated with this chronic disorder. Sinuses and scars result.

Fig. 1.61 Pustular psoriasis. Typical clusters of pustules arise in intertriginous areas and spread outward, forming 'lakes' of pus at the periphery of the eruption. Patients are febrile and ill, though the pustules are sterile. This form of psoriasis is relatively rare but may be precipitated by systemic corticosteroid therapy.

setting in which to diagnose this disease. The circinate balanitis (*Fig. 1.62*) may appear as nonscaly erythematous plaques, or the eruption may be more pustular, crusted, and scaly. On nongenital skin, it is very similar in appearance to pustular psoriasis (*Fig. 1.63*). Arthritis is also a typical feature, and conjunctivitis also may be seen. Patients with Reiter's disease usually have histocompatibility antigen HLA-B27, with a high risk of developing ankylosing spondylitis. A link to infections such as *Chlamydia* has been postulated. Fortunately, skin lesions often respond to low-potency topical corticosteroids. The arthritis may be more difficult to treat and can be disabling.

Benign familial pemphigus (*Hailey–Hailey disease*) presents as pustules and erosions in intertriginous areas (*Fig. 1.64*), but this inherited disorder can easily become superinfected with *Candida* or bacteria, which may obscure the initial diagnosis. The familial occurrence and chronicity, as well as a typical histologic picture, make diagnosis relatively easy, although the varied spectrum of lesions from hyperkeratotic papules to erosions may mislead the clinician who looks for fluid-filled vesicles in this so-called 'bullous disease'.

Nodules and Tumors

Epidermoid cysts are firm, yellow, subcutaneous nodules that may occur singly or, in some cases, prolifically over the vulva or scrotum (*Fig. 1.65*). Treatment usually is sought when the cysts rupture or become secondarily infected.

Although cutaneous crusting and erosion may be present over the cyst, the nodular nature of the lesion is unlike other sexually transmitted genital ulcers, which are more superficial. Antistaphylococcal antibiotics and sitz baths usually resolve the secondary infection, and, if necessary, the cyst may later be removed. In most cases, the patient is aware of the diagnosis, although with multiple lesions one also should consider the possibility of *steatocystoma multiplex*. The latter cysts extrude a clear to yellowish gel-like material when punctured, and often appear on the face, neck, upper trunk, and axillae as well. This condition is a hereditary disorder, primarily of cosmetic concern.

Fox–Fordyce disease is characterized by aggregations of tiny 1–2 mm papules in the groin or axilla. This hereditary condition affects the apocrine sweat ducts and is much more common in women than in men. The most common complaint is severe pruritus, which may respond to systemic estrogen therapy.

Keloids (*Fig. 1.66*) are irregular, often linear, firm nodules, seen most often in patients with recurrent episodes of folliculitis or hidradenitis. They should be differentiated from epidermoid cysts, for they will often respond to intralesional steroid therapy, and excision may worsen the condition.

Seborrheic keratoses are elevated 'stuck-on' growths that may be pigmented or flesh-colored, which most often appear on the trunk (*Fig. 1.67*) but may occur on the genitalia. These warty growths are quite benign, and similar lesions are usually found elsewhere on the body. They require removal only if they occur in areas where friction from clothing causes irritation. In

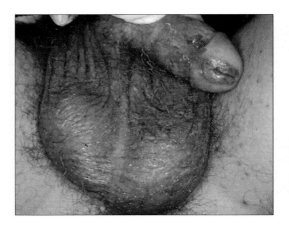

Fig. 1.62 Reiter's disease of the penis. The typical erythema and scale are seen producing the psoriasis-like picture of circinate balanitis. This disorder is associated with HLA-B27, and symptoms of arthritis are extremely common.

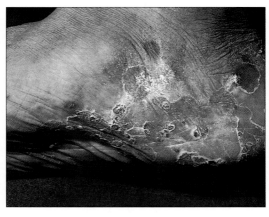

Fig. 1.63 Reiter's disease. Scaly papules cover the instep and heel. Palmar and plantar involvement is termed keratoderma blenorrhagica.

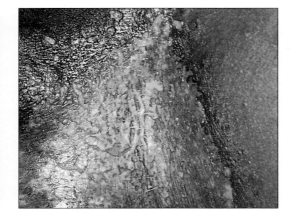

Fig. 1.64 Erosive lesions of benign familial pemphigus (Hailey–Hailey disease) on the scrotum and groin. Traumatic loss of the blister roof in an intertriginous area may cause an otherwise typical bullous disease to appear as multiple erosions.

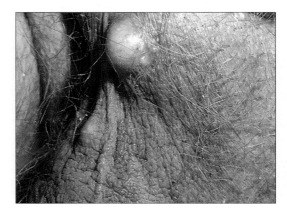

Fig. 1.65 Epidermoid cysts of the scrotum. Generally asymptomatic, these lesions occasionally may rupture and cause discomfort to the patient. They should be differentiated from steatocystoma multiplex, which contain a gel-like material rather than the thick, yellow, sebaceous substance typical of the epidermoid cyst.

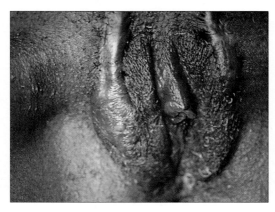

Fig. 1.66 Vulvar keloids. Thickened, linear nodular scars are present on both labia majora. Inciting factors in susceptible individuals include any inflammation or infectious or traumatic insult to skin.

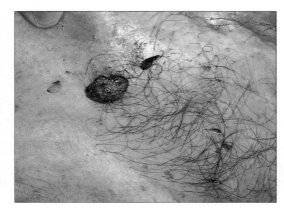

Fig. 1.67 Seborrheic keratosis. This thickened, warty lesion has a typical 'stuck-on' appearance. Similar lesions may be found elsewhere on the trunk.

intertriginous areas, seborrheic keratoses or even simple *acrochordons* (skin tags) may, with time, become pedunculated and prominent (*Fig. 1.68*). When one of these lesions becomes twisted on its stalk the entire lesion may infarct, becoming black and alarming the patient.

Hyperkeratotic or ulcerated lesions that are asymmetrically located on the genitalia should be evaluated carefully for the possibility of *squamous cell carcinoma* (*Figs. 1.69* and *1.70*). The lesions may be asymptomatic, and patients may be unaware of them or deny the chronicity of the problem. Biopsy is recommended for suspicious lesions, and mulitple biopsies should be taken of all suspicious areas. In some forms of squamous cell carcinoma, such as Bowen's disease of the vulva and Bowenoid papulosis, the presence of certain human papillomaviruses (HPV 16 and 18) has been reported (*see Chapter 12*). Evaluation of the patient with a suspicious lesion should include palpation of regional lymph nodes. It may be appropriate to refer the patient directly to a specialist for evaluation and biopsy, although physicians should be aware that apprehension may make the patient reluctant to seek appropriate and timely health care. For this reason it may be expeditious to perform a biopsy on the first visit so that the correct diagnosis may be made (*Fig. 1.71*).

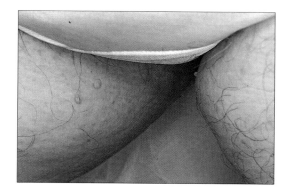

Fig. 1.68 Acrochordons. 'Skin tags' are often found in intertriginous areas. They usually are asymptomatic unless traumatized.

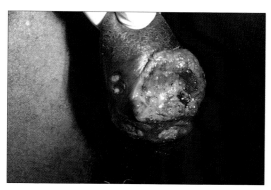

Fig. 1.69 Squamous cell carcinoma of the penis. This large chronic ulcer had been present for over a year. Patients may delay consultation with a physician because they are afraid that a malignancy will be diagnosed.

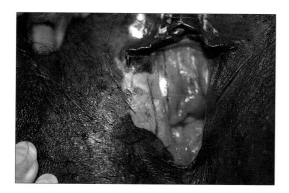

Fig. 1.70 Carcinoma *in situ* of the vulva. Note the asymmetric, rough, whitish, eroded, thickened appearance of this malignancy on the labium.

Fig. 1.71 Needle shave technique for skin biopsy.

(a) Using a small (27–30 gauge) needle, a wheal is formed under and around the lesion with local anesthetic (generally less than 1 ml of 1% xylocaine with epinephrine). For the biopsy, a half-inch 25-gauge needle is preferable, as a 30-gauge needle tends to bend when lifting up on the skin. Place the needle on a syringe for better control.

(b) The orientation of needle insertion is not critical, but a good guide might be the direction of what is to be the long axis of the biopsy. The needle is inserted just proximal to the lesion, advanced just under it, and exited just distal to it.

(c) The scalpel blade (#15 is small and manageable) should also be mounted on a handle for good control. The long axes of the scalpel and the needle are maintained at approximate right angles to one another, and the blade is inserted under the point of the needle, with the back of the blade actually touching the distal needle shaft. The biopsy incision is begun slightly distal to the exit point of the needle, and is directed toward the hub for maximum control.

(d) The angle of the blade should be determined before beginning the incision — a shallow angle for a superficial incision and a wider angle for a deeper specimen. The blade angle (depth of cut) should be maintained as consistently as possible, as the scalpel is drawn toward the hub of the syringe. Running the blade along the undersurface of the needle should be avoided as the incision will be too shallow and tissue immobilization will be lost as the specimen shifts off the needle. 'Scooping' with the blade also should be avoided since the incision will then be wider and deeper than necessary, and wound edges will be ragged.

(e) The incision is begun and ended slightly beyond the needle entrance and exit. The skin is lifted gently with the needle, as the blade slices underneath; the specimen on the needle should not 'pop' free as the biopsy is completed. The biopsy specimen should come smoothly free of the surrounding skin, impaled neatly on the needle for ease of handling. The biopsy specimen may be left on the needle and set aside briefly until bleeding is stopped, or it may be placed directly into fixative.

(f) To remove the biopsy specimen from the needle, use the *back* of the scalpel blade to slide the specimen off into the bottle of fixative.

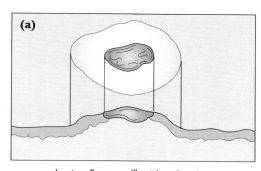

Lesion "pumped" with xylocaine

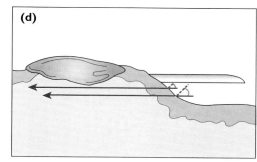

Needle inserted through/under lesion

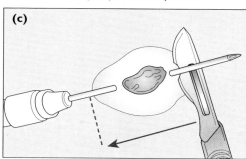

Begin and end incision slightly beyond needle

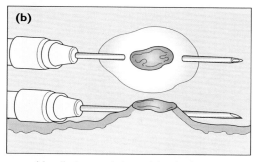

Angle of blade determines depth

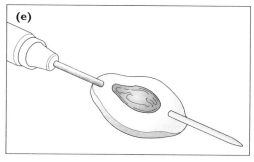

Biopsy specimen stays on needle for easy transport

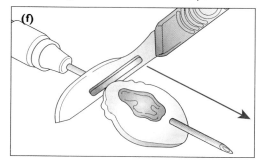

Back of scalpel is used to slide specimen off needle

Erosions and Ulcers

An erosion is defined as the loss of epidermis, while an ulcer extends through the epidermis into the dermis. The lack of a primary lesion makes evaluation of erosions and ulcers extremely difficult for most physicians, and biopsies rarely are helpful unless taken from the edge of a fresh lesion. Infectious ulcers will be covered in other chapters, so this discussion will be limited to noninfectious genital erosions and ulcers.

Bullous Diseases

The fragility of a blister roof in an intertriginous area makes erosions the most common presentation of the bullous diseases, which classically appear as blisters elsewhere on the skin. *Erythema multiforme* (EM) typically appears as 'target' or 'bull's-eye' lesions on the extremities (*Fig. 1.72*). Involvement of the oral mucosa (*Fig. 1.73*), palms, soles, and glans penis (*Fig. 1.74*) is seen most often in the bullous form called the Stevens–Johnson syndrome. EM often is associated with ingestion of drugs or a preceding HSV infection; however, other infections such as mycoplasma, pneumonia, or other viral or bacterial infections may be associated with the occurrence of this disorder. Recurrent episodes are not uncommon and may be limited to mucous membranes such as the mouth and genitalia. It is important to ask the patient whether or not there has been an episode of HSV preceding the outbreak of EM, for control of HSV recurrences with acyclovir may lead to control of EM as well.

As mentioned previously in the section on pustular dermatoses, *benign familial pemphigus* is most commonly seen as localized erosions in the groin. *Pemphigus vulgaris*, however, also may present with similar ulcers or erosions. Chronic pemphigus may even result in somewhat heaped-up, friable papules (*pemphigus vegetans*).

Ulcerative Dermatoses

Ulcerative forms of dermatoses may occur when a dermatologic condition makes the skin exceptionally fragile and easily traumatized. When these conditions occur in the genitalia, their presentation may be obscured by their erosive appearance.

Seen most commonly on the glans penis or hands, the *fixed drug eruption* (*Fig. 1.75*) has been linked with tetracycline therapy, phenolphthalein found in certain laxatives, and several other drugs (*Fig. 1.76*). Typically appearing as a hyperpigmented round macule on the skin, acute lesions may be eczematous, bullous, or erosive in appearance. The appearance of genital lesions in a patient who is being treated with tetracycline for an STD may cause that patient to believe that he or she is experiencing a relapse of the disease or has another STD (*see Chapter 2, Differential Diagnosis*).

Lichen planus was discussed under its most typical presentation as a papulosquamous disorder, but ulcerative forms of this disorder do occur on mucous membranes (*Figs. 1.77* and *1.78*) and can be extremely difficult to manage.

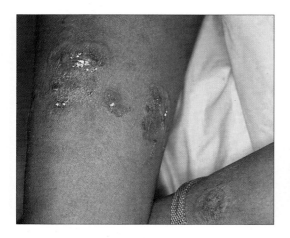

Fig. 1.72 Erythema multiforme (EM) on the arms. The concentric shape ('target' lesions) and presence of bullae are helpful clues to the recognition of this skin disorder, in which many different morphologic types of lesions may be present.

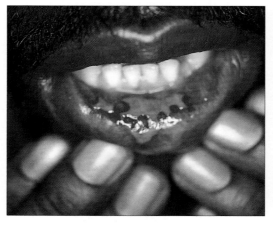

Fig. 1.73 Oral erythema multiforme (Stevens–Johnson syndrome). This patient's lips exhibit painful erosions and crusting. There were multiple tender erythematous plaques on the palms and soles.

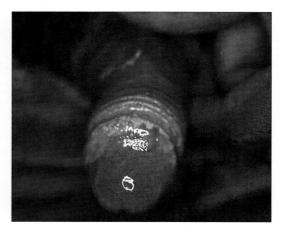

Fig. 1.74 Penile erosion in erythema multiforme. These painful shallow erosions developed after a herpesvirus infection of the mouth — a relatively common association.

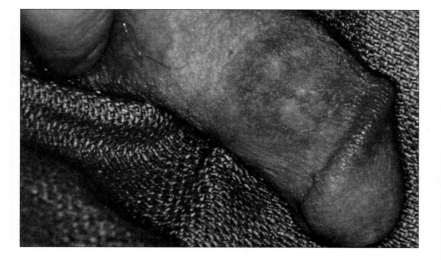

Fig. 1.75 Fixed drug eruption of the penis. Lesions may appear elsewhere on the body as hyperpigmented round macules or bullae that flare with readministration of the offending drug.

DRUGS COMMONLY CAUSING FIXED DRUG ERUPTIONS

Barbiturates

Chlordiazepoxide

Dapsone

Oxyphenbutazone

Phenolphthalein

Quinine and derivatives

Sulfonamides

Tetracycline

Fig. 1.76 Drugs commonly causing fixed drug eruptions.

Vulvovaginal erosions may be extensive, and their chronicity may cause the physician to consider the possibility of malignancy. Superinfection with *Candida* may also occur in this disorder, and should be considered and treated, if present. Treatment for ulcerative lichen planus generally is symptomatic, and topical steroids may be necessary.

Lichen sclerosus was discussed under the category of atrophy (page 12), but the extreme friability of the epidermis in this condition makes the presence of erosions, petechiae, and purpura a common occurrence. The patient should be examined carefully for the typical white atrophic epidermis occurring symmetrically around the rectum and perineum in this condition.

Cutaneous trauma is an often overlooked source of genital ulceration. A relatively innocuous dermatitis on the genitalia may be extremely pruritic and bothersome, and may result in the patient's traumatizing the skin during bouts of itching and scratching. *Erosions* can be deep and severe (*Fig.1.79*), and secondary infection may make evaluation difficult. Questioning the patient about his underlying symptoms will frequently evoke an admission of intractable pruritus, and therapy should be directed toward alleviation of symptoms. Trauma induced by the patient's sexual partner also should be considered, especially with oral sex. *Human bites* (*Fig. 1.80*) are notoriously infectious, and cultures may be necessary to determine appropriate broad-spectrum antibiotic therapy. The presence of symmetric bruises or cuts encircling the penis should lead the physician to suspect cutaneous trauma as a likely etiology; this becomes especially important in the evaluation of children for possible sexual abuse.

Systemic Diseases

Systemic diseases also may lead to secondary genital ulcers. *Behçet's disease* is a multisystem disorder that may present with skin involvement in a majority of cases. In the full-blown syndrome, oral and genital ulcerations are present (*Figs. 1.81* and *1.82*), as well as a pustular eruption, which may involve the genitals. A spectrum of ocular involvement includes conjunctivitis, photophobia, uveitis, and optic neuritis. Central nervous system changes are variable and can be severe, thus frequently dominating the clinical picture. Fever, arthralgias, and cardiac or pulmonary involvement also may be present. The mucosal ulcerations are nonspecific, and more common causes should be excluded before a diagnosis of Behçet's is made on the basis of oral and genital ulcers alone.

Pyoderma gangrenosum (*Fig. 1.83*) is a shaggy, painful, 'dirty' looking ulcer with a bluish overhanging border. The name reflects the exceptionally infectious appearance of this actually noninfectious ulcer. It is seen most commonly in patients with inflammatory bowel disease, but also may be seen with multiple myeloma or other hematologic or immunologic disorders.

Although pyoderma gangrenosum may be seen with gastrointestinal disease, *cutaneous Crohn's disease* classically presents long 'knife-cut' ulcers along the intertriginous groin folds. Flares of these cutaneous lesions often parallel the course of the gastrointestinal disease, and control of one often will lead to control of the other.

Asymmetric ulcers of the genitalia that do not heal with appropriate therapy should be biopsied to rule out carcinoma. Biopsies should be multiple

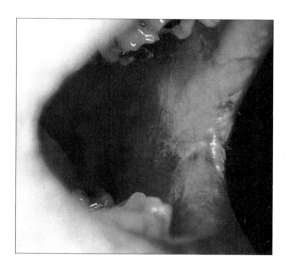

Figs. 1.77 and **1.78** Erosive lichen planus on the oral mucous membrane. **Fig. 1.77 (above)** The lips and buccal mucosa are seen.

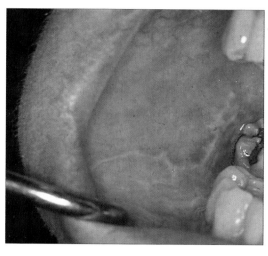

Fig. 1.78 The buccal mucosa is seen.

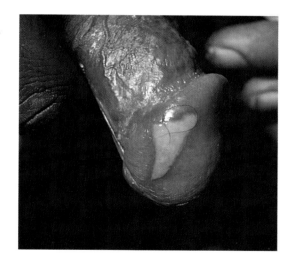

Fig. 1.79 Traumatic ulcer of the penis. The sharply angled borders of this lesion are a clue to its traumatic rather than infectious etiology.

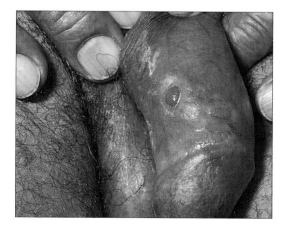

Fig. 1.80 Ulcer secondary to human bite of the penile shaft. Secondary infection is a common sequela of human bite wounds and cultures may be necessary for appropriate antibiotic therapy.

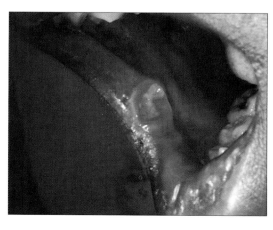

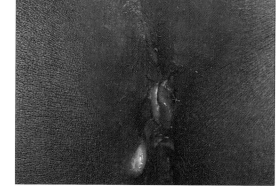

Figs. 1.81 and **1.82** Behçet's disease. Nonspecific painful recurrent ulcers of the oral and genital mucosa were the presenting complaints in this young woman in whom Behçet's disease was diagnosed.

and taken from the thickest part of a lesion and the edge of an ulcer. *Squamous cell carcinoma* was discussed under nodules and tumors (p. 17). *Extramammary Paget's disease* may have a remarkably eczematous appearance on first examination. Hallmarks of this diagnosis are its chronicity, asymmetry, and lack of response to topical therapy.

Itching (Pruritus Ani, Scroti, Vulvae)

Acute-onset perineal itching or burning should take the physician through a standard differential diagnosis, including *Candida* infection, irritant and contact dermatitis, urinary tract infection, hemorrhoids, pinworms, and condylomata. It is a different challenge to evaluate chronic cutaneous symptomatology, and this problem is not within the scope of this text. However, a few points should be made: lichen simplex chronicus (LSC) (see earlier section on dermatitis/eczema, *p. 6*) is thickening of the skin in response to chronic scratching, and several underlying causes of pruritus must be considered. On the genitalia, maceration and intertriginous rubbing contribute to flares and continuation of symptoms, and infections are particularly likely to initiate itching. Cultures should be done for yeast and fungus as tinea and *Candida* are the most common offenders, and may be primary or secondary to the process. Vigorous scratching or eczematous change disturbs the skin barrier, allowing the development of secondary bacterial infection. In many cases of LSC, the initiating cause cannot be identified; the patient should be reassured that this is probably of no consequence, because the problem is now only the secondary change which has developed as a result of scratching.

In childhood, genital pruritus is often the result of irritant dermatitis, although STDs are an obvious consideration. Young girls may have fecal contamination of the vulva from careless hygiene, or conversely may irritate the skin from vigorous scrubbing or soaping. Pinworms are more common in childhood and typically involve the anus, but may also be seen at the vaginal opening. Vaginal or rectal discharge in childhood should be evaluated for evidence of possible sexual abuse, and genital lesions should be examined carefully. Lichen sclerosus (*see below*) can occur in childhood, and traumatic-appearing purpuric lesions are typical with the fragile epithelium of this cutaneous condition.

The symptomatic patient should be asked about pre-existing dermatoses (including oral mucosal lesions), *Candida*, condylomata, methods of cleansing, and the use of topical and systemic medications. Previous treatments should be explored, especially if they resulted in a clearly allergic response (vesicles or erosions lasting for two weeks) rather than local irritation (stinging and burning on application). The patient should be asked specifically about risk factors: for example, the *Candida*-prone patient may receive frequent rounds of antibiotics for sinusitis, urinary tract infections, or acne; steroids or other immunosuppressants may be prescribed for a variety of disorders. Estrogen deficiency may be important if the patient is perimenopausal. On the genitalia, erythematous papules and pustules develop as a complication of topical steroid use, as well as with cutaneous infections.

While some patients will describe elements of itching and burning, the two conditions can usually be differentiated on physical examination. Cutaneous changes of lichenification (leathery thickening) or excoriation (scratch marks) are more typical of pruritus, because the patient with burning skin rarely rubs or scratches the affected area. Without evidence of scratching, the patient with cutaneous burning or dysesthesia may appear to have a normal examination.

Picture credits for this chapter are as follows: Figs. 1.4, 1.8, and 1.9 courtesy of Stevens A, Lowe J, Histology. London, Mosby, 1992; Figs 1.7 and 1.10 courtesy of Mr Peter Greenhouse; Figs. 1.30, 1.31, 1.77 and 1.78 courtesy of Emory University School of Dentistry; Figs. 1.93 and 1.74 courtesy of Heidi Watts; Figs. 1.27, 1.32 and 1.33, 1.46, 1.57, 1.58, 1.59 and 1.60 courtesy du Vivier A.: Atlas of Clinical Dermatology. New York, Gower Medical Publishing, 1986.

BIBLIOGRAPHY

Ackerman AB, Kornberg R: Pearly penile papules — acral angiofibromas. *Arch Derm* **108**:673, 1973.

Bergeron C, Ferenczy A, Richart RM, et al: Micropapillomatosis labialis appears unrelated to human papillomavirus. *Obstet Gynecol* **76**:281, 1990.

Betterle C, Caretto A, DeZio A, et al.: Incidence and significance of organ-specific autoimmune disorders (clinical, latent, or only autoantibodies) in patients with vitiligo. *Dermatologica* **171**:419, 1985.

Brewerton DA, Nicholls A, Oates JK, et al.: Reiter's disease and HL-A 27. *Lancet* **996**, 1973.

Fischer A: *Contact Dermatitis*, 3rd ed. Philadelphia, Lea and Febiger, pp 195–198, 1986.

Fitzpatrick B, Eisen A, Wolff K, et al.: *Dermatology in General Medicine*, 3rd ed. New York, McGraw-Hill, 1987.

Friedrich EG Jr: The vulvar vestibule. *J Reprod Med* **28**:773, 1983.

Friedrich EG Jr: *Vulvar Disease*, 2nd ed. Philadelphia, WB Saunders Co., 1983.

Growdon WA, Fu YS, Lebherz TB, et al.: Pruritic vulvar squamous papillomatosis: evidence for human papillomavirus etiology. *Obstet Gynecol* **66**:564, 1985.

Hall J, Moreland A, Cox J, et al.: Oral acanthosis nigricans: Report of a case and comparison of oral and cutaneous pathology. *Am J Dermatopathol* **10**:68, 1988.

Jorizzo JL, Abernathy JL, White WL et al.: Mucocutaneous criteria for the diagnosis of Behçet's disease: an analysis of clinicopathologic data from multiple international centers. *J Amer Acad Dermatol* **32**:968, 1995.

Landthaler M, Braun-Falco O, Richter K, et al.: Malignant melanomas of the vulva. *Dtsch Med Wochenschr* **110**:789, 1985.

Lemak MA, Duvic M, Bean SF: Oral acyclovir for the prevention of herpes-associated erythema multiforme. *J Am Acad Derm* **15**:50, 1986.

Lyell A, Gordon A, Dide H, et al.: Mycoplasma and erythema multiforme. *Lancet* ii:1116, 1967.

McKay M: Pruritus vulvae and vulvodynia: itching and burning. In: Hurst JW (ed): *Medicine for the Practicing Physician*, 3rd ed. Boston, Butterworth–Heinemann, chap 10–15, pp 678–680, 1992.

Moyal-Barracco M, Leibowitch M, Orth G: Vestibular papillae of the vulva. Lack of evidence for human papillomavirus etiology. *Arch Dermatol* 126:1594, 1990.

Nethercott JR, Choi BC: Erythema multiforme (Stevens–Johnson syndrome) — Chart review of 123 hospitalized patients. *Dermatologica* **171**:383, 1985.

Powell FC, Schroeter AL, Su WPD, et al.: Pyoderma gangrenosum: A review of 86 patients. *Q J Med* **55**:173, 1985.

Reyman L, Milano A, Demopoulos R, et al.: Metastatic vulvar ulceration in Crohn's disease. *Am J Gastro* **81**:46, 1986.

Rook A, Wilkinson DS, Ebling FJG, et al.: *Textbook of Dermatology*, 4th ed. Boston, Blackwell Scientific Publications, 1986.

Sehgal VH, Gangwani OP: Genital fixed drug eruptions. *Genitourin Med* **62**:56, 1986.

Sheagren JN: Staphylococcal infections of the skin and skin structures. *Cutis* **36**:2, 1985.

Slaney G, Muller S, Clay J, et al.: Crohn's disease involving the penis. *Gut* **27**:329, 1986.

Strauss WB, Maibach HI: Bacterial interference, treatment of recurrent furunculosis: *JAMA* **208**:861, 1969.

Tokoro Y, Seto T, Abe Y, et al.: Skin lesions in Behçet's disease. *Int J Derm* **16**:227, 1977.

Wilkinson EJ: Normal histology and nomenclature of the vulva, and malignant neoplasms, including VIN. *Dermatol Clin* **10**:283, 1992.

Wolska H, Jablonska S, Langner A, et al.: Etretinate therapy in generalized pustular psoriasis (Zumbusch type). *Dermatologica* **171**:297, 1985.

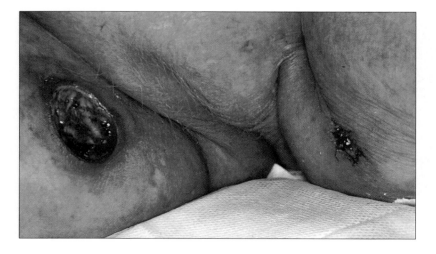

Fig. 1.83 Pyoderma gangrenosum. Multiple deep necrotic ulcers with dusky overhanging margins are characteristic of pyoderma gangrenosum. These lesions may be seen in patients with various systemic diseases.

CHAPTER TWO

Syphilis

S Thompson, S Larsen, and A Moreland

INTRODUCTION

Syphilis is a chronic systemic infectious disease that is transmitted during sexual intercourse or other intimate contact; it also can be transmitted from a pregnant woman to her fetus *in utero* or by the infant having contact with a maternal lesion during birth. The causative agent of syphilis is *Treponema pallidum* subspecies *pallidum*, a spirochete (*Fig. 2.1*). This agent has never been cultured successfully on artificial media, and does not take up the Gram stain. Three other treponemes (subspecies *pertenue*, subspecies *endemicum*, and *T. carateum*) are also pathogenic for humans (*Fig. 2.2*). Infection with these organisms will cause serologic tests for syphilis to be reactive, though the infections are not sexually transmitted.

EPIDEMIOLOGY

Syphilis is a disease of worldwide importance (*Fig. 2.3*). In the USA, primary and secondary (infectious) syphilis rates were at a peak in 1947, declined sharply over the following 10 years, and then gradually increased over each succeeding decade to reach a post-World War II peak of 50,578 in 1990 (*Fig. 2.4*). Many factors have undoubtedly contributed to this increase, including an earlier age of first intercourse and large numbers of lifetime partners.

In the 1970s, syphilis was predominantly a disease of homosexual men, but the advent of AIDS and the subsequent practice of safer sex has led to a decrease in the incidence of syphilis in this population. A shift of syphilis to the heterosexual population began in 1984 and can be most probably attributed to the practice of exchanging sex with multiple partners for drugs, particularly for crack cocaine. The spread of acquired syphilis to heterosexual populations, with poorer access to medical treatment, has been paralleled by an increase in the number of cases of congenital syphilis. Although there has been a true increase in the incidence of congenital syphilis, a new reporting system for congenital syphilis begun in 1989 has artificially inflated the numbers.

Individuals are infectious for their sex partners during the primary and secondary stages, when skin or mucosal lesions are present. Women are most likely to transmit the infection to their unborn infants during the early stages of the disease when they are spirochetemic, but infection of the fetus during early latency is also possible.

Fig. 2.1 Transmission electron micrograph of *Treponema pallidum* subspecies *pallidum* in tissue.

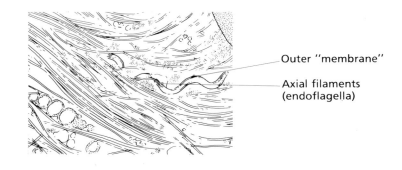

Outer "membrane"

Axial filaments (endoflagella)

Fig. 2.2 Pathogenic treponemes of humans.

PATHOGENIC TREPONEMES OF HUMANS				
	SYPHILIS	YAWS	BEJEL	PINTA
ORGANISM	*T. pallidum* subspecies *pallidum*	*T. pallidum* subspecies *pertenue*	*T. pallidum* subspecies *endemicum*	*T. carateum*
TRANSMISSION	Sexual contact	Skin contact	Skin contact, oral	Skin contact
LESION TYPE				
PRIMARY	Chancre	Crusted papules	Oral mucosal lesions	Crusted papules and plaques
SECONDARY	Macular or papulosquamous	Papillomatous, and scarring	Mucous patches and condylomata lata	Scaly plaques
LATE	Gummata and endarteritis	Gummata of bone and skin	Gummata of cartilage, bone, and skin	Dyschromia

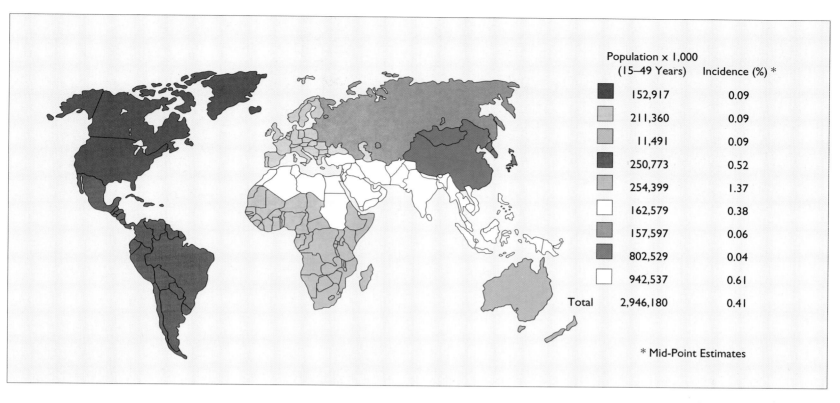

Fig. 2.3 Incidence of syphilis: estimates by region.

	Population x 1,000 (15–49 Years)	Incidence (%) *
	152,917	0.09
	211,360	0.09
	11,491	0.09
	250,773	0.52
	254,399	1.37
	162,579	0.38
	157,597	0.06
	802,529	0.04
	942,537	0.61
Total	2,946,180	0.41

* Mid-Point Estimates

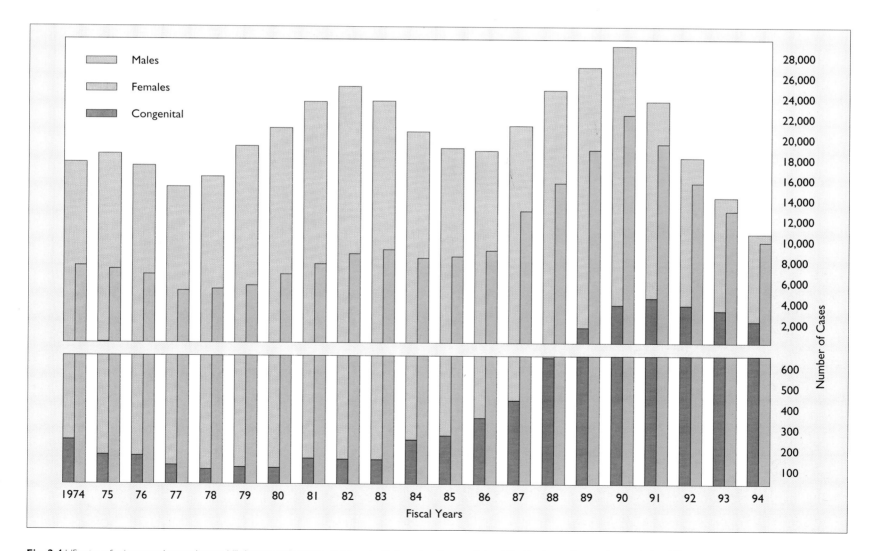

Fig. 2.4 US rates of primary and secondary syphilis in men and women compared with the rates of congenital syphilis. Numbers of cases of congenital syphilis are a highly sensitive indicator of the amount of infectious syphilis in a population and the need for control activities. In 1989, in addition to the reporting of symptomatic cases of congenital syphilis, asymptomatic babies born to mothers with reactive serologic tests for syphilis and without a history of adequate treatment for syphilis, and syphilitic stillborns were included in the surveillance case definition.

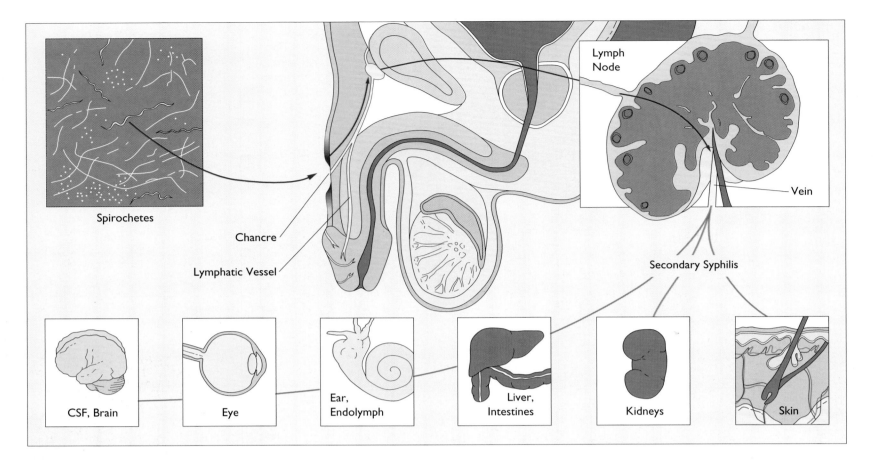

Fig. 2.5 Schematic diagram to show how spirochetes enter regional lymph nodes from a skin chancre, and then enter the bloodstream. Organ systems that are involved are shown: CSF, brain, eye, ear endolymph, liver, intestines, kidneys, skin.

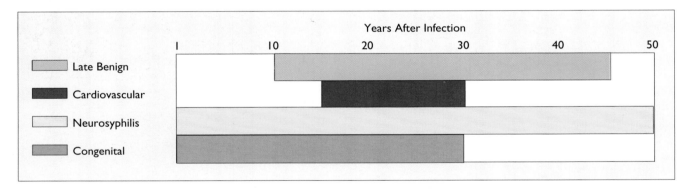

Fig. 2.6 The clinical course of untreated syphilis.

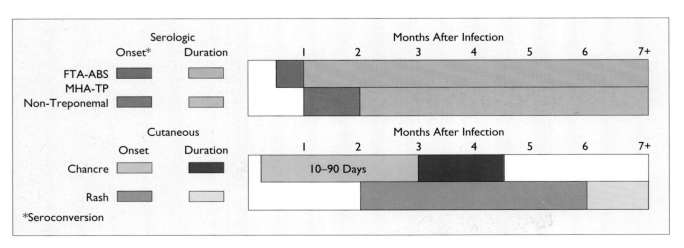

Fig. 2.7 Correlation of serologic and cutaneous changes in untreated syphilis.

CLINICAL MANIFESTATIONS

Untreated, syphilis is a chronic disease that is spread throughout the body hematogenously and which can produce manifestations in virtually every organ system (*Fig. 2.5*). The infectious, clinically manifest stages of the disease — primary and secondary syphilis — are transient events. During latency, by definition, there are no clinical signs or symptoms of infection, despite the fact that *T. pallidum* can be demonstrated in some tissues. Serology is the only available method for accurate diagnosis during this stage of the disease. The clinical course and serologic changes of untreated syphilis are summarized in *Figs. 2.6 –2.7*.

PRIMARY SYPHILIS

The first clinical manifestation of syphilis, the chancre, develops on average about 3 weeks after infection (10–90 days). The chancre appears at the site where treponemal invasion of the dermis first occurred, usually on or near the genitals. However, it may occur on any skin or mucous membrane. Chancres are usually single lesions and are painless (*Fig. 2.8*) unless superinfected; hence, they may be missed by the patient if they occur in an inaccessible region, such as the cervix, pharynx, or rectum. Nontender regional adenopathy is also common. If untreated, the chancre will persist for 2–6 weeks and heal without scarring. Occasionally, a relapsing chancre will occur at the same site. Motile spirochetes should be demonstrable in untreated chancres during most stages of their evolution. They may be difficult to demonstrate in late, healing lesions, and are usually absent if the patient has applied local medications or taken antibiotics.

The typical chancre is indurated, has a clean base, and rolled edges (*Fig. 2.9*). Secondary infection with bacteria or even herpesviruses occasionally occurs, and may cause the ulcer to appear somewhat atypical (*Fig. 2.10*). The differential diagnosis includes chancroid, granuloma inguinale, and occasionally herpes. The labia and fourchette are the most typical areas for chancres to occur in women (*Fig. 2.11*). Perianal, anal or rectal chancres occur primarily in homosexual men, and in women who have a history of rectal intercourse (*Fig. 2.12*). While single lesions are seen most commonly, multiple primary chancres are not uncommon (*Fig. 2.13*). Healing lesions may present problems in diagnosis, particularly in their later stages when they are dark-field negative, and adenopathy may not be prominent (*Fig. 2.14*). Acquired syphilis can occur in infants and children (*Fig. 2.15*). Syphilitic chancres occasionally may occur in extragenital sites, such as the fingers (*Fig. 2.16*) or oral cavity (*Fig. 2.17*). Clinical findings of primary syphilis are summarized in *Fig. 2.18*.

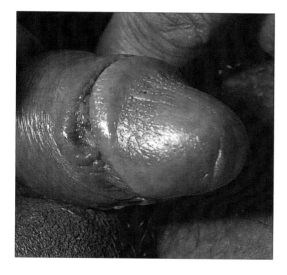

Fig. 2.8 Typical syphilitic chancre of the coronal sulcus. This early asymptomatic chancre in the coronal sulcus shows characteristic induration and a 'clean' base. Dark-field examination will almost always be positive if no medication has been given or applied topically.

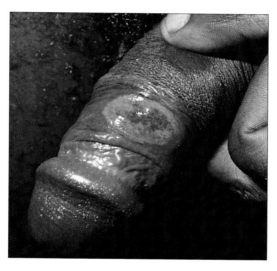

Fig. 2.9 Large, indurated primary chancre of the penile shaft. This penile chancre has been present for several weeks, but it is still painless and large. The induration produces a cartilaginous quality.

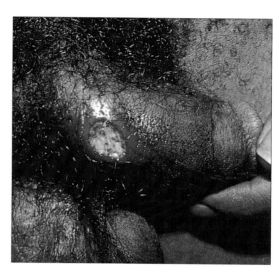

Fig. 2.10 Atypical penile chancre. This chancre appears atypical because it has become secondarily infected with bacteria. Dark-field examination may be difficult because of the presence of nonpathogenic treponemes.

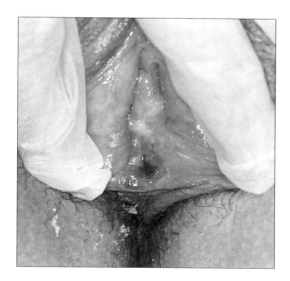

Fig. 2.11 Painless button-like syphilitic chancre of the posterior forchette, a common site for chancres in women.

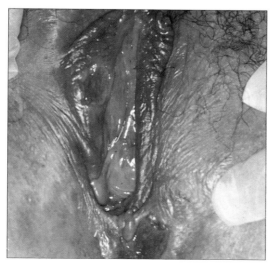

Fig. 2.12 Multiple primary syphilitic chancres of labia and perineum. Typical induration and edema of the chancres is easily seen.

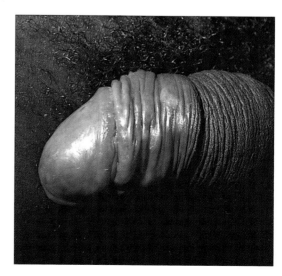

Fig. 2.13 Multiple chancres of primary syphilis. Multiple primary chancres are not uncommon in primary syphilis. They occur most frequently on the penis and vulva.

SECONDARY SYPHILIS

Onset of the secondary stage of disease ranges from 6 weeks to 6 months after infection in the untreated patient. The primary chancre may still be present when clinically apparent secondary lesions occur. In this phase of the disease, spirochetes enter the bloodstream from their dermal and lymph node foci and are distributed to most tissues and organs (*see Fig. 2.5*). After a suitable multiplication period, generalized but nonspecific symptoms occur, such as fever, malaise, headache, sore throat, arthralgias, and anorexia. Generalized adenopathy occurs in more than 50% of patients. Hepatomegaly and occasionally splenomegaly may also occur. There may be leukocytosis, anemia, and an elevated erythrocyte sedimentation rate. Syphilitic hepatitis is characterized by mild derangement of liver enzymes and a markedly elevated alkaline phosphatase. An acute, 'viral type' of meningitis may complicate the picture.

A rash, which is sometimes called a syphilid, occurs in about 75% of patients and is extremely variable in appearance. It may be localized or generalized. Symmetric discrete erythematous, brown or hyperpigmented macules are the earliest generalized syphilid (*Fig. 2.19*). This eruption commonly begins on the trunk. The macules may enlarge or become annular; and scaling and pruritus are absent. As the eruption progresses, some of the macules may become thickened and papular (*Fig. 2.20*), and thus macular syphilid may coexist with

the papular forms (*Fig. 2.21*). Papular syphilids (*Fig. 2.22*) appear to be more common than macular eruptions, perhaps because they are easier to see. If the disease remains untreated for several weeks, the papules may develop a dry, thin collarette of scale, which peels off easily (*Figs. 2.23* and *2.24*).

Frequent involvement of the palms and soles in macular and papular syphilids may help to distinguish them from other dermatoses (*see Fig. 2.25* and the following section on *Differential Diagnosis*). Many varieties of papular syphilids have been described, and include, among others, the papulosquamous (*Fig. 2.26*), annular (*Fig. 2.27*), lenticular (*Fig. 2.28*) syphilis cornee, in which the lesions resemble clavi (*see Figs. 2.24* and *2.25*), psoriasiform (*Fig. 2.29*), and framboesiform (*Fig. 2.30*) types.

Moist hypertrophic papular lesions, condylomata lata, occur in intertriginous areas, such as the genitals (*Figs. 2.31* and *2.32*) and gluteal folds (*Fig. 2.33*). Occasionally, they may become hyperplastic or verrucous, and as such may very closely resemble condylomata acuminata (*Fig. 2.34*). These lesions may also be seen in extragenital areas (*Fig. 2.35*). Condylomata lata are usually covered with a grayish exudate containing numerous spirochetes, making them much more infectious than other secondary syphilids. Another variant of papular syphilis is the so-called split papules found in the postauricular area (*Fig. 2.36*) or in the oral commissures. Nonspecific superficial erosions

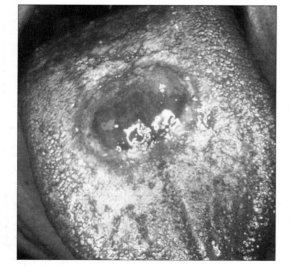

Fig. 2.14 Healing chancre. Primary chancres heal spontaneously, as seen here in this almost resolved penile chancre.

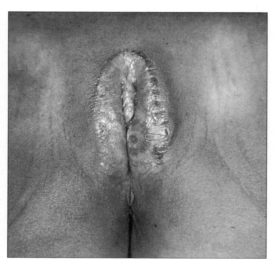

Fig. 2.15 Vulvar chancre in a child. A painless ulcer found on the genitals of a child should always raise the possibility of syphilis, but also may be acquired through nonsexual means.

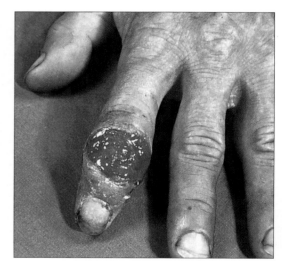

Fig. 2.16 Digital syphilitic chancre. Occupational exposure of health care workers may be the cause of chancres on the hands.

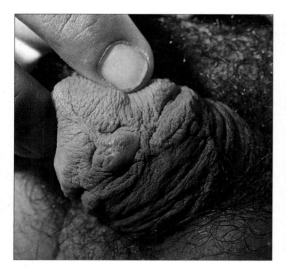

Fig. 2.17 Chancre of the tongue. Dark-field examination of mouth lesions may not be reliable due to the presence of saprophytic spirochetes. However, the direct FA test is useful in this situation.

SYNOPSIS OF CLINICAL FINDINGS OF PRIMARY SYPHILIS

I. ULCER
    Single genital ulcer most common
    Diameter of lesion usually > 0.5 cm
    Nonpainful
    Indurated, rolled edges
    Clean lesion base
    Dark-field (+) for motile spirochetes

II. ADENOPATHY
    Inguinal, ipsilateral to ulcer
    Nontender
    Nonfluctuant

III. CONSTITUTIONAL SYMPTOMS
    None

Fig. 2.18 Synopsis of clinical findings of primary syphilis.

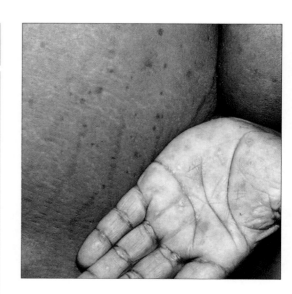

Fig. 2.19 Oval hyperpigmented macules of the trunk and extremities in early secondary syphilis. The eruption was generalized, but not readily visible, and therefore unnoticed by the patient.

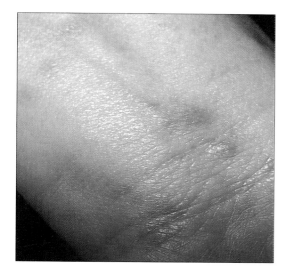

Fig. 2.20 Early papular syphilis. The lack of scale suggests that this is an early form of papular syphilis. Erythema and firmness of the papules on palpation are characteristic.

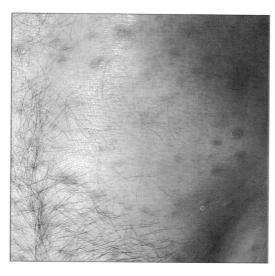

Fig. 2.21 Macular and papulosquamous forms of syphilis coexisting in syphilis of 1 month's duration. This eruption was completely asymptomatic.

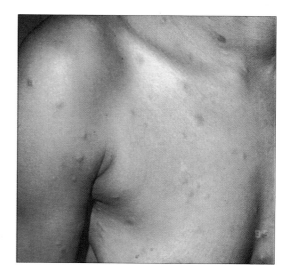

Fig. 2.22 Papular secondary syphilis. The generalized erythematous papules are quite obvious to both patient and physician.

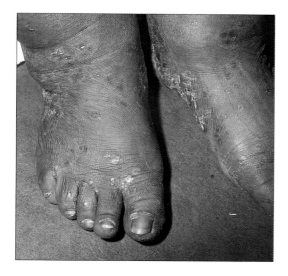

Fig. 2.23 Papulosquamous secondary syphilis. The annular scaling seen here had been present for several weeks. It is quite common.

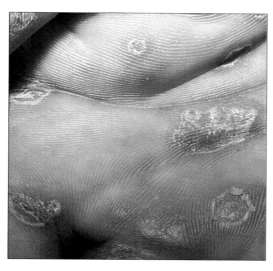

Fig. 2.24 A close-up view of the characteristic colarette of scale and hyperpigmentation seen in untreated secondary syphilis.

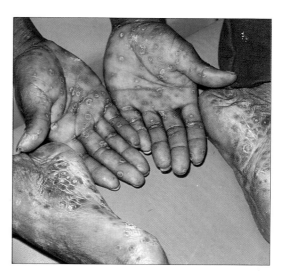

Fig. 2.25 Palmar and plantar papulosquamous secondary syphilis.

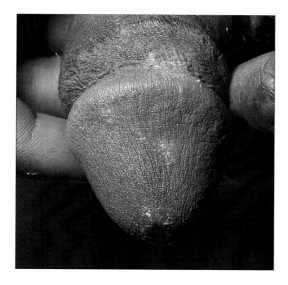

Fig. 2.26 Papulosquamous syphilids are typically flat papules, which are red, indurated, and slightly scaly. Lesions may be limited to the genital region.

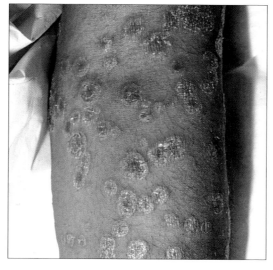

Fig. 2.27 Annular syphilids are florid annular scaly plaques, some with a targetoid hyperpigmented center.

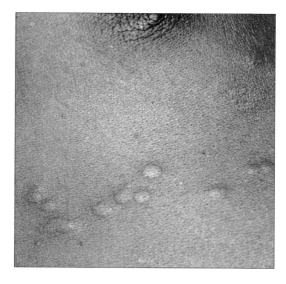

Fig. 2.28 Smooth firm pea-sized brown papules characterize the lenticular form of secondary syphilis.

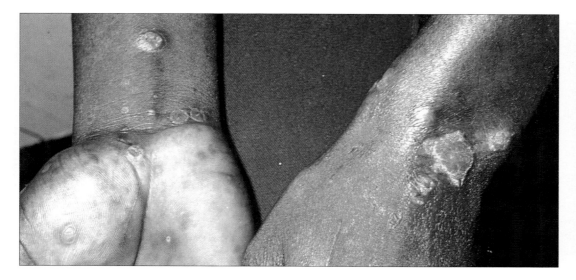

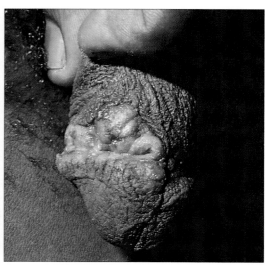

Fig. 2.29 Large and small psoriasiform plaques with thick scale and an irregular shape in late secondary syphilis.

Fig. 2.30 Verrucous and eroded (framboesiform) lesions of late secondary syphilis in the coronal sulcus.

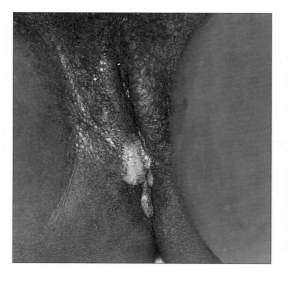

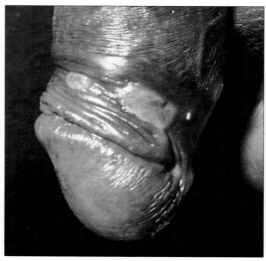

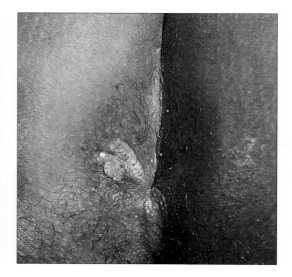

Fig. 2.31 Condylomata lata. Typical condylomata lata on the labia and perineum are moist gray plaques and papules.

Fig. 2.32 Condylomata lata. Flat, broad-based dark-field positive plaques are seen in the folds of the foreskin.

Fig. 2.33 Condylomata lata. Perianal condylomata detected in a patient who sought help because of a palmar rash.

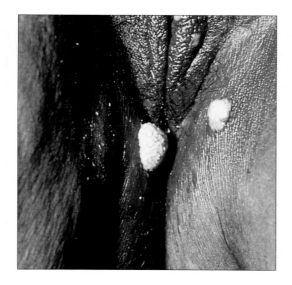

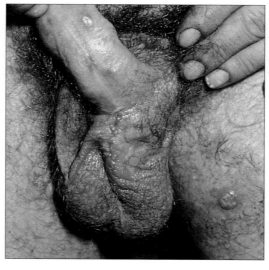

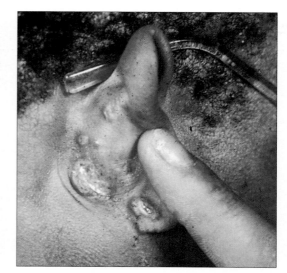

Fig. 2.34 Condylomata lata. Unusually verrucous condylomata lata resembling condylomata acuminata in a patient who presented with a generalized macular eruption.

Fig. 2.35 Condylomata lata. Broad-based moist, dark-field-positive condylomata lata on the thigh. Note the other erosive lesions of secondary syphilis on the penile shaft.

Fig. 2.36 Split papules, seen here on the posterior auricular fold, may also be present at the angles of the mouth.

of the oral or genital mucous membranes, called mucous patches, are another common manifestation of secondary syphilis. These round or oval lesions appear as grayish or denuded patches on the buccal or labial mucosa (*Fig. 2.37*), on the tongue (*Figs. 2.38* and *2.39*), or on the palate or tonsils.

Alopecia may occur during secondary syphilis as a patchy thinning (*Fig. 2.40*) or as a more diffuse loss of hair (*Fig. 2.41*). Eyebrows, beard hair, or any other hairy body areas may be involved. The alopecia regrows in both treated and untreated patients.

The signs and symptoms of secondary syphilis usually last only a few weeks. Relapses may occur in the untreated patient, usually within the first year or two after infection, but are rare after adequate penicillin therapy.

Differential Diagnosis

The eruptions of secondary syphilis are almost infinitely varied and mimic many common dermatoses. In this section, examples of common presentations of secondary syphilis are compared to the nonsyphilitic dermatoses that resemble them.

The brown-red hyperpigmentation and fine scale seen in cases of secondary syphilis (*Fig. 2.42*) may closely resemble the characteristically oval, slightly scaly, brown-red eruptions of pityriasis rosea (*Fig. 2.43*). However,

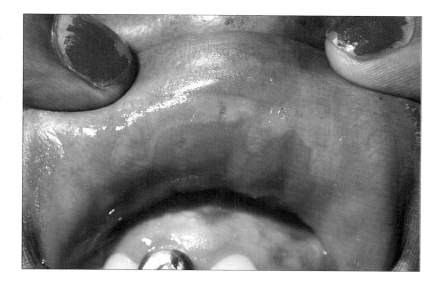

Fig. 2.37 Serpiginous mucous patches on the labial mucosa and tongue were the presenting sign of syphilis in this patient.

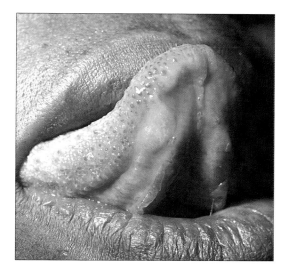

Fig. 2.38 Mucous patches are seen on the ventral tongue.

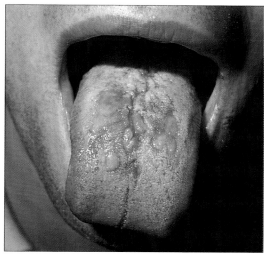

Fig. 2.39 Mucous patches are seen on the dorsum of the tongue.

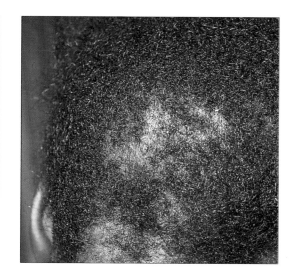

Fig. 2.40 The patchy or 'moth-eaten' alopecia may not be noticed by the patient, but can be found by the alert examiner.

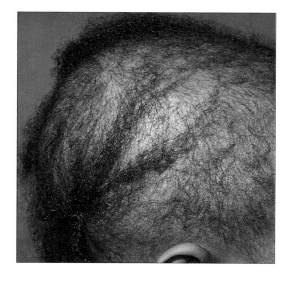

Fig. 2.41 Occasionally a more diffuse alopecia accompanies secondary syphilis.

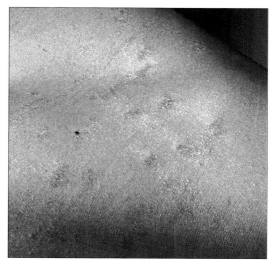

Fig. 2.42 Differential diagnosis in secondary syphilis. Early papulosquamous form of syphilis.

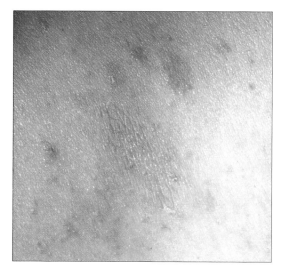

Fig. 2.43 Differential diagnosis in secondary syphilis. Pityriasis rosea (compare with **2.42**).

generalized adenopathy is absent and serologic tests for syphilis are negative in pityriasis rosea.

The appearance of hyperpigmented oval plaques of secondary syphilis on the upper back (*Fig. 2.44*) resembles a common form of hyperpigmented tinea versicolor. Tinea versicolor is usually found in this location and has adherent KOH-positive scales, which may not be readily visible (*Fig. 2.45*).

The generalized macular and papular eruptions of syphilis (*Fig. 2.46*) may at first glance resemble generalized scabies (*Fig. 2.47*). However, the pruritus in scabies is pronounced, and the lesions are often excoriated. Lack of these signs and symptoms should suggest syphilis in eruptions of this sort.

Occasionally, the scattered papulosquamous eruptions of secondary syphilis (*Fig. 2.48*) resemble the guttate variety of psoriasis (*Fig. 2.49*). However, psoriatic scaling is frequently quite thick and adherent. In addition, involvement of the scalp and extensor surfaces in psoriasis may offer further clues to the correct diagnosis. Adenopathy and alopecia, common in syphilis, are generally absent in psoriasis. Involvement of the genitals may occur in either disorder (*see Chapter 1*).

Secondary syphilis may be the cause of fairly large erythematous plaques on the penis, which resemble fixed drug eruptions (*Fig. 2.50*). The

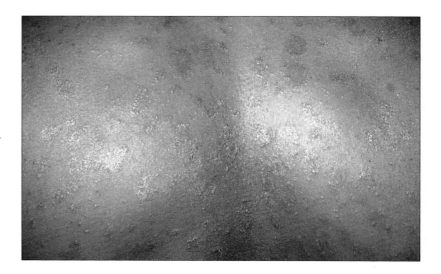

Fig. 2.44 Differential diagnosis in secondary syphilis. Hyperpigmented oval macules of secondary syphilis.

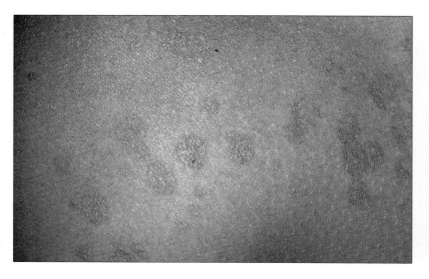

Fig. 2.45 Differential diagnosis in secondary syphilis. Tinea versicolor (compare with **2.44**).

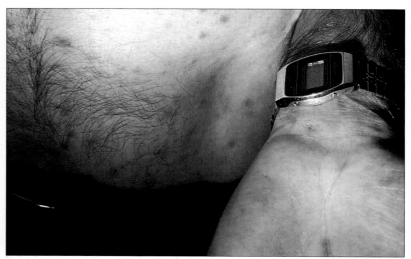

Fig. 2.46 Differential diagnosis in secondary syphilis. Generalized papular form of secondary syphilis.

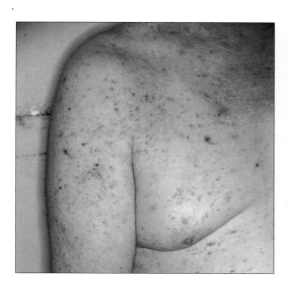

Fig. 2.47 Differential diagnosis in secondary syphilis. Generalized scabies (compare with **2.46**).

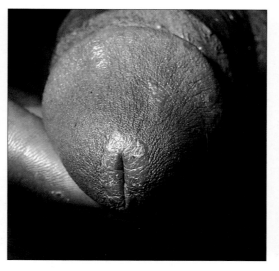

Fig. 2.48 Differential diagnosis in secondary syphilis. Papulosquamous secondary syphilis of the penis.

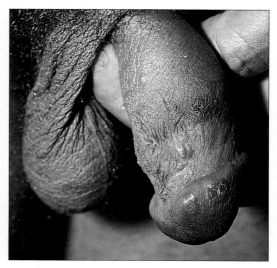

Fig. 2.49 Psoriasis involving the genitals (compare with **2.48**).

latter has a predilection for the genitals and hands. The erythematous plaques of early fixed drug eruptions (*Fig. 2.51*), which later become scaly and hyperpigmented, can closely resemble the eruptions of secondary syphilis. Tetracycline, a commonly prescribed antibiotic in the STD clinic, is one of the drugs most frequently implicated as a causative agent of fixed drug eruptions (*see Chapter 1*).

Annular palmar or plantar macules or plaques in some cases of syphilis (*Fig. 2.52*) may resemble the characteristic 'target' or 'iris' lesions of erythema multiforme (*Fig. 2.53*). However, erythema multiforme is usually not scaly and may even become bullous. Bullae do not occur in acquired secondary syphilis. Serologic tests for syphilis help differentiate the two, in most cases.

Plantar or palmar eruptions of syphilis that have developed very little scale (*Fig. 2.54*) may resemble entities such as pityriasis lichenoides chronica (*Fig. 2.55*), a chronic, mildly scaly skin disorder, or even viral exanthems. If serologic testing is not definitive, biopsies may be necessary.

Annular syphilids with central hyperpigmentation on sun-exposed skin (Fig. 2.56) resemble discoid lupus erythematosus (Fig. 2.57). False-positive syphilis serologies in lupus may confuse the picture. However, rapid plasma reagin titers are generally of high titer in secondary syphilis (1:16 or greater) and low in lupus (1:8 or less).

LATENT SYPHILIS

Latent syphilis is the period of quiescence after completion of the secondary stage of disease, during which there are no clinical manifestations. An exposure history and a reactive serologic test for syphilis is the only way of establishing the diagnosis. Not infrequently, no history of syphilis can be obtained, and, in such a case, a true-positive serology must be distinguished from a false-positive one (*see* laboratory section on interpretation of test results).

Latency is divided into early and late phases. Early latency encompasses the first year after secondary infection. It is during this period that relapses of secondary disease are most apt to occur in the untreated patient. Occasionally, infection of a partner may occur during early latency, and the pregnant woman is at risk of transmitting the disease to her fetus. The patient in late latency (more than 1 year into the latent period) has a decreasing risk of transmission to partner or fetus as latency progresses.

LATE SYPHILIS

The late manifestations of syphilis fall into three main types: cardiovascular, gummatous, and meningovascular (neural). In general, these manifestations occur decades after infection, but some of the meningeal and cerebrovascular

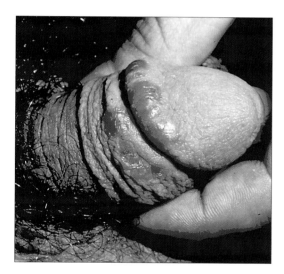

Fig. 2.50 Differential diagnosis in secondary syphilis. Erythematous penile plaques of secondary syphilis.

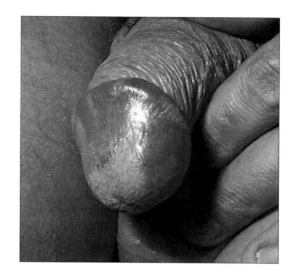

Fig. 2.51 Differential diagnosis in secondary syphilis. Fixed drug eruption (compare with **2.50**).

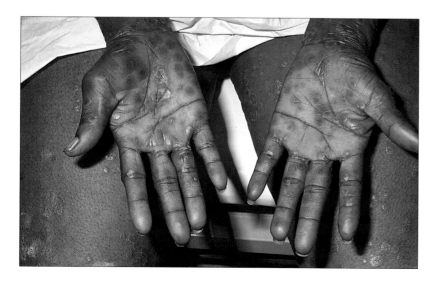

Fig. 2.52 Differential diagnosis in secondary syphilis. Targetoid annular papulosquamous secondary syphilis of the palms.

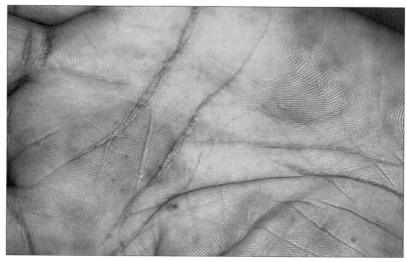

Fig. 2.53 Differential diagnosis in secondary syphilis. Erythema multiforme on the palm of the hand (compare with **2.52**).

forms can occur within a year after initial infection. The common underlying pathophysiologic event appears to be an endarteritis and periarteritis of small and medium-sized vessels (*Fig. 2.58*).

Cardiovascular Syphilis

This form of late syphilis is uncommon today, but still needs to be considered in the evaluation of aortic aneurysm and aortic valvular disease (*Fig.*

2.59). Cardiovascular syphilis has been estimated to occur in approximately 10% of cases of untreated syphilis, and may affect black patients more commonly than white ones.

The major pathologic changes in cardiovascular syphilis are dilatation of the aortic ring with incompetence of the valve, left ventricular hypertrophy, aortic root dilatation with aneurysm formation, and stenosis of the coronary artery ostia (*Fig. 2.60*).

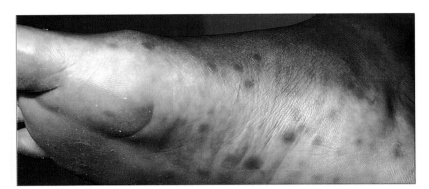

Fig. 2.54 Differential diagnosis in secondary syphilis. Papular secondary syphilis of the plantar surface of the foot.

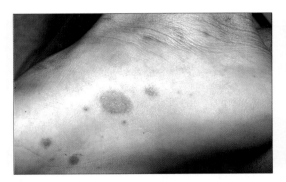

Fig. 2.55 Differential diagnosis in secondary syphilis. Pityriasis lichenoides chronica involving the leg and plantar aspect of the foot (compare with **2.54**).

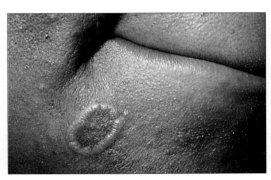

Fig. 2.56 Differential diagnosis in secondary syphilis. Discoid secondary syphilis of the face.

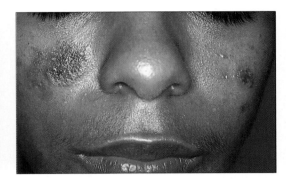

Fig. 2.57 Differential diagnosis in secondary syphilis. Discoid lupus erythematosus (compare with **2.56**).

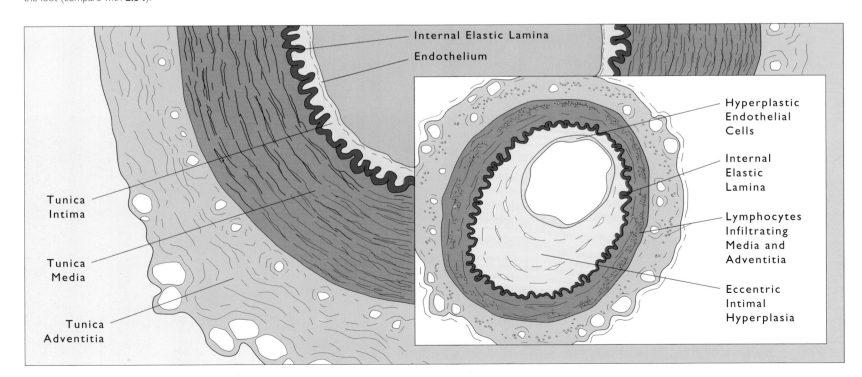

Fig. 2.58 The primary pathologic lesions of neurosyphilis. Schematic diagram showing the endarteritis of cerebral blood vessels, with lymphocytic infiltration and obliteration of the vessel lumen.

Late Benign Syphilis

The gummatous lesion probably represents a severe inflammatory response to treponemal antigens, but the exact mechanism of pathogenesis is not known. Microscopically, the active lesions are granulomas. Older lesions show extensive fibrosis and the lesions heal with deep scarring and fibrosis. Treponemes are difficult to detect in gummata.

Virtually any organ system may be affected by this inflammatory process, but the skin and bones are affected most commonly (*Fig. 2.61*). Skin lesions may be nodular, noduloulcerative, or gummatous (*Figs 2.61–2.64*). The nodules appear in groups, and are usually asymmetric in distribution. They are chronic, painless, and slowly progressive, and are found most often on the face, trunk, and extremities. Over time the nodules may break down into ulcers, which heal slowly centrally, leaving a characteristic arciform scar. Gummata of the skin are usually deep in the dermis and are solitary. They evolve into a granulomatous ulcer, with areas of spontaneous healing and scar formation. The most common lesion in bone is an osteitis, usually with periosteal changes. Radiographically, it may be indistinguishable from bacterial osteomyelitis. Characteristic areas of involvement are the hard palate, leading to perforation, and the nasal bones and nasal septum. Any mucous

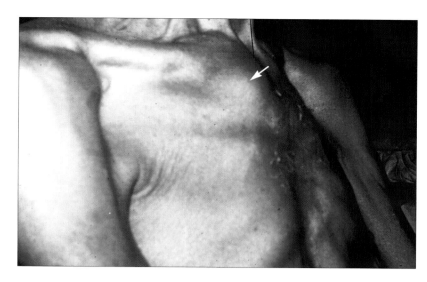

Fig. 2.59 Cardiovascular syphilis. Syphilitic aortic aneurysm with erosion through the chest wall (arrowed).

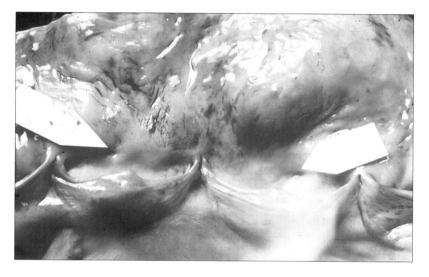

Fig. 2.60 Cardiovascular syphilis. Narrowing of the coronary ostia in syphilitic aortitis.

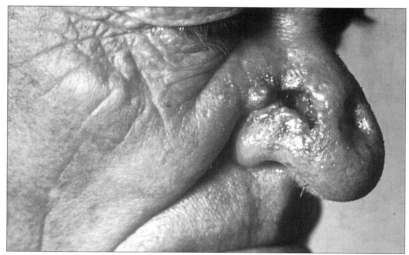

Fig. 2.61 Benign tertiary or gummatous syphilis. Ulcerating facial gummata such as these are now unusual in the USA, though they are still common in other parts of the world.

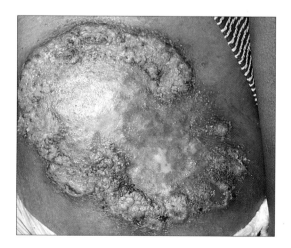

Fig. 2.62 Benign tertiary or gummatous syphilis. The crusted serpinginous border contrasts with the central flatter scarred areas which demonstrate partial spontaneous resolution.

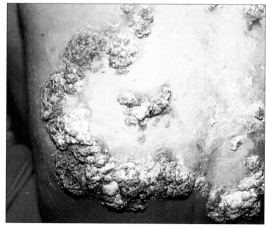

Fig. 2.63 Late nodular syphilis before treatment.

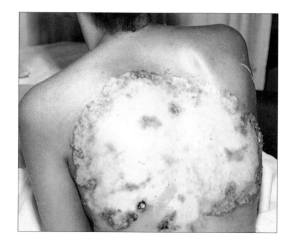

Fig. 2.64 Late nodular syphilis (as seen in **2.63**) after treatment with 10 million units of benzathine penicillin.

membrane surface may also be affected (*Fig. 2.65*). The digestive system may also be involved, especially the stomach, liver, and esophagus. These lesions are usually misdiagnosed initially as carcinomas.

Neurosyphilis

T. pallidum invades meninges and neural tissue during the secondary stage of the disease. Spirochetes may be seen in CSF, and in ocular and middle-ear fluid. There are basically two types of histopathologic lesions found in CNS syphilis:
- A chronic, low-grade meningitis with lymphocytic infiltration of meninges
- An endarteritis of small vessels of the brain and spinal cord.

Most often, the two lesion types coexist, accounting for the complex constellation of signs and symptoms in the various forms of neurosyphilis. With suitable stains, spirochetes may be demonstrated in the neural tissue of patients with neurosyphilis (Fig. 2.66). A general classification of neurosyphilis is presented in Fig. 2.67.

SYPHILIS AND HUMAN IMMUNODEFICIENCY VIRUS (HIV) COINFECTION

Most HIV-infected persons who also are infected with *T. pallidum* seem to have typical clinical signs and symptoms as well as serologic tests for syphilis.

However, exceptions have been noted (*Fig. 2.68*), and there are sundry problems in diagnosing syphilis in the HIV-positive person. Syphilis, the great imitator, can masquerade in the HIV-seropositive person as hairy leukoplakia (*Figs. 2.69* and *2.70*), Kaposi's sarcoma or gastric carcinoma (*Figs. 2.71–2.74*). However, most unusual clinical signs and symptoms appear to be associated with a rapid progression to the late stages of syphilis (*Figs. 2.75–2.77*), and to neurologic involvement (*Figs. 2.78–2.80*) even after treatment of primary or secondary syphilis, though neurologic symptoms may also occur in HIV-seronegative patients with secondary syphilis. Reported aberrant serologic responses in syphilitic patients seem to be related to abnormally low absolute CD4 cell counts and are relatively rare.

The failure of nontreponemal test titers to decline after treatment with standard therapy has been documented for both HIV-seronegative and HIV-seropositive persons treated during latent-stage or late-stage syphilis and in persons treated for reinfection; thus the reported failure of the titer to decline with treatment of the HIV-infected person is probably related to the stage of syphilis rather than to HIV status. The disappearance of reactivity in the treponemal tests after treatment and over time has been reported in the past, before the identification of HIV-1. Schroeter *et al.* reported that 14% of the patients with early syphilis lost their reactivity in the fluorescent treponemal

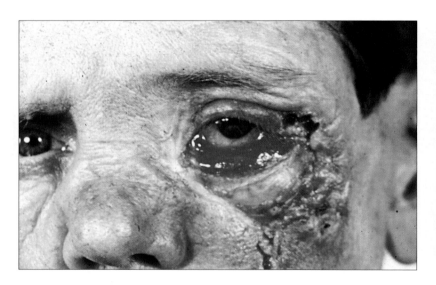

Fig. 2.65 Gummatous involvement of conjunctiva. Note also a noduloulcerative gumma over the right malar surface.

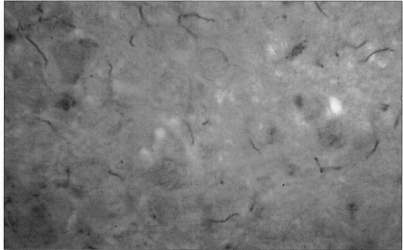

Fig. 2.66 Spirochetes demonstrated in neural tissue (Dieterle's silver stain).

NEUROSYPHILITIC SYNDROMES

I. MENINGEAL SYPHILIS
   a. Acute syphilitic meningitis
   b. Spinal pachymeningitis

II. MENINGOVASCULAR SYPHILIS
   a. Cerebrovascular syphilis
   b. Meningovascular syphilis of the spinal cord

III. PARENCHYMATOUS NEUROSYPHILIS
   a. General paresis
   b. Tabes dorsalis

IV. CNS GUMMATA

V. ISOLATED NEURAL EVENTS
   a. Optic neuritis/atrophy
   b. Sensorineural hearing loss

VI CONGENITAL NEUROSYPHILIS

Fig. 2.67 Neurosyphilitic syndromes.

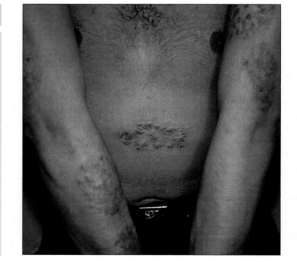

Fig. 2.68 Although an atypically severe rash occurred in this HIV-positive person with secondary syphilis, the serologic results for this individual were typical: VDRL titer of 2048 and a reactive FTA-ABS test result.

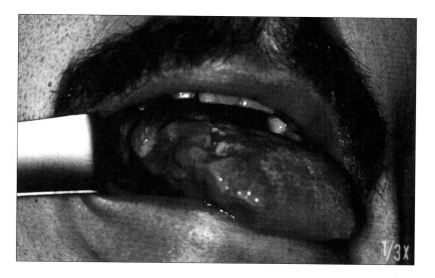

Fig. 2.69 Secondary syphilis resembling hairy leukoplakia.

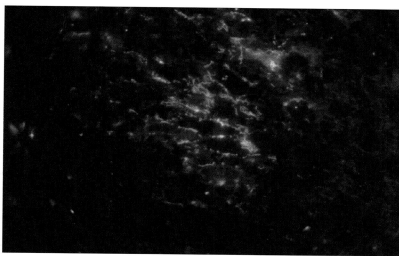

Fig. 2.70 *T. pallidum* observed in biopsy material of tongue shown in **2.69**, using fluorescein-labeled monoclonal antibody.

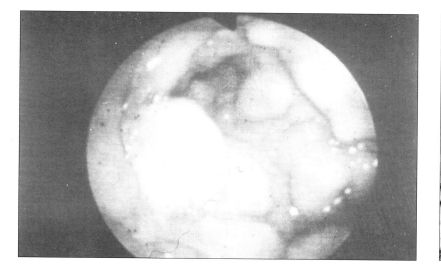

Fig. 2.71 Esophagogastroduodenoscopy demonstrating prominent gastric rugae and multiple polypoid masses with areas of friable mucosa and superficial ulcerations in patient with RPR titer of 512 and a reactive MHA-TP result.

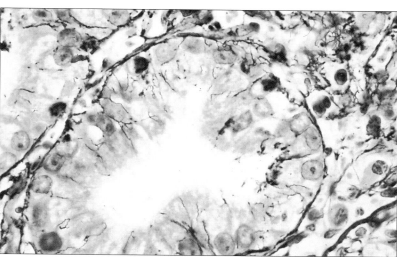

Fig. 2.72 On microscopic examination of gastrointestinal tract biopsy specimen from patient in **2.71**, numerous treponemes were observed (Steiner stain).

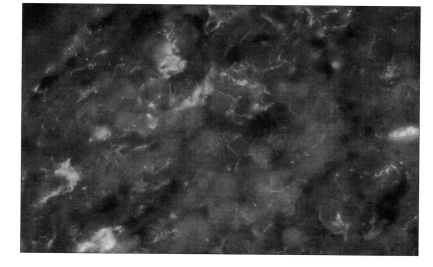

Fig. 2.73 *T. pallidum* observed in gastrointestinal tract biopsy specimen from patient in **2.71**, using fluorescein-labeled monoclonal antibody.

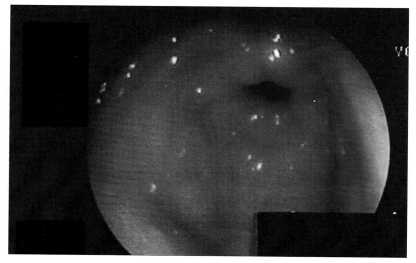

Fig. 2.74 Esophagogastroduodenoscopy of patient in **2.71** repeated at 3 months following a 10 day course of IV penicillin G, demonstrating normal-appearing gastric mucosa. The patient's RPR titer at 3 months, was 64.

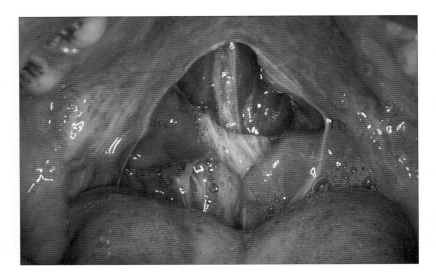

Fig. 2.75 Erosion of hard palate in a patient with a VDRL test titer of 4096.

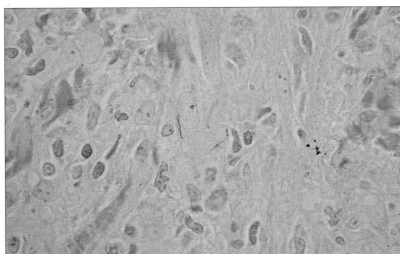

Fig. 2.76 On microscopic examination of erosion in **2.75**, an abscess and intense inflammatory cell infiltrates were observed, as well as abundant ill-defined, confluent granulomas, accompanied by large numbers of plasma cells. The Steiner stain revealed an occasional spirochete.

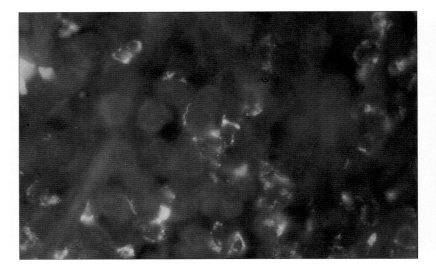

Fig. 2.77 The presence of *T. pallidum* in lesion in **2.75** was confirmed by DFAT-TP. Five months after treatment with 10 days of IV penicillin, the VDRL titer was 256.

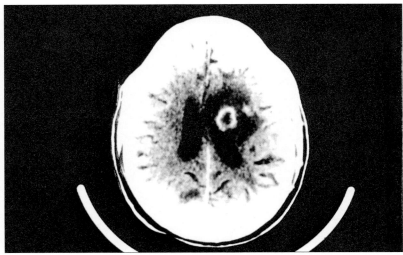

Fig. 2.78 Cranial CT scan demonstrating multiple ring enhancing lesions with a hyperdense nodule in the left centrum semiovale with surrounding edema. Additional lesions were noted in the right parietal area. Patient's serum RPR titer was 8; FTA-ABS results were reactive; CSF showed elevated (11) lymphocytes, increased protein (178mg/dl), and a titer of 2 in the VDRL CSF test.

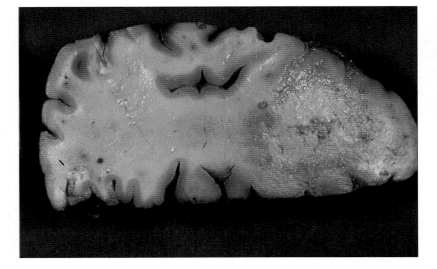

Fig. 2.79 Two lesions in the parietal lobe observed at autopsy of the patient in **2.78** had rubbery central firm greenish cores surrounded by a darker area. Similar lesions were observed in the white matter; and the presence of treponeme confirmed by PCR.

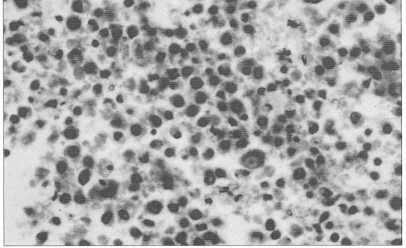

Fig. 2.80 Areas of coagulative necrosis with a marked chronic inflammatory exudate of lymphocytes and plasma cells were observed by microscopic examination (hematoxylin and eosin) of the lesions in **2.79**.

antibody absorption (FTA-ABS) test within 2 years after treatment. A more recent study found that over 20% of specimens from HIV-positive patients with acquired immunodeficiency syndrome (AIDS), with AIDS-related conditions (ARC), or without symptoms but with histories of treatment for syphilis, became nonreactive in the treponemal tests, whereas the treponemal tests results of HIV-seronegative persons remained reactive. Loss of reactivity in the treponemal tests was related to decreased total CD4 lymphocytes and CD4:CD8 ratios, and a nontreponemal test titer of less than 32 at the time of treatment. In the second study, the loss of reactivity could not be related to HIV status, CD4 count, or stage of syphilis. However, an initial low nontreponemal test titer was weakly associated with the loss of treponemal test reactivity. The unusually high titers in nontreponemal tests occasionally reported in the HIV-seropositive person are perhaps the result of B-cell activation. It is still unclear whether problems in diagnosing syphilis occur more frequently in HIV-seropositive persons than in HIV-seronegative persons.

Even though most HIV-seropositive persons treated with standard regimens for syphilis appear to respond to treatment, one cannot totally disregard the role of cell-mediated immunity in protecting the person against the progression of syphilis or the interaction of an intact immune system with therapeutic agents. Although still within the normal ranges, early findings in our most recent study indicated that the percentage of CD4 cells was significantly lower (p = <0.001) and CD8 cells higher (p = 0.03) among patients with syphilis than in the uninfected population. Thus, infection with *T. pallidum* in the HIV-positive person may exacerbate the depletion of CD4 receptor cells and result in less effective treatment of syphilis in the HIV-seropositive patient with standard regimens.

Recommendations for diagnosing and treating syphilis among HIV-infected persons have been made by the Centers for Disease Control and Prevention (CDC), Atlanta, Georgia. These include:

- the increased usage of direct microscopic examinations of lesion or biopsy material when clinical findings suggest syphilis, but serologic test results are nonreactive
- careful serologic and physical examination follow-up to ensure adequacy of treatment
- a CSF examination of patients in whom syphilis is latent and in whom the duration, if known, is less than 1 year
- the treatment of neurosyphilis among HIV-infected patients, with at least 10 days of aqueous crystalline penicillin G or aqueous procaine penicillin G plus probenecid
- the reporting of unusual manifestations of syphilis to state epidemiologists.

TREATMENT SCHEDULES FOR SYPHILIS*

A   EARLY SYPHILIS

(primary, secondary, latent <1 year's duration)
1. Benzathine penicillin G: 2.4 million U, im stat.
2. For the penicillin-allergic patient: a) tetracycline HCl : 500 mg po qid for 15 days, or b) doxycycline: 100 mg po bid for 15 days.

B   SYPHILIS OF MORE THAN ONE YEAR'S DURATION

(latent syphilis of indeterminate or >1 year's duration, cardiovascular, or late benign syphilis, NOT neurosyphilis)
1. Benzathine penicillin G: 2.4 million U, im once a week for 3 successive weeks (7.2 million U total).
2. Penicillin-allergic patients: Same as early syphilis (A), except the duration of therapy is 30 days.

C   CSF EXAMINATION

Cerebrospinal fluid examination should be done for patients with clinical symptoms or signs consistent with neurosyphilis. This examination is desirable in all patients with syphilis of indeterminate age to rule out asymptomatic neurosyphilis. However, this is not always practical. Patients who are treated without spinal fluid examination should be followed carefully.

D   NEUROSYPHILIS

1. Aqueous crystalline penicillin G: 12 million U every 4 hours for 10 days + benzathine penicillin G: 2.4 million U im weekly for 3 consecutive weeks.
2. Aqueous procaine penicillin G: 2.4 million U im daily for 10 days + 3 weeks of benzathine penicillin as above.
3. Regimen for penicillin-allergic patients: there are no recommended regimens. Consult with an infectious disease specialist.

E   SYPHILIS DURING PREGNANCY

1. For the nonpenicillin-allergic woman, penicillin prescribed in the doses recommended for nonpregnant patients appropriate for the stage of syphilis should be administered.
2. There are no proven alternatives to penicillin. A pregnant woman with a history of penicillin allergy should be treated with penicillin after desensitization, if necessary. Skin testing may be helpful for some patients and in some settings.
3. Patients should have monthly quantitative nontreponemal serologic tests for the remainder of the pregnancy. Women with a fourfold rise in titer should be retreated.

F   SYPHILIS AMONG HIV-INFECTED PATIENTS

1. When clinical findings suggest that syphilis is present, but serologic tests are nonreactive or confusing, it may be helpful to perform direct fluorescent antibody staining of lesion or biopsy material.
2. Neurosyphilis should be considered in the differential diagnosis of neurologic disease among HIV-infected persons.
3. a) Early syphilis. Treatment as for individuals without HIV infection is recommended. However, some experts recommend additional treatments such as multiple doses of benzathine penicillin G as suggested for late syphilis, or other supplemental antibiotic in addition to benzathine penicillin G 2.4 million U im. b) Latent syphilis. Patients who have both latent syphilis and HIV infection should undergo CSF examination before treatment. A patient with latent syphilis, HIV infection, and a normal CSF examination can be treated with benzathine penicillin G 7.2 million U (as 3 weekly doses of 2.4 million U each).

* Specimens for dark-field examination and blood for serologic tests for syphilis should always be collected and preferably interpreted together with clinical findings prior to instituting therapy for syphilis.

Fig. 2.81 Treatment schedules for syphilis.

TREATMENT

Penicillin is the mainstay of syphilotherapy. Although alternative drugs are listed, their efficacy has never been proven in clinical trials. The recommendations presented in *Fig. 2.81* are a synopsis of those provided by the CDC.

LABORATORY TESTS

COLLECTION OF SPECIMENS

Specimens for dark-field microscopy can be collected from genital lesions or from lymph nodes. In addition, specimens for the direct immunofluorescent antibody test for *T. pallidum* (DFA-TP) can be collected from oral and anal lesions. The ideal specimen for direct examination is serous fluid with minimal red blood cells. To collect serous material from the chancre, any scab or crust should first be gently removed using a scalpel blade, a tongue blade, or a needle. A gauze sponge soaked in 0.9% nonbacteriostatic saline should be used to remove tissue debris and superficial bacteria from the lesion only if

necessary. The first few drops of exudate, which may contain blood, are then wiped away. Relatively clear fluid should be collected, either by applying a clean microscope slide or coverslip to the lesion, or by transferring the fluid, using a bacteriologic loop, to the microscope slide. The coverslip is then pressed onto a clean glass slide and examined on a dark-field microscope. The steps for properly collecting this material are demonstrated in *Figs. 2.82–2.84*. Specimens collected for dark-field can be examined by DFA-TP simply by removing the cover slip and letting the slide air dry, or specimens can be collected in capillary tubes. Material collected from the lesion's depths is more likely to contain motile treponemes than surface material. Healing skin lesions merit examination as well. They should be abraded with a sharp instrument, or fluid may be collected from the lesion by injecting a drop of sterile saline into the base of the lesion and aspirating with a small-gauge needle and syringe.

Collection of lesion material in the cervix or vaginal vault for direct examination follows the same principles, but must always be by direct visualization through a speculum. Aspiration of lymph nodes is done by injecting 0.2 ml or less of sterile saline into the node through sterilized skin, followed by aspiration of the tissue material. The dark-field examination must be performed immediately after specimen collection; however the specimen for DFA-TP can be held until staining can be conveniently performed. For all

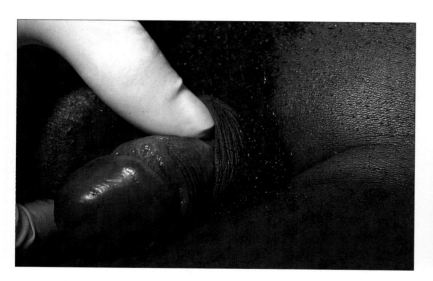

Fig. 2.82 Collection of specimen for dark-field microscopy or DFA-TP test. Penile ulcer after cleaning with gauze.

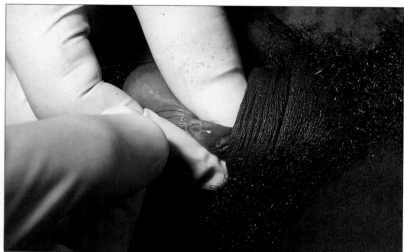

Fig. 2.83 Collection of specimen for dark-field microscopy or DFA-TP test. Squeezing the ulcer to obtain exudate.

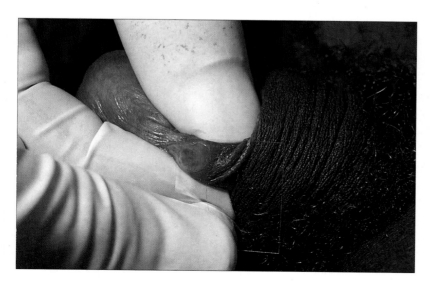

Fig. 2.84 Collection of specimen for dark-field microscopy or DFA-TP test. Touching coverslip to ulcer to obtain fluid for dark-field examination.

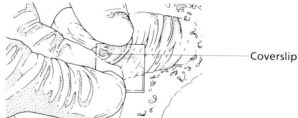

Coverslip

serologic tests for syphilis, blood is collected into dry tubes without anti-coagulant, allowed to clot, and the serum separated by centrifugation (*Fig. 2.85*). If the test is not to be performed immediately, sera should be removed from the clots and either stored at refrigerator temperature (4°C) or frozen.

DIRECT DIAGNOSIS

The most specific method for the diagnosis of the early stages of syphilis is direct microscopy of material taken from the lesion or lymph node aspirates. These tests are usually the first to become positive. The demonstration of treponemes with characteristic morphology and motility, or staining with a fluorescent-labeled conjugate specific for *T. pallidum* is diagnostic of primary, secondary, and congenital syphilis, and of relapses during early latent syphilis, provided yaws, bejel, and pinta have been excluded.

Direct microscopy is useful in establishing a diagnosis of reinfection as well. In addition, direct microscopy is often used to rule out syphilis as the cause of lesions associated with other sexually transmitted diseases. When specimens have been properly collected and the patient has not been treated locally or systemically with antimicrobials, direct methods are at least 95% sensitive.

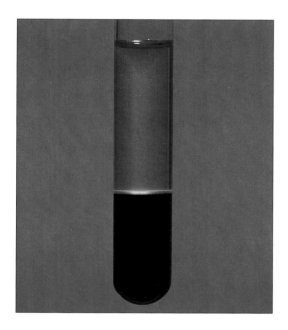

Fig. 2.85 Centrifuged blood clot ready for removal of serum after centrifugation. Serum is collected by venipuncture into a 'red top' vacutainer tube without anticoagulant, centrifuged, and if necessary, separated from clot for storage.

Dark-field Microscopy

In dark-field microscopy, light rays strike organisms or particles at such an oblique angle that no direct light enters the microscope, except that reflected from the organisms or particles. Thus, anything in the light path appears luminous against a dark background (*Fig. 2.86*). The non-pathogens *T. refringens* and *T. denticola* are usually found in the gastrointestinal tract and are easily confused with *T. pallidum* on dark-field examination.

Direct Fluorescent Antibody Test for T. pallidum

The DFA-TP is an immunofluorescent antibody test in which an anti-*T. pallidum* monoclonal or absorbed polyclonal antibody is labeled with a fluorochrome dye, fluorescein isothiocyanate (FITC) to identify the organism. Motility of the organism is not required in the DFA-TP. As the conjugates used are specific for pathogenic strains of *Treponema*, the DFA-TP is applicable to samples collected from both oral and rectal lesions. Samples collected as for dark-field examination are air-dried, fixed in methanol or acetone, and then stained with the FITC conjugate (*Fig. 2.87*). The use of the DFA-TP test has been extended to include the staining of tissue sections (DFAT-TP). Any tissue can be used (*Figs. 2.70–2.77*), but tissue for paraffin-embedded sections are collected most often from the brain, gastrointestinal tract, placenta, umbilical cord, or skin. Often DFAT-TP is used to diagnose late-stage adult syphilis or congenital syphilis or to distinguish skin lesions of secondary or late syphilis from those of Lyme disease.

Polymerase chain reaction

The methods used for PCR have not been standardized, but one group of investigators has successfully used the method briefly described here. Samples to be examined by PCR are prepared by alkaline lysis extraction of the treponemal DNA in the sample. The primers and probe for detection of *T. pallidum* are prepared from the 47 kDa gene. After a 40-cycle series of denaturing, annealing, and extension, the PCR products are visualized by electrophoresis, Southern blot hybridization with a ^{32}P-labeled probe and then autoradiography. At least one commercial company has incorporated *T. pallidum* primers in a PCR for genital ulcer disease. PCR offers the advantage over dark-field microscopy and DFA of detecting low numbers, or even portions, of treponemes that may be in the lesion even after the patient has been treated. PCR should be of greatest value in the diagnosis of neurosyphilis and congenital syphilis, since the current serologic tests are inadequate in these areas.

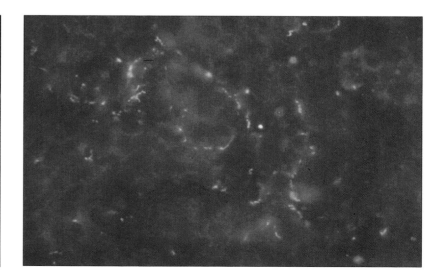

Fig. 2.86 Positive dark-field examination. Treponemes are recognized by their characteristic corkscrew shape and deliberate forward and backward movement with rotation about the longitudinal axis.

Fig. 2.87 DFA-TP positive tissue section. The DFA-TP has the following advantages over the dark-field examination: motile organisms are not required; pathogenic treponemes can be differentiated from nonpathogenic treponemes in oral lesions; and tissue sections for biopsy can be examined as well as autopsy material.

INDIRECT DIAGNOSIS USING NONTREPONEMAL SEROLOGIC TESTS

The serologic tests for syphilis are divided into screening tests and confirmation tests, based on the specific antigen used. Nontreponemal (reagin) tests may be used either as qualitative or quantitative tests. Qualitative nontreponemal tests are used as screening tests to measure IgM and IgG antibodies to lipoidal material released from damaged host cells, as well as to lipoprotein-like material released from the treponemes. The antilipoidal antibodies are antibodies that are produced not only as a consequence of syphilis and other treponemal diseases, but also in response to nontreponemal diseases of an acute and chronic nature in which tissue damage occurs.

In primary syphilis, reactivity in these tests does not develop until 1–4 weeks after the chancre first appears. For this reason, patients with suspected lesions and nonreactive nontreponemal tests should have repeat tests performed at 1-week, 1-month, and 3-month intervals from the time of initial testing. Nonreactive tests during the 3-month period exclude the diagnosis of syphilis.

The nontreponemal tests are reactive in secondary syphilis almost without exception, and usually in titers of 16 or greater regardless of the test method used. Less than 2% of sera will exhibit a prozone (*Fig. 2.88*). Nontreponemal test titers in early latent syphilis are similar to those of secondary syphilis. However, as the duration of the latent stage increases the titer decreases.

The nontreponemal cerebrospinal fluid veneral disease research laboratory (CSF VDRL) test (*Fig. 2.89*) is the only serologic test recognized as a standard test for the diagnosis of neurosyphilis. Asymptomatic neurosyphilis should not be diagnosed by a reactive CSF VDRL alone. CSF criteria for the diagnosis of neurosyphilis are:
• Reactive CSF VDRL
• Reactive serum treponemal test
• Five or more lymphocytes/mm³ CSF
• CSF total protein of ≥ 45 mg/dl.
Symptomatic neurosyphilis is diagnosed by clinical symptoms and signs, supplemented with reactive results in the above diagnostic procedures.

Serial quantitative nontreponemal tests can be used to measure the adequacy of therapy. Titers should be obtained at 3-month intervals for at least 1 year. A fourfold drop in titer is frequently noted by 3 months, in adequately treated early syphilis.

In congenital syphilis, the role of nontreponemal tests is to monitor the antibody titer. Titers will decrease with treatment; however, a rising titer in monthly tests from an infant over a 6-month period is diagnostic for congenital syphilis. If an infant has not been infected *in utero*, passively transferred antibodies should no longer be detected by 3 months postpartum with nontreponemal tests. All nontreponemal tests will occasionally give false-positive results. In general populations, this occurs in 1–2% of tests. *Acute false-positive* reactions lasting less than 6 months usually occur after febrile diseases or immunizations, or during pregnancy. However, false-positive rates may exceed 10% in populations with a high prevalence of intravenous drug use. The titers of false-positive reactions are usually less than 8. Since titers are also low in latent syphilis, not all low titers are false positives. In addition, not all high titers are true positives. In intravenous drug users, approximately 12% of false-positive titers are 8 or greater. *Chronic false-positive* reactions are more often associated with autoimmune disorders, such as rheumatoid arthritis and systemic lupus erythematosus, or with chronic infections such as leprosy. Titers in chronic false-positive reactions also are low, usually less than 8.

Specific Nontreponemal Serologic Tests

Standard nontreponemal tests for syphilis are listed in *Fig. 2.89*. All four tests use the VDRL antigen (cardiolipin, cholesterol, and lecithin) as the principal component. The VDRL slide test is the only test using an antigen that has not been stabilized by the addition of EDTA, and which does not contain choline chloride to eliminate the need for heat-inactivation of the serum. The rapid plasma reagin (RPR) test is the most widely used test. The CSF VDRL slide test is the only recognized procedure for the serodiagnosis of neurosyphilis. All four tests use similar equipment (*Fig. 2.90*).

STANDARD NONTREPONEMAL TESTS

MICROSCOPIC TESTS

Venereal Disease Research Laboratory (VDRL) Slide Test

Unheated Serum Reagin (USR) Test

MACROSCOPIC TESTS

Rapid Plasma Reagin (RPR) Test

Toluidine Red Unheated Serum Test (TRUST)

Fig. 2.89 Standard nontreponemal tests.

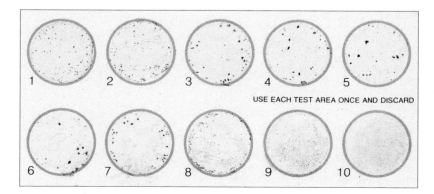

Fig. 2.88 The prozone phenomenon. Some high-titered sera, such as this one at 1:256, when tested undiluted may appear to give rough nonreactive or minimally reactive (circle 1) results. However, upon dilution, the flocculation intensifies (circle 5) and then progressively decreases to become nonreactive (circle 10). The prozone phenomenon may be due not only to an antibody excess, but also to blocking or incomplete antibody formation.

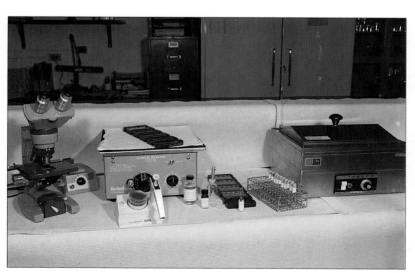

Fig. 2.90 This is an example of equipment required to perform the nontreponemal tests for syphilis. Shown here are a mechanical rotator, a water bath, a microscope, a safety pipetter, and reagents.

VDRL SLIDE TEST Because of the nature of the VDRL antigen, when the antigen is reacted with antibody, the antigen-antibody complex remains suspended rather than precipitating or agglutinating as in most serologic tests (*Fig. 2.91*). The resulting antigen-antibody complex in the VDRL antigen based tests results from flocculation, and because the complex particles are usually small, they must be viewed with a microscope.

UNHEATED SERUM REAGIN (USR) TEST is a microscopic test like the VDRL. The principle of the USR is identical to that of the VDRL, although the antigen for the USR has been stabilized. The USR has two advantages over the VDRL: firstly, the antigen is ready for use once it reaches room temperature; and secondly, the sera do not require heating before testing. In all other aspects, the test is performed and read like the VDRL slide test (*see Fig. 2.91*).

RPR CARD TEST AND TRUST The principle of the TRUST and RPR card tests is the same as that of the VDRL slide test. However, in these two tests sized particles (charcoal for the RPR and red paint pigment for the TRUST) are added to the USR antigen to enhance antigen-antibody visualization (*Fig. 2.92*). The particles become entrapped within the antigen-antibody

lattice of a positive reaction, yielding flocculation that is visible to the naked eye (*Figs. 2.93–2.94*). No microscope is needed, which makes these macroscopic tests more convenient than the VDRL or USR, accounting for their present popularity.

VDRL-EIA A new format for a nontreponemal test is the enzyme immunoassay (EIA). In the VISUWELL™ Reagin Test, VDRL antigen coats the well of the microtiter plate. Anticardiolipin antibodies in the patient's serum adhere to the antigen in the wells and this antibody reaction is detected by an antihuman IgG antibody, labeled with urease as the enzyme.

INDIRECT DIAGNOSIS USING TREPONEMAL SEROLOGIC TESTS

In contrast to the nontreponemal tests, the treponemal tests should be reserved for confirmatory testing when the clinical signs and/or history disagree with the reactive nontreponemal test results. Treponemal tests are based on the detection of antibodies formed specifically to the antigenic determinants of the treponemes. They are qualitative procedures, which therefore cannot be used to monitor the efficacy of treatment. Like

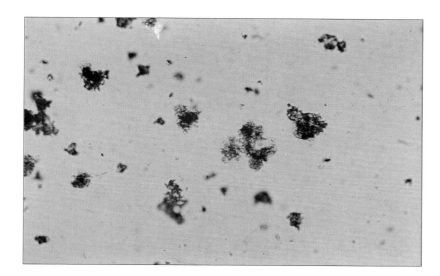

Fig. 2.91 Reactive VDRL or USR result. Specimens exhibiting medium and/or large flocculation particles are reported as reactive (R). Those with small particles are reported as weakly reactive (W), while those with complete dispersion of antigen particles or slight roughness are reported as nonreactive (NR). Sera exhibiting slight roughness should be quantitated to check for the prozone phenomenon.

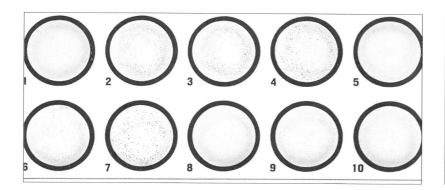

Fig. 2.93 Qualitative RPR card test. Specimens exhibiting medium to large flocculation are reported as reactive (circles 4 and 7). Specimens with definite but small flocculation are read as reactive minimal (Rm) (circle 2 and 3). Specimens with an even dispersion of antigen particles (circles 1, 5, 8, and 10) or specimens that are slightly rough (circle 6) are reported as nonreactive.

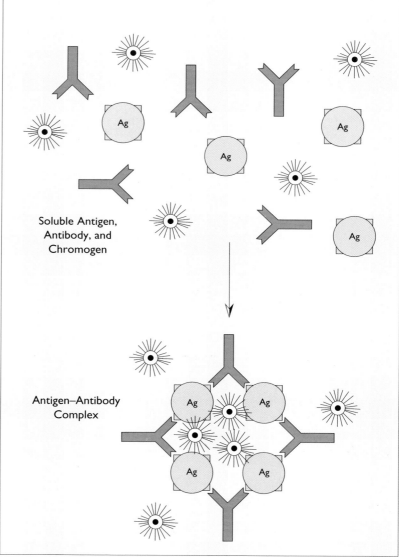

Fig. 2.92 In the macroscopic nontreponemal tests, sized colored particles become entrapped in the antigen-antibody formation. Results for these card tests are reported as reactive or nonreactive; there is no weakly reactive report.

the nontreponemal tests, treponemal tests are almost always reactive in secondary and latent syphilis. For most cases, once the treponemal tests are reactive, they remain so for the patient's lifetime. In fact, in some patients with late syphilis, a reactive treponemal test may be the only means of confirming the suspected diagnosis. Currently, none of the treponemal tests are recommended for use with CSF.

The greatest value of the treponemal tests is to differentiate true-positive nontreponemal test results from false-positive results. However, false-positive treponemal test results do occur with about the same frequency (1%) as false-positive nontreponemal test results. Although some false-positive results in the treponemal tests are transient and of unknown cause, they have been associated with connective tissue diseases. When unexplained reactive tests occur in elderly patients, attempts should be made to rule out acquired or congenital syphilis, or infections with other treponemes, before a diagnosis of false-positive serology is made.

Specific Treponemal Serologic Tests

Standard treponemal tests for syphilis are listed in *Fig. 2.95*.

FTA-ABS AND FTA-ABS DS Both of these indirect immunofluorescence tests are based on the same principle (*Fig. 2.96*). The two tests differ in that the double-stain test employs a FITC-labeled conjugate as a direct stain for *T. pallidum* and a tetramethyl rhodamine isothiocyanate (TMRITC)-labeled antihuman IgG conjugate to detect the antibody in the patient's serum. This eliminates the need for first having to use dark-field microscopy on the smear to find treponemes (*Figs. 2.97* and *2.98*). Both tests are reported as shown in *Fig. 2.99*.

MHA-TP Passive hemagglutination of erythrocytes sensitized with antigen is an extremely simple method for the detection of antibody (*Fig. 2.100*). The antigen used in the procedure is formalized, tanned sheep erythrocytes sensitized with ultrasonicated material from *T. pallidum* (Nichols strain). Unsensitized cells are used as a control for nonspecific reactivity. Hemagglutination results are read and reported as in *Figs. 2.101* and *2.102*.

TREPONEMAL EIA Several commercial EIA tests have been designed to replace the FTA-ABS tests and MHA-TP as confirmatory tests for syphilis. These tests are relatively similar in that a treponemal antigen, either cloned or sonicated, coats the plate. The patient's serum is added and the mixture is then incubated and washed. An enzyme-labeled antihuman immunoglobulin conjugate and enzyme substrate are then added to detect the initial antigen-antibody reaction. Initial evaluations of several of these EIA tests have found that they all have sensitivities and specificities similar to those of other treponemal tests, but more extensive evaluation is necessary.

T. PALLIDUM WESTERN BLOT Another test format that has been used frequently in the research laboratory is the Western blot for *T. pallidum* (*Fig. 2.103*). The test using IgG conjugate appears to be at least as sensitive and specific as the FTA-ABS tests and efforts have been made to standardize the procedure. To date, many investigators agree that the presence of antibodies to the immunodeterminants with molecular weights of 15.5, 17, 44.5 and 47 appear to be diagnostic for acquired syphilis. Several studies have found the Western blot for *T. pallidum* to have its greatest value as a diagnostic test for congenital syphilis when an IgM-specific conjugate is used.

SENSITIVITY AND SPECIFICITY OF SEROLOGIC TESTS

While the overall sensitivity of the nontreponemal tests (*Fig. 2.104*) is approximately 90%, up to 28% of patients with early primary syphilis will have nonreactive nontreponemal test results on the initial visit. In addition, patients will present with nonreactive nontreponemal tests in about

Fig. 2.94 Quantitative TRUST. The reading of the TRUST is identical to that of the RPR card test.

STANDARD TREPONEMAL TESTS

Fluorescent Treponemal Antibody Absorption (FTA-ABS) Test

FTA-ABS double-staining (DS) Test (FTA-ABS DS)

Microhemagglutination Assay for Antibodies to *T. pallidum* (MHA-TP)

Fig. 2.95 Standard treponemal tests.

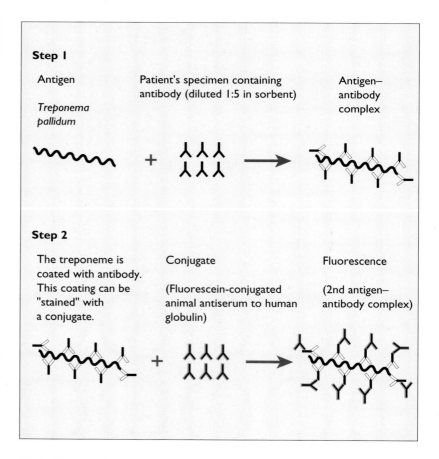

Step 1

| Antigen | Patient's specimen containing antibody (diluted 1:5 in sorbent) | Antigen– antibody complex |

Treponema pallidum

Step 2

The treponeme is coated with antibody. This coating can be "stained" with a conjugate.

Conjugate

(Fluorescein-conjugated animal antiserum to human globulin)

Fluorescence

(2nd antigen– antibody complex)

Fig. 2.96 Theory of FTA test – reactive reaction. To perform the FTA-ABS tests, the patient's serum, which has been diluted with sorbent, is layered on a microscope slide to which *T. pallidum* has been fixed. If the patient's serum contains antibody, it will coat the treponeme. Next fluorochrome-labeled antihuman IgG conjugate is used to detect the initial antigen–antibody reaction.

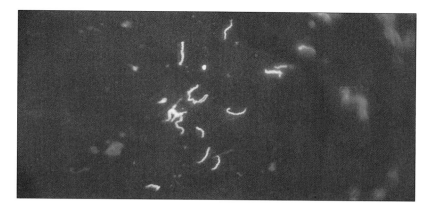

Fig. 2.97 Example of the FTA-ABS DS. In reading the FTA-ABS DS, the treponemes are easily located, since the antigen is counterstained with the direct-staining FITC-labeled antitreponemal globulin component. If the patient's serum does not contain anti-*T. pallidum* antibodies, when the slide is read using the rhodamine filter set, no treponemes will be observed.

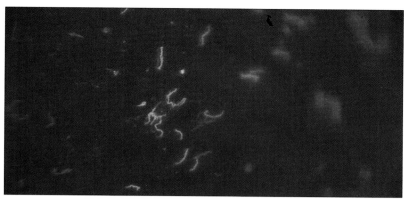

Fig. 2.98 Reactive FTA-ABS DS test. If the patient's serum contains antibodies to *T. pallidum*, the treponemes will appear reddish-orange when the rhodamine filters are used, due to the TMRITC-labeled antihuman IgG globulin used as the indicator stain or indirect component of the system.

INTERPRETATION AND REPORTING OF FTS-ABS AND FTA-ABS DS TESTS

INTERPRETATION OF FLUORESCENCE

INITIAL TEST	REPEAT TEST	REPORT
2+ to 4+		Reactive
1+	>1+	Reactive
1+	=1+	Reactive minimal*
<1+		Nonreactive
−		Nonreactive

* In the absence of historical or clinical evidence of treponemal infection, the test result should be considered equivocal. A second specimen should be submitted for serologic testing.

Fig. 2.99 Interpretation and reporting of FTA-ABS and FTA-ABS DS tests.

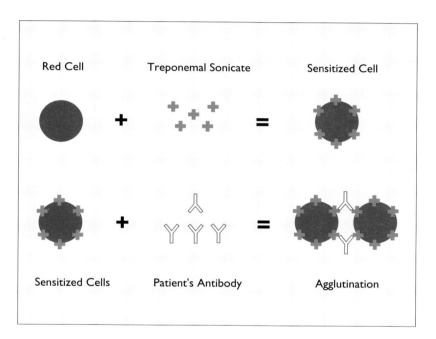

Fig. 2.100 To perform the MHA-TP, the patient's serum is first mixed with absorbing diluent made from nonpathogenic Reiter treponemes and other absorbents and stabilizers. The serum is then placed in a microtiter plate and sensitized sheep red cells are added. Serum that contains antibodies reacts with these cells to form a smooth mat of agglutinated cells in the microtiter plate.

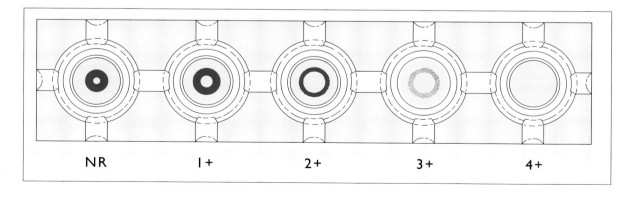

Fig. 2.101 Hemagglutination test results. Results for the MHA-TP are reported as reactive (1+, 2+, 3+, 4+) or nonreactive (±, −). Completely negative readings vary in pattern from a solid compact button of cells to a circle of cells with a small central hole, as seen in this drawing.

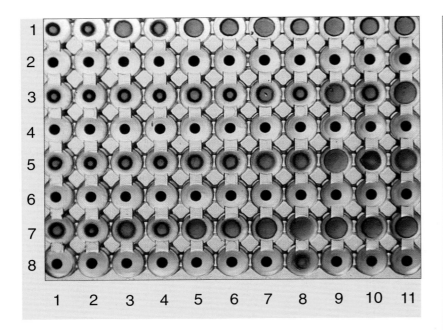

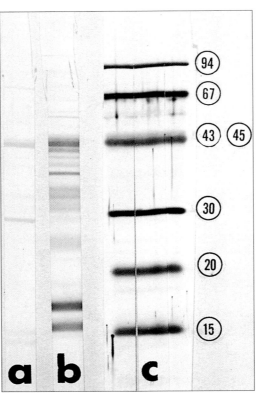

Fig. 2.102 Example of a microhemagglutination test result. (Rows are horizontal and wells are vertical.) Agglutination patterns vary from 1+ (well 5, row 3) to 4+ (well 5, row 1). An example of a 2+ is seen in well 7, row 5, while an example of a 3+ appears in well 7, row 7. A ± reading appears in well 3 of row 3. Heterophile reactions can occur in the MHA-TP procedure; an example of a heterophile reaction is seen in well 8, row 8.

Fig. 2.103 To perform Western blots, the antigen is first electrophoresed through polyacrylamide gel, and then the proteins are electrophoretically blotted to nitrocellulose. The blot is cut into strips and incubated with the patient's serum. If antibody is present, this antigen–antibody reaction is detected using a second antibody, such as in other indirect tests such as EIA. In lane a, there is a serum sample from an individual without syphilis (negative control), while in lane b there is a reactive control and in lane c the molecular weight standard. To be considered reactive in the Western blot, the patient's serum must react with bands of 15.5 kDa, 17 kDa, and 47 kDa.

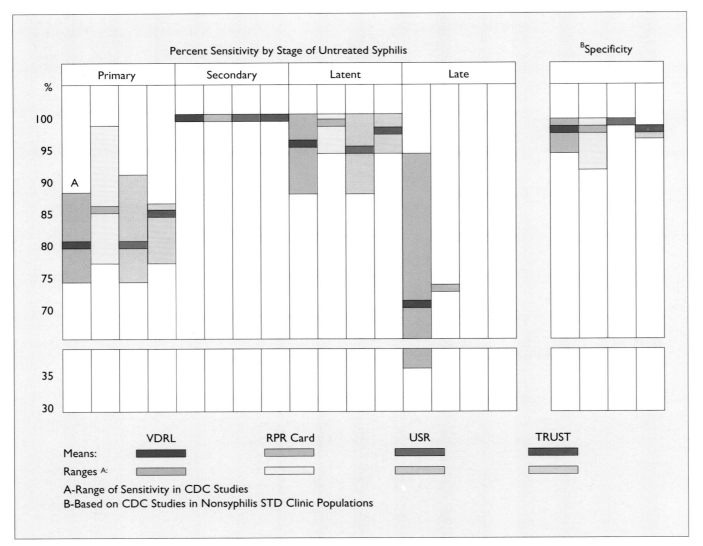

Fig. 2.104 Sensitivity and specificity of nontreponemal tests.

30% of cases of late untreated syphilis. Specificity for the nontreponemal tests is 98%. However, the specificity of the test is greatly influenced by the population being tested. In intravenous drug users, the specificity may be as low as 79% for the VDRL slide test and approximately 89% for the RPR test. The VDRL CSF test is 90% sensitive and 100% specific in symptomatic cases of neurosyphilis, but it is only about 10% sensitive in asymptomatic neurosyphilis.

The overall sensitivity (about 98%) of the FTA-ABS test is greater than that of the other three major treponemal tests (each of which has a sensitivity of approximately 95%) (*Fig. 2.105*). The major difference in the sensitivities of these tests is found in primary syphilis. However, if data are analyzed according to the diagnosis of primary syphilis based on dark-field positive lesions alone, and primary cases are separated into those with reactive nontreponemal test results, then the sensitivities of the four treponemal tests are almost identical and are greater than 99%. False positives can occur in the treponemal tests, but only rarely do false positives occur in both treponemal and nontreponemal tests for the same patient. Individuals with connective tissue diseases may present difficult serodiagnostic problems.

Serologic tests must be interpreted according to the disease stage, possible underlying disease conditions, and the possibility of false-positive test results. Ideally, all sera in suspected cases of syphilis should be tested first with a nontreponemal procedure and reactive results verified with a second specimen and quantification. Cases in which clinical or epidemiologic evidence is counter to the diagnosis of syphilis should be confirmed with a treponemal test. With the proper use of serologic tests, a reactive nontreponemal test with a reactive treponemal test gives a positive predictive value of approximately 97%, or only a 3% error factor. In contrast, if any one test is used, the positive predictive value, regardless of the method, is less than 50% in a low-prevalence disease such as syphilis.

Misinterpretation of test results for nontreponemal tests most often results from:
* The failure to recognize the variation of plus or minus one dilution inherent in most serologic tests
* The failure to establish the true positivity of test results
* The failure to recognize reactivity due to nonvenereal treponematoses.

In summary, serologic testing for syphilis often plays a crucial role in making a diagnosis of syphilis. Many tests are commercially available and are of high quality. All tests require rigid standardization with negative and positive control sera before being used to test sera from patients. Finally, the serologic tests should be interpreted carefully by an experienced clinician, in the light of a thorough history, physical, and, if possible, dark-field examination, before a diagnosis of syphilis is made.

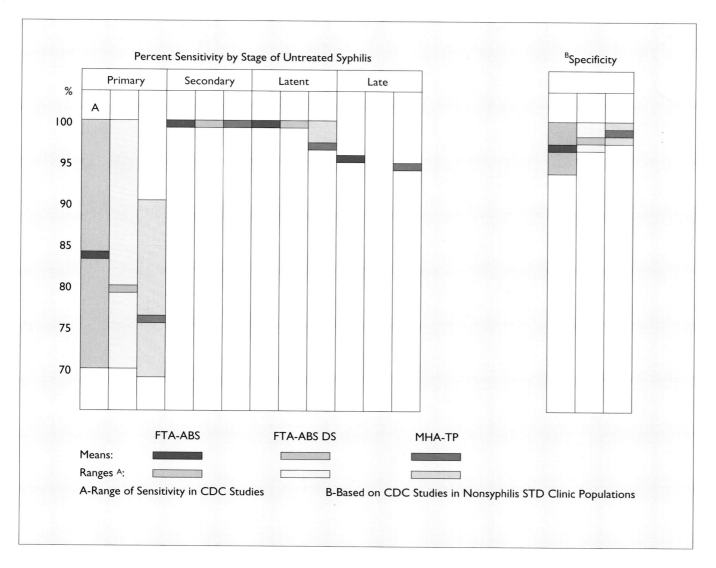

Fig. 2.105 Sensitivity and specificity of treponemal tests.

Picture credits for this chapter are as follows: Fig. 2.3 courtesy of JPA, WHO; Figs. 2.6 and 2.7 adapted from the unpublished work of Hans Ristow, MD; Figs. 2.11 and 2.12 courtesy of Barbara Romanowski, M.D.; Fig. 2.30 courtesy of Heidi Watts; Fig. 2.58 adapted from a drawing by Karlene Hewan-Lowe, MD; Fig. 2.86 courtesy of Ralph Ramsey; Figs. 2.62 to 2.64 courtesy of Professor Norma Saxe; Figs. 2.15 to 2.17, 2.36, 2.59, 2.60, 2.62, 2.66, 2.85, 2.87, 2.88, 2.90, 2.91, 2.93, 2.97, 2.98, and 2.102 from the collection of the Centers for Disease Control in Atlanta, Georgia; Fig. 2.68 courtesy of Jeffrey Gilbert, M.D., Briarcliff Manor, New York; Figs. 2.69 and 2.70 courtesy of Gregory Mertz, M.D., Department of Medicine, University of New Mexico; Figs. 2.71 to 2.74 courtesy of John F. Turner, M.D., Dennis B. Weiserbs, M.D., and James B. Francis, M.D., Roanoke Memorial Hospital, Roanoke, Virginia; Figs. 2.75 to 2.77 courtesy of Wesley Wong, Jennifer Flood, M.D., and Joseph Engelman, M.D., San Francisco City Clinic, San Francisco, California; Figs. 2.78 to 2.80 courtesy of Harold Horowitz, M.D., New York Medical College, Valhalla, New York, reprinted by permission of the *New England Journal of Medicine* **331**:1488–1492, 1884; Fig. 2.103 courtesy of Robert George M.S., Centers for Disease Control and Prevention, Atlanta, Georgia.

BIBLIOGRAPHY

Bayne LL, Sidley JW, Goodin DS: Acute syphilitic meningitis: Its occurrence after clinical and serologic cure of secondary syphilis with penicillin G. *Arch Neurol* **43**:137, 1986.

Brown ST, Zaidi A, Larsen SA, Reynolds GH: Serologic response to syphilis treatment: A new analysis of old data. *JAMA* **253**:1296, 1985.

Centers for Disease Control: Recommendations for diagnosing and treating syphilis in HIV-infected patients. *MMWR* **37**:600–602, 607–608, 1988.

Clark EG, Dunbolt N: The Oslo study of the natural course of untreated syphilis: An epidemiologic investigation based on a re-study of the Boeck–Bruusgaard material. *Med Clin North Am* **48**:613, 1964.

Fiumara NJ: Treatment of primary and secondary syphilis: Serologic responses. *JAMA* **243**:2500, 1980.

Heggtveit HA: Syphilitic aortitis: A clinicopathologic autopsy study of 100 cases, 1950 to 1960. *Circulation* **29**:346, 1964.

Hooshmand H, Escobar MR, Kopf SW: Neurosyphilis: A study of 241 patients. *JAMA* **219**:726, 1972.

Kampmeier RH: The late manifestations of syphilis: Skeletal, visceral and cardiovascular. *Med Clin North Am* **48**:667, 1964.

Larsen SA, Hambie EA, Pettit DE, Perryman MW, Kraus SJ: Specificity, sensitivity and reproducibility among the fluorescent antibody absorption test, the microhemagglutination assay for *Treponema pallidum* antibodies, and the hemagglutination treponemal test for syphilis. *J Clin Microbiol* **14**:441, 1981.

Larsen SA, Hunter EF, Kraus SJ (eds): *A Manual of Tests for Syphilis*, 8th ed. Washington, D.C. American Public Health Association, 1990.

Larsen SA, Steiner BM, Rudolph AH: Laboratory diagnosis and interpretation of tests for syphilis. *Clinical Microbiology Reviews*, **8**:1, 1995.

Norgard MV: Clinical and diagnostic issues of acquired and congenital syphilis encompassed in the current syphilis epidemic. *Current Opinion Infect Dis* **6**:9–16, 1993.

Olansky S: Late benign syphilis. *Med Clin North Am* **48**:653, 1964.

Schroeter AL, Lucas JB, Price EV, Falcone VH: Treatment of early syphilis and reactivity of serologic tests. *JAMA* **221**:471, 1972.

Stokes JH, Beerman H, Ingraham NR: *Modern Clinical Syphilology: Diagnosis, Treatment, Case Study*, 3rd ed. Philadelphia, WB Saunders, 1944.

World Health Organization: *Treponemal Infections*. Technical Report Series No. 674. Geneva, WHO, 1982.

Chancroid

R Ballard and S Morse

INTRODUCTION

Chancroid, or soft chancre (ulcus molle), is characterized by one or more genital ulcers and often by painful inguinal lymphadenopathy. The disease was differentiated clinically from syphilis by Bassereau in France in 1852. In 1889, Ducrey in Italy showed the infectious origin of the disease by inoculating the forearm skin of human volunteers with purulent material from their own genital ulcers. At weekly intervals, he inoculated a new site with material from the most recent ulcer and, following the fifth or sixth reinoculation in each patient, he found a single microorganism in the ulcer exudate. The organism described was a short, compact, streptobacillary rod. Ducrey could not, however, isolate the causative bacterium that now bears his name, *Haemophilus ducreyi*. Isolation was accomplished by other workers by 1900.

EPIDEMIOLOGY

Chancroid is particularly common in parts of Africa, Asia, and Latin America where its incidence may exceed that of syphilis as a cause of genital ulceration (*Fig. 3.1*). However, chancroid is considered an uncommon sexually transmitted infection in the United States. Based on data forwarded to the Centers for Disease Control and Prevention (CDC), the reported number of chancroid cases peaked in 1947 at 9515 cases before beginning a decline which lasted until the mid-1980s (*Fig. 3.2*). During the 20-year period between 1965 and 1984, the number of reported cases averaged 925 cases a year. However, beginning in 1985, the number of reported cases of chancroid increased dramatically, with 4986 cases reported in 1987. Since 1987, the number of reported cases of chancroid has decreased steadily.

Chancroid cases are not evenly distributed throughout the United States (*Fig. 3.3*). Most cases are reported among minorities living in eastern cities and in the South. In 1993, five states (Florida, Georgia, Louisiana, New York, Texas) accounted for 83% of the reported cases of chancroid. Recent data suggest that chancroid is a common cause of genital ulcers in some areas of the United States. For example, *H. ducreyi* was detected in 37 of 101 consecutive men presenting at a New Orleans sexually transmitted disease (STD) clinic with genital ulcers.

The increase in the incidence of chancroid in the mid-1980s occurred at the same time that the incidence of primary and secondary syphilis increased among minority heterosexual men and women (see *Fig. 3.4*). The increase in syphilis was associated with cocaine use in both men and women and, among men, with the exchange of drugs or money for sexual favors. It has been postulated that similar factors might also be responsible for the increase in chancroid.

The persistence of chancroid in a population depends on several factors, which can be expressed mathematically by the equation $R_0 = \beta Dc$ where R_0 is the reproductive rate and is defined as the average number of secondary cases generated by one primary case in a susceptible population of defined density; β is the average probability that the infection is transmitted per sexual partner contact per unit time; D is the average duration of infectiousness of an infected individual; and c is the average number of sexual partners per unit time. If $R_0 < 1$ the infection will not persist and no epidemic will occur. It has been estimated that the probability of transmitting chancroid from an infected male to an uninfected female during a single sexual exposure is 0.35, whereas the probability of transmitting chancroid from an infected female to an uninfected male during a single sexual exposure is 0.30. The duration of infectivity is estimated to be 45 days. The observation that some chancroid outbreaks in the United States have been associated with prostitution suggests that the number of sexual partners (c) is a critical factor in the spread of chancroid. This may also help explain the association of chancroid with certain risk factors such as crack cocaine and alcohol use since individuals who abuse cocaine or alcohol have more sexual partners and are more likely to engage in high-risk sexual behavior.

The majority of cases occur in males (*Fig. 3.4*). This is probably the result of a combination of factors: more easily visible male anatomy; small numbers of infected prostitutes having sexual relations with many men; women with cervical ulcers who are asymptomatic; and spontaneous healing of lesions in women which occur in dry areas such as the inner thighs.

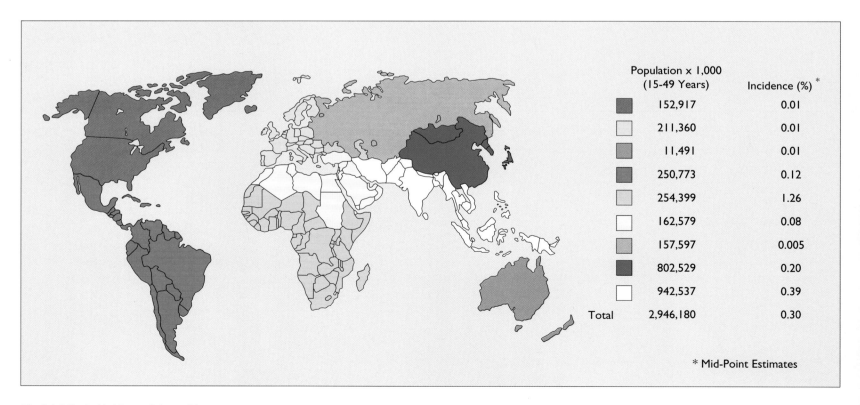

Fig. 3.1 Estimated incidence of chancroid.

STDs in general, and genital ulcerative diseases in particular, have been risk factors in the heterosexual transmission of HIV. Two mechanisms have been proposed to explain how genital ulcers enhance the transmission of HIV. Chancroid and other genital ulcerative diseases could facilitate the transmission of HIV by increasing the shedding of virus through the ulcer. In fact, HIV has been detected in chancroidal ulcers. The presence of an ulcer could also increase suscepti-bility to HIV infection by disrupting the epithelial barrier and perhaps by increasing the number of HIV-susceptible cells at the point of entry. An infiltrate of T-lymphocytes and macrophages in the dermis is characteristically seen in biopsy specimens of chancroidal lesions from persons experimentally infected with *H. ducreyi*. The proportion of these cells that are CD4 lymphocytes, and susceptible to infection with HIV, remains to be determined.

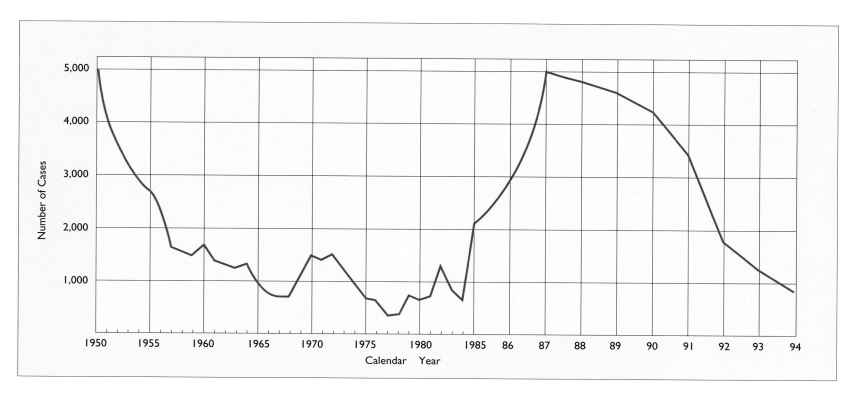

Fig. 3.2 Numbers of reported cases of chancroid in the USA from 1950 to 1994.

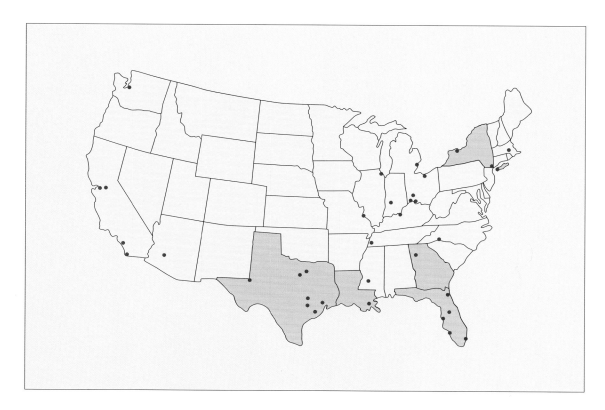

Fig. 3.3 Selected (>200,000 population) cities in the USA where at least three culture-confirmed or clinically diagnosed cases of chancroid were reported from 1989 to 1994. In 1994, five states (Florida, Georgia, Louisiana, New York, Texas) accounted for more than 80% of reported cases of chancroid.

CLINICAL MANIFESTATIONS

The incubation period is usually 4–10 days, but longer incubation periods are not uncommon. The lesions begin as a tender, erythematous papule or pustule at the site of inoculation (*Fig. 3.5*); some patients do not recall a papule but describe an initial erythematous, shallow ulcer. The early lesion may be described simply as a 'sore'. Over the next 1–2 days, the papule erodes into a painful ulcer. Some ulcers may be quite superficial (*Fig. 3.6*), but most are deep (*Figs. 3.7–3.10*); the ulcers are excavated into the skin and often have a beefy, granular base. The edge of the ulcer is usually irregular, has a red margin, and is not indurated. The tenderness of the ulcer often makes examination difficult. The ulcer is sometimes masked by dried or crusted exudate that, when gently removed by saline-soaked gauze, will reveal the ulceration. In men, ulcers often occur on the prepuce, resulting in phimosis, a painful inability to retract the prepuce (*Figs. 3.11* and *3.12*).

As the disease progresses, as many as 50% of cases develop unilateral or bilateral inguinal lymphadenopathy, which is characteristically painful even though nodes may be small (*Fig. 3.13*). Adenopathy ranges from being barely palpable — yet quite painful — to quite large. Buboes (large,

fluctuant lymph nodes) may occur, a finding that is not seen with syphilis or genital herpes. In the absence of effective treatment and prophylactic needle drainage, buboes often suppurate, leaving fistulas or secondary ulcers at the drainage site (*Fig. 3.14*). A variant form of ulcer known as chancre mou volant (transient chancre) has been described, which involutes spontaneously after 4–6 days but may be followed by diagnostically puzzling inguinal adenopathy.

Ulcers in women usually occur in the vulvar area; carriage of *H. ducreyi* without any sign of infection appears to be uncommon (*Figs. 3.15–3.20*).

There are several differences in disease expression between men and women (*Fig. 3.19*). In about one-half of individuals, there is more than one ulcer. Men are invariably symptomatic, but an occasional woman may not be symptomatic due to the presence of asymptomatic ulcers on the cervix or in the vagina. Anal ulcers in women are thought to be the result of drainage or autoinoculations and not necessarily anal intercourse. Transient ulcers may frequently be seen on the inner thighs of infected women. The relative infrequency of adenopathy in women is presumably due to differences in lymphatic drainage between males and females.

Ulcers may occur in the mouth as a result of oral intercourse and, rarely, elsewhere on the body because of autoinoculation. Colonization of the mouth, cervix, and penis in the absence of signs or symptoms has been

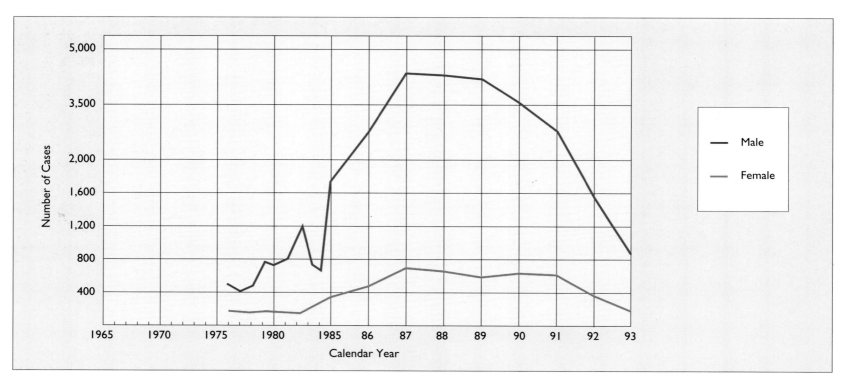

Fig. 3.4 Reported cases of chancroid by gender in the USA from 1966 to 1993.

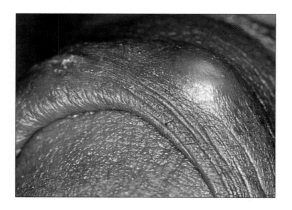

Fig. 3.5 A pustule, the first sign of infection, at the site where an ulcer will appear.

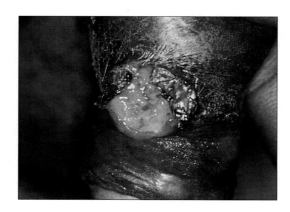

Fig. 3.6 Pustules and a newly erupted ulcer on shaft of penis.

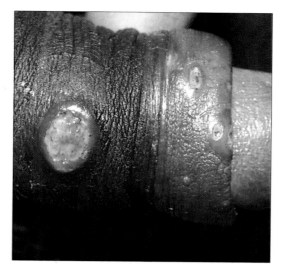

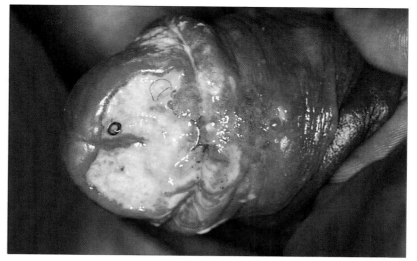

Fig. 3.8 Extensive
ulceration may occur. The
base of the ulcer is granular
and friable

Fig. 3.7 Ulcer on the penile shaft with small ulcers on
foreskin.

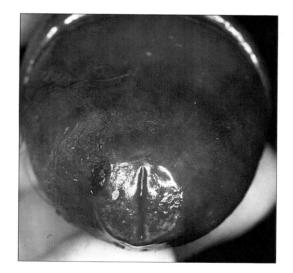

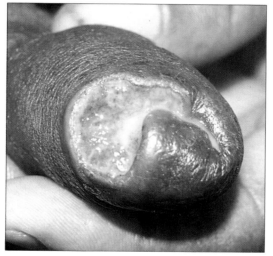

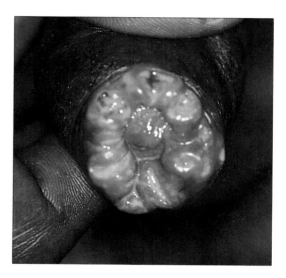

Fig. 3.9 Although most ulcers in men occur on the foreskin
or shaft, ulcers can occur on the glans.

Fig. 3.10 Another example of extensive ulceration, in which
the base of the ulcer is granular and friable.

Fig. 3.11 Lesions occurring on the prepuce are commonly
associated with swelling of the prepuce, and retraction of the
foreskin may be impossible.

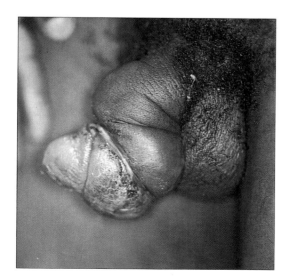

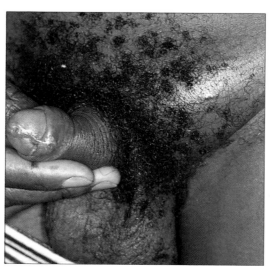

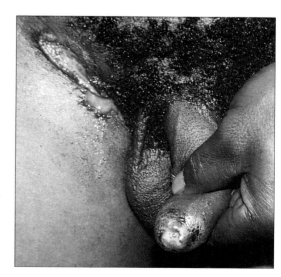

Fig. 3.12 Ulcer on the retracted prepuce with secondary
edema.

Fig. 3.13 Ulcer on the prepuce, with visibly enlarged inguinal
lymph nodes showing overlying erythema of the skin.

Fig. 3.14 Buboes may spontaneously suppurate and
subsequently form draining, chronic fistulas.

described. Unfortunately chancroid ulcers often have an atypical clinical appearance which results in misdiagnosis and thus failure to provide appropriate therapy. Chancroid can mimic genital herpes (*Fig. 3.21*), gonorrhea (*Fig. 3.22*) and donovanosis (*Fig. 3.23*). The situation is further complicated by changes in clinical presentation, which may occur as a result of concomitant infection of *H. ducreyi* and HIV. Lesions may become less vascular and more closely resemble those of syphilis (*Figs. 3.24* and *3.25*). Alternatively, they may spread locally with large numbers of painful lesions (*Figs. 3.26* and *3.27*).

DIFFERENTIAL DIAGNOSIS

The two diseases that most commonly have to be differentiated from chancroid are syphilis and genital herpes; one of these diseases coexists with chancroid in about 10% of chancroid cases. In contrast to the ulcers of syphilis, the ulcers of chancroid are almost invariably tender and, in contrast to the ulcers of genital herpes, they tend to be deeper and not grouped (*Fig. 3.28*). A dark-field examination of the lesion and a serologic test for syphilis should always be performed. Ideally, a follow-up serologic test for syphilis should be performed, as current therapy for chancroid cannot be relied upon to treat syphilis successfully. Lymphogranuloma venereum (LGV) may occasionally need to be differentiated from chancroid, particularly when lymphadenopathy is the prominent feature of the clinical presentation. The ulcer sometimes associated with LGV, however, is not a prominent part of the illness, is transitory and precedes the appearance of lymphadenopathy. LGV is characterized by a longer incubation period. Granuloma inguinale (donovanosis), though causing destructive lesions in the genital area, is not associated with acute, painful ulcerations or lymphadenopathy. However, lesions in the inguinal area can occur.

LABORATORY TESTS

HISTOPATHOLOGY

The biopsy of ulcers, though not studied in recent years, was formerly described as being diagnostically useful. A biopsy specimen 3 mm in diameter from the

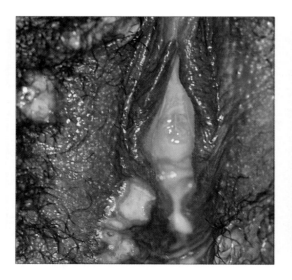

Fig. 3.15 Multiple vulvar lesions.

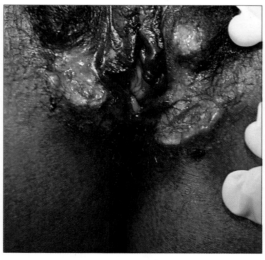

Fig. 3.16 Another example of multiple vulvar lesions.

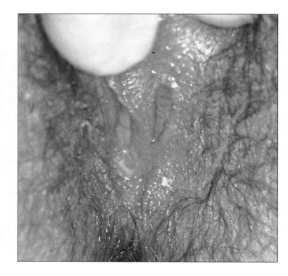

Fig. 3.17 Single ulcer with granular base of the vaginal fourchette; ulcers are commonly found also in the perineum.

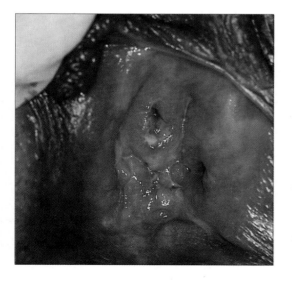

Fig. 3.18 Single periurethral lesion.

CLINICAL FEATURES OF CHANCROID IN MEN AND WOMEN

FEATURES	MEN	WOMEN
Genital ulcers	Multiple ulcers Usually on prepuce (uncircumcised) or coronal sulcus (circumcised) Painful ulcers	Multiple ulcers Usually vulvar, but anal and cervical ulcers may occur Painful ulcers on vulva or anus; Cervical ulcers asymptomatic
Inguinal lymphadenopathy	Up to 50% of cases painful Large nodes suppurate May be bilateral	Occasionally painful Suppuration not common May be bilateral

Fig. 3.19 Clinical features of chancroid in men and women.

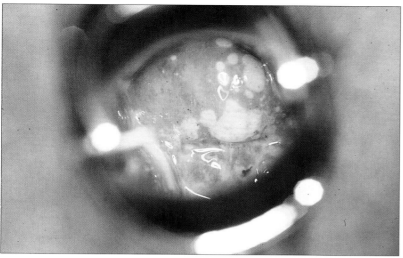

Fig. 3.20 Multiple cervical lesions.

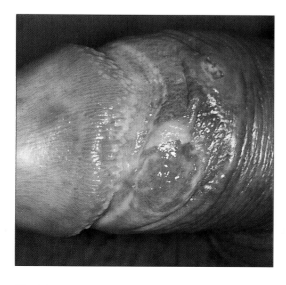

Fig. 3.21 Cluster of small lesions which clinically resemble genital herpes lesions.

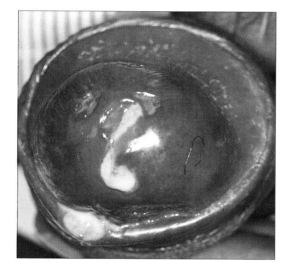

Fig. 3.22 Endourethral lesions which may be misdiagnosed as gonorrhea.

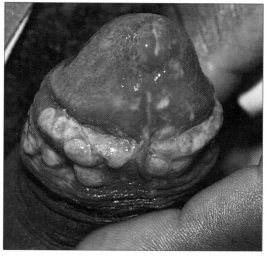

Fig. 3.23 Exuberant chancroid lesions clinically resembling those of donovanosis.

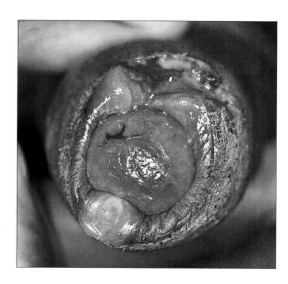

Fig. 3.24 Atypical lesion of chancroid in HIV-positive patients. Lesions are often less purulent in HIV-positive cases

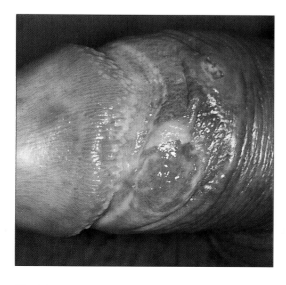

Fig. 3.25 Another example of an atypical lesion of chancroid in an HIV-positive patient.

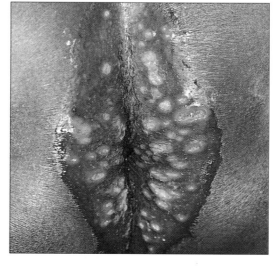

Fig. 3.26 Extensive lesions of chancroid between the buttocks in an HIV-positive patient.

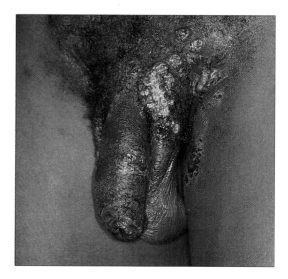

Fig. 3.27 Penile lesions of chancroid in an HIV-positive patient.

ulcer base or bubo wall, which can be obtained without anesthesia, is adequate for study. Three histologic zones occur in lesions of 2–3 weeks' duration (*Figs. 3.29–3.32*). The first, from the base of the ulcer, is shallow and consists of polymorphonuclear leukocytes, fibrin, red blood cells, and necrotic tissue. Below this surface zone is a wide cellular zone in which the predominant cells are proliferating endothelial cells, both within existing vessels and by cells involved in new vessel formation. Near the surface zone, vessels may be infiltrated with neutrophils and may be undergoing necrosis. The supporting connective tissue is edematous and, in contrast to the endothelial cell proliferation, there is a marked lack of fibroblast proliferation. The interstitium is infiltrated by neutrophils near the surface zone and more deeply by lymphocytes and plasma cells. Finally, the deep zone of the ulcer is characterized by a marked infiltration of plasma cells and, less so, by lymphocytes. Some endothelial proliferation within the vessel lumen may be seen, but there is neither infiltration of the vessel walls by inflammatory cells nor endothelial necrosis. Occasionally, organisms morphologically compatible with *H. ducreyi* may be seen in the first or the upper middle zone.

SPECIMEN COLLECTION

Before obtaining Gram-stain and culture material, the ulcer base should be exposed and free of pus. If necessary, crusted pus can be removed by gentle soaks with sterile saline; otherwise, the ulcer does not need cleaning. Gram-stain material should be obtained from the base or margins with a cotton or calcium alginate swab and rolled over the slide to preserve cellular morphology, which might be disturbed by smearing the material. Culture material should be obtained from the base or margins of the ulcer with either a swab or a wire loop. The ability of transport media to maintain *H. ducreyi* has not been well studied, and it is best to inoculate culture plates directly with the swab or loop. Also, primary isolation plates frequently have only small numbers of colonies. It is conceivable that the dilution effect of liquid transport media might cause some cultures to be falsely negative.

GRAM-STAIN CHARACTERISTICS

H. ducreyi is a small, Gram-negative, nonmotile rod, 0.5–0.6 mm in width by 1.6–2.0 mm in length. Examination of Gram-stained smears of human

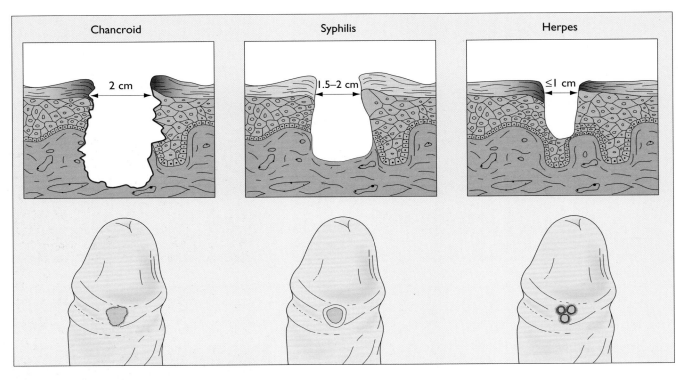

Fig. 3.28 Differences in clinical appearance among chancroid, syphilis, and genital herpes, the three most common infectious diseases manifested by genital ulcers.

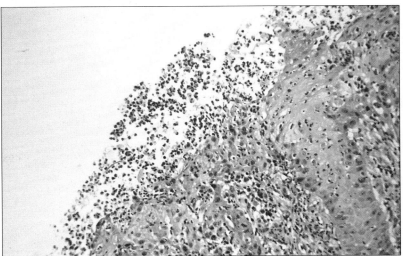

Fig. 3.29 Ulcer biopsy demonstrating the three cellular zones (*see also* **3.30–3.32**). At the surface, there is an inflammatory exudate with partial ulceration of the skin (hematoxylin and eosin).

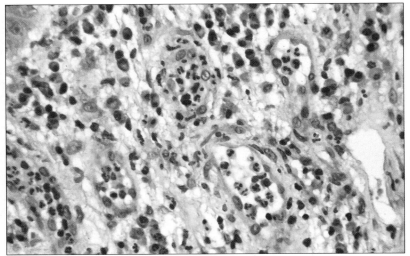

Fig. 3.30 Below the base of the ulcer, there is a wide cellular zone, with proliferating blood vessels (hematoxylin and eosin).

genital lesion material reveals groups or clumps of *H. ducreyi* cells with occasional short streptobacillary chains among the lesion debris (*Fig. 3.33*). Sometimes organisms forming long trails within mucous strands are seen, the so-called 'railroad tracks', which are felt to be characteristic of *H. ducreyi* (*Fig. 3.34*). The utility of the Gram stain in diagnosing chancroid is unclear. A sensitivity of 40–60% has been generally accepted, but the specificity has not been well defined, as organisms with a similar morphology that might be mistaken for *H. ducreyi* may be found in genital secretions. Thus, the Gram stain from lesion material should be used as a presumptive means of diagnosis only (*Fig. 3.35*). Gram stains of material aspirated from buboes are more specific, but the organism is difficult to find in such smears.

GROWTH CHARACTERISTICS

H. ducreyi is a fastidious organism that requires microbiologists experienced in working with *H. ducreyi* to obtain optimal isolation rates. The isolation of *H. ducreyi* as the primary means of diagnosis has been a difficult task. Most isolation rates of *H. ducreyi* from patients who are suspected

of having chancroid have been less than 60%, though studies in Kenya and South Africa have reported higher rates. Isolation of *H. ducreyi* from buboes, for reasons that are unclear, is even less successful than isolation from ulcers.

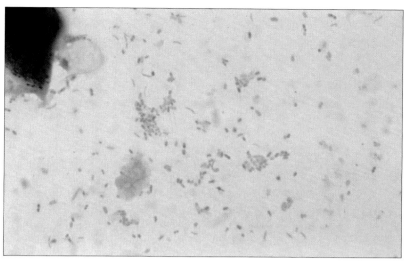

Fig. 3.33 Gram-stained human genital lesion material showing groups of organisms (oil immersion × 1,000).

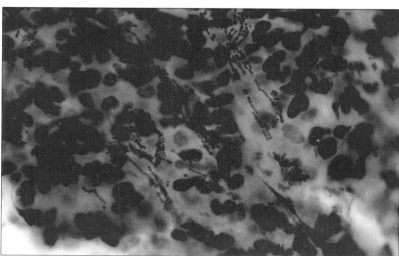

Fig. 3.34 Gram-stained human genital lesion material showing the 'railroad track' appearance (oil immersion × 1,000).

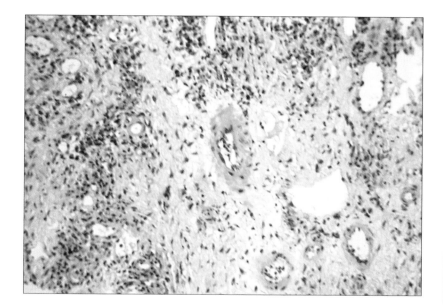

Fig. 3.31 In the cellular zone, there is granulation tissue with edema of the connective tissue (hematoxylin and eosin).

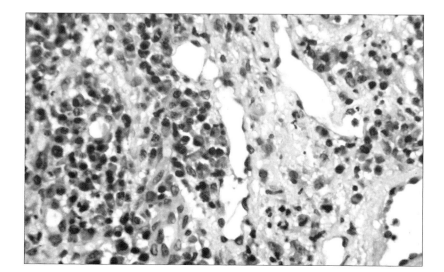

Fig. 3.32 Deeper cellular zone, composed of plasma cells and lymphocytes (hematoxylin and eosin).

DIAGNOSTIC METHODS IN CHANCROID

PRESUMPTIVE	DIAGNOSTIC
Gram stain of material from genital lesion	Culture
Immunofluorescence of organisms in ulcer smears using monoclonal antibody	

Fig. 3.35 Diagnostic methods in chancroid.

Growth temperatures of 33–35°C are recommended. Inoculated plates are incubated in a humid atmosphere (about 100%) with 5% CO_2 or in a microaerophilic atmosphere; these conditions are met by the use of a candle jar with a moist, but not dripping, paper towel in the bottom of the jar, or a commercial anerobic jar from which the catalyst has been removed plus gas generating packets.

H. ducreyi can be cultivated on an enriched medium containing supplements such as IsoVitaleX (BBL), Vitox (Oxoid), or CVA (Gibco); the organism requires the X (hemin) factor, but not the V (NAD) factor for growth. A variety of media have been devised for the cultivation of *H. ducreyi*, but no single medium appears able to support the growth of all strains from clinical material (*Fig. 3.36*). To increase isolation rates, most workers recommend that two media are used: a blood agar and a chocolated agar plate are usually chosen. The addition of vancomycin (3 µg/ml) greatly enhances the ability to recover *H. ducreyi* from clinical specimens by suppressing the growth of other microorganisms, and its effect can be quite dramatic (*Figs. 3.37* and *3.38*).

Colonies growing on rabbit blood agar are semiopaque, translucent, and yellow–light gray (*Fig. 3.39*). The colonies are nonmucoid and can easily be pushed intact across the agar surface with an inoculating loop. The removal of colonies may show slight pitting of the agar surface.

Recently, a transport medium, comprising agar, hemin, thioglycolate and balanced salts supplemented with bovine albumin and glutamine, has been developed which will maintain the viability of *H. ducreyi* in swabs taken from clinical lesions for up to 1 week, provided the specimens are stored at 4°C.

PRESERVATION

H. ducreyi can be removed from the agar surface with a swab, suspended in one of several freezing solutions, and stored at varying temperatures (*Fig. 3.40*). All solutions can be stored in liquid nitrogen at −70, −35, or −20°C. The latter two temperatures should be used only for short-term storage because marked losses in viability may occur.

CULTURE CHARACTERIZATION

On primary isolation media, growth may be visible at 24 hours, but identifiable colonies of *H. ducreyi* may not be seen until 48–72 hours of incubation. Plates should not be discarded as negative, however, until after at least 5 days of incubation.

Colonies of *H. ducreyi* are almost invariably smaller than colonies of other bacteria isolated from the genital tract. A unique characteristic of colonies of *H. ducreyi* is that they can be pushed along the agar surface with a wire loop, a useful diagnostic clue. A Gram stain should be performed on colonies suspected of being *H. ducreyi* (*Fig. 3.41*). Various arrangements of Gram-negative bacilli may be present, depending upon the age of the culture and the media from which a colony is isolated. These include individual organisms, 'school-of-fish' arrangements (cells lined up parallel with one another, suggesting a school of fish swimming in one direction), 'fingerprint' swirls (a variation of the 'school-of-fish' pattern), and short streptobacillary chains.

Gram-negative bacilli from colonies compatible with *H. ducreyi* should be biochemically tested. Carbohydrate fermentation tests are not useful in

ISOLATION OF *H. DUCREYI* ON SELECTIVE MEDIA FROM PATIENTS WITH A CLINICAL DIAGNOSIS OF CHANCROID*

MEDIUM †	COMMENTS	CULTURE SENSITIVITY
GC agar base (Difco)‡ + 1% hemoglobin + 1% IsoVitaleX (BBL)	Relatively low sensitivity	56%
Heart infusion agar (BBL) + 10% fetal bovine serum (FBS)	The addition of FBS resulted in an increase in colony size; medium has not been extensively evaluated	81%
GC agar base (Gibco) + 1 or 2% hemoglobin + 5% FBS + 1% CVA enrichment (Gibco) (GcHbFBS)	Best medium when only a single medium is used to isolate *H. ducreyi*	67–84%
Mueller Hinton agar (BBL) + 5% chocolatized horse blood + 1% IsoVitaleX (BBL) (MH-HB)	Not as sensitive as GcHbFBS However, some isolates will grow on MH-HB that do not grow on GcHbFBS	53–65%
GcHbFBS and MH-HB	Can be used in a single biplate	75–81%
Modified Bieling agar §	More complicated to prepare than either GcHbFBS or MH-HB if a commercial source of yeast dialysate is not available *H. ducreyi* colonies are easily recognized on this medium	77%
GcHbFBS (2 cultures, 48 h apart)	A 48 h delay in initiating therapy may preclude use of this technique	85%
Columbia agar base + 5% fetal bovine serum + 1% hemoglobin + 1% IsoVitaleX (BBL) + 0.2% activated charcoal	Able to detect stains which grow on GcHbFBS and those which grow on MH-HB	90%

Most of the cited studies were performed on patient populations having a high prevalence of chancroid.

† *All media contained vancomycin (3 µg/ml).*

‡ *The manufacturer is given where the composition of the medium may vary with the manufacturer.*

§ *Modified Bieling agar is comprised of Columbia agar base (2 parts) and hemolized horse blood (1 part) that is supplemented with 2.5% yeast dialysate and 1% CVA enrichment.*

Fig. 3.36 Isolation of *H. ducreyi* on selective media from patients with a clinical diagnosis of chancroid. Culture sensitivity tends to be overestimated due to the inaccuracy of a clinical diagnosis of chancroid.

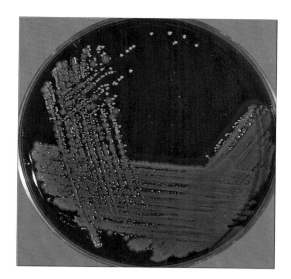

Fig. 3.37 Growth of microorganisms from human genital lesion material on heart infusion agar containing 5% rabbit blood, 1% IsoVitaleX, and 10% fetal bovine serum.

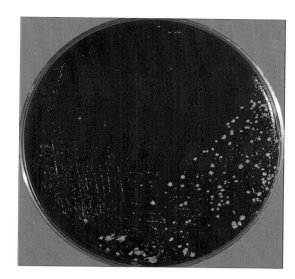

Fig. 3.38 The same medium as described in **3.38** has been used, but with the addition of vancomycin (3.0 mg/ml). On the left side of this plate, there is almost pure growth of *H. ducreyi*.

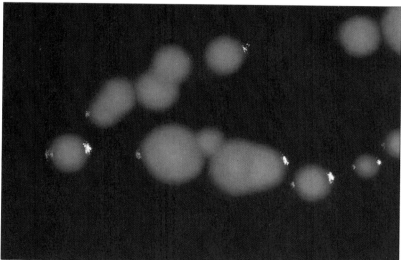

Fig. 3.39 Colonies of *H. ducreyi* growing on heart infusion agar, 5% rabbit blood, 1% IsoVitaleX, and 10% fetal bovine serum.

METHODS OF PRESERVING *H. DUCREYI*

SOLUTIONS

Heart infusion broth, trypticase soy broth, or bovine serum albumin, containing 10% glycerol and 10% fetal bovine serum (filter sterilized)
Skim milk, with or without 10% glycerol (filter sterilized)
Defibrinated rabbit blood
Serum-inositol (for lyophilization)

STORAGE CONDITIONS

Liquid nitrogen
   −70°C
   −35°C
   −20°C
Lyophilization

Fig. 3.40 To preserve *H. ducreyi*, growth is removed from the agar surface, mixed into any one of the listed freezing solutions, and then immediately frozen.

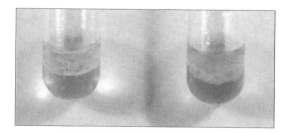

Fig. 3.42 Porphyrin test viewed in room light. A negative result with *H. ducreyi* is shown on the left.

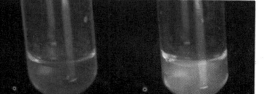

Fig. 3.43 Porphyrin test viewed with a Wood's lamp. A negative result for *H. ducreyi* is shown on the left.

Fig. 3.41 Gram stain of *H. ducreyi* colony removed intact from agar medium.

identifying *H. ducreyi*, and differentiation from other *Haemophilus* species depends upon biochemical testing. As *H. ducreyi* requires X factor (hemin) for growth, it is negative in the porphyrin test (*Figs. 3.42* and *3.43*). *H. ducreyi* is also negative in the catalase test (*Fig. 3.44*). Positive reactions are obtained from alkaline phosphatase (*Fig. 3.45*) and nitrate reductase (*Fig. 3.46*) tests. In the oxidase test, a positive reaction is only observed using tetramethyl-*p*-phenylenediamine; it is important not to use the dimethyl reagent, which will result in a negative test (*Fig. 3.47*).

Nonculture Diagnostic Tests

There are no commercially available nonculture tests for the diagnosis of chancroid. However, recent studies have indicated that PCR is more sensitive than culture; an assay which will detect *H. ducreyi*, *Treponema pallidum* and herpes simplex virus type 2 in a single specimen is currently under commercial development.

Monoclonal antibodies have been developed and used in immunofluorescence assays to detect *H. ducreyi*. The organism has been detected in human genital lesion specimens by an indirect immunofluorescence assay.

The test is performed by incubating a fixed smear of lesional material with a mouse monoclonal antibody specific for *H. ducreyi*. After washing, the bound antibody is detected by adding fluorescein-labeled antimouse immunoglobulin and examining the slide (*Fig. 3.48*).

PATHOGENICITY

The virulence of *H. ducreyi* has been studied by injecting pus from human genital lesions into the skin of rabbits. Within 48 hours, a lesion 1–2 cm in diameter occurred. After 24 hours, the lesion subsided, and healing was complete within 1 week. Some strains of *H. ducreyi* failed to produce lesions after serial passage on laboratory media, suggesting that these strains may have lost one or more as yet unidentified virulence factors. *H. ducreyi* produces lesions that appear more rapidly and are larger than lesions produced by *Treponema pallidum*, subspecies *pallidum* in the rabbit model (*Fig. 3.49*).

HUMAN IMMUNE RESPONSE AND SEROLOGY

Delayed-type hypersensitivity to *H. ducreyi* antigens and complement fixation were formerly used as aids in the diagnosis of chancroid. However, their

Fig. 3.44 Catalase test. A negative result with *H. ducreyi* is shown on the right.

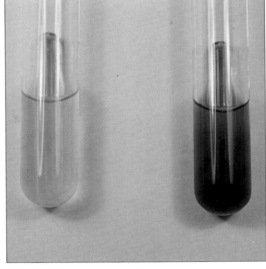

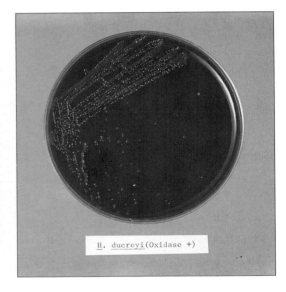

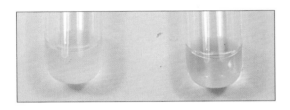

Fig. 3.45 Alkaline phosphatase test. A positive result with *H. ducreyi* is shown on the right.

Fig. 3.46 Nitrate reductase test. A positive result with *H. ducreyi* is shown on the right.

Fig. 3.47 Oxidase test. A positive result with *H. ducreyi*, showing dark colonies where oxidase reagent has been placed.

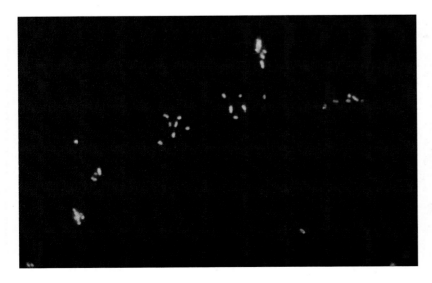

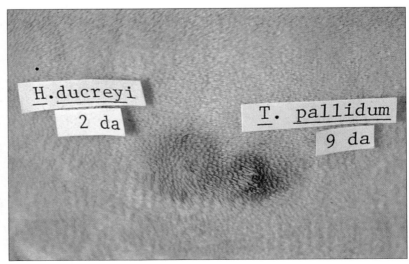

Fig. 3.48 Indirect immunofluorescence assay of human genital lesion material with a monoclonal antibody directed against *H. ducreyi*.

Fig. 3.49 Induction of skin lesions in a normal rabbit by injectiion of *H. ducreyi* and *T. pallidum*. The *T. pallidum* lesion is shown as a smaller pustule requiring 9 days for induction, compared with the larger lesion of *H. ducreyi*, which requires only 48 hours for lesion formation.

poor sensitivity and specificity precludes their current use in diagnosis. Increased knowledge of the antigenic composition of *H. ducreyi* and the human immune response to infection has led to the development of serologic tests for chancroid. The specificity of these tests is improved by the removal of cross-reacting antibodies by adsorption; the *H. ducreyi*-specific antibodies are to outer membrane protein and lipooligosaccharide antigens. Studies have shown that the sensitivity of these tests is reduced when acute phase serum specimens are used and in younger patients; however, sensitivity is increased with increased duration of infection. Moreover, the sensitivity of the serologic tests are antigen-dependent and antibody levels remain elevated for extended periods of time. Thus, their use in diagnosis is problematic. However, these assays have been used successfully to measure the prevalence of chancroid in various individuals or groups for targeting and evaluating control efforts, as part of larger interventions designed to reduce the transmission of HIV (*Fig. 3.50*).

STRAIN TYPING

H. ducreyi has very limited biochemical activities which can be used to characterize individual strains. A typing system with a high degree of discrimination could accomplish the following:

- Address unanswered questions concerning the geographic distribution of strains and mode of transmission
- Discriminate between treatment failure and reinfection
- Identify strains of differing virulence
- Provide a means to study the genetic diversity of *H. ducreyi*.

The outer membrane protein profile of *H. ducreyi* can be differentiated from the outer membrane proteins profiles of *Haemophilus influenzae* or *Haemophilus parainfluenzae* using sodium dodecyl sulfate polyacrylamide gel electrophoresis (SDS-PAGE) (*Fig. 3.51*). Similar, but not identical, outer membrane protein profiles of *H. ducreyi* strains isolated from different geographic locations in the USA may provide a useful epidemiologic tool (*Fig. 3.52*).

Ribotyping, based on restriction fragment length polymorphisms of ribosomal RNA genes, provides a reproducible method to discriminate between different strains of *H. ducreyi*. Ribosomal RNA genes are highly conserved and are usually present in multiple copies on the genome of microorganisms. DNA isolated from *H. ducreyi* is first digested with an endonuclease such as *Hinc*II or *Hind*III; the resulting fragments are separated by agarose gel electrophoresis and transferred onto nylon membranes. The ribosomal DNA-containing fragments are visualized by hybridization with a labeled probe consisting of ^{32}P-labeled 16S and 23S RNA from *Escherichia coli* followed

PREVALENCE (%) OF ANTIBODIES TO *H. DUCREYI* IN DIFFERENT POPULATIONS

POPULATION	N	*H. DUCREYI* ANTIBODY PREVALENCE (%)		
		IgM	IgG	Ig A
Patients with culture-proven chancroid				
Kigali, Rwanda	114	41	54	64
Nairobi, Kenya	66	48	90	75
Bangkok, Thailand	42	20	46	46
Populations at low risk for chancroid				
STD patients (Antwerp, Belgium)	563	<1	<1	<1
Couples (Nairobi, Kenya)	96	1	9	3
Men (Banjul, The Gambia)	96	1	7	2
Pregnant women (Banjul, The Gambia)	96	1	8	3

*Adapted from: Roggen EL, Hoofd G, Van Dyck E, Piot :. Enzyme immunoassays (EIAs) for the detection of anti-Haemophilus ducreyi serum IgA, IgG, and IgM antibodies. Sex Transm Dis 1994 **21**: 35–42.*

Fig. 3.50 Prevalence (%) of antibodies to *H. ducreyi*.

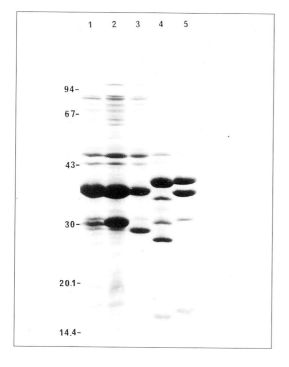

Fig. 3.51 SDS-PAGE of outer membrane preparations of two strains of *H. ducreyi* isolated in the USA (lanes 1 and 2), *H. ducreyi* strain CIP 542 (lane 3), *H. influenzae* ATCC 8143 (lane 4), and *H. parainfluenzae* ATCC 7857 (lane 5).

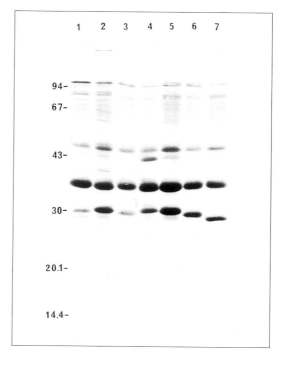

Fig. 3.52 SDS-PAGE of USA *H. ducreyi* outer membrane preparations (lanes 1 to 6) and an outer membrane preparation of *H. ducreyi* strain CIP 542 (lane 7).

by autoradiography (*Fig. 3.53*). Ribotypes obtained using *Hin*dIII can differentiate between strains isolated from different geographic areas (*Fig. 3.54*). Plasmid profiles (*see Fig. 3.58*) can be used to differentiate further between strains belonging to a single ribotype.

ULTRASTRUCTURE

H. ducreyi ultrastructure viewed by transmission electron microscopy shows the typical streptobacillary chains with cells adhering to each other end to end (*Figs. 3.55* and *3.56*). Organisms also appear to adhere at the sides or from end to side, which may explain the appearance of clumps of cells that are frequently observed in Gram-stained smears. The cell envelope is typical of

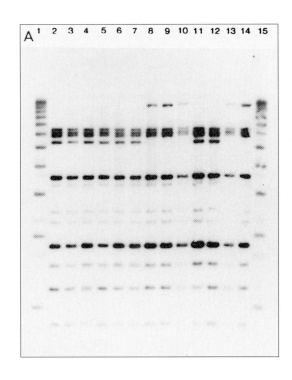

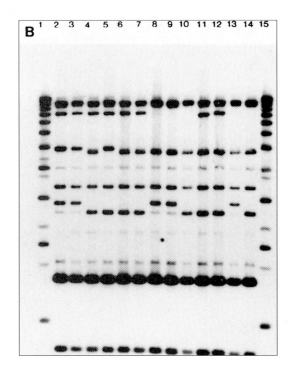

Fig. **3.53** Southern blots of *H. ducreyi* DNA, digested with *Hin*cII (A) or *Hin*dIII (B), separated by agarose gel electrophoresis, and hybridized with ^{32}P-labeled 16S and 23S *E. coli* rRNA. Lanes: 1 and 15, 1-kb DNA ladder labeled with ^{32}P by nick translation; isolates of *H. ducreyi* from different geographic areas.

GEOGRAPHIC SOURCE AND *HINDIII* RIBOTYPES OF 130 ISOLATES OF *HAEMOPHILUS DUCREYI*

SOURCE	YEAR	1	2	3	4	5	6	7	8	9	10	11	12
						HINDIII RIBOTYPE							
Hanoi, Vietnam	1954	1											
Winnipeg, Canada	1975	1											
Seattle, WA	1979		1										
Orange County, CA	1981–1982					17		1					
Atlanta, GA	1982				2								
Nairobi, Kenya	1982		2										
	1984		5	1	2		5		1				
	1990		4	2	2					1			
West Palm Beach, FL	1984		2										
Bangkok, Thailand	1984		13		11							5	1
Tampa, FL	1989				1								
San Francisco, CA	1989–1990		4		4	13				8	2	1	
New Orleans, LA	1990				17								
Total		2	31	3	39	30	5	1	1	9	2	6	1

Fig. **3.54** Geographic source and *Hin*dIII ribotypes of 130 isolated of *H. ducreyi*.

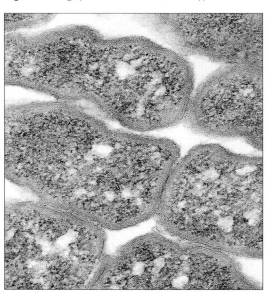

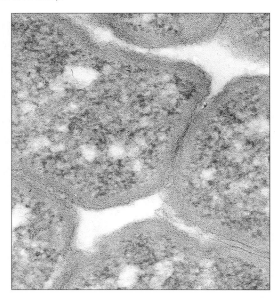

Fig. **3.55** Thin-section electron micrograph of *H. ducreyi* from agar medium (× 90,000).

Fig. **3.56** Thin-section electron micrograph of *H. ducreyi* from agar medium (× 175,000).

Gram-negative bacteria and is bordered on the outside by an outer membrane and on the inside by a cytoplasmic membrane, between which is a layer of medium electron-dense material (peptidoglycan). Regions of distinct nuclear material are not evident.

TREATMENT

Over the past decade, *H. ducreyi* has developed resistance to penicillins, sulfonamides, and tetracyclines by acquiring plasmids encoding resistance to these drugs; resistance to tetracycline in some cases is chromosomally mediated. The plasmids in *H. ducreyi* have varying functions (*Fig. 3.57*). The 3.2 MDa and 5.7 MDa plasmids encode for β-lactamase, conferring resistance to penicillins, while the 4.9 MDa plasmid encodes for sulfonamide resistance. Many strains from East Africa contain a 7.0 MDa plasmid that encodes for β-lactamase. The 3.2 MDa, 5.7 MDa, and 7.0 MDa β-lactamase plasmids are related to one another as well as to the β-lactamase plasmids found in *Neisseria gonorrhoeae*. Plasmid analysis with *H. ducreyi*, as with other microorganisms, may offer an epidemiologic tool for distinguishing

similarities among strains isolated in varying geographic areas. Geographic variation in plasmids has been reported (*Fig. 3.58*).

Little variability in minimum inhibitory concentrations (MIC) to currently recommended antimicrobials occurs in isolates from around the world (*Fig. 3.59*). Ceftriaxone, cefotaxime, erythromycin, and members of the quinolone family are highly active *in vitro*. *H. ducreyi* resistance to trimethoprim-sulfamethoxazole (TMP-SMX) has been reported in Rwanda where the prevalence of resistant strains has increased dramatically between 1988 and 1991. All of the TMP-SMX-resistant isolates were resistant to TMP (MIC, >4.0μg/ml). Strains resistant to TMP-SMX have also been isolated in the United States, South Africa, Thailand, and Kenya. These data suggest that TMP-SMX should no longer be recommended for the treatment of chancroid.

Currently, treatment with erythromycin is recommended by both the US Public Health Service and the World Health Organization, though the daily dosage is different (*Fig. 3.60*). Fleroxacin (400mg as a single oral dose) has also been shown to be effective in the treatment of culture-proven chancroid. Single-dose therapy is advantageous because it avoids problems with

---

ANTIBIOTIC RESISTANCE CONFERRED BY VARIOUS PLASMIDS OF *H. DUCREYI*

SIZE (MDa)	ANTIBIOTIC	COMMENTS
3.1	Streptomycin and kanamycin	Encodes for two APH; enzyme modifying kanamycin appears to be a type I 3', 5''-APH.
3.1	Sulfonamide, streptomycin, and kanamycin	Encodes for type II Su^r dihydropteroate synthase (*SulI*) and Sm^r determinant, StA, similar to those found on plasmid RSF1010: Km^r gene similar to that found on Tn *903*.
3.2	Ampicillin	Encodes for a TEM-1-type β-lactamase; plasmid is identical to the 3.2-MDa gonococcal Ap^r plasmid and carries about 40% of the TnA sequence.
3.5	Ampicillin	Encodes for ROB-1-type β-lactamase; plasmid is identical to the ROB-1 β-lactamase plasmid originally isolated in *Actinobacillus pleuropneumoniae*.
4.9	Sulfonamide	Plasmid is related to the enteric streptomycin and sulfonamide resistance plasmid RSF1010.
5.7	Ampicillin	Encodes for TEM-1-type β-lactamase; plasmid is homologous to the 3.2-MDa gonococcal Ap^r plasmid and contains the complete TnA sequence; it differs from the 7.0-MDa Ap^r plasmid by the absence of a 1.3-MDa insertion element.
7.0	Ampicillin	Encodes for a TEM-1-type β-lactamase; plasmid is homologous to the 4.4-MDa gonococcal Ap^r plasmid and contains the complete TnA sequence.
30	Tetracycline	A conjugative plasmid; will not mobilize 7.0-MDa Ap^r plasmid; appears to be related to a Tc^r plasmid found in *H. influenzae*
34	Tetracycline and chloramphenicol	A conjugative plasmid; can mobilize Ap^r plasmids; 70–80% homologous to pRI234 from *H. influenzae*; encodes for a type II CAT and possesses a class B Tc^r determinant.
34	Tetracycline	A conjugative plasmid; will not mobilize Ap^r plasmids; carries most, if not all, of the TetM transposon.
23	None	Able to mobilize nonconjugative R plasmids; it can cross species and generic lines.

Ap^r, ampicillin resistant; APH, Aminoglycoside phosphotransferase; CAT, chloramphenicol acetyltransferase; Cm^r, chloramphenicol resistant; Km^r, kanamycin resistant; Sm^r, streptomycin resistant; Su^r, sulfonamide resistant, Tc^r, tetracycline resistant.

Fig. 3.57 Antibiotic resistance conferred by various plasmids of *H. ducreyi*.

PLASMID PROFILES OF SELECTED *H. DUCREYI* ISOLATES, WORLDWIDE FROM 1952 TO 1990

LOCATION	YEAR OF ISOLATION	N	PLASMID CONTENT(MDa)*					
			NONE	7.0	5.7	4.9,5.7	3.2	1.8*
United States	1985	26	-	2	4	-	-	-
New York, NY	1989	1	-	-	1	-	-	-
Chicago, IL	1989–1990	2	-	-	2	-	-	-
Columbus, OH	1988	1	1	-	-	-	-	-
Elkins Park, PA	1989	4	1	-	-	-	-	-
Nashville, TN	1952–1958	8	8	-	-	-	-	-
Atlanta, GA	1980–1989	16	1	4	1	9	1	-
Augusta, GA	1990	1	-	-	1	-	-	-
Jacksonville, FL	1986–1990	4	1	-	3	-	-	-
Belle Glade, FL	1983	3	-	-	3	-	-	-
Fort Meyers, FL	1990	1	1	-	-	-	-	-
Orlando, FL	1985	2	-	-	2	-	-	-
Tampa, FL	1987–1990	159	76	-	83	-	-	-
New Orleans, LA	1989–1990	51	2	-	37	12	-	-
Houston, TX	1989	3	-	-	3	-	-	-
Orange County, CA	1981–1982	22	3	-	-	-	19	-
Long Beach, CA	1987	17	2	-	6	-	9	-
Los Angeles, CA	1987	6	1	-	3	-	2	-
San Francisco, CA	1989–1990	32	10	-	2	5	14	1
Winnipeg, Canada	1978	19	16	-	3	-	-	-
Nairobi, Kenya	1980–1982	274	7	157	110	-	-	-
Johannesburg, South Africa	1988	29	-	4	21	4	-	-
Bangkok, Thailand	1984	30	-	-	1	-	-	29

*MDa = megadalton
Combination of the 1.8-, 2.6-. 2.8-, and 3.2-, 5.7- or 7.0-MDa β-lactamase plasmids.

Fig. 3.58 Plasmid profiles of selected *H. ducreyi* isolates, worldwide from 1952 to 1990.

SUSCEPTIBILITY OF STRAINS OF *H. DUCREYI* TO CLINICALLY USEFUL ANTIMICROBIALS

COUNTRY	N	ANTIMICROBIAL*		
		ERYTHROMYCIN	CEFTRIAXONE/CEFOTAXIME	TRIMETHOPRIM
United States				
Orange County, CA	38	0.004–0.016 (0.004)	≤ 0.001	0.032–16(4)
New York, NY	22	< 0.008–0.064 (< 0.064)	≤ 0.001–0.008 (0.004)	0.25–4(2)
San Francisco, CA	25	0.002–0.25 (0.015)	0.06–0.125 (0.06)	Not tested
Kenya	35	Not tested	Not tested	0.125–2.0 (2)
Thailand	100	0.007–0.06 (0.03)	0.0007–0.007 (0.003)	0.12–>16(4)
France	29	0.002–0.032 (0.016)	0.004–0.016 (0.008)	Not tested
South Africa	122	0.002–0.125 (0.06)	0.002–0.008 (0.004)	< 0.12–16(4)

* Expressed as µg/ml
Figure in parentheses indicates minimum inhibitory concentration of 90% of strains.

Fig. 3.59 Susceptibility of strains of *H. ducreyi* to clinically useful antimicrobials.

THERAPEUTIC REGIMENS FOR CHANCROID

Fig. 3.60 Therapeutic regimens recommended by the US Public Health Service and the World Health Organisation.

US PUBLIC HEALTH SERVICE
RECOMMENDED

Azithromycin, 1 g po in a single dose

Ceftriaxone, 250 mg im once

Erythromycin base, 500 mg po qid for 7 days

ALTERNATIVES

Amoxicillin, 500 mg plus clavulanic acid 125 mg tid for 7 days

* Ciprofloxacin, 500 mg po bid for 3 days

WORLD HEALTH ORGANIZATION
RECOMMENDED

Erythromycin base or stearate, 500 mg po tid for 7 days

ALTERNATIVES

Ceftriaxone, 250 mg im once

* Ciprofloxacin, 500 mg po in a single dose

Spectinomycin, 2 g im in a single dose

* Ciprofloxacin is contraindicated for pregnant and lactating women, children, and adolescents ≤17 years of age.

compliance; however, cost is a major consideration in developing countries where chancroid is prevalent. A subjective response to eventually successful therapy is almost always present within 48 hours of starting treatment, and complete healing usually takes 10–11 days. The response of lymph nodes generally parallels that of ulcers, though some nodes progress to fluctuance in spite of otherwise successful therapy, and this is not a sign of treatment failure. Fluctuant nodes should be aspirated by needle through normal skin. Sexual partners of affected persons should be examined and treated whether or not lesions are present.

Several factors affect treatment efficacy. Concurrent HIV infection was found to increase the probability of treatment failure following a single dose of either ceftriaxone (250mg IM) or fleroxacin (400mg PO); treatment failure was not due to infection with an antibiotic-resistant strain. Increasing the duration of fleroxacin treatment (400mg PO once daily for 5 days) appears promising and should be studied further as a possible treatment regimen for HIV-infected men.

Picture credits for this chapter are as follows: Fig. 3.1 courtesy of Global Program on AIDS, World Health Organization; Fig. 3.18 courtesy of the American Academy of Dermatology; Figs. 3.30–3.33 courtesy of Bhagirath Majmudar, MD; Fig. 3.49 courtesy of the University of Chicago Press; Gi. 3.53 courtesy of the American Society for Microbiology.

BIBLIOGRAPHY

Blackmore CA, Limpakarnianarat K, Rigau-Perez JC, et al.: An outbreak of chancroid in Orange County, California: Descriptive epidemiology end disease control measures. J Infect Dis 151:840, 1985.

Dangor Y, Ballard RC, Miller SD, Koornhof HJ: Antimicrobial susceptibility of Haemophilus ducreyi. Antimicrob Ag Chemother 34:1303, 1990.

Dangor Y, Ballard RC, Miller SD, Koornhof HJ: Treatment of chancroid. Antimicrob Ag Chemother 34:1308, 1990.

Dangor Y, Radebe F, Ballard RC: Transport media for Haemophilus ducreyi. Sex Transm Dis 20:5, 1993.

Dangor Y, Ballard RC, Expasto F da L, Fehler G, Miller SD, Koornhof HJ: Accuracy of clinical diagnosis of genital ulcer disease. Sex Transm Dis 17:184, 1990.

Hammond GW, Lian CJ, Witt JC, Ronald AR: Comparison of specimen collection and laboratory techniques for the isolation of Haemophilus ducreyi. J Clin Microbiol 7:39, 1978.

Hammond GW, Slutchuk M, Scatliff J, Sherman E, Wilt JC, Ronald AR: Epidemiologic, clinical, laboratory and therapeutic features of an urban outbreak of chancroid in North America. Rev Infect Dis 2:867, 1980.

Kaplan W, Deacon WE, Olansky S, Albritton DC: VDRL Chancroid Studies II: Experimental chancroid in the rabbit. J Invest Dermatol 26:407, 1956.

Kilian M, Theilade J: Cell wall ultrastructure of Haemophilus ducreyi and Haemophilus piscium. Int J System Bacteriol 25:351, 1975.

Kinghorn GR. Hafiz S, McEntegart MG: Oropharyngeal Haemophilus ducreyi infection. Br Med J 287:650, 1983.

McNicol PJ, Ronald AR: The plasmids of Haemophilus ducreyi. J Antimicrob Chemother 14:561, 1984.

Morse SA: Chancroid and Haemophilus ducreyi. Clin Microbiol Rev 2:137, 1989.

Museyi K, Van Dyck E, Vervoort T, Taylor D, Hoge C, Piot P: Use of an enzyme immunoassay to detect serum IgG antibodies to Haemophilus ducreyi. J Infect Dis 157:1039, 1988.

Nsanze H, Plummer FA, Maggwa ABN, Martha G, Dylewski J, Piot P, Ronald AR: Comparison of media for the isolation of Haemophilus ducreyi. Sex Transm Dis 11:6, 1984.

Oberhofer TR, Back AE: Isolation and identification of Haemophilus ducreyi. J Clin Microbiol 15:625, 1982.

Plummer FA, D'Costa LI, Nsanze H, Karasira P, Maclean IW, Plot P, Ronald AR: Clinical and microbiologic studies of genital ulcers in Kenyan women. Sex Transm Dis 12:193, 1985.

Ronald AR, Plummer FA: Chancroid and Haemophilus ducreyi. Ann Intern Med 102:705, 1985.

Schalla WO, Sanders LL, Schmid GP, Tam MR, Morse SA: Use of dot-immunobinding and immunofluorescence assays to investigate clinically suspected cases of chancroid. J Infect Dis 153:879, 1986.

Schmid GP, Sanders LL Jr, Blount JH, Alexander ER: Chancroid in the United States: Reestablishment of an old disease. JAMA 258:3265, 1987.

Sheldon WH, Hayman A: Studies on chancroid: Observations on the histology with an evaluation of biopsy as a diagnostic procedure. Am J Pathol 22:415, 1945.

Sottnek FO, Biddle JW, Kraus SJ, Weaver RE, Stewart JA: Isolation and identification of Haemophilus ducreyi in a clinical study. J Clin Microbiol 12:170, 1980.

Taylor DN, Duangmani C, Suvongse C, O'Connor R, Pitarangsi C, Panikabutra K, Echeverria P: The role of Haemophilus ducreyi in penile ulcers in Bangkok, Thailand. Sex Transm Dis 11:148, 1984.

Trees DL, Morse SA: Chancroid and Haemophilus ducreyi: An update. Clin Microbiol Rev 8: 357, 1995.

CHAPTER FOUR

Infections Caused by Chlamydia trachomatis

J Schachter and R Barnes

INTRODUCTION

Chlamydia trachomatis is a bacterium with a limited metabolic capability that restricts its growth to within the intracellular environment of parasitized host cells. The organism is distributed worldwide and apparently is restricted to human hosts, unlike the distantly related *Chlamydia psittaci*, which has a broad host range among nonhuman vertebrates. The first recognition that *Chlamydia* organisms were responsible for STDs occurred before 1910 when the association with inclusion conjunctivitis of the newborn and nongonococcal urethritis (NGU) and cervicitis was described. Then, a relationship with LGV was noted in the 1930s. Sexually acquired LGV is rare in the USA (*Fig. 4.1*) but occurs frequently in the tropics. The pathogenic role of *C. trachomatis* in STDs other than LGV has been widely recognized only within the past three decades. *C. psittaci* is responsible for the zoonotic disease *ornithosis* (formerly 'psittacosis'), which is characterized by res-

piratory disease in humans who become accidental hosts for avian strains of the organism. Recently, respiratory illness in humans has been associated with the so-called TWAR organism, now recognized as a separate species, *Chlamydia pneumoniae*. This organism appears to be found worldwide, and is a very common pathogen with seroprevalence rates often exceeding 50% in adult populations.

C. trachomatis has been successfully propagated only within embryonated chickens' eggs, or in cell or tissue culture. This has impeded study of both the biology and clinical manifestations of infection. Until the recent recognition of the high prevalence of sexually transmitted chlamydial infections within developed countries, cell culture methods for the isolation and identification of *Chlamydia* were limited to research laboratories.

Because of their small size and obligate intracellular parasitism, *Chlamydia* were considered viruses from their original description until the 1960s. However, they possess a characteristic bacterial cell wall, ribosomes, both DNA and RNA, and metabolic functions that confirm their bacterial nature (*Fig. 4.2*).

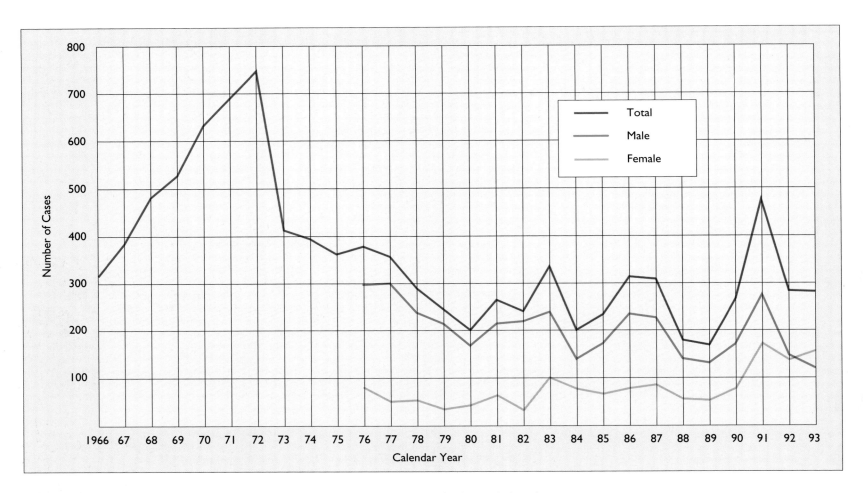

Fig. 4.1 Reported cases of lymphogranuloma venereum (LGV) by year in the USA. The accuracy of such reporting is not known.

DISTINGUISHING FEATURES OF CHLAMYDIAE

Fig. 4.2 Distinguishing features of chlamydiae.

Obligate intracellular parasites
Deficient in endogenous ATP production
Contain DNA, RNA, and typical prokaryotic ribosomes
Outer membrane similar to other Gram-negative bacteria
Dimorphic developmental cycle which takes place in an intracellular cytoplasmic inclusion
Small genome size (ca. $^1/_8$ of *Escherichia coli*)
Extremely diverse in DNA homology

Knowledge of the distinctive intracellular development cycle of the chlamydial organism is important in understanding parasite–host interaction (*Fig. 4.3*). Much of what is known has been obtained through studies of chlamydiae grown in mammalian cell culture. These studies expanded information generated through observation of the growth cycle of the organism as interpreted from conjunctival scrapings obtained from individuals with trachoma or inclusion conjunctivitis of the newborn, or experimentally infected nonhuman primates. The organism is dimorphic. The infectious form, the elementary body (EB), is a condensed, sporelike spheroid with a diameter of 200–400 nm (*Figs. 4.4* and *4.5*). It is metabolically inactive, and contains a tightly compressed nucleoid and an outer membrane composed primarily of lipopolysaccharide and proteins that are highly disulfide-linked. Upon contact with a suitable host cell, the EB appears to induce its own entry by a process of receptor-mediated endocytosis. The ingested EB resides within a membrane-limited phagosome, which is able to avoid fusion and destruction by the primary lysosomes of the parasitized cell by an unknown mechanism.

Several hours following invasion of the host cell, the EB undergoes conversion to the vegetative form, the reticulate body (RB). The RB is metabolically active, and competes with the host cell for metabolic precursors. It is less electron-dense, suggesting relaxation of the condensed DNA, and has a diameter of 500–900 nm (*Fig. 4.6*). Approximately 12 hours following invasion of the host cell, the RB begins to replicate by binary fission. By

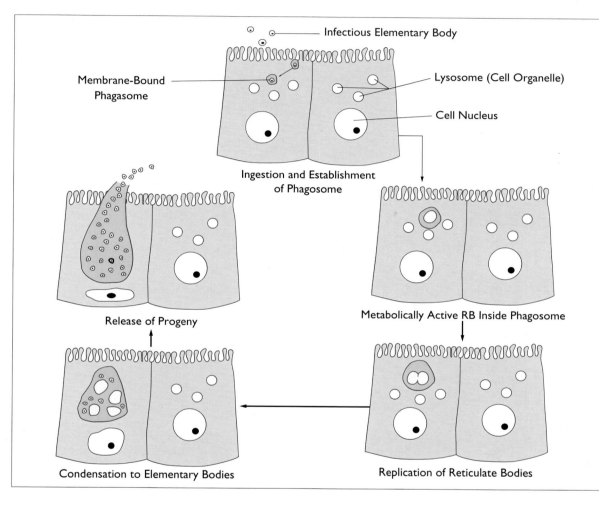

Fig. 4.3 Chlamydial development cycle. The infectious elementary body (EB) attaches to the host cell and is ingested by a process that is poorly understood. The EB resides within a membrane-bound endosome. The normal process of fusion with lysosomes is aborted, and transformation to the metabolically active reticulate body (RB) begins. Synthesis of chlamydial constituents and replication of the RBs through binary fission occurs next. A chlamydial inclusion body containing numerous replicative forms can be seen 24–48 hours following infection. At 48–72 hours following infection, RBs condense to the sporelike EBs. The inclusion body contains several hundred infectious particles at the peak of its maturation. The infectious progeny EBs are released from the infected host cell by extrusion of the inclusion body and/or by lysis of the host cell.

Figure labels:
- Infectious Elementary Body
- Membrane-Bound Phagasome
- Lysosome (Cell Organelle)
- Cell Nucleus
- Ingestion and Establishment of Phagosome
- Release of Progeny
- Metabolically Active RB Inside Phagosome
- Condensation to Elementary Bodies
- Replication of Reticulate Bodies

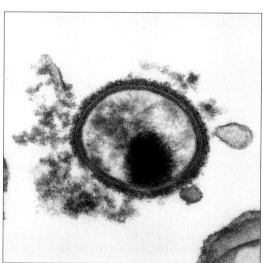

Fig. 4.4 Transmission electron micrograph of single *C. trachomatis* elementary body (× 120,000).

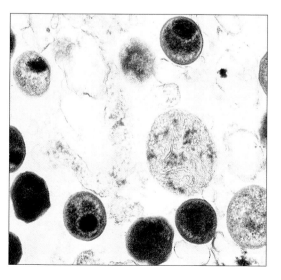

Fig. 4.5 Transmission electron micrograph of *C. trachomatis* elementary bodies outside the host cell. A single, electron-lucent reticulate body and a mitochondrion are also seen (× 67,500).

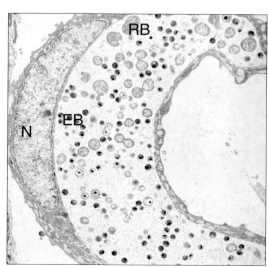

Fig. 4.6 A mature *C. trachomatis* inclusion displaces the host cell nucleus and includes various chlamydial developmental forms. N, nucleus; EB, elementary bodies; RB, dividing reticulate bodies.

24 hours, the RBs appear to form visible 'inclusions' within the membrane-limited phagosome (*Fig. 4.7*), each inclusion containing up to several hundred organisms. During the next 24–36 hours, the RBs condense into EBs, such that by 60–72 hours the inclusion contains primarily EBs.

After 48–60 hours of development, polysaccharide components within the inclusion may be seen following iodine staining. This staining distinguishes *C. trachomatis* from *C. psittacia* and *C. pneumoniae*, which do not produce large quantities of glycogen or glycogenlike deposits and do not stain with iodine. Other biologic properties that distinguish these species are illustrated in *Figure 4.8*. The processes by which EBs egress from the host cell are unclear, and may include both lysis of the host cell and extrusion of intact inclusions without the immediate death of the host cell. Most serotypes of *C. trachomatis* are unable to establish multiple cycles of infection *in vitro* in mature cell monolayers, greatly limiting their ability to propagate to high concentrations.

The infectious EB possesses a distinct outer membrane with protein and lipopolysaccharide components. A single major outer membrane protein (MOMP) comprises the bulk of outer membrane protein. The MOMP has an approximate subunit mass of 40,000 Da, though the mass appears to differ among the various serotypes of *C. trachomatis*. Structural rigidity of the organism appears to be maintained by disulfide bonds among three cysteine-rich proteins. MOMP and an approximately 60 kDa cysteine-rich protein are highly immunogenic. Another protein of approximately 60 kDa is not a structurally important protein but is related to common heat-shock proteins and may have an important immunopathogenic role. The MOMP has genus, species, subspecies, and serotype-specific epitopes, and is antigenic in humans. Other prominent antigens in human infections appear with apparent molecular masses of 62 kDa, 60 kDa, 28 kDa, and less than 12kDa. The most prominent genus-specific antigen is the chlamydial lipopolysaccharide that resembles the rough lipopolysaccharide of Re ('deep rough') mutants of *Salmonella minnesota*.

C. trachomatis strains can be classified by antiserum or monoclonal antibodies into 18 readily distinguished serotypes. Endemic trachoma is usually associated with infection by serotypes A, B, Ba, and C, while nontrachomatous oculogenital infection is usually caused by serotypes B and D–K. Lymphogranuloma venereum infections (*see Clinical Manifestations*) are caused by the invasive LGV biovar strains of serotypes L1–L3 (*Fig. 4.9*). Chlamydial genital infection by multiple serotypes has been reported, and can be observed *in vitro* (*Fig. 4.10*). *C. trachomatis* EBs contains a plasmid

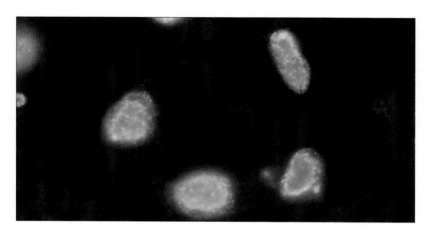

Fig. 4.7 Chlamydial inclusions in cell monolayer stained with fluorescein-labeled monoclonal antibody specific for *C. trachomatis*.

DISTINGUISHING CHARACTERISTICS OF C. TRACHOMATIS, C. PSITTACI, AND C. PNEUMONIAE

	C. TRACHOMATIS	*C. PSITTACI*	*C. PNEUMONIAE*
HOST RANGE	Humans, mice	Non-human vertebrates	Humans
INCLUSION MORPHOLOGY	Granular, vacuolar	Lucent, dense	Dense
INCLUSION STAINING	Iodine +	Iodine –	Iodine –
ELEMENTARY BODY SHAPE	Coccoid	Coccoid	Pear-shaped
FOLATE ANTAGONISTS	Sensitive	Resistant	Resistant

Fig. 4.8 Distinguishing characteristics of *C. trachomatis, C. psittaci,* and *C pneumoniae.*

DISEASES COMMONLY ASSOCIATED WITH SEROTYPES OF C. TRACHOMATIS

SEROTYPE	DISEASE
A, B, Ba, C	Endemic trachoma
B, D–K	Genitourinary disease
LI, L2, L3	LGV

Fig. 4.9 Diseases commonly associated with serotypes of *C. trachomatis.*

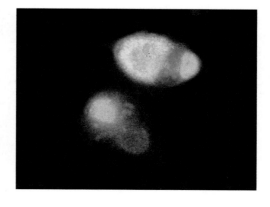

Fig. 4.10 HeLa cells infected simultaneously with two serotypes of *C. trachomatis* and stained with two type-specific monoclonal antibodies, each labeled with a different fluorochrome. The upper cell shows two inclusions, one containing both serotypes, illustrating that multiple serotypes can coexist within the same host cell. Clinical examples of chlamydial infection by two serotypes have been reported.

that exhibits considerable similarity among the serotypes (*Fig. 4.11*). This plasmid is approximately 7 500 base pairs in size, and has several open reading frames capable of encoding polypeptide products. Although the ubiquitous nature of this cryptic plasmid suggests that it may be functionally important, no clear functions have been ascribed to it.

EPIDEMIOLOGY

Chlamydial infections are the most frequently occurring STDs in the USA (*Figs. 4.12* and *4.13*), and probably in most developed countries. As they are not uniformly reported in the USA, only crude estimates of the incidence of these infections are available, based on extrapolation of data from particular clinics. The US Public Health Service estimates that 3–5 million cases occur each year (*Fig. 4.14*). Data from private health care reports suggest that although cases of urethritis due to *Neisseria gonorrhoeae* have been decreasing in the past decade, office visits by men with NGU — due in large part to *C. trachomatis* infection — have been increasing (*Fig. 4.15*). Risk factors for chlamydial genitourinary infection are shown in *Figure 4.16*.

The classic venereal disease caused by *Chlamydia* is lymphoganuloma venereum, or LGV. This disease is rare in the USA but common in developing countries, especially in central Africa. *Figure 4.1* illustrates the number of cases of LGV reported to the CDC between 1966 and 1993.

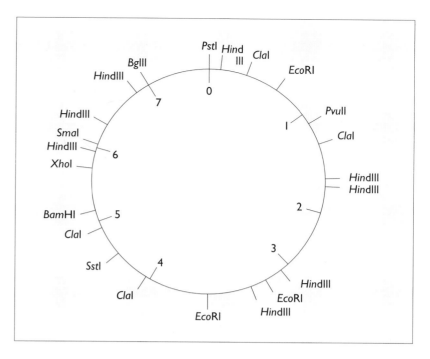

Fig. 4.11 Restriction endonuclease map of the 7.5 kB cryptic plasmid from *C. trachomatis* serotype L2. The same or a similar plasmid has been found in all serotypes investigated.

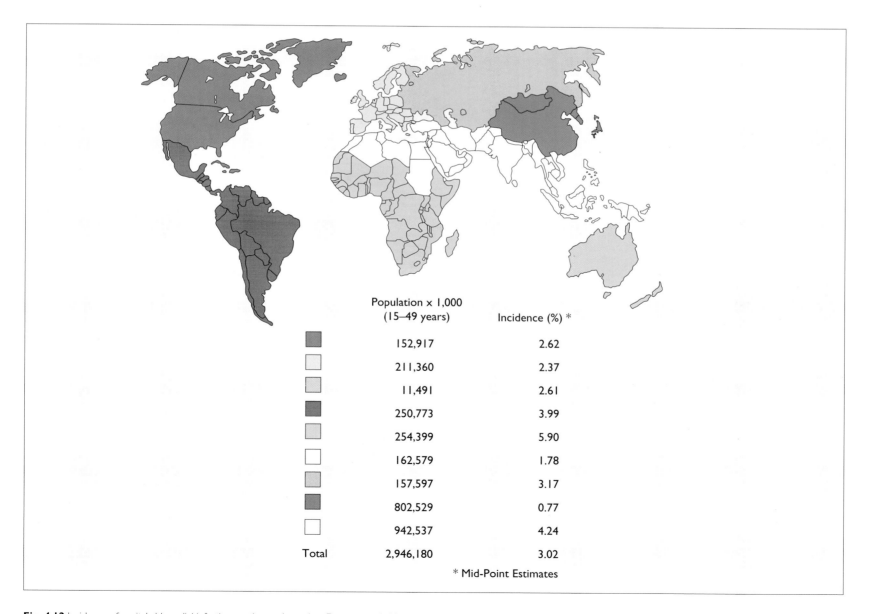

	Population x 1,000 (15–49 years)	Incidence (%) *
	152,917	2.62
	211,360	2.37
	11,491	2.61
	250,773	3.99
	254,399	5.90
	162,579	1.78
	157,597	3.17
	802,529	0.77
	942,537	4.24
Total	2,946,180	3.02

* Mid-Point Estimates

Fig. 4.12 Incidence of genital chlamydial infections: estimates by region. Data are probably underestimates due to the relative insensitivity of most diagnostic tests used.

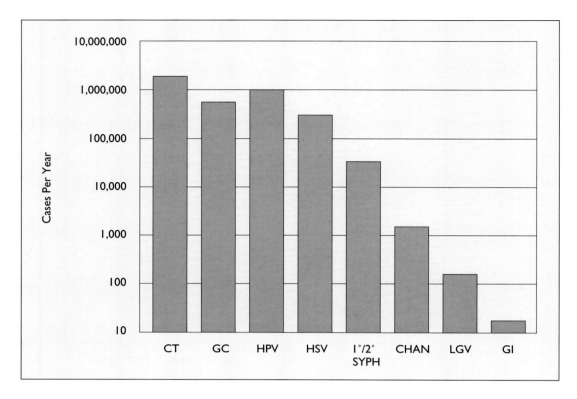

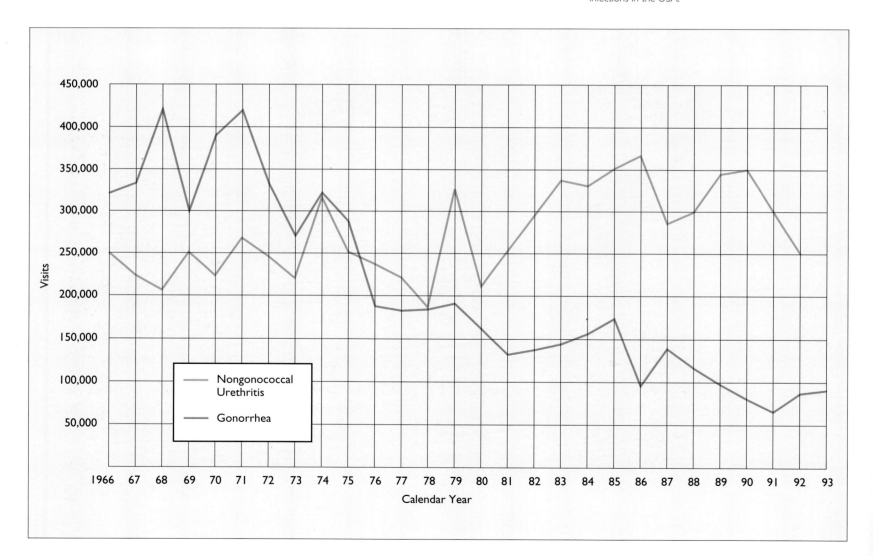

**ESTIMATED ANNUAL INCI-
DENCE OF *C. TRACHOMATIS*
INFECTIONS IN THE USA**

INFECTION	INCIDENCE
MALE	
Nongonococcal urethritis	1,550,000
Epididymitis	250,000
FEMALE	
Asymptomatic cervical infection	700,000
Symptomatic cervical infection	300,000
Pelvic inflammatory disease	300,000
NEONATAL	
Total infections	247,000
Conjunctivitis	74,000
Pneumonia	37,000

Fig. 4.13 Estimated incidence of non-HIV STDs in the USA. Note the logarithmic scale.

Fig. 4.14 Estimated annual incidence of *C. trachomatis* infections in the USA.

Fig. 4.15 Number of physicians' office visits for urethritis in the USA, from 1966 to 1993. Although visits by men with urethritis due to *Neisseria gonorrhoeae* have decreased, there has been a substantial increase in the number of visits for nongonococcal urethritis. These data suggest that chlamydial genitourinary infection may be increasing.

Genital infection in adults occurs through sexual intercourse. In recent years, the USA has witnessed substantial increases in ectopic pregnancy (*Fig. 4.17*) and involuntary infertility, particularly among populations at high risk for prior chlamydial infection. Studies of antibody prevalence to *Chlamydia* have shown that chlamydial exposure is approximately three times more common among women with tubal factor infertility or women having ectopic pregnancies as compared to control populations. *C. trachomatis* is recognized as a major cause of pelvic inflammatory disease (PID). It is likely that these conditions result from tubal damage caused by chlamydial salpingitis. Many of the women suffering from tubal factor infertility or ectopic pregnancy have no prior history of PID. It is likely that they have had a silent salpingitis. Ocular infection may accompany genital infection. In neonates, infection most commonly occurs through exposure to chlamydial organisms in the birth canal. Although infection of the genitals and conjunctivae are common, the mucosal surfaces of the pharynx, urethra, and rectum are also sites of chlamydial colonization. *C. trachomatis* may reside for years within the genital tracts of infected patients who have not been treated with antimicrobials. Some infants born to infected mothers may have a clinically inapparent infection for years following birth.

As the causative agent of endemic trachoma, *C. trachomatis* is one of the most frequent infections leading to blindness in the developing world.

CLINICAL MANIFESTATIONS

Infection by *C. trachomatis* can occur at several anatomic locations and cause a variety of distinct disease syndromes. Several animals models of *C. trachomatis* genital infection have been used to explore the pathophysiology of chlamydial infection. Several models of pneumonitis have been developed in the mouse. Models of upper and lower genital tract infection have been developed using mice, guinea pigs, and nonhuman primates (*Figs. 4.18–4.22*). The latter have also been used as an animal model for *C. trachomatis* rectal infections.

PATIENT GROUPS AT HIGH RISK FOR CHLAMYDIAL STDs

Patients with other STDs
Patients with chlamydia-associated syndromes
Sexual partners of patients with gonorrhea or chlamydia-associated syndromes
Younger patients
Patients with multiple sexual partners
Neonates born to infected mothers

Fig. 4.16 Patient groups at high risk for chlamydial STDs.

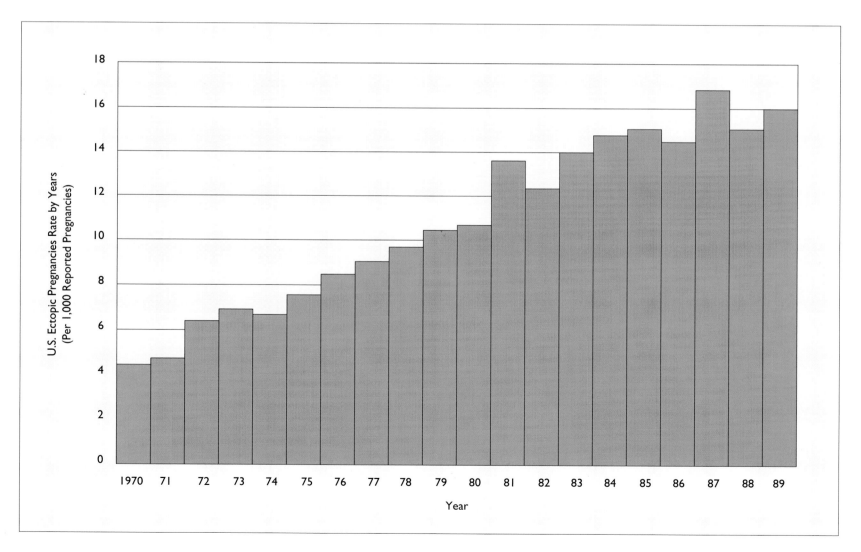

Fig. 4.17 Incidence of ectopic pregnancy in the USA, 1970–1989.

LYMPHOGRANULOMA VENEREUM

After genital inoculation, there is apparently systemic spread of the organism until localization in the genital or rectal lymph node tissues occurs. This infection of the lymphatics becomes locally invasive, and is characterized by induration, multifocal suppuration, and fistula formation. Involvement of both femoral and inguinal lymph node groups, more frequent among infected men than women, can produce swelling on both sides of the inguinal ligament. The resulting 'groove sign' (*Fig. 4.23*) has been said to be pathognomonic of LGV, but occurs in only 10–15% of infected patients. LGV can produce chronic scarring and lymphedema, particularly if the rectum is infected. Cicatricial scarring can produce long fibrotic narrowings of the colonic lumen.

URETHRITIS AND PROCTITIS IN MEN

Chlamydia causes about a third to a half of the infections in men presenting to STD clinics with urethral inflammation from which *N. gonorrhoeae* cannot be identified. The majority of men with chlamydial infection of the urethra have symptoms of urethral discharge, dysuria, or pruritus of the urethra. Up to 25% of men found upon culture screening to have urethral infection by

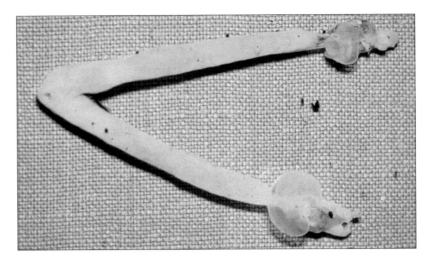

Fig. 4.18 Salpingitis in animal models. Resected reproductive tract from a mouse experimentally infected with *C. trachomatis*. Bilateral hydrosalpinx is seen at the distal extremities of both uterine horns.

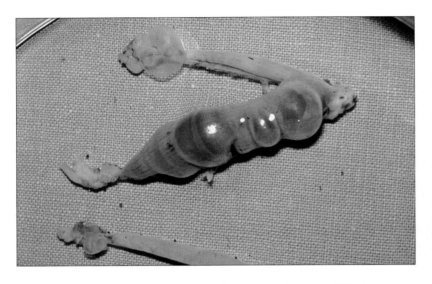

Fig. 4.19 Salpingitis in animal models. Specimen from a mouse impregnated following unilateral hydrosalpinx development. Embryos are implanted in the normal horn, while the hydrosalpinx side is unimplanted.

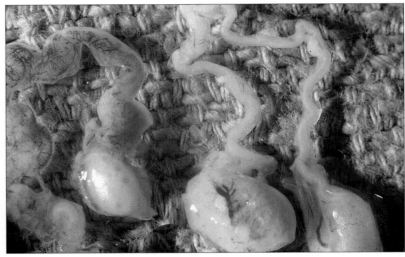

Fig. 4.20 Salpingitis in animal models. Resected fallopian tubes from guinea pigs, showing tubes inflamed and swollen with acute salpingitis due to chlamydial infection (left) compared with the uninfected control (right).

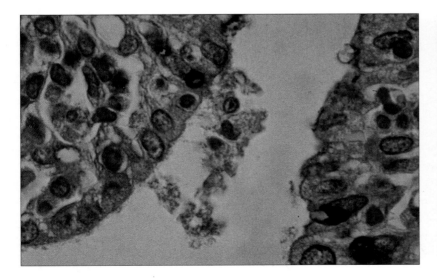

Fig. 4.21 Salpingitis in animal models. Immunoperoxidase stain of *C. trachomatis* inclusions (dark black) in a segment of monkey fallopian tube transplanted subcutaneously and stained 5 days following infection.

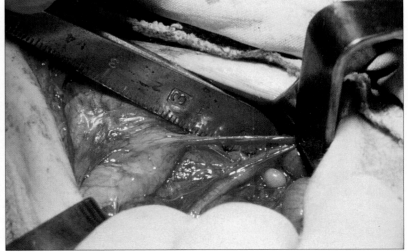

Fig. 4.22 Salpingitis in animal models. Adhesions seen at laparotomy in a monkey following experimentally induced *C. trachomatis* salpingitis. Such experimental animal models provide knowledge regarding mechanisms of scarring following salpingitis.

C. trachomatis are asymptomatic. *Chlamydia* may cause acute epididymitis (*Fig. 4.24*), apparently due to infection ascending from the urethra. *Chlamydia* causes most cases of epididymitis in young heterosexual men without anatomic anomalies of the genitourinary system.

In homosexual men, infection of the rectal mucosa by *C. trachomatis* can result in a severe proctocolitis (*Figs. 4.25* and *4.26*). Although infection is usually asymptomatic, infection by organisms of the more virulent LGV strains can produce a severe and symptomatic form.

CERVICITIS AND URETHRITIS IN WOMEN

In women, *Chlamydia* has been isolated from the cervix, the urethra, Bartholin's duct, the fallopian tubes, the uterus, and the rectal mucosa. However, up to 70% of genital infections in women are asymptomatic. When symptoms of cervicitis and urethritis are described in association with proven infection of the cervix, they are nonspecific, and may include dysuria, vaginal discharge, or vaginal pruritus, though several studies have failed to associate specific symptoms with endocervical chlamydial infection. Upon examination of the infected patient, a mucopurulent cervical discharge and/or easily induced bleeding of the cervix (*Figs. 4.27–4.33*) may be noted, though these signs are also neither sensitive nor specific for chlamydial infection. Sampling from the endocervical canal can produce gross evidence of purulent inflammation (*Figs. 4.34–4.36*). *C. trachomatis* has been isolated from the urethra of women presenting with dysuria; it is also responsible for a proportion of abacteriuric pyuria in sexually active young women — the 'acute urethral syndrome.'

SALPINGITIS AND PERIHEPATITIS

The most serious complication of chlamydial genital infection in women is acute salpingitis, presumably caused by ascent of the organism from the lower genital tract to the endometrium and fallopian tubes (*Fig. 4.37*). The clinical manifestations of upper reproductive tract infection by *C. trachomatis* are nonspecific, but can be severe, with fever, lower abdominal pain, prostration, and tenderness of the uterus and adnexae. Silent salpingitis may also be a result of chlamydial infection. A severe inflammatory response can be observed on laparoscopy to involve the fallopian tubes and peritoneum (*Figs. 4.38–4.39*). Peritoneal inflammation can result in hepatic capsular adhesions, which may produce the Fitz–Hugh–Curtis syndrome: pain, tenderness in the right upper quadrant, and occasionally a hepatic friction rub on auscultation (*Fig. 4.40*). In addition to the acute morbidity of PID, scarring of the tubal transport system following chlamydial salpingitis may lead to infertility and/or ectopic pregnancy (*Figs. 4.41* and *4.42*).

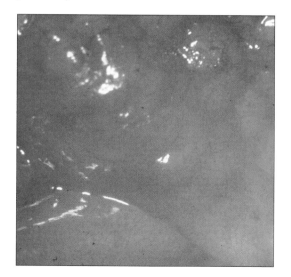

Fig. 4.23 'Groove sign' in a man with lymphogranuloma venereum (LGV). Although often said to be pathognomic for LGV, this sign is seen infrequently in LGV patients and may be produced by other conditions.

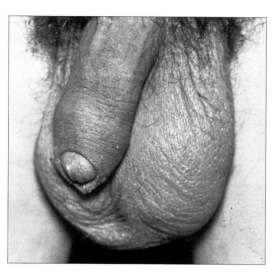

Fig. 4.24 Red, swollen scrotum of a man with chlamydial epididymitis.

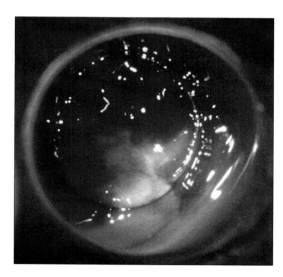

Fig. 4.25 Anoscopic view of rectal mucosa with area of focal purulence in a man with chlamydial proctitis.

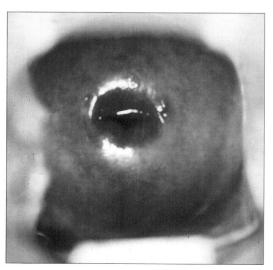

Fig. 4.26 Lymphoid follicular proctitis seen in a case of *C. trachomatis* rectal infection.

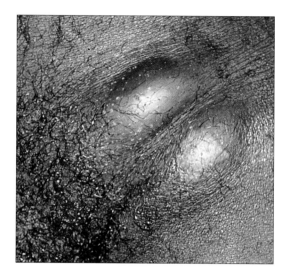

Fig. 4.27 Normal nulliparous cervix of a postmenarchal female, showing no cervical ectopy.

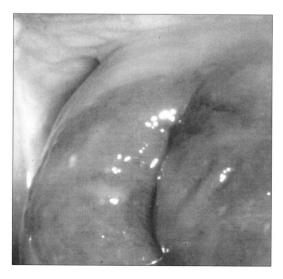

Fig. 4.28 Colposcopic view of early metaplastic changes in the cervical epithelium. This is a normal finding with sexual maturity.

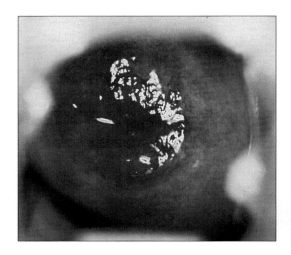

Fig. 4.29 Cervix showing effacement of the transitional zone (squamocolumnar junction) as might be observed in a young patient or in an oral contraceptive user.

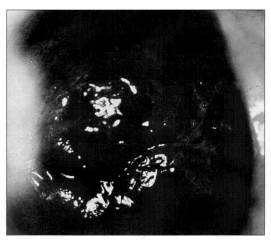

Fig. 4.30 Beefy red mucosa of columnar epithelium in chlamydial infection.

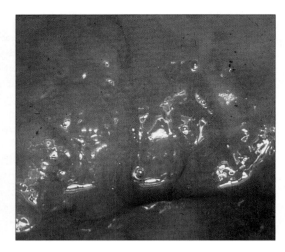

Fig. 4.31 Columnar epithelium cobblestoned by follicular changes of chlamydial infection.

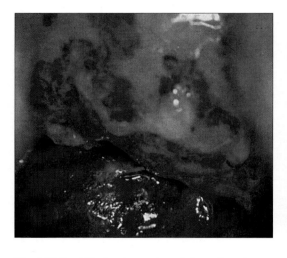

Fig. 4.32 Cervicitis showing purulent discharge from the os. Focal bleeding at areas previously touched during external cleansing of the cervix is evidence of friability.

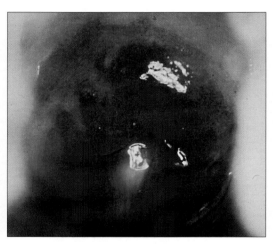

Fig. 4.33 Mucopurulent discharge seen coming from the cervical os following removal of ectocervical mucus. Endocervical swab from this patient was culture-positive for *C. trachomatis*.

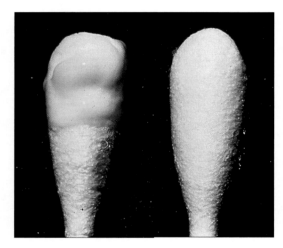

Fig. 4.34 Swab from the endocervical canal of a *Chlamydia*-infected woman (left) compared with fresh swab. The yellow–green exudate may reflect infection of the endocervix or endometrium.

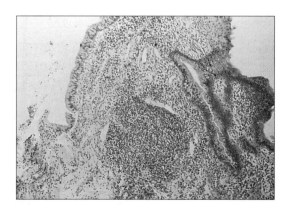

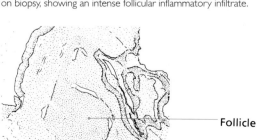

Fig. 4.35 Histologic image of *Chlamydia*-infected human cervix on biopsy, showing an intense follicular inflammatory infiltrate.

Follicle

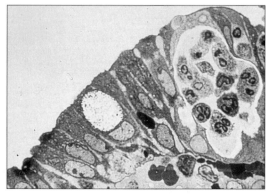

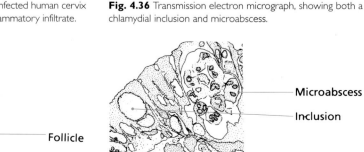

Fig. 4.36 Transmission electron micrograph, showing both a chlamydial inclusion and microabscess.

Microabscess

Inclusion

Fig. 4.37 Fluorescence micrograph showing chlamydial inclusions developing in an experimentally infected monkey fallopian tube. Chlamydial infection may ascend from the endocervix to the endometrium and fallopian tube epithelium.

PERINATAL INFECTIONS

Exposure to *C. trachomatis* during passage through an infected birth canal can cause infection in newborns (*see Chapter 14*). The most common symptomatic illness of these children is a self-limited purulent conjunctivitis (*Fig. 4.43*), which usually occurs within several weeks following birth. About 20–30% of children born to infected mothers develop this infection. Approximately 10–20% of exposed children develop a distinct pneumonitis syndrome.

The incubation period of the pneumonitis is variable, ranging from 2 weeks to 3 months. Infants generally show failure to thrive. Respiratory disease has an insidious onset, is afebrile and is characterized by a hacking nonproductive cough. The radiographic picture is not distinctive, but frequently shows hyperaeration and generalized interstitial changes (Fig. 4.44). C. trachomatis is the most commonly identified cause of infant pneumonitis in the first 6 months of life.

OTHER CHLAMYDIAL INFECTIONS IN ADULTS

Ocular infection by *C. trachomatis* is not limited to perinatally acquired infection. Although not an STD, endemic trachoma is one of the most common causes of visual impairment in the developing worrld, causing millions of cases of blindness (*Figs. 4.45* and *4.46*). Similarly, ocular infection in sexually active adults can occur frequently, probably as a consequence of genital–ocular autoinoculation. This infection is usually self-limited and without severe sequelae, though a distinctive follicular conjunctivitis can result (*Fig. 4.47*).

Genital infection by *C. trachomatis* has been associated in serologic studies with the development of reactive arthropathy in Reiter's syndrome, which consists of conjunctivitis (*see Fig. 10.31*), urethritis, and arthritis (*Fig. 4.48*). Recently, chlamydial particles have been seen in joint aspirates from patients with this postinfectious arthropathy, suggesting that direct infection of the joint space may produce this complication. Reiter's syndrome is a chronic, fluctuating disease that may have striking rheumatologic and dermatologic presentations (*Figs. 4.49* and *4.50*).

In humans, uncomplicated genital infection by *C. trachomatis* produces few diagnostic symptoms and signs. Similarly, a number of organisms can be responsible for PID. The lack of specific clinical criteria in the diagnosis of chlamydial infection mandates laboratory diagnosis in almost all cases of infection.

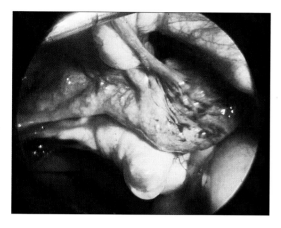

Fig. 4.38 Acute salpingitis. The fallopian tube is congested and swollen. A dense adhesion has formed between the ampulla of the tube and the pelvic sidewall.

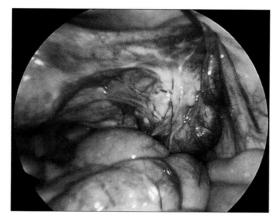

Fig. 4.39 Acute salpingitis. Hydrosalpinx with adhesions. Dye has been instilled into the grossly swollen fallopian tube on the right. Dense adhesions obscure the ovary.

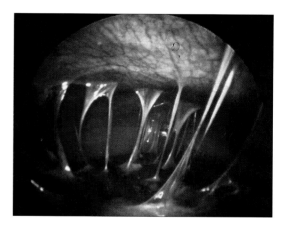

Fig. 4.40 Acute salpingitis. Laparoscopic view of 'violin-string' adhesions in a patient with perihepatitis (Fitz–Hugh–Curtis syndrome).

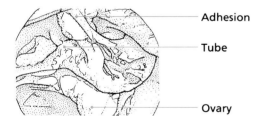

Adhesion

Tube

Ovary

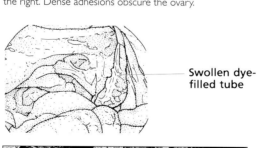

Swollen dye-filled tube

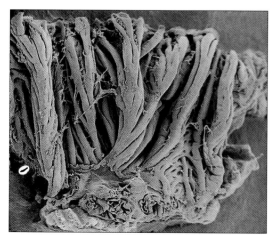

Fig. 4.41 Scanning electron micrograph of a monkey fallopian tube ampulla following experimental infection with *C. trachomatis*. Adhesions such as seen on both low power and magnified (**4.42**) images are presumably responsible for the development of tubal obstruction with infertility and/or ectopic pregnancy.

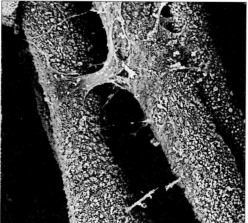

Fig. 4.42 Scanning electron micrograph of a monkey fallopian tube ampulla following experimental infection with *C. trachomatis* (see also **4.41**).

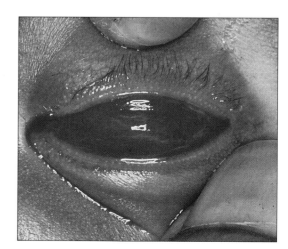

Fig. 4.43 Chlamydial ophthalmia. Erythematous conjunctiva is seen in this infant.

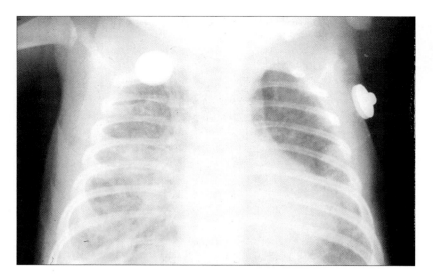

Fig. 4.44 Chlamydial pneumonitis. X-ray of a neonate showing the generalized patchy infiltrates.

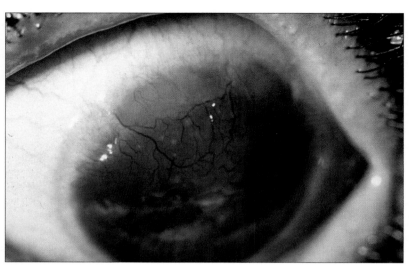

Fig. 4.45 Inflammatory infiltration and neovascularization of the cornea (pannus). Similar destructive lesions are infrequently observed in ocular infection by genital strains of *C. trachomatis* (paratrachoma).

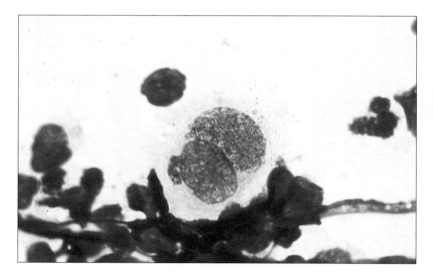

Fig. 4.46 Giemsa stain of an ocular scraping from a patient with trachoma, showing a *C. trachomatis* intracellular inclusion.

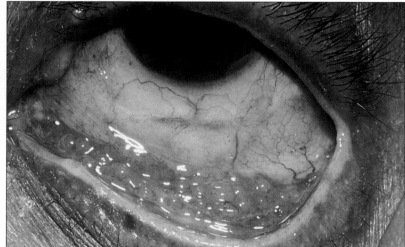

Fig. 4.47 Follicular conjunctivitis. Infection of the palpebral conjunctiva with lymphocytic follicle formation by *C. trachomatis*.

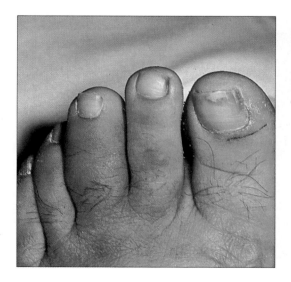

Fig. 4.48 A red and swollen third toe is seen in this photograph of the foot of a man presenting with Reiter's syndrome arthritis.

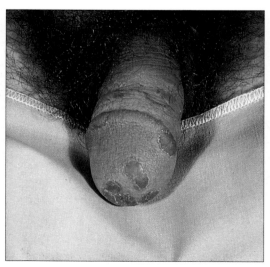

Fig. 4.49 Scaling erythematous plaques on the penis. Circinate balanitis of Reiter's syndrome. This is one of the infrequent but distinctive cutaneous findings associated with this syndrome.

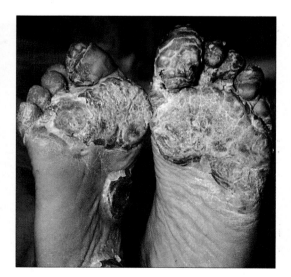

Fig. 4.50 Keratodermea blenorrhagica in Reiter's syndrome. Note the thick scales and crusts on the feet of this patient.

LABORATORY TESTS

The diagnosis of endemic trachoma can usually be made by an experienced clinician on the basis of patient history and physical examination. The diagnosis of *C. trachomatis* genital infection, however, is dependent upon specific laboratory identification. Infection is asymptomatic in the majority of infected women, and a substantial proportion of infected men. In addition, the symptoms and signs of infection are highly variable when present, and may be caused by other infectious agents or by noninfectious processes. The medical history and physical examination, while necessary in every instance, are neither sensitive nor specific enough to identify infected patients.

Isolation of *Chlamydia* in cell culture or eggs was originally the only practical method for detection of infection. Thereafter, the development of monoclonal antibodies directed against the organism and increased knowledge about the components of the EB resulted in new tests capable of detecting the presence of chlamydial antigen in clinical specimens. Since 1982, there has been a dramatic increase in the use of antigen detection tests in clinical laboratories. DNA amplification tests, such as PCR and ligase chain reaction (LCR), appear to be more sensitive and specific than other nonculture diagnostic tests.

PATHOLOGY

Gram stains

The diagnosis of NGU in men is usually based on the clinical presentation of scanty urethral discharge (*Fig. 4.51*) and a Gram stain of urethral exudate. The Gram stain is sensitive and specific for the diagnosis of gonorrhea (*Fig. 4.52*). Many men with gonococcal urethritis also have chlamydial infection. Thus only the absence of intracellular Gram-negative diplococci (*Fig. 4.53*) is useful in microscopically distinguishing NGU from gonorrhea.

Histopathology

Histopathologic characteristics of chlamydial infection include chronic inflammation and fibrotic changes with granulation. In many sites, the response to infection includes follicle formation. Left untreated, these processes lead to morbid complications regardless of location of the infection. In LGV, there is local acute and granulomatous inflammation in involved lymph nodes, often with gross formation of stellate abscesses (*Fig. 4.54*).

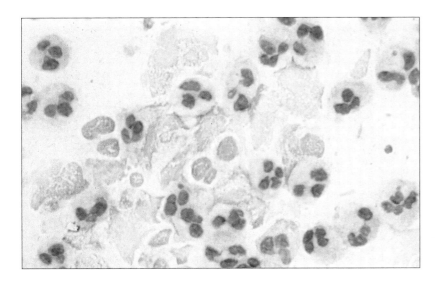

Fig. 4.51 Chlamydial urethritis. Mucoid, penile discharge with meatal erythema. *C. trachomatis* was isolated whereas *N. gonorrhoeae* was not.

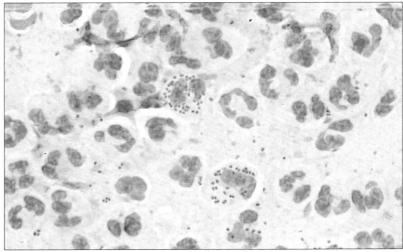

Fig. 4.52 Gonorrhea. A Gram stain of penile urethral exudate shows inflammatory cells containing gonococci.

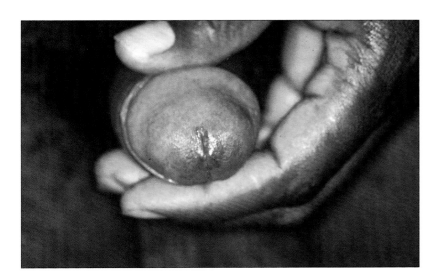

Fig. 4.53 Nongonoccal urethritis. The Gram stain of penile urethral exudate show inflammatory cells without visible gonococci.

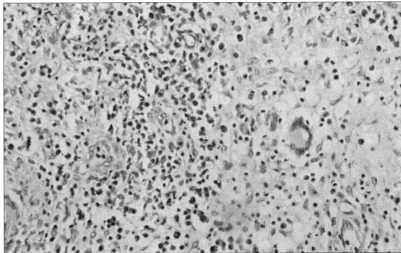

Fig. 4.54 Biopsy specimen of a lymph node in lymphogranuloma venereum showing acute and chronic inflammation with occasional multinucleate giant cells.

SPECIMEN COLLECTION

Isolation of *C. trachomatis* in cell culture remains a preferred method for identifying an infected patient. Proper collection of a specimen for culture is essential for successful results. A fiber-tipped swab is the most commonly used instrument for collection of a clinical specimen. Swab shafts should be made of inert material, preferably plastic or metal. Soluble components eluting from wooden shafts may be cytotoxic in chlamydial culture systems. Swab tips made of cottton or dacron appear to be less inhibitory to propagation than tips of nylon or alginate; however, individual lots of swabs should be tested to assure a lack of toxicity to the cell monolayer and lack of growth inhibition. Recently, collection devices resembling biopsy brushes have been developed to improve the sensitivity of sample collection from the endocervix. For enzyme immunoassays and DNA detection tests, it is imperative that manufacturers' instructions concerning appropriate collection methods are followed. There may be specific requirements for swab types to assure optimal performance of the tests. Typical sample collection instruments are shown in *Figure 4.55*.

Transport media for chlamydial culture may contain buffered salt solution, sucrose, and antibiotics that do not inhibit *Chlamydia* such as vancomycin, gentamicin, and nystatin. Many laboratories add fetal bovine serum to the media to enhance specimen recovery.

The organism may be difficult to isolate from specimens containing excess mucus or inflammatory cells, such as from bubo aspirates in patients with LGV. Likewise, components in semen are toxic to cell culture systems (*Fig. 4.56*). *C. trachomatis* can exhibit direct cytotoxicity to cell monolayers when inoculated at high multiplicities of infection. Cytopathic effects seen in clinical specimens are unlikely to be due to *Chlamydia*, as the number of organisms in clinical samples is probably never sufficient to produce this effect. Cytotoxicity, due to collection or transport system components or due to semen components, inflammatory cells, or genital microorganisms other than *Chlamydia*, may interfere with cell culture identification of *Chlamydia* in up to 5% of specimens from STD clinics. Dilution of such specimens prior to attempting cell culture has improved organism recovery.

C. trachomatis in clinical specimens has limited viability at temperatures above −70°C. Once collected, specimens should be refrigerated on ice or at 4°C and inoculated into cell culture within 48 hours. If specimens must be stored for longer periods prior to culture, they should be frozen at temperatures below −70°C.

CELL CULTURE

The typical procedure for isolation of *C. trachomatis* by cell culture is seen in *Figure 4.57*. If frozen, specimens to be cultured are thawed at 37°C and mixed. The specimen is inoculated onto the surface of confluent monolayers of susceptible cells. Commonly used cells include McCoy, HeLa 229, and BHK lines. The inoculated cell monolayers are centrifuged at 30–35°C at 2,000–3,000 g to improve the sensitivity of the culture. Following inoculation and centrifugation, the monolayer is overlaid with growth medium. Cycloheximide is included at a predetermined concentration to increase the number and size of chlamydial inclusions by inhibiting host cell protein synthesis.

After incubation of the inoculated cell monolayer for 48–72 hours, characteristic inclusions may be observed. The inclusion of *C. trachomatis* is surrounded by a distinct membrane and is visible under direct microscopic examination, particularly using phase microscopy. The inclusions may be visualized by staining with iodine, Giemsa, acridine orange, fluorescein-conjugated monoclonal or polyclonal antibody preparations, or with immunochemical stains using enzyme-conjugated antichlamydial monoclonal antibodies (*Figs. 4.58–4.65*). The most common stains used are iodine and fluorescein-labeled antibodies. Staining with fluorescein-labeled monoclonal antibodies to the MOMP of *C. trachomatis* is more sensitive and specific than iodine staining. Iodine stains intracellular glycogen, which is maximal at 40–60 hours following infection. Although inexpensive and easily performed, iodine stains are more subject to artifact formation due to staining of nonchlamydial material.

Several studies have indicated that isolation of *Chlamydia* in cell culture is relatively insensitive. Studies using multiple sampling in the same patient or repeated passage of inoculated host cells have suggested that a single endocervical swab may detect infection in only 70% of infected women. Additional sampling of women using a urethral swab has been shown to improve the sensitivity substantially.

DIRECT FLUORESCENT ANTIBODY DETECTION·

Detection of *C. trachomatis* infection by nonculture methods (antigen detection) became feasible with the recent development of immunologic reagents specific for chlamydial outer membrane components. Direct fluorescent antibody (DFA) detection uses one or more monoclonal antibodies (MAbs) conjugated to fluorescent molecules as shown in *Figure 4.66*. Monoclonal antibodies directed against species, subspecies, and genus (lipopolysaccharide) specific antigens have been developed for this method. Data to date suggest that monoclonal antibodies reacting to the chlamydial MOMP produce superior staining and characteristic morphology compared with antilipopolysaccharide antibodies. As with *Chlamydia* culture, proper technique in the collection of the clinical specimen is necessary to ensure adequate

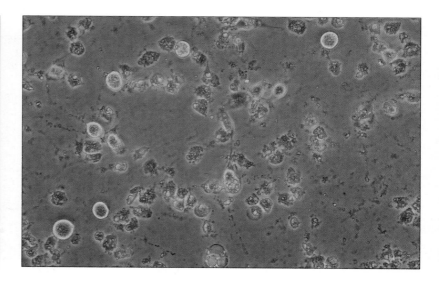

Fig. 4.55 *Various instruments available for sampling for chlamydia from the genitourinary tract. Left to right: The large-diameter cotton or dracon swab on a nontoxic plastic shaft and the brush-like device are satisfactory for endocervical sampling, though the latter is more traumatic. Urethral specimens may be obtained with the rigid aluminum-shafted swab or a flexible, steel, cotton-tipped device. An example of a swab for urethral enzyme immunoassay is seen on the far right.*

Fig. 4.56 *Cytotoxicity in cell culture. Cells exhibit a round morphology and have sloughed from the coverslip, resulting in a diffuse cytopathic effect.*

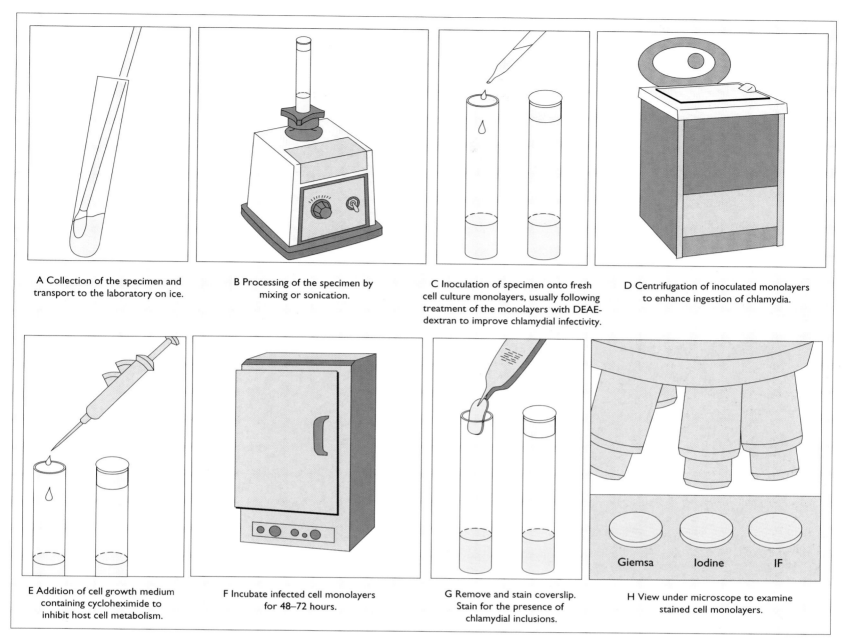

A Collection of the specimen and transport to the laboratory on ice.

B Processing of the specimen by mixing or sonication.

C Inoculation of specimen onto fresh cell culture monolayers, usually following treatment of the monolayers with DEAE-dextran to improve chlamydial infectivity.

D Centrifugation of inoculated monolayers to enhance ingestion of chlamydia.

E Addition of cell growth medium containing cycloheximide to inhibit host cell metabolism.

F Incubate infected cell monolayers for 48–72 hours.

G Remove and stain coverslip. Stain for the presence of chlamydial inclusions.

H View under microscope to examine stained cell monolayers.

Giemsa   Iodine   IF

Fig. 4.57 Culture method of *Chlamydia* isolation. Although recognized as the standard method for sensitive and specific laboratory identification of *C. trachomatis* organisms, the required skill and laboratory resources, coupled with the 2–7 days' turnaround for results, has made less demanding techniques generally more acceptable for routine clinical diagnosis.

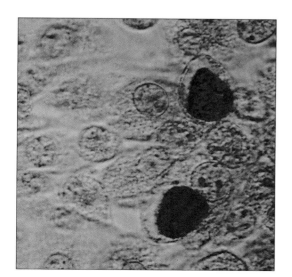

Fig. 4.58 Cell monolayer infected with *C. trachomatis*. Dark-red inclusions are positive in this specimen stained with Jones' iodine.

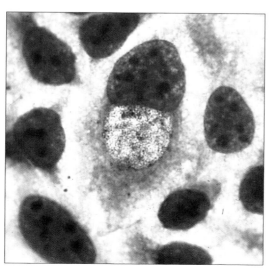

Fig. 4.59 Giemsa-stained inclusions (bright-field) showing the open, granular nature of an intracellular inclusion of *C. trachomatis*. Compare this with the dense inclusions seen with TWAR and *C. psittaci* (**4.61**).

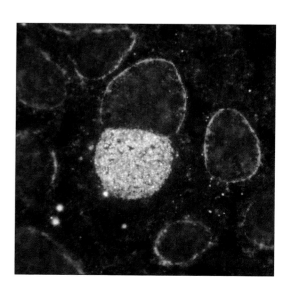

Fig. 4.60 Giemsa-stained inclusions (dark-field) showing the open, granular nature of an intracellular inclusion of *C. trachomatis*. Compare this with the dense inclusions with TWAR and *C. psittaci* (**4.61**).

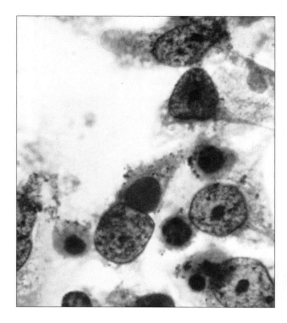

Fig. 4.61 Giemsa-stained inclusions (bright-field) showing the dense inclusion seen in TWAR and *C. psittaci* following staining.

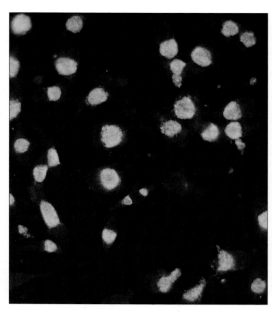

Fig. 4.62 Chlamydial inclusions in cycloheximide-treated McCoy cell monolayers stained with a fluorescein-labeled genus-specific monoclonal antibody. *C. trachomatis* inclusions occur individually.

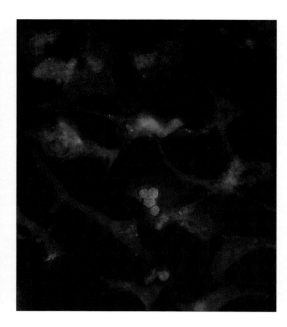

Fig. 4.63 Chlamydial inclusions in cycloheximide-treated McCoy cell monolayers stained with a fluorescein-labeled genus-specific monoclonal antibody. *C. psittaci* or TWAR may produce multiple or multilobed inclusions within a single infected cell.

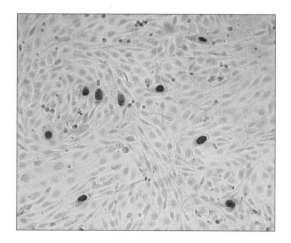

Fig. 4.64 Distinct red chlamydial inclusions detected using an alkaline-phosphatase monoclonal antibody method with naphthal-AS chromogenic substrate (original magnification × 250).

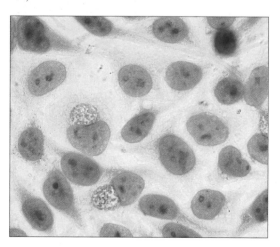

Fig. 4.65 Black, granular *C. trachomatis* inclusion produced using peroxidase-labeled monoclonal antibody and 1-chloro-4-naphthol chromogenic substrate (original magnification × 400).

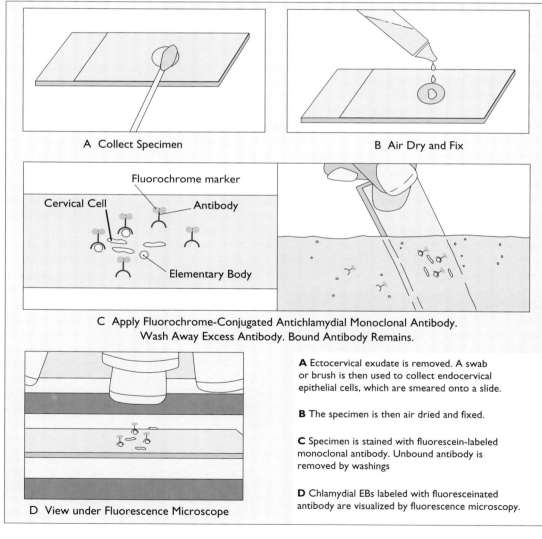

A Collect Specimen

B Air Dry and Fix

Fluorochrome marker

Cervical Cell

Antibody

Elementary Body

C Apply Fluorochrome-Conjugated Antichlamydial Monoclonal Antibody. Wash Away Excess Antibody. Bound Antibody Remains.

D View under Fluorescence Microscope

A Ectocervical exudate is removed. A swab or brush is then used to collect endocervical epithelial cells, which are smeared onto a slide.

B The specimen is then air dried and fixed.

C Specimen is stained with fluorescein-labeled monoclonal antibody. Unbound antibody is removed by washings

D Chlamydial EBs labeled with fluoresceinated antibody are visualized by fluorescence microscopy.

Fig. 4.66 Direct fluorescent antibody detection of *C. trachomatis*.

test performance. Upon addition to a specimen smear, these reagents bind to chlamydial EBs, producing brightly fluorescent and morphologically distinctive dots. Several to several hundred organisms may be seen in any smear (*Fig. 4.67*). The sensitivity of the DFA method in comparison with cell culture has varied in published studies, but averages 80–90% in women and symptomatic men. When a cutoff value for positive test results of 10 EBs is used, the test specificity will be approximately 97–98% in experienced expert laboratories.

A significant advantage of the DFA method is the lack of necessity for rapid transporting of specimens to the laboratory and storage of specimens in the cold, since slides can be fixed and mailed to a central area for staining and interpretation. In addition, the cellular background observed on the smear allows the microscopist to reject slides without sufficient cellular material from the endocervix (*Figs. 4.68–4.70*). Some studies have shown that up to 10% of all specimens are inadequate for the DFA method, suggesting that inadequate specimen collection contributes significantly to the insensitive nature of all *Chlamydia* detection methods. Disadvantages of the DFA method include the need for a trained microscopist, who must devote several minutes to the interpretation of each specimen, and the need for a fluorescence microscope. Some artefacts have been noted to occur due to

cross-reactivity of reagents with nonchlamydial organisms (*Figs. 4.71* and *4.72*), but an experienced microscopist is rarely confused by these.

ENZYME IMMUNOASSAY

Other methods for the rapid detection of chlamydial components use *Chlamydia*-specific or second antibodies labeled with an enzyme. Following incubation of a specimen with the antibody preparation, an enzyme substrate is added to generate a colored product, which can be detected visually or photometrically (*Figs. 4.73* and *4.74*). These enzyme immunoassay (EIA) tests can be designed to allow testing of numerous specimens for chlamydial antigen. EIA tests, like the DFA method, are less sensitive than culture methods; they are also somewhat less specific than the DFA method. The advantages of EIA include the high throughput capability for screening large numbers of patients, and due to the objective nature of the test results, the lack of requirement for highly skilled personnel to interpret the information. The reagents for EIA are expensive, costing $3–$7 per test. Tests based upon the reactivity of polyvalent antisera with chlamydial lipopolysaccharide may cross-react with those bacteria of the gastrointestinal tract that share common lipopolysaccharide antigenic determinants. For this reason, these tests are limited to those sites not potentially contaminated by gastrointestinal flora. The

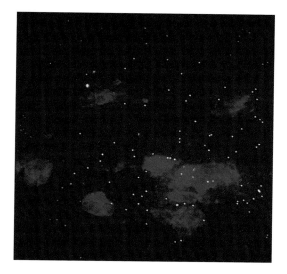

Fig. 4.67 Direct fluorescent antibody stain of chlamydia elementary bodies from a smear of cervical exudate (× 630).

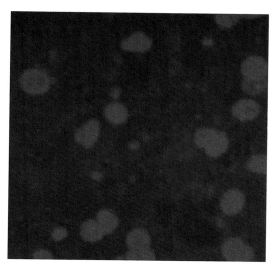

Fig. 4.68 Normal endocervical epithelial cells stained with a commercial chlamydial DFA reagent. The presence of such cells indicates the satisfactory quality of the sample collection to the microscopist (× 630).

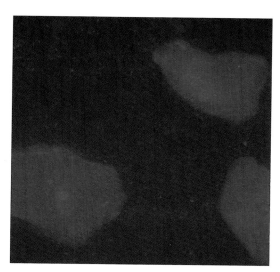

Fig. 4.69 An abundance of squamous cells is seen in this genital specimen from a women. This indicates that specimen collection has been unsatisfactory (× 630).

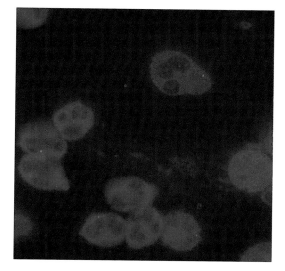

Fig. 4.70 Inflammatory cells stained as in **4.68** (× 630).

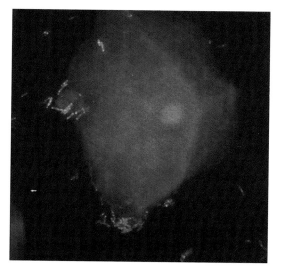

Fig. 4.71 Example of cross-reacting microorganisms seen in a clinical specimen stained with a chlamydial MOMP-specific monoclonal antibody. Such artifacts are uncommon and are not confusing to an experienced microscopist.

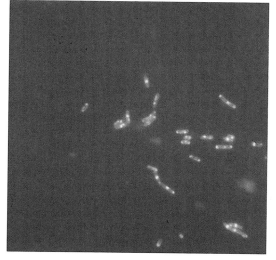

Fig. 4.72 Another artifactual example of cross-reacting microorganisms in a clinical specimen stained with a chlamydial MOMP-specific monoclonal antibody.

specificity of the EIA tests has been improved by the introduction of confirmatory blocking tests. In these procedures, all positive results are repeated in the presence of antibodies that will inhibit specific chlamydial reaction. If the EIA test result is adequately reduced, the initial positive result is accepted.

According to current guidelines, positive nonculture EIA and DFA test results in high-risk populations, such as in STD clinics, are accepted. In all other settings, confirmatory tests (either blocking tests or use of other tests aimed at a different antigen or molecule) are needed. Thus, all positive results are considered presumptive until confirmed in low to moderate prevalence screening situations. In cases where there are legal ramifications, such as child abuse, incest, rape, etc., the use of culture is mandated and nonculture tests should not be used.

SEROLOGY

Although not occurring in every case of uncomplicated genital infection, antibody to *C. trachomatis* usually occurs following infection and persists for years. IgM responses can be seen in first episodes of infection. These antibody responses have been used for decades to diagnose chlamydial infection.

Complement Fixation
With the availability of high-quality antigen in the 1940s, the chlamydial group complement fixation (CF) test was developed. The CF test uses the chlamydial 'group' antigen to detect serum antibody to any of the members of this genus. This test is still used in the diagnosis of LGV, in which a negative single-serum test rules out the disease, and in ornithosis, in which a change in titer between acute and convalescent sera can be diagnostic.

Microimmunofluorescence
The limited sensitivity and genus specificity of the CF test limits its use in seroepidemiologic studies. The development of the microimmunofluorescence (MIF) test in the 1970s allowed studies of the clinical epidemiology

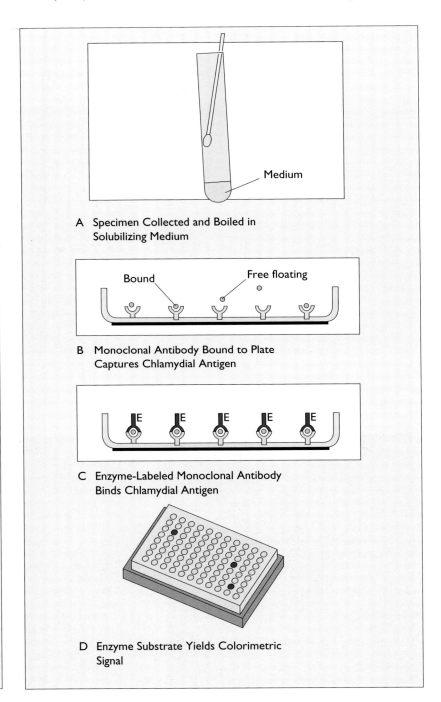

Fig. 4.73 Detection of *Chlamydia* by enzyme immunoassay (EIA), using direct antigen capture technique.

Fig. 4.74 Detection of *Chlamydia* by enzyme immunoassay (EIA), using the MAb sandwich antigen capture technique.

of chlamydial infection. The MIF uses fixed, purified chlamydial antigens, which are dotted onto a glass slide and reacted with the patient serum (*Figs. 4.75* and *4.76*). The test is sensitive, and usually provides information regarding the infecting serotype in *C. trachomatis* infections. It is also capable of determining IgM responses characteristic of acute infection, and is of particular use in the diagnosis of infant chlamydial pneumonia. However, the technique is laborious and technically demanding, and interpretation requires extensive experience. Less demanding ELISA tests or inclusion—indirect immunofluorescent tests using a single serovar have been described or are available commercially, but have not been critically examined in large clinical trials. Several studies have indicated the association

of local antibody in acute chlamydial disease, and serum IgA has been suggested to predict infection; however, these tests have not been sufficiently researched to be recommended. Due primarily to the background prevalence of chlamydial infections, serologic diagnosis of *C. trachomatis* infection has limited utility (*Fig. 4.77*).

PAPANICOLAOU SMEAR

Another method advocated by some for the laboratory diagnosis of chlamydial infection is examination of Papanicolaou-stained cervical smears (Pap smear). The detection of intact chlamydial inclusions in the Pap smear is insensitive. In addition, the cytologic changes that accompany *C. trachomatis*

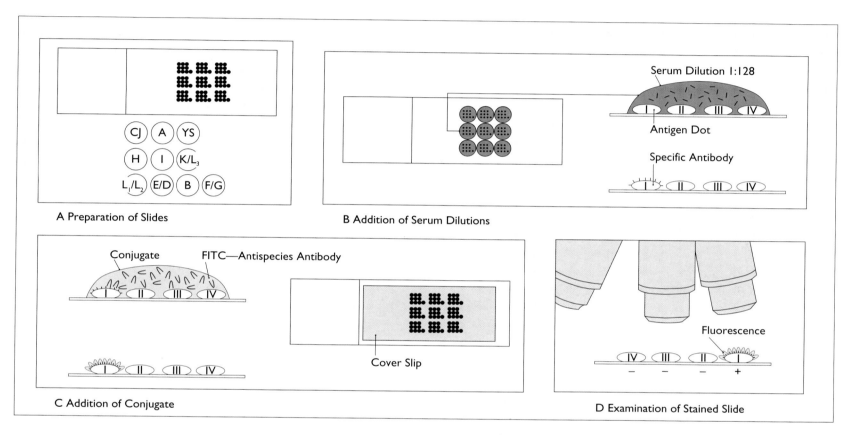

Fig. 4.75 Microimmunofluoresence assay.

Fig. 4.76 Fluorescent chlamydial EBs suspended in egg yolk sac material as viewed by the microimmunofluorescence method. The laborious nature of this test and the degree of skill required for proper interpretation have limited its acceptance outside research laboratories.

USES OF SEROLOGY IN CHLAMYDIAL DIAGNOSIS

TEST	DIAGNOSTIC USE	PERFORMANCE
Complement fixation	LGV Ornithosis	Sensitive but not specific. Can rule out LGV if-negative.
Microimmunofluorescence	Trachoma Genital infection Infant pneumonia	Sensitive and specific. Type responses in majority of infections.
ELISA	Unknown	Sensitivity and specificity undefined. Various methods not standardized.

Fig. 4.77 Uses of serology in *Chlamydia* diagnosis.

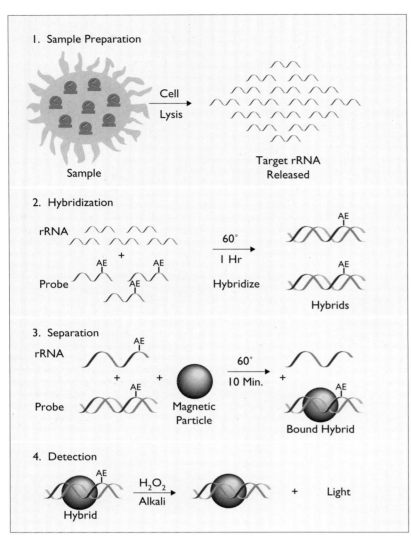

1. Sample Preparation

Sample

Cell Lysis →

Target rRNA Released

2. Hybridization

rRNA
+
Probe

60°
1 Hr
Hybridize →

Hybrids

AE

3. Separation

rRNA
+
Probe
+
Magnetic Particle

60°
10 Min. →

+

Bound Hybrid

AE

4. Detection

Hybrid

H₂O₂
Alkali →

+ Light

Fig. 4.78 Assay principles of a nonamplified DNA probe test for the detection of *C. trachomatis* rRNA (Gen-Probe Pace ® 2 Assay System). DNA probes labeled with acridinium ester (AE) are allowed to hybridize with target rRNA released during cell lysis. Hybrids are captured on magnetic particles and the unhybridized single-stranded DNA probe chemically inactivated. Captured hybrids are detected by chemiluminescence in the presence of hydrogen peroxide and a strong alkali.

cervical infection are nonspecific. For these reasons, the Pap smear cannot be used to diagnose chlamydial endocervical infection; however, the finding of inflammatory cells may indicate the need for specific chlamydial testing.

NUCLEIC ACID PROBE AND AMPLIFICATION TESTS

Straightforward detection of nonamplified chlamydial nucleic acid, including commercially available probes, which detect ribosomal RNA, is less sensitive than culture. These tests (*Fig. 4.78*) appear to have a sensitivity of the same order as the modern EIAs. The amplified DNA tests (PCR and LCR), in contrast, are more sensitive than culture for detection of urethral *C. trachomatis* infection in men and cervical infection in women (*Figs. 4.79* and *4.80*). In some studies, there have been problems with inhibitors of Taq polymerase which may be present in cervical specimens. These technologies involve detection of specific chlamydial nucleotide sequences, and using different technologies amplify the detected sequence exponentially. In addition, the nucleotide sequences being sought are those present in the common chlamydial plasmid, which is present at 7–10 copies per elementary body. These tests are capable of detecting less than one chlamydial particle. Although there is not as yet widespread experience using these techniques, the preliminary data are convincing. These tests, though expensive, will greatly increase our ability to diagnose infection with *C. trachomatis*.

Urine as a Diagnostic Specimen

The use of urine as a specimen for chlamydial diagnosis has been explored. Chlamydial lipopolysaccharide antigens can be detected by EIA in urine sediment from men with symptomatic urethritis; however, these assays are

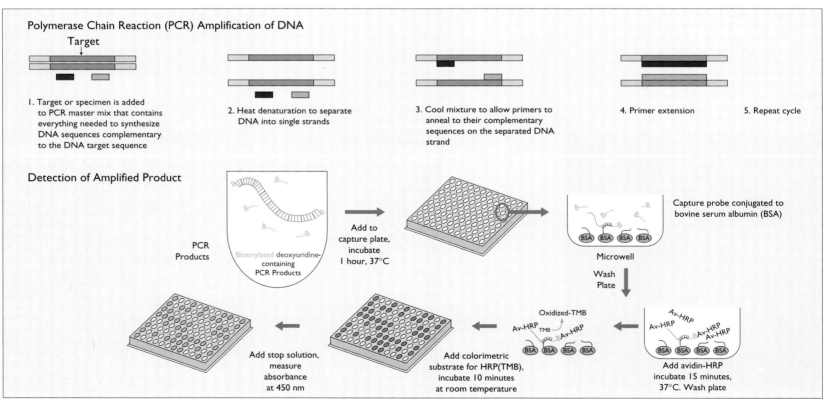

Polymerase Chain Reaction (PCR) Amplification of DNA

Target

1. Target or specimen is added to PCR master mix that contains everything needed to synthesize DNA sequences complementary to the DNA target sequence

2. Heat denaturation to separate DNA into single strands

3. Cool mixture to allow primers to anneal to their complementary sequences on the separated DNA strand

4. Primer extension

5. Repeat cycle

Detection of Amplified Product

PCR Products

Biotinylated deoxyuridine-containing PCR Products

Add to capture plate, incubate 1 hour, 37°C →

Microwell

Capture probe conjugated to bovine serum albumin (BSA)

Wash Plate ↓

Add avidin-HRP incubate 15 minutes, 37°C. Wash plate

← Add colorimetric substrate for HRP(TMB), incubate 10 minutes at room temperature

← Add stop solution, measure absorbance at 450 nm

Fig. 4.79 Assay principles of the Roche Amplicor™ PCR assay for the detection of *C. trachomatis*. PCR technology amplifies a selected region of DNA. All PCR assays involve three steps per cycle: 1. heat denaturation, wherein the two strands of DNA are separated; 2. annealing of a biotinylated primer pair; and 3. primer extension in which a heat-stable DNA polymerase (*Taq* polymerase) adds complementary nucleotides to the growing strand of DNA. The cycle is repeated over and over leading to an exponential increase in the number of copies of DNA; millions of copies are produced after only 20 cycles and billions of copies, after only 30 cycles. Amplified product is detected in a microwell plate assay. Target-specific oligonucleotide probes are attached to the surface of the microwells. The amplified target DNA, biotin-labeled, hybridizes to the immobilized probe and the product detected colorimetrically with a conjugate of streptavidin-horseradish peroxidase.

relatively insensitive for detecting infection in asymptomatic men and may give false positive results with urine specimens from women. Protocols have been developed by the manufacturers of DNA amplification tests, such as LCR and PCR, for use with urine specimens. Urine sediment can be used to diagnose chlamydial infection in men with an efficiency that is equal to or greater than the use of urethral swabs. While urine testing for women is probably less sensitive than doing a pelvic examination and then performing tests on cervical and urethral swabs, the noninvasive nature of the specimen collection makes it likely that urine will ultimately become the specimen of choice for screening purposes.

TREATMENT

Treatment of chlamydial infection in the acute stages of disease is straightforward; chlamydiae are susceptible to many antibiotics, and acquired resistance to antimicrobials has not yet been recognized (*Fig. 4.81*). As the cell wall differs from that of many bacteria, β-lactam antibiotics such as penicillin lack bactericidal activity against these organisms. The tetracyclines and macrolides of the erythromycin class are the currently recommended choices for proven or suspected chlamydial infection. Sulfonamides have activity against *C. trachomatis*, as does rifampin and its derivatives. Quinolones have variable activity *in vitro* against *C. trachomatis*. Long-acting cogeners of erythromycin are effective for use against infection in short-term therapeutic regimens. The currently recommended therapy is presented in *Figure 4.82*.

Picture credits for this chapter are as follows: Figs. 4.4 and 4.5 courtesy of Elizabeth H. White; Fig. 4.6 courtesy of Wyrick PB, Gutman LT, Hodinka RL. Chlamydiae, in Joklik W, *et al.* (eds): Zinsser Microbiology, ed. 19. New York: Appleton-Lange, 1983, p 609–616; Fig. 4.12 courtesy of JPA, WHO; Fig. 4.14 courtesy of NIH, NIAID Study Group of Sexually Transmitted Disease: 1980. Status report. Summaries and panel recommendations. Washington D.C.: U.S. Government Printing Office 1981: 215–264; and courtesy of Washington AE, Johnson RE, Sanders LL, Barnes RC, Alexander ER: Incidence of Chlamydia trachomatis in the United States: Using reported Neisseria gonorrhoeae as a surrogate, in Oriel D, Ridgway G, Schachter J, Taylor-Robinson D, Ward M (eds): Chlamydial Infections. Cambridge: Cambridge University Press, 1986, pp 487–490; Figs. 4.15 to 4.17 courtesy of Centers for Disease Control; Fig. 4.23 courtesy of P. Morel, Hôpital Saint-Louis, Paris; Fig. 4.54 courtesy of Woodruff JD, Parmley TH: Atlas of Gynecologic Pathology. New York, Gower Medical Publishing, 1988; Fig. 4.24 courtesy of Richard E. Berger, MD, University of Washington; Fig. 4.25 courtesy of Walter E. Stamm, MD, University of Washington; Figs. 4.26 and 4.31 courtesy of Bingham JS: Pocket Picture Guide to Clinical Medicine. Sexually Transmitted Diseases. London, Gower Medical Publishing Ltd., 1984; Figs. 4.29 and 4.30 courtesy of Paul Weisner, MD; Fig. 4.28 courtesy of Fernando Guijon, MD; Fig. 4.33 courtesy of Lourdes Frau, MD; Fig. 4.34 courtesy of George Schmid, MD; Fig. 4.35 courtesy of Robert Branham, MD, (Kunimoto, *et al.*) Rev Infect Dis 1985; 7(5):666; Fig. 4.36 courtesy of John Swanson, MD. J Infect Dis 1975; (3):678–687; Figs. 4.37, 4.41, 4.42, and 4.50 courtesy of Dorothy Patton, PhD; Fig. 4.40 courtesy of Richard Sweet, MD, University of California; Figs. 4.48 to 4.50 courtesy of Robert Wilkens, MD; Fig. 4.42 courtesy of Am J O G 1968;100:422–431; Fig. 4.44 courtesy of E.R. Alexander, MD; Fig. 4.45 courtesy of Spalton DJ, Hitchings RA, Hunter PA: Atlas of Clinical Ophthalmology. London, Gower Medical Publishing Ltd, 1984; Fig. 4.47 courtesy of George Waring, MD, Emory University; Figs. 4.18 to 4.20 courtesy of Julius Schachter, PhD; Fig. 4.56 courtesy of Francisco J. Candal; Figs. 4.59 and 4.61 courtesy of Billie R. Bird; Fig. 4.60 courtesy of C.C. Kuo, PhD; Figs. 4.62 and 4.63 courtesy of Shannon Mitchell and Janice C. Bullard; Fig. 4.64 courtesy of James Mahoney, PhD; Fig. 4.65 courtesy of Robert Suchland; Fig. 4.67 courtesy of Howard Soule, PhD, Kallestad Diagnostics; Figs. 4.68, 4.69, 4.71, and 4.76 courtesy of Janice C. Bullard, Centers for Disease Control; Fig. 4.72 courtesy of Linda Cles; Fig. 4.81 adapted from (1) Schachter J: Chlamydial Infection. N Engl J Med 1978; 298:428,490,540, (2) Bowie WR, Shaw CE, Chan DGW, Black WA: AAC 1987; 31:470–472, (3) Walsh M, Kappus EW, Quinn TC: AAC 1987; 31:811–812; Fig. 4.82 adapted from (1) Centers for Disease Control. MMWR 1985; 32[suppl]:535–735, (2) MMWR 1985; 34[4S]:4–21, (3) Med Letter 1988; 30:5–10.

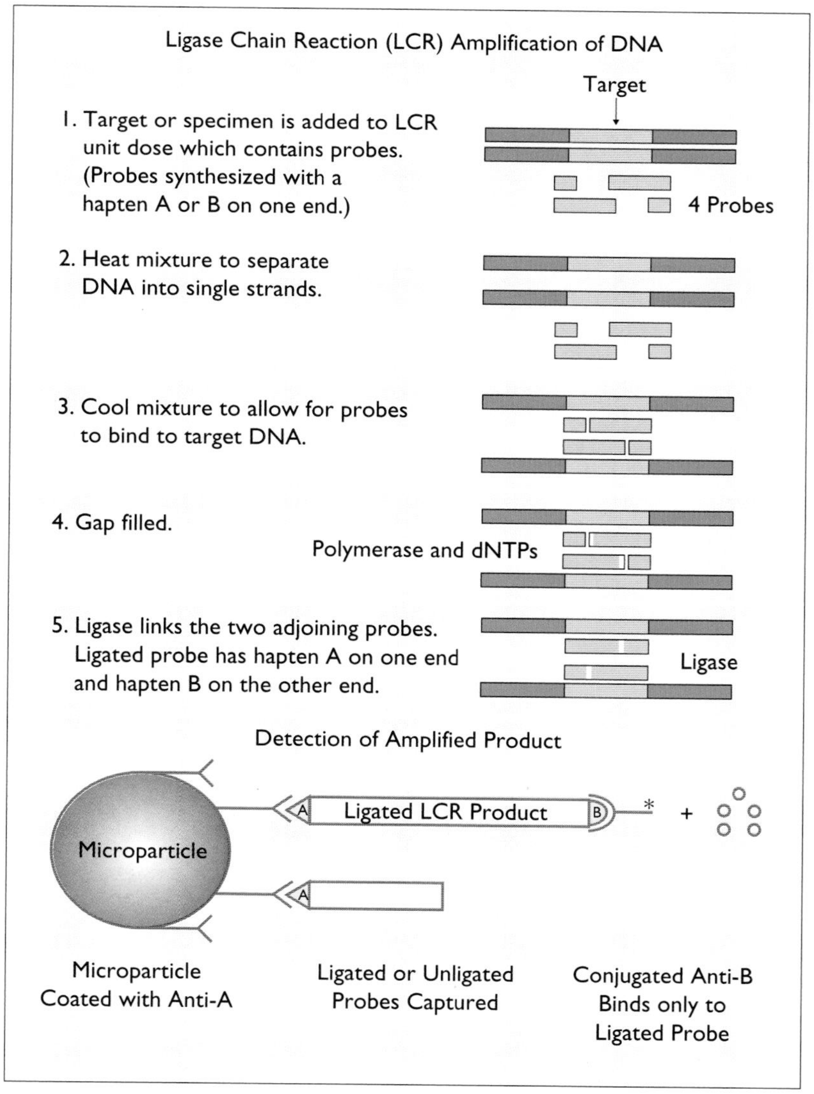

Ligase Chain Reaction (LCR) Amplification of DNA

1. Target or specimen is added to LCR unit dose which contains probes. (Probes synthesized with a hapten A or B on one end.)

2. Heat mixture to separate DNA into single strands.

3. Cool mixture to allow for probes to bind to target DNA.

4. Gap filled.
   Polymerase and dNTPs

5. Ligase links the two adjoining probes. Ligated probe has hapten A on one end and hapten B on the other end.

Detection of Amplified Product

Microparticle Coated with Anti-A | Ligated or Unligated Probes Captured | Conjugated Anti-B Binds only to Ligated Probe

Fig. 4.80 Assay principles of the Abbott ligase chain reaction amplification test (LCx Assay™) for the detection of *C. trachomatis*. If the specimen being analyzed contains the target nucleic acid sequence of interest, two LCR probes will bind to each strand of the target sequence. Two enzymes, polymerase and ligase, acting sequentially, will join probes that hybridize at adjacent positions on a given strand of target DNA, creating copies of the target. Amplified product is detected by a microparticle enzyme immunoassay.

REPRESENTATIVE VALUES OF *C. TRACHOMATIS* MICS

ANTIMICROBIAL	MIC (μg/ml)
Tetracycline	0.03–0.50
Doxycycline	0.02–0.03
Azithromycin	0.25–1.0
Erythromycin	0.50–2.0
Clindamycin	2.0–16.0
Rifampicin	0.005–0.25
Sulfamethoxazole	0.50–4.0

Variability of strains and methods used in the determination of chlamydial susceptibilities limits the clinical utility of these in vitro data.

Fig. 4.81 Representative values of *C. trachomatis* MICs.

TREATMENT REGIMENS FOR CHLAMYDIAL INFECTIONS AND CHLAMYDIA-ASSOCIATED CONDITIONS

PATIENT	CONDITION	THERAPY	COMMENTS
Adults	Uncomplicated urethral, endocervical, or rectal infections	Doxycycline 100 mg po bid for 7 days or Azithromycin 1g po in a single dose	Alternatives: Erythromycin base 500 mg po qid for 7 days. or Sulfisoxazole 500mg qid for 10 days or Ofloxacin 300 mg bid for 7 days or Erythromycin ethylsuccinate 800 mg po qid for 7 days
Pregnant women	Urogenital infection	Erythromycin base 500 mg po qid for 7 days	If 2 g daily dose not tolerated, decrease to 250 mg po qid for 14 days; or erythromycin ethylsuccinate either 800 mg po qid for 7 days or 400 mg qid for 14 days. If the patient cannot tolerate erythromycin, use amoxicillin 500 mg po tid for 7–10 days
Neonates or infants	Conjunctivitis or pneumonitis	Erythromycin syrup 12.5 mg/kg po qid for 10–14 days	Concurrent gonococcal conjunctival infection must be ruled out in conjunctivitis. Topical therapy not beneficial.
Young men	Epididymitis (in presence of urethritis and absence of bacteriuria)	Doxycycline 100 mg po bid for 10 days or Ofloxacin 300 mg po bid for 10 days	Given in conjunction with effective antigonococcal therapy. Oflaxacin is contraindicated in persons ≤17 years of age
Women	PID*	*	*
Adults	LGV	Doxycycline 100 mg po bid for 21 days or Erythromycin 500 mg po qid for 21 days. or Sulfisoxazole 500 mg po qid for 21 days or equivalent sulfonamide course	

* See Chapter 8 (PID)

Fig. 4.82 Treatment regimens for chlamydial infections and chlamydial-associated conditions.

BIBLIOGRAPHY

Centers for Disease Control: Recommendations for the Prevention and Management of *Chlamydia trachomatis* Infection. MMWR **42**: RR–12; **34** (suppl.):53S–74S, 1993.

Chernesky MA, Jang D, Lee H, Burczak JD, Hu H, Sellors J, Tomazic-Allen SJ, Mahony JB. Diagnosis of *Chlamydia trachomatis* infections in men and women by testing first-void urine by ligase chain reaction. J Clin Microbiol **32**:2682–2685, 1994.

Grayston JT: *Chlamydia pneumoniae*, strain TWAR. *Chest* **95**:664–669, 1989.

Schachter J: Biology of *Chlamydia trachomatis*. In: Holmes KK, Mårdh P–A, Sparling PF, Wiesner PJ (eds). *Sexually Transmitted Diseases*, 2nd ed. New York, McGraw–Hill, pp 167–180, 1990.

Schachter J: Chlamydial infections. *N Engl J Med* **298**:428–435, 490–495, 540–549, 1978.

Schachter J, Dawson CR: *Human Chlamydial Infections*. Littleton, MA, Publishing Sciences Group, 1978.

Stamm WE: Diagnosis of *C. trachomatis* genitourinary infections. *Ann Intern Med* **108**:710–717, 1988.

Thompson SE, Washington AE: Epidemiology of sexually transmitted *C. trachomatis* infections. *Epidemiol Rev* **5**:96–123, 1983.

CHAPTER FIVE

Granuloma Inguinale

R Ballard and B Majmudar

INTRODUCTION

Donovanosis (granuloma inguinale, granuloma venereum) was first described in India (1882) as 'serpiginous ulcer'. Donovanosis is a progressive inflammatory disease of the skin and subcutaneous tissues of the genital and anal regions. Although the disease has been considered an STD, nonvenereal transmission has been documented. Diagnosis relies on clinical findings and the demonstration of intracellular 'Donovan bodies' in cytologic and tissue preparations. These bodies are generally not seen unless special stains are employed. This requirement could be partly responsible for the reported low incidence and the paucity of information regarding this disease. Once the diagnosis is established, the treatment is usually simple and effective.

The etiologic agent is *Calymmatobacterium granulomatis*, a coccobacillus (0.5–1.5 mm by 1–2 mm) that is Gram-negative, non-motile, asporogenic, and encapsulated. It is classified as an unassigned genus associated with the family Enterobacteriaceae. Morphologically and antigenically, it resembles members of the genus *Klebsiella*, in particular *K. rhinoscleromatis*. It has been cultured only under microaerophilic to anaerobic conditions. It will not grow on the surface of ordinary laboratory media, simple or complex. It has been grown in special liquid media, egg yolk slant fluid and yolk sacs of 5-day-old chicken embryos. Optimal growth temperature is 37°C. Electron microscopy confirms ultrastructural characteristics similar to all Gram-negative rods. It has also demonstrated possible bacteriophage-like particles in the Donovan bodies. *C. granulomatis* may be a normal intestinal organism that can be modified by a bacteriophage into a pathogenic organism.

EPIDEMIOLOGY

Donovanosis is found primarily in tropical and subtropical countries, most commonly in India, Brazil, West Indies, New Guinea, and Australia and has emerged as a minor cause of genital ulceration in parts of southern Africa (*Fig. 5.1*). Case reporting is incomplete in some areas and nonexistent in others. In the USA, an average of 30 cases have been reported annually for the past 10 years (*see References, STD Summary*). It is considered a venereal disease because there is a preponderance of cases in the 20–30-year-old group, coinciding with the peak ages for STDs. However, only 1–50% of marital partners of infected patients contract the disease and it is also found, though only infrequently, in the very young and the elderly. The male-to-female ratio is 2.5:1. Most cases in the USA occur in the black population of the southeast and among immigrants from the West Indies. No resistance to the disease has been documented and no spontaneous regressions of well-developed lesions have occurred without therapy, even in the presence of high levels of circulating antibodies.

A bacterium resembling *C. granulomatis* has been isolated from feces, suggesting *C. granulomatis* might be a member of the family Enterobacteriaceae normally residing in the intestine. Presumably, as a result of minor trauma, such as a break in the skin or mucosa, the organisms are inoculated subcutaneously and produce the clinical lesions of donovanosis. This suggests the possibility of transmission by either intercourse or close physical contact to the anogenital region.

Two possible modes of transmission of this disease are:
- Direct contact during rectal intercourse
- Indirect contact through vaginal contamination by feces or fecal organisms.

The latter might explain the rarity of the disease in prostitutes, most of whom douche regularly, which would tend to reduce any fecal contamination of the vaginal tract. In addition, those who develop clinical donovanosis, particularly the disseminated form, are possibly deficient in some way in their cellular immune response.

CLINICAL MANIFESTATIONS

Donovanosis is an acute or chronic infection manifested by ulcerating necrotizing lesions of the skin and subcutaneous tissues in the genitoanal areas. In most patients the period from exposure to lesion is between 7 and 30 days. The initial lesion is a small papule that erodes the skin surface, breaking down to ulcers that progressively enlarge. Similar lesions are seen in both males

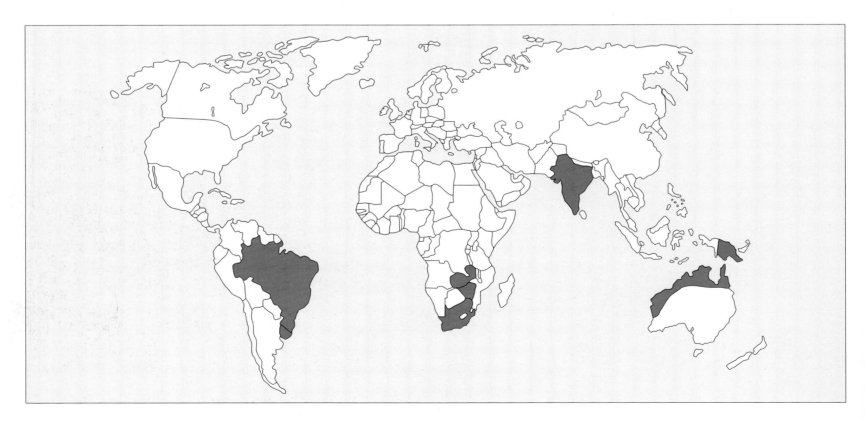

Fig. 5.1 Principal areas from which donovanosis has been reported.

(*Figs. 5.2–5.6*) and females (*Figs. 5.7–5.10*). Late lesions appear as hypertrophic, velvety, beefy red, indurated granulation tissue (*Figs. 5.4–5.6, 5.8, and 5.10*). Uncomplicated lesions are painless, but secondary infection induces pain and an exudate (*Figs. 5.11–5.13*). Lesions most commonly occur on the inner aspect of the labia or the fourchette in the female (*Fig. 5.14*) and on the penis in the male. The disease progresses by extension to adjacent skin (*Figs. 5.15 and 5.16*) and frequently spreads by autoinoculation and lymphatic or systemic dissemination.

In women, massive swelling of the labia is common. The lymphatics are widely dilated, but unobstructed, as dye injected into the tissues rapidly reaches the regional lymph nodes. Even in extensive donovanosis, the regional lymph nodes are not enlarged, painful, or tender. Absence of lymphadenopathy is a diagnostic characteristic; however, secondary infection produces inguinal adenopathy. These inguinal swellings appear as indurated masses or fluctuant abscesses, which eventually break down to be replaced by ulcers. They are called 'pseudobuboes' because they represent subcutaneous granulation tissue and not enlarged lymph nodes (*Figs. 5.17 and 5.18*). Large and massively destructive lesions (*Figs. 5.19–5.29*) may be mistaken for malignancy. A combination of biopsy and cytology is necessary to rule out malignancy in these cases. Proper treatment results in healing and finally total resolution of lesions (*Figs. 5.30–5.37*). In general, the response to treatment is very satisfactory, but in long-standing cases genital deformities may occur, such as residual hypopigmentation of the skin (*Fig. 5.38*), stenosis of the urethral, vaginal, and anal orifices (*Figs. 5.39 and 5.40*), and massive edema (*Fig. 5.41*).

Extragenital lesions have been reported on the face, neck, mouth, and throat. Metastatic lesions involving the bones, joints, and viscera have been found. In these cases, there was an associated cervical or uterine lesion, and in some a history of a prior pregnancy or operative procedure. There is no evidence for congenital transmission of this disease.

DIFFERENTIAL DIAGNOSIS

The diagnosis of donovanosis is often overlooked because several genital infections are similar clinically, prior antibiotic therapy alters presentation, and there may be a failure to consider it as a diagnosis because of its low incidence in the USA. At present, the only conclusive method of diagnosis is to demonstrate Donovan bodies in large mononuclear cells in biopsy or cytology of the lesion.

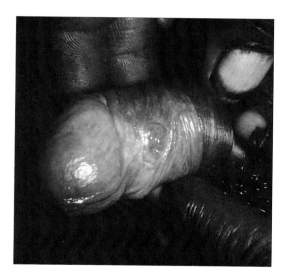

Fig. 5.2 Donovanosis, penile lesion in a male. A well-punched-out, clean, and shallow ulcer is seen upon retraction of the foreskin.

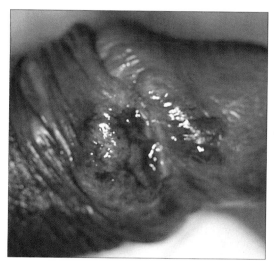

Fig. 5.3 Donovanosis, penile lesion in a male. Occasionally the ulcer can be large but with an elevated appearance.

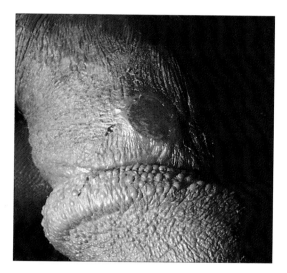

Fig. 5.4 Donovanosis, penile lesion in a male. An ulcer exhibiting red granulation tissue in the ulcer base.

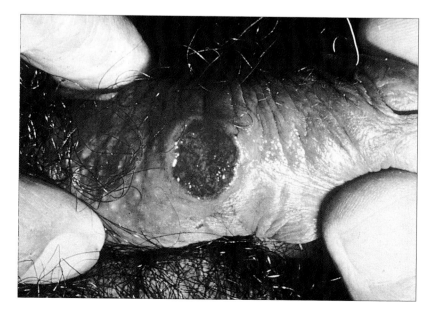

Fig. 5.5 Donovanosis, penile lesion in a male. A penile ulcer, as seen here, can mimic a hard chancre of syphilis. The latter can be diagnosed by dark-field examination, revealing spirochetes. Donovanosis will show the characteristic intracellular *C. granulomatis*.

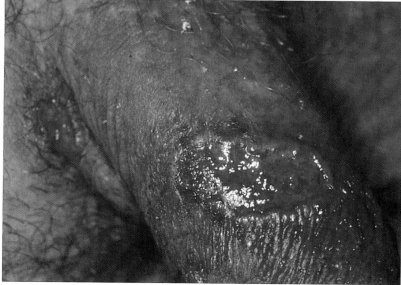

Fig. 5.6 Donovanosis, penile lesion in a male. A large ulcer with raised and indurated margins. The floor of the ulcer is granular and red due to granulation tissue.

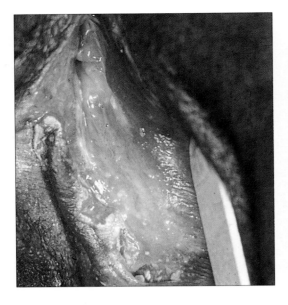

Fig. 5.7 Donovanosis lesion in a female. The morphology of the ulcers is similar in males and females. Retraction of the left labium shows a shallow, clean ulcer.

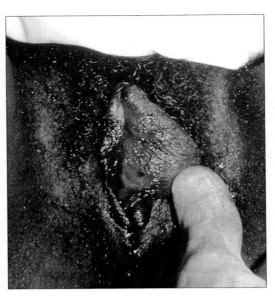

Fig. 5.8 Donovanosis lesion in a female. Retraction of the left edematous labium partially reveals a beefy red, ulcerating lesion.

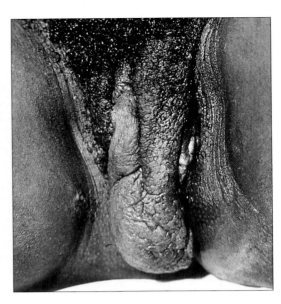

Fig. 5.9 Donovanosis lesion in a a female. A large ulcer is partially obscured by markedly edematous labium majus. The patient was pregnant.

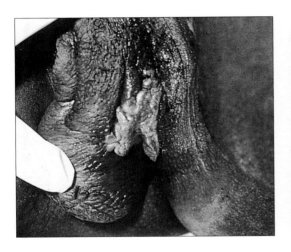

Fig. 5.10 A clearer view of the same lesion in **5.9**. Association of pregnancy and donovanosis can cause considerable therapeutic problems due to the contraindication of chloramphenicol and streptomycin in pregnancy.

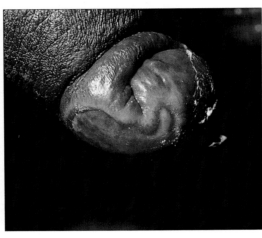

Fig. 5.11 Secondary infection in donovanosis. An irregular penile ulcer with an angry-red border and purulent floor suggesting a secondary infection. The lesion of donovanosis becomes painful when infected. Also note the marked edema of the surrounding skin.

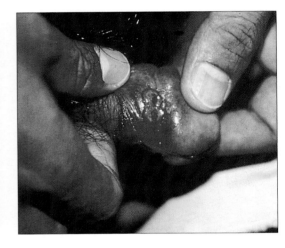

Fig. 5.12 Secondary infection of penile donovanosis makes the lesion painful, red, and vascular.

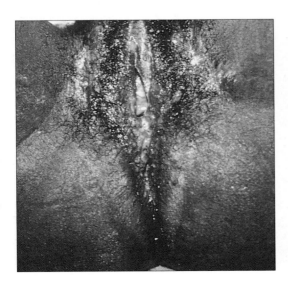

Fig. 5.13 Multiple, shallow ulcers seen on the vulvar skin. Secondary infection made them painful. Multiple lesions are usually caused by autoinoculation.

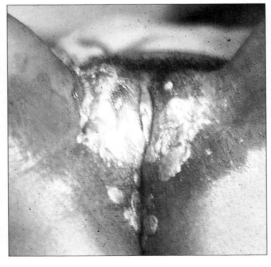

Fig. 5.14 The labia and fourchette are the common sites of donovanosis in the female.

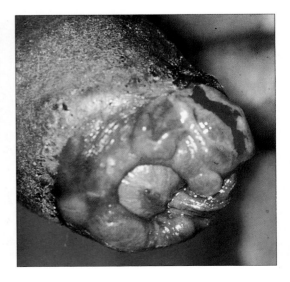

Fig. 5.15 The disease spreads by formation of satellite lesions in adjacent skin.

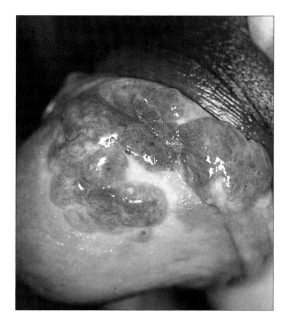

Fig. 5.16 Similar lesions to those in **5.15** undergoing spread on the glans penis.

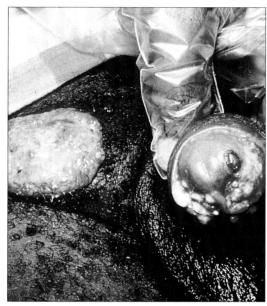

Fig. 5.17 Pseudobuboes. Penile donovanosis seen as an ulcerating, nodular lesion with marked tissue destruction. There is a large, inguinal ulcer indicating soft tissue breakdown in the area secondary to donovanosis. This is known as a 'pseudobubo.'

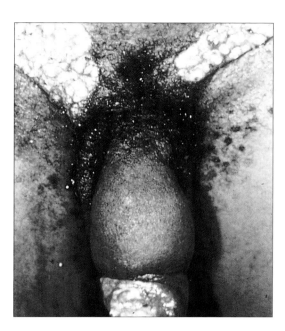

Fig. 5.18 A large necrotic ulcer is seen in the glans penis. Note the secondary edema of the penile shaft. Bilateral inguinal pseudobuboes are also seen.

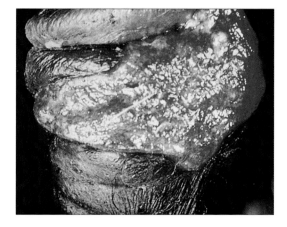

Fig. 5.19 Destructive donovanosis penile lesion in a male. A large and necrotic ulcer mimicking carcinoma. Note that the floor of the ulcer is clean, shallow, and smooth, unlike what one expects to see in a malignant ulcer.

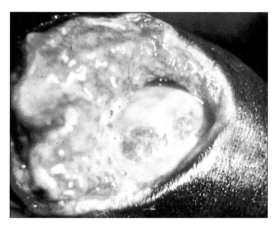

Fig. 5.20 Destructive donovanosis penile lesion in a male. The glans penis is completely destroyed by donovanosis. Such a lesion simulates malignancy.

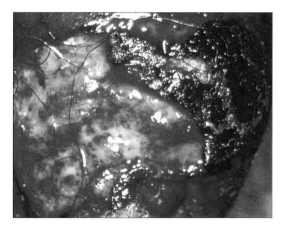

Fig. 5.21 Destructive donovanosis penile lesion in a male. A necrotic ulcer with an uneven, granular, and bleeding surface may closely mimic carcinoma.

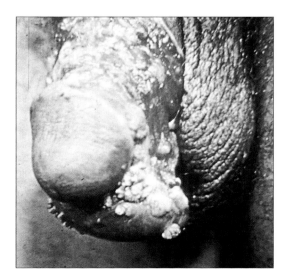

Fig. 5.22 Destructive donovanosis penile lesion in a male. Skin at the margin of this large ulcer shows multiple nodules composed of granulation tissue.

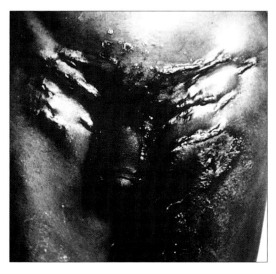

Fig. 5.23 Destructive donovanosis penile lesion in a male. Severe donovanosis with extensive scarring in the inguinal region.

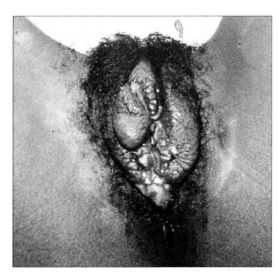

Fig. 5.24 Destructive donovanosis lesion in a female, showing a large, fungating ulcer obscured by edematous labia.

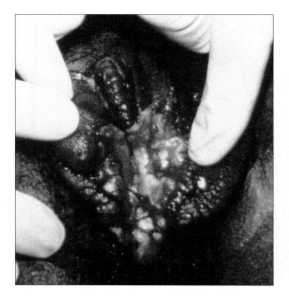

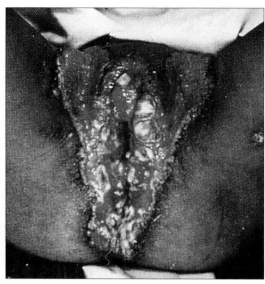

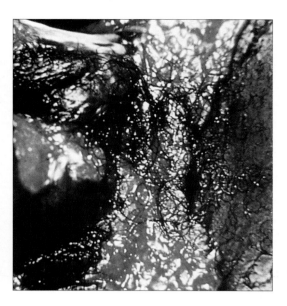

Fig. 5.25 The same patient as in **5.24**, with the labia drawn back.

Fig. 5.26 Destructive donovanosis lesion in a female. The entire vulva is destroyed by a large, fungating, necrotic ulcer. A biopsy and cytology are necessary to rule out malignancy in such cases.

Fig. 5.27 Destructive donovanosis lesion in a female, showing an irregular stellate vulvar ulcer. Exuberant granulation tissue is seen in the floor of the ulcer.

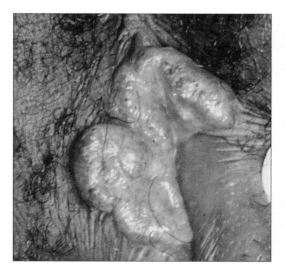

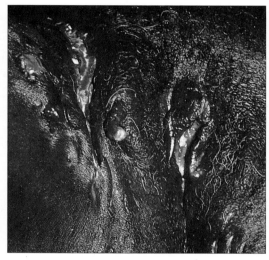

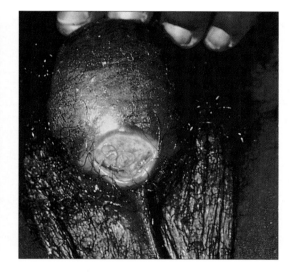

Fig. 5.28 Destructive donovanosis lesion in a female. There is an irregular, large vulvar ulcer with indurated, edematous, and partly everted margins mimicking carcinoma.

Fig. 5.29 Destructive donovanosis lesion in a female. Extensive scarring of the vulva and inner thighs associated with progressive disease.

Fig. 5.30 Earlier healing stages in donovanosis in a male. A chronic ulcer seen at the penoscrotal junction. The floor of the ulcer is grayish-white due to fibrosis, indicating attempts at healing.

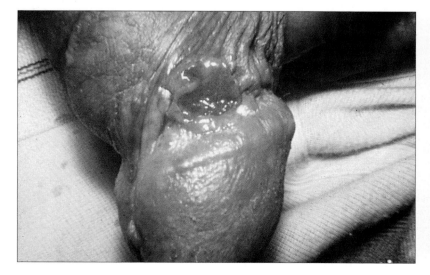

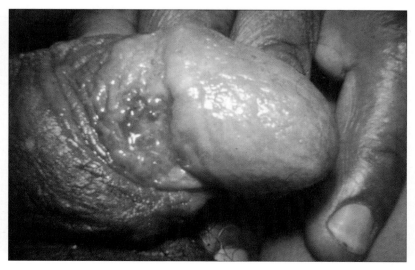

Fig. 5.31 Earlier healing stages in donovanosis in a male. A partially healing ulcer seen at the coronal sulcus.

Fig. 5.32 Earlier healing stages in donovanosis in a male. An ulcer showing pale granulation tissue in the floor. The borders are grayish-white. These changes indicate healing.

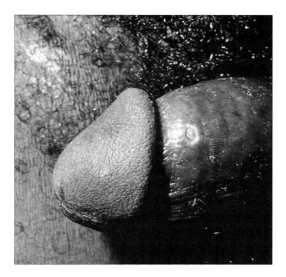

Fig. 5.33 Later healing stages in donovanosis in a male. Penile ulcer at an advanced stage of healing.

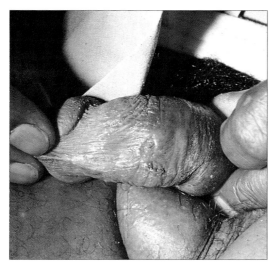

Fig. 5.34 Later healing stages in donovanosis in a male. Penile ulcer at an advanced stage of healing.

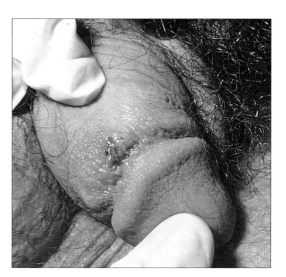

Fig. 5.35 Later healing stages in donovanosis in a male. This lesion is almost completely healed, leaving behind a small, red area.

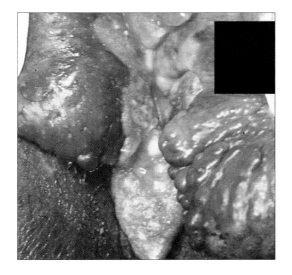

Fig. 5.36 Healing stages in donovanosis in a female. A vulvar ulcer indicating early attempts at healing. The granulation tissue is relatively pale and avascular compared with **5.28**.

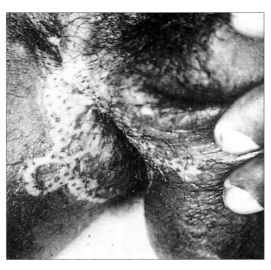

Fig. 5.37 Healing stages in donovanosis in a female. Fibrosis and re-epithelialization of a healed lesion.

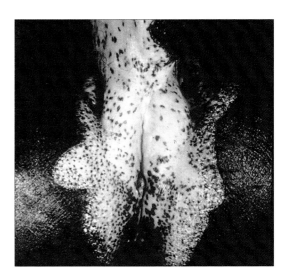

Fig. 5.38 Residual hypopigmentation of a healed lesion.

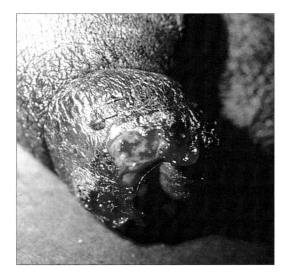

Fig. 5.39 Fibrosis and edema causing a marked penile deformity. The patient had a large, long-standing lesion, which healed after antibiotic therapy.

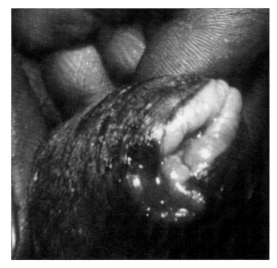

Fig. 5.40 Urethral stenosis in a case of healed donovanosis.

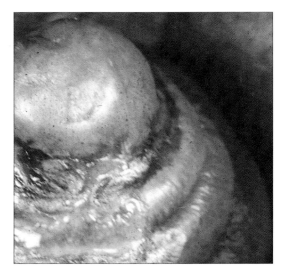

Fig. 5.41 Massive edema, phimosis, and ulceration in a case of advanced donovanosis. The ulcer shows evidence of healing by fibrosis, which can further act as a constricting band.

Syphilis

The chancre of early syphilis may be confused with early lesions of donovanosis. Its exclusion is usually done by negative serology and dark-field examination of the lesion for spirochetes.

Lymphogranuloma Venereum

This disease is characterized by bilateral tender, inguinal nodes (buboes) that often become suppurative. Elephantiasis of the external genitalia may be seen. Exclusion is aided by serology with chlamydial micro-IF titers greater than 1:256.

Chancroid

Chancroid is manifested by shallow, painful, exudate-filled ulcers and tender inguinal adenopathy. The causative agent (*Haemophilus ducreyi*) can be cultured on a modified selective chocolate agar medium. Nodes will heal spontaneously.

Herpes Simplex Virus type 2

This is characterized by symptomatic initial vesicles that quickly break down to form shallow, clean-based ulcers. Local edema and enlargement of inguinal lymph nodes may be present. Exclusion is by detection of intranuclear inclusions and multinucleated giant cells in smears or culture of the herpesvirus.

Vulvar Cancer/Cervical Cancer

Both cancers are usually excluded by biopsy. Exophytic lesions or large necrotic ulcers of granuloma inguinale may closely simulate carcinoma on clinical examination. Parametrial involvement may add to this confusion.

Donovanosis can coexist with other venereal diseases. It should always be considered when genital lesions have a history of considerable duration and slow progression (weeks to months).

LABORATORY TESTS

BIOPSY AND CYTOLOGY

Biopsy and cytologic smears of the lesion are the most dependable tools to diagnose donovanosis. Biopsy shows that the affected skin is usually infiltrated by a dense mixed cellular infiltrate composed predominantly of mononuclear cells with occasional foci of neutrophils and histiocytes (*Figs. 5.42* and *5.43*). Vascular proliferation of granulation tissue is evident. Fibrosis sets in later in the process. The epithelial border of the lesions frequently shows acanthosis, epidermal microabscesses, elongation and intercommunication of the rete pegs, and pseudoepitheliomatous hyperplasia. Caseation, suppuration, and epithelioid giant cells are not typical. Both in biopsy and cytology, there is a striking intracellular inclusion of *C. granulomatis* within histiocytes resulting in the diagnostically characteristic 'pathognomonic cells'. These enlarged cells (20–90 mm) have an eccentric nucleus and contain individual or groups of organisms in capsular or cystlike compartments of the cytoplasm (*Fig. 5.44*). Polymorphonuclear leukocytes are rarely seen except on the surface aspects of the lesion. Pathognomonic cells are scattered in variable numbers in the upper half of the granulation tissue particularly near the margins of the ulcer. They are abundant in exuberant granulation tissue. The capsules are thought to protect the organism from degradation. The only currently effective laboratory procedure for the diagnosis of donovanosis is a properly prepared and stained tissue or smear.

Specimen Collection

An area of granulation tissue near the periphery of the lesion is carefully cleaned with several saline-soaked gauze squares and carefully dried with dry gauze. The appearance of blood does not affect specimen character. Using a punch biopsy, forceps, or small curette secure a small piece of tissue (about the size of a matchhead).

Specimen Preparation and Staining

Smear the underside of the specimen over the surface of a glass slide. Do not respread any area and cease spreading when the specimen begins to dry. The dry area will contain rubbed, broken cells of no use as diagnostic material. The slide specimen is air dried, fixed in 95% ethanol for five minutes, and stained in a routine way. Special stains discussed below can be employed whenever possible. The tissue should be submitted for histopathologic examination. Hematoxylin and eosin stain will show marked acute and chronic inflammation with granulation tissue formation. Donovan bodies can be seen by this stain infrequently and only when present in large numbers (*Fig. 5.43*). For special stains, in both tissue and smear, use either Wright (*Fig. 5.44*), Giemsa (*Fig. 5.45*), Pinacyanole, or

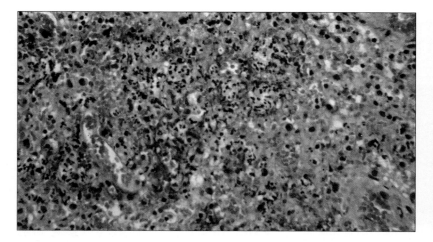

Fig. 5.42 Microscopic section of the ulcer in **5.41** to show acute inflammation with microabscess formation and granulation tissue (hematoxylin and eosin × 50).

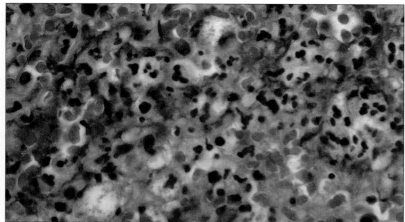

Fig. 5.43 Donovan bodies when abundant in tissue can be seen intracellularly even by hematoxylin and eosin stain (× 120).

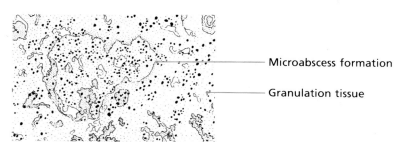

— Microabscess formation

— Granulation tissue

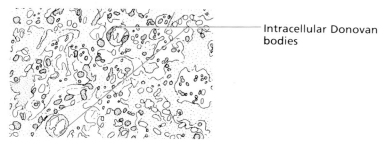

— Intracellular Donovan bodies

Warthin–Starry (*Figs. 5.46–5.48*) stains by the usual procedures, except for the Wright stain. With the latter stain, allow the dye to remain on the preparation for 1.5 minutes before diluting with phosphate buffer at pH 6.4. A positive specimen will exhibit large mononuclear cells whose cytoplasm contains small, straight, or curved dumbell-shaped ('closed safety pin') rods having a blue-to-deep purple color and surrounded by pink capsules (*Fig. 5.44*). Broken tissue cells are not satisfactory for examination since there are many other extracellular objects of similar size and character in the specimen. The large 'pathognomonic cells' can be detected with low magnification (x 450) with some experience and confirmed at a higher magnification (x 1 000) (*Figs. 5.49* and *5.50*).

CULTURE SPECIMEN AND EXAMINATION

A specimen obtained as above is placed between two sterile glass slides and mashed between them with a twisting motion. Separate the slides and add 0.2–0.5 ml of sterile saline to each slide surface. Emulsify the tissue debris with a sterile toothpick or loop.

For isolation of *C. granulomatis* in chick embryos, inoculate 0.2 ml of the tissue debris into the yolk sac of a 5-day-old chicken embryo and incubate at 37°C for 72 hours. Growth of *C. granulomatis* will occur in the yolk sac fluid and will demonstrate the characteristic 'safety pin' morphology of this organism.

For isolation of *C. granulomatis* on 'Dulaney slants,' inoculate 0.2 ml of the tissue debris suspension onto the coagulated egg yolk slants, then cover three-quarters of the surface of the slant with Locke's salt solution. Close the tubes and incubate upright at 37°C for 48–72 hours. Slants made of egg yolks from range-fed chickens (ducks, geese, and turkeys) are effective, whereas those made from egg yolks obtained from diet-fed birds are ineffective: the reasons for this are still unknown, but may be due to the presence of antibiotics in animal feed.

IMMUNOLOGY AND PATHOGENICITY

Serologic methods for the diagnosis of donovanosis are not widely used because cultured organisms are not freely available. Recently an indirect immunofluorescence test, employing Donovan-rich tissue sections obtained from typical lesions, was found to be both sensitive and specific in detection of antibody to *C. granulomatis*. Antibodies have been detected in human sera by complement fixation procedures when isolates of *C. granulomatis* were available. Significant serum titers were found only in sera from patients in whom the duration of a lesion exceeded 3 months. The lack of protection by

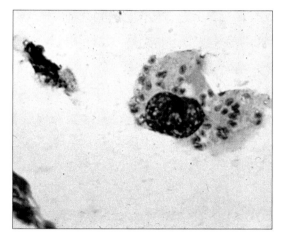

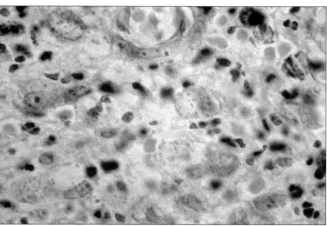

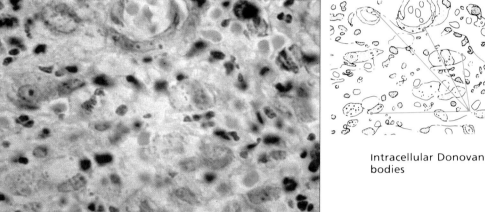

Fig. 5.44 A fragmented mononuclear cell containing Donovan bodies. Bipolar staining creating a closed safety pin appearance is seen (Wright–Giemsa × 1,000).

Fig. 5.45 Giemsa stain of a tissue to show intracellular Donovan bodies (× 320).

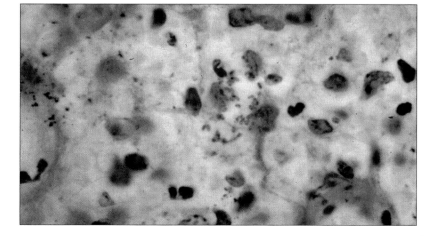

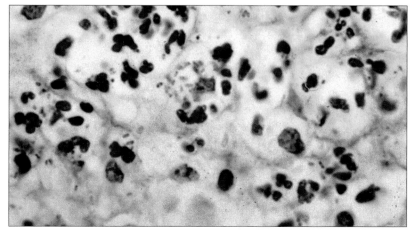

Fig. 5.46 Warthin–Starry stain in tissue to show intracellular Donovan bodies (× 320).

Fig. 5.47 Intracellular Donovan bodies. Another view of the same tissue as in **5.46** (× 320).

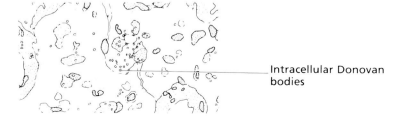

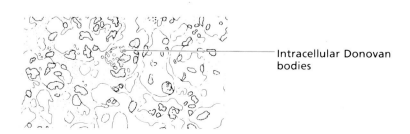

circulating antibodies is similar to other diseases in which the organism is found intracellularly, e.g., lepromatous leprosy, tuberculosis, and chronic mucocutaneous candidiasis. *C. granulomatis* exhibits antigenic cross-reactivity with *Klebsiella pneumoniae* and *Klebsiella rhinoscleromatis*. This observation lends some support to the proposed similarity between *K. rhinoscleromatis* and *C. granulomatis*. Other than the chick embryo, *C. granulomatis* is pathogenic only for humans.

TREATMENT

The treatment of choice is tetracycline (500 mg po qid), doxycycline (100 mg po bid), or erythromycin base or stearate (500 mg po qid) for a minimum of 2–3 weeks until the lesions have healed completely. The disease tends to relapse after successful treatment and healing, so prolonged follow-up is necessary. In severe cases any of the above regimens may be supplemented by streptomycin (1g im bid for 10 days). The combination of lincomycin and erythromycin has been satisfactory for the treatment of pregnant patients. Penicillin is not efficacious and ampicillin has given inconsistent results.

PROGNOSIS

As a rule, the lesions resolve satisfactorily following proper treatment. They commence epithelialization from the edges of active lesions towards the center. Hypopigmentation is often a consequence of successful treatment (*Figs. 5.51* and *5.52*). Untreated lesions will distort, mutilate, and destroy involved tissues and spread to other areas of the body by either contiguity or systemic dissemination. Mortality is rare and its occurrence has been due to secondary causes, such as pneumonia, cardiac failure, and hemorrhage.

ASSOCIATION WITH CARCINOMA

An association of donovanosis with genital carcinoma changes the treatment and therefore should be recognized early in the process. This association has been suspected for the following reasons:

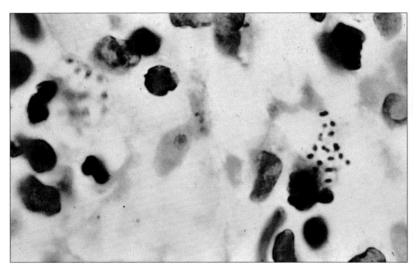

Fig. 5.48 Intracellular Donovan bodies. Higher magnification of same tissue as in **5.46** (× 1,000).

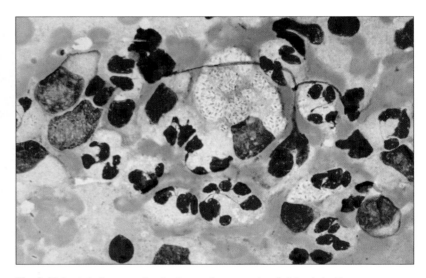

Fig. 5.49 A cytologic preparation to show pathognomonic cell distended with numerous Donovan bodies (Giemsa eosin stain × 1,000).

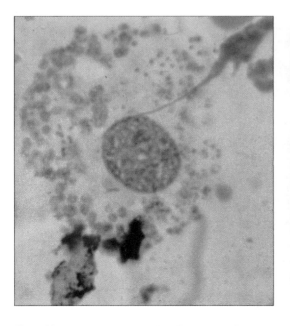

Fig. 5.50 Pathognomonic intracellular Donovan bodies (methylene blue stain × 1,500).

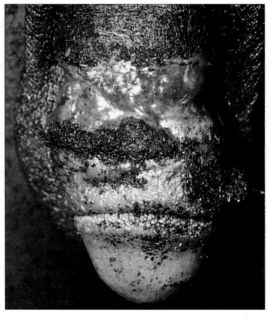

Fig. 5.51 Active donovanosis in a male prior to initiation of therapy.

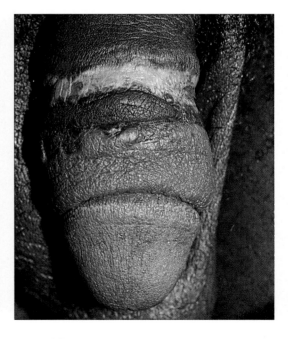

Fig. 5.52 The same patient as in **5.51**, following complete healing as a result of tetracycline therapy. There is marked depigmentation.

- There is a higher incidence of genital carcinoma where donovanosis is endemic
- Carcinoma has occurred within hypopigmented areas of healed donovanosis
- There has been concurrence of carcinoma and donovanosis in the same lesion.

Vulvar ulcers, lesions on the cervix or vaginal vault that appear as necrotizing and proliferating masses of granulation tissue, and the thickening of the parametrial tissues seen with donovanosis are often mistaken for carcinoma.

Donovanosis is differentiated from carcinoma on the basis of dense dermal infiltration with microabscesses, plasma cells, and macrophages containing capsulated intracytoplasmic Donovan bodies. Acanthosis as well as pseudoepitheliomatous hyperplasia is present in donovanosis, but nuclear hyperplasia, hyperchromasia, individual cell keratinization, and

other characteristics of malignancy are absent. When a biopsy from a large, necrotic lesion clinically suspicious of carcinoma shows only inflammatory changes, a possibility of donovanosis should be considered and special stains obtained to demonstrate the diagnostic organisms. On the other hand, when the lesion remains unaltered or grows in spite of treatment, multiple biopsies should be obtained to rule out malignancy. An association between donovanosis and carcinoma, though reported, is distinctly uncommon.

Picture credits for this chapter are as follows: Figs. 5.5 and 5.6, 5.21, and 5.30 courtesy of American Academy of Dermatology; Figs. 5.2, 5.7, 5.14, 5.18, 5.22, 5.27, and 5.28, 5.31,and 5.32, 5.36, 5.38, 5.40, and 5.41 courtesy of the Centers for Disease Control; Figs. 5.3 and 5.4, 5.11, and 5.12, 5.33 to 5.35, and 5.39 courtesy of Adele Moreland, MD; Fig. 5.26 courtesy of McGraw-Hill Publishing Co.; Figs. 5.17 and 5.19 courtesy of Bingham JS: Pocket Picture Guide to Sexually Transmitted Diseases, London, Gower Medical Publishing, 1984; Figs. 5.28 and 5.46 to 5.48 courtesy of the Journal of Reproductive Medicine.

BIBLIOGRAPHY

Arya O: *Tropical Venerology*. New York, Churchill Livingstone Press, 1980.

Bergys Manual of Systematic Bacteriology. Washington DC, American Society of Microbiology, Vol.1, pp 585–587, 1984.

Cannefax GR: The technique of the tissue spread method for demonstrating Donovan bodies. *J Vener Dis Info* **19**:201–204, 1948.

Davis C: Granuloma inguinale. *JAMA* **211**:632–636, 1970.

Freinkel AL, Dangor Y, Koornhof HJ, Ballard RC: A serological test for granuloma inguinale. *Genitourin Med* **68**:269–272, 1992.

Fritz GS, Hubert WR, Dodson RE, et al.: Mutilating granuloma inguinale. *Arch Dermatol* **111**:1464–1465, 1975.

Goens JL, Schwartz RA, DeWolf K: Mucocutaneous manifestations of chancroid, lymphogranuloma venereum, and granuloma venereum. *Am Fam Physician* **49**:415–418, 423–425,1994.

Goldberg J: Studies on granuloma inguinale IV. Growth requirements of *Donovania granulomatis* and its relationship to the natural habitat of the organism. *Br J Vener Dis* **35**:266–268,1959.

Goldberg J: Studies on granuloma inguinale V. Isolation of a bacterium resembling *Donovania granulomatis* from the feces of a patient with granuloma inguinale. *Br J Vener Dis* **38**:99–102,1964.

Goldberg J: Studies on granuloma inguinale VII. Some epidemiological considerations of the disease. *Br J Vener Dis* **40**:140–145,1964.

Goldberg J, Weaver RH, Packer H: Studies on *Granuloma inguinale* II. The complement fixation test in the diagnosis of granuloma inguinale. *Am J Syph Gonorrhea Vener Dis* **37**:71–76,1953.

Goldberg J, Annamunthodo H: Studies on granuloma inguinale VIII. Serological reactivity of sera from patients with carcinoma of the penis when tested with *Donovania* antigens. *Br J Vener Dis* **42**:205–209,1966.

Greenblatt RB, Barfield WE: Newer methods in the diagnosis and treatment of granuloma inguinale. *Br J Vener Dis* **28**:123–128,1952.

Janovski NA: *Diseases of the Vulva*, 1st ed. Hagerstown, IN, Harper & Row, 1972.

Joseph AK, Rosen T: Laboratory techniques used in the diagnosis of chancroid, granuloma inguinale, and lymphogranuloma venereum. *Dermatol Clin* **12**:1–8,1994.

Kalstone B, Howell JA Jr, Cline FX: Granuloma inguinale with hematogenous dissemination to the spine. *JAMA* **176**:152–154,1961.

Kirkpatrick DJ: Donovanosis (granuloma inguinale): A rare cause of osteolytic bone lesions. *Clin Radiol* **21**:101–105,1970.

Kuberski T: Granuloma inguinale (donovanosis). A review. *Sex Transm Dis* **7**:29–36,1980.

Kuberski T, Papadimitriou JM, Phillips P: Ultrastructure of *Calymmatobacterium granulomatis* in lesions of granuloma inguinale. *J Infect Dis* **142**:744–749,1980.

Lal S, Nicholas C: Epidemiological and clinical features in 165 cases of granuloma inguinale. *Br J Vener Dis* **46**:461–463,1980.

Maddocks I, Anders EM, Dennis E: Donovanosis in Papua New Guinea. *Br J Vener Dis* **52**:190–196,1976.

Mitchell KM, Roberts AN, Williams VM, Schneider J: *Genitourin Med* **62**:191–195,1986.

Nayar M, Chandra M, Saxena HM, et al.: Donovanosis — a histopathological study. *Indian J Pathol Microbiol* **24**:71–76,1981.

O'Farrell N: Clinico-epidemiological study of donovanosis in Durban, South Africa. *Genitourin Med* **69**:108–111,1993.

Pund ER, Greenblatt RB: Specific histology of granuloma inguinale. *Arch Pathol* **23**:224–229,1937.

Richens J: The diagnosis and treatment of donovanosis (granuloma inguinale). *Genitourin Med* **67**:441–452,1991.

Robertson DH: *Clinical Practice in Sexually Transmissible Diseases*, 1st ed. Baltimore, IN, University Park Press, 1980.

Schwartz R: Chancroid and granuloma inguinale. *Clin Obstet Gynecol* **26**:138–142,1983.

Sexually Transmitted Diseases Summary. Atlanta, GA, US Department of Health and Human Services, Technical Information Services, 1986.

Spagnola DV, Coburn PR, Cream JI, Azadian BS: Extragenital granuloma inguinale (donovanosis) diagnosed in the United Kingdom: A clinical, histological, and electron microscopical study. *J Clin Pathol* **37**:945–949,1984.

Stewart DB: The gynecological lesions of lymphogranuloma venereum and granuloma inguinale. *Med Clin North Am* **48**:773–786,1964.

Wysoki RS, Majmudar B, Willis D: Granuloma inguinale (donovanosis) in women. *J Reprod Med* **33**:709–713,1988.

CHAPTER SIX

Gonorrhea

W Whittington, C Ison, and S Thompson

INTRODUCTION

The clinical syndrome of gonorrhea was described by biblical authors, but the etiologic agent, *Neisseria gonorrhoeae*, was not described until 1879, when Albert Neisser observed the organism in smears of purulent exudates from urethritis, cervicitis, and ophthalmia neonatorum. The genus *Neisseria* includes the pathogenic species *N. gonorrhoeae* and *N. meningitidis*, as well as species that are normal flora of the oropharynx and nasopharynx. Strains of the commensal *Neisseria* spp. may occasionally be isolated in clinical specimens from anogenital sites and observed intracellularly in polymorphonuclear leukocytes, and are morphologically indistinguishable from the pathogenic *Neisseriae*. Thus, accurate laboratory identification of the gonococcus is essential because of the social and medicolegal consequences of misidentifying strains of nonpathogenic *Neisseria* spp. as *N. gonorrhoeae*.

Because of the fastidious growth requirements of *N. gonorrhoeae*, it was difficult to culture the organism until the development of chocolatized blood agar supplemented with growth factors. In the 1960s, the development of selective media containing antimicrobial and antifungal agents (such as Thayer-Martin medium), which enhanced the isolation of the gonococcus by inhibiting not only Gram-positive bacteria but also the closely related *Neisseria* spp., further simplified the laboratory diagnosis of gonorrhea. Recently, rapid biochemical and serologic tests have been developed, allowing identification of the gonococcus within a few hours of its isolation.

Although technological advances have reduced the problems involved in isolating the gonococcus, strains of some commensal *Neisseria* and related species may be isolated on gonococcal selective media and may be misidentified as *N. gonorrhoeae* in rapid tests. Thus the accurate laboratory identification of *N. gonorrhoeae* remains of paramount importance.

EPIDEMIOLOGY

Gonorrhea is a disease of worldwide importance (*Fig. 6.1*) and is the most frequently reported infectious disease in the USA (*Fig. 6.2*). Between 1977 and 1993, the number of reported cases decreased 56%, from 1 million to 439,000 per annum, which represents a decrease from 468/100,000 to 176/100,000 population. There is also at least one unreported case for every reported case of gonorrhea.

Gonorrhea is transmitted almost exclusively by sexual contact. Persons under 25 years of age who have multiple sexual partners are at highest risk. Rates of gonorrhea are higher in males and in minority and inner-city populations.

Often, gonorrhea is acquired from a sexual partner who is either asymptomatic or who has only minimal symptoms. Transmission efficiency (a measure of transmission through one sexual exposure) is estimated to be 50–60% from an infected man to an uninfected woman and 20% from an infected woman to an uninfected man. More than 90% of men with urethral gonorrhea will develop symptoms within 5 days of infection. Most men with symptomatic urethritis will seek health care. Infections at other anatomic sites in men and infections in women are far less likely to produce early symptoms that will encourage the seeking of health care. The rationale of public health measures, such as screening and contact tracing, is to identify and treat patients with asymptomatic or minimally symptomatic infections, thus shortening the infectious period and preventing further transmission of the disease. Additionally, because all women with lower genital tract gonococcal infection are at risk for PID, the early identification and treatment of infected women is important.

The evolution of antimicrobial resistance in *N. gonorrhoeae* has, in both developed and developing countries, potential negative implications for the control of gonorrhea (*Fig. 6.3*). Resistance to new therapeutic agents has generally developed within a few years of an agent's introduction.

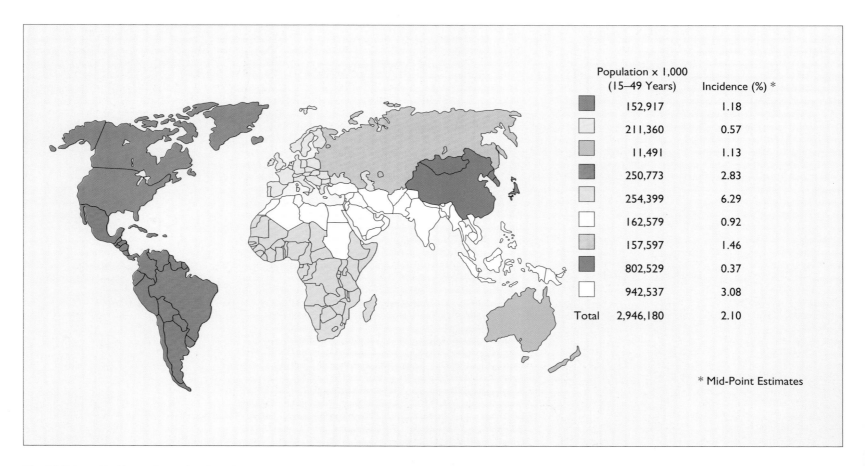

Fig. 6.1 Estimated incidence of gonorrhea; by region.

Strains with chromosomal resistance to penicillin, tetracycline, erythromycin, and cefoxitin, as well as decreased susceptibility to ceftriaxone, have been identified in the USA and most of the world, especially southeast Asia. Sporadic high-level resistance to spectinomycin has also been reported. Resistance to broad-spectrum cephalosporins has not been described in *N. gonorrhoeae*. Recent reports from Asia, Australia, the UK, and North America have described gonococcal organisms with high-level decreased susceptibility to fluoroquinolones. Although there is little data available on the outcome of treatment, strains with MICs of 2 μg/ml to ciprofloxacin and ofloxacin are unlikely to be treated successfully with a fluoroquinolone. The mechanisms of fluoroquinolone resistance have not been definitively established, but are probably the results of one or more mutations in genes encoding gonococcal DNA gyrase and/or changes in membrane permeability.

Penicillinase-producing *N. gonorrhoeae* (PPNG) strains, which inactivate penicillins and other β-lactams, were first described in 1976. Four β-lactamase plasmids of different sizes have been identified in PPNG strains and have been used to follow the spread of PPNG geographically (*Fig. 6.4*). PPNG strains cause one-half of all gonococcal infections in parts of Africa and Asia, and became endemic in the USA in 1981. In the USA, PPNG accounted for 9.6% of gonococcal isolates evaluated in the Gonococcal Isolate Surveillance Project (GISP) during 1993. An additional 6.1% of isolates were resistant to penicillin due to apparent chromosomal mutations. These levels of penicillin resistance make penicillins inappropriate agents for gonococcal therapy.

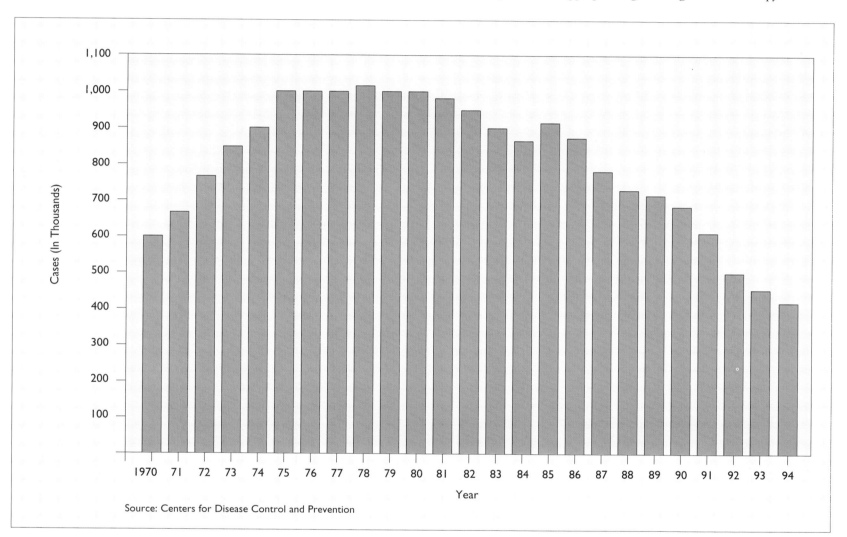

Source: Centers for Disease Control and Prevention

Fig. 6.2 Reported cases of gonorrhea in the USA, 1977–1994.

TYPES OF ANTIMICROBIAL RESISTANCE IN *NEISSERIA GONORRHOEAE*

Fig. 6.3 Types of antimicrobial resistance in *N. gonorrhoeae*.

TYPE OF RESISTANCE	ANTIMICROBIAL AGENT
Chromosomal (genes located on the chromosome)	Penicillin Tetracycline Spectinomycin Fluoroquinolones Broad spectrum cephalosporins (decreased susceptibility)
Plasmid-mediated (genes located on plasmids)	Penicillin (β-lactam antibiotics)—PPNG Tetracycline—TRNG

Plasmid-mediated, high-level resistance to tetracycline was reported in *N. gonorrhoeae* (TRNG) in 1985. This plasmid has also been detected in strains of *N. meningitidis* and *Kingella denitrificans*. It may be transferred between gonococcal strains and strains of other *Neisseria* spp. by conjugation (*Fig. 6.5*) and also mobilizes β-lactamase plasmids. Isolates with plasmid-mediated tetracycline resistance have also possessed β-lactamase plasmids. During 1993, TRNG phenotypes accounted for 7.3% of isolates tested through the US GISP system. An additional 13.1% of isolates were tetracycline resistant due to chromosomal mutations. Like the penicillins, tetracyclines are inappropriate sole therapies for gonococcal infections.

Vancomycin-susceptible strains of *N. gonorrhoeae* occasionally occur and may not grow on selective media containing 4 μg vancomycin/ml, which was routinely used for the isolation of the gonococcus. Selective media have been modified to contain 2 μg or 3 μg vancomycin/ml in order to overcome this problem. Vancomycin-susceptible gonococci should be suspected in a community when false-negative cultures are obtained, as evidenced by a discrepancy between Gram-stain positivity and culture-positivity rates for urethral gonorrhea in men; these should agree for at least 95% of cases.

CLINICAL MANIFESTATIONS

In the majority of cases, gonococcal infections are limited to mucosal surfaces. Infection occurs in areas of columnar epithelium including the cervix, urethra, rectum, pharynx, and conjunctiva. Squamous epithelium is not susceptible to infection by the gonococcus. However, the prepubertal vaginal epithelium which has not been keratinized under the influence of estrogen, may be infected. Hence, gonorrhea may present in a young girl as a vulvovaginitis. In mucosal infections, there is usually a brisk, local neutrophilic response manifested clinically as a purulent discharge (*Fig. 6.6*).

In women, untreated cervical infection may lead to endometritis and salpingitis, a sign–symptom complex more commonly known as pelvic inflammatory disease, or PID. In approximately 1–3% of patients with mucosal infection, hematogenous spread occurs, causing disseminated gonococcal infection (DGI).

GONORRHEA

The most common symptom of gonorrhea in men is urethral discharge that may range from a scanty, clear, or cloudy fluid to one that is copious and purulent (*Figs. 6.7* and *6.8*). Dysuria is usually present. However, men with asymptomatic urethritis may be an important reservoir for transmission. Although most men with gonorrhea develop symptoms, those who ignore their symptoms or have asymptomatic infection are at risk of developing complications (*see Fig. 6.6*). Endocervical infection is the most common type of uncomplicated gonorrhea in women (*Figs. 6.9* and *6.10*).

At least one-half of infected women are asymptomatic or have symptoms that are mild to nonspecific. Cervical infections may be accompanied by vaginal discharge, abnormal vaginal bleeding, or dysuria. Local complications include abscesses in Bartholin's and Skene's glands (*Fig. 6.11*). Asymptomatic infections are found most often in women who are screened

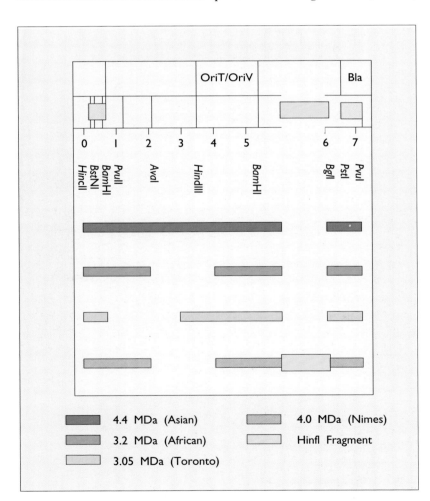

Fig. 6.4 Restriction endonuclease digestion maps of four β-lactamase plasmids described in *N. gonorrhoeae*. The 3.2 MDa 'African' and 3.05 MDa 'Toronto' β-lactamase plasmids appear to have been formed by deletions of segments from the 4.4 MDa β-lactamase 'Asian' plasmid. The 4.0 MDa 'Nimes' β-lactamase plasmid appears to have been formed by the insertion of a *Hinfl* fragment into the 3.2 MDa plasmid. Recent studies have shown that the Toronto plasmid is identical to the 2.9 MDa plasmid detected in strains from Brazil ('Rio' plasmid). Bla is the structural gene for β-lactamase, OriT is the origin of transfer of the plasmid, and OriV is the origin of replication of the plasmid.

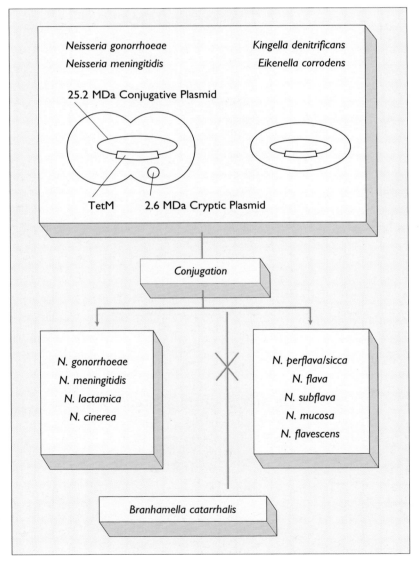

Fig. 6.5 Conjugative transfer of 25.2 MDa TetM-containing plasmids from *N. gonorrhoeae*, *N. meningitidis*, *Kingella denitrificans*, and *Eikenella corrodens* to *Neisseria* and related spp.

CLINICAL MANIFESTATIONS OF GONOCOCCAL INFECTIONS

SITE OF INFECTION	UNCOMPLICATED	COMPLICATED

Urethra	Symptomatic
	    Scant, clear discharge
	    Copious purulent discharge
	Asymptomatic
		(Epididymitis) *
		
		(Penile edema)
		(Abscess of Cowper's, Tyson's glands)
		(Seminal vesiculitis)

Various		DGI
		    Bacteremia
		    Fever
		    Skin lesions: macular, erythematous pustular,
		        necrotic, hemorrhagic
		    Tenosynovitis
		    Joints: septic arthritis
		    Endocarditis
		    Meningitis

Cervix	Symptomatic
	    Red, friable cervical os
	    Purulent discharge from os
	    Bilateral or unilateral lower abdominal
	    tenderness
	Asymptomatic
		PID
		    Endometritis
		    Salpingitis
		    Tubo-ovarian abscess
		    Ectopic pregnancy
		    Infertility
		DGI

Rectum	Symptomatic
	    Copious, purulent discharge
	    Burning/stinging pain
	    Tenesmus
	    Blood in stools
	Asymptomatic
		DGI

Pharynx	Symptomatic
	    Mild pharyngitis
	    Mild sore throat
	    Erythema
	Asymptomatic
		DGI

Conjunctiva	Symtomatic Copius purulent discharge	Keratitis and corneal ulceration: perforation, extrusion of lens Scarring: opacification of lens Blindness

* Syndromes listed in parenthesis occur infrequently

Fig. 6.6 Clinical manifestations of gonococcal infections.

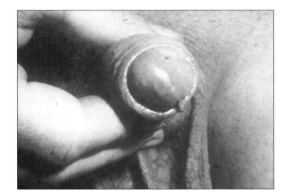

Fig. 6.7 Symptomatic gonococcal urethritis. Scanty urethral discharge obtained after urethral stripping.

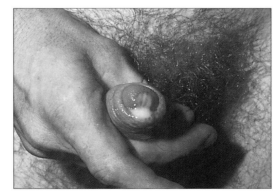

Fig. 6.8 Symptomatic gonococcal urethritis. Copious spontaneous urethral discharge.

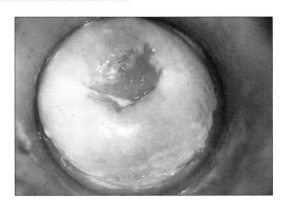

Fig. 6.9 Endocervical gonorrhea. A small amount of purulent discharge is visible in the endocervical canal.

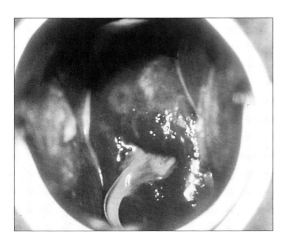

Fig. 6.10 Signs of endo-cervical gonorrhea: cervical edema and erythema as well as discharge.

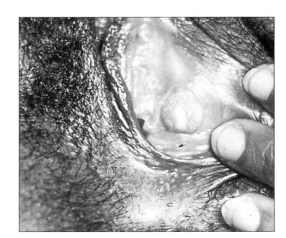

Fig. 6.11 Urethral gonorrhea in the female. Purulent discharge is visible, with involvement of Bartholin's gland.

for gonorrhea in routine gynecologic examinations or who are seen as sexual contacts of men with gonorrhea. On examination, the cervical os may be erythematous and friable, with a purulent exudate (*Figs. 6.10* and *6.12*), or may be normal.

Rectal infections, which occur in 30% of women with cervical gonorrhea, probably represent colonization from cervical discharge and are symptomatic in less than 5% of women. Infections in homosexual men, however, result from anal intercourse and are more often symptomatic (18–34%). Symptoms and signs range from mild burning on defecation to itching to severe tenesmus, and from mucopurulent discharge to frank blood in the stools.

Pharyngeal 'infections' are diagnosed most often in women and homosexual men with a history of fellatio. There has never been a convincing demonstration of a relationship between pharyngeal infection (or colonization, as some would put it) and the signs and symptoms of a sore throat or tonsillitis.

Ocular infections occur in newborns who are exposed to infected secretions in the birth canal of an infected mother (*Fig. 6.13*). Occasionally, keratoconjunctivitis is seen in adults (*Fig. 6.14*). Conjunctival infection, tearing, and lid edema occur early, followed rapidly by the appearance of a frankly purulent exudate. Prompt diagnosis and treatment are important because corneal scarring or perforation may result (*Fig. 6.15*).

DISSEMINATED GONOCOCCAL INFECTION

Disseminated gonococcal infection (DGI) is the result of gonococcal bacteremia. The sources of infection are primarily asymptomatic infections of the pharynx, urethra, or cervix. The most common form of DGI is the 'dermatitis–arthritis' syndrome in which the patient develops fever, chills, skin lesions, and arthralgias, usually involving the hands, the feet (or, less often, ankles), and the elbows over a few days. Skin lesions, which are distributed sparsely on the extensor surfaces of the distal extremities, may be macular, pustular, centrally necrotic, or hemorrhagic (*Figs. 6.16–6.18*). On careful examination, the areas of tenderness and erythema are due to

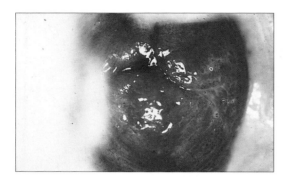

Fig. 6.12 Gonococcal cervicitis with mucoid discharge and marked cervical erythema and edema. This is indistinguishable clinically from chlamydial cervicitis.

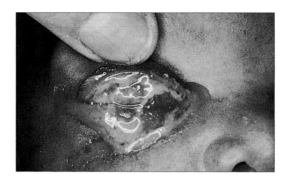

Fig. 6.13 Gonococcal ophthalmia neonatorum. Lid edema, erythema, and marked purulent discharge are seen. The Gram-stained smear was loaded with Gram-negative diplococci within neutrophils.

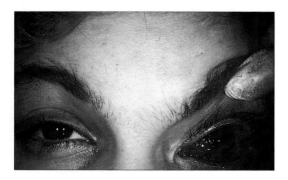

Fig. 6.14 Early gonococcal ophthalmia in an adult showing marked chemosis and tearing with no discharge.

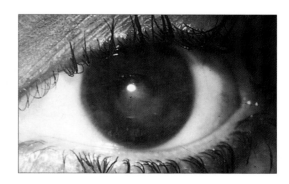

Fig. 6.15 Corneal clouding following gonococcal ophthalmia in an adult.

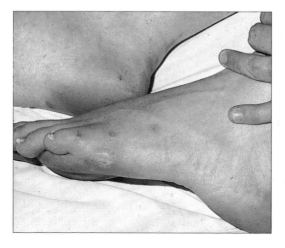

Fig. 6.16 Skin lesions of disseminated gonococcal infection. Papular and pustular lesions on the foot.

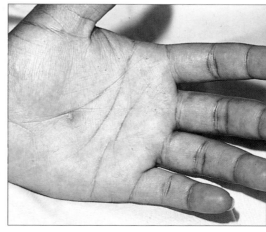

Fig. 6.17 Skin lesions of disseminated gonococcal infection. Small painful midpalmar lesion on an erythematous base.

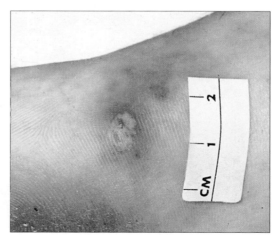

Fig. 6.18 Skin lesions of disseminated gonococcal infection. Classic large lesions with a necrotic, grayish central lesion on an erythematous base.

periarticular inflammation of the tendon sheaths rather than true arthritis. A minority of cases develop septic joints with effusion. Gonococci may be isolated from the synovial fluid in about 50% of cases, while blood cultures are positive in less than 50% of DGI cases. Rarely, patients may develop endocarditis or meningitis. Patients with a congenital deficiency in one of the late-acting complement components (C7, C8, C9) may experience recurrent DGI infections.

DGI must be distinguished from Reiter's syndrome, meningococcemia, acute rheumatoid arthritis, other septic arthritides, and the immune complex-mediated arthritides caused by hepatitis B virus and HIV (*Figs. 6.19* and *6.20*). A diagnosis of DGI may be based on the identification of gonococci from synovial fluid, blood, or CSF. Gonococci are rarely isolated from skin lesions, but a Gram-stained smear or purulent material taken from an unroofed lesion should be examined whenever possible because the presence

of Gram-negative diplococci within polymorphonuclear leukocytes (*Fig. 6.21*) assists in making the diagnosis. If available, a direct fluorescent antibody (FA) stain of the smear is even better.

In one-half of cases, gonococci cannot be isolated from blood, CSF, or synovial fluid, even with the best laboratory techniques. A presumptive diagnosis of DGI can be made based upon a combination of two of the following three criteria, provided other diagnoses have been eliminated:

- The isolation of gonococci from a mucosal site of the patient or the patient's sexual partner (in the case of an infant, isolation from the conjunctiva or a nasogastric specimen)
- The finding of pustular, hemorrhagic, or necrotic skin lesions on the extremities
- Rapid resolution of signs and symptoms on appropriate antimicrobial therapy (*Fig. 6.22*).

DIFFERENTIAL DIAGNOSIS OF DERMATITIS–TENOSYNOVITIS SYNDROME (POLYARTICULAR)

Meningococcemia
Staphylococcal sepsis or endocarditis
Other bacterial septicemias (rare)
HIV infection: Acute thrombocytopenia and arthritis
Hepatitis B prodrome
Acute Reiter's syndrome
Juvenile rheumatoid arthritis
Lyme disease

Fig. 6.19 Differential diagnosis of disseminated gonococcal infection. Dermatitis—tenosynovitis syndrome.

DIFFERENTIAL DIAGNOSIS OF MONARTICULAR ARTHRITIS

INFECTIOUS

Bacterial
  Adults
    Gonococcus*
    Staphylococcus
    Pneumococcus
    Streptococcus
  Children
    Staphylococcus
    Streptococcus
    Pneumococcus
    Haemophilus influenzae
    Gram-negative rods

Tuberculosis

Fungal

* *Most common*

NONINFECTIOUS

Gout, pseudogout*
Rheumatoid arthritis (especially juvenile rheumatoid arthritis)
Trauma
Tumors
Hemarthrosis
Osteochondritis
Palindromic
Pigmented/villonodular syndrome

Fig. 6.20 Differential diagnosis of disseminated gonococcal infection. Monarticular arthritis.

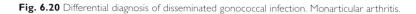

Fig. 6.21 Gram-negative diplococci visible in one neutrophil in a smear of a pustular skin lesion from a patient with disseminated gonococcal infection. Meningococci cannot be distinguished from gonococci with this method.

CRITERIA SUPPORTING A CLINICAL DIAGNOSIS OF DISSEMINATED GONOCOCCAL INFECTION

Gonococci are demonstrated in synovial fluid, blood, cerebrospinal fluid, or skin lesions by culture

Observation of diplococci in Gram- or methylene blue-stained smear

Clinical diagnosis of DGI may be based on two of the following three criteria:
  Isolation of gonococci from urogenital, rectal, pharyngeal, or conjunctival sites of the patient or the patient's sexual partner
  Infection is manifested as pustular, hemorrhagic, or necrotic skin lesions distributed on the extremities
  Patient responds rapidly to appropriate antimicrobial therapy

Fig. 6.22 Criteria supporting a clinical diagnosis of disseminated infection.

Pelvic Inflammatory Disease (PID, Salpingitis)

The gonococcus (or chlamydia) may ascend from the endocervical canal through the endometrium to the fallopian tubes and ultimately to the pelvic peritoneum (*Fig. 6.23*), resulting in endometriosis, salpingitis, and finally peritonitis. Patients may report pelvic and abdominal pain, fever, and chills. Adnexal, fundal, and cervical motion tenderness are found on examination. Acute pyogenic complications of PID include tubo-ovarian abscesses, pelvic peritonitis (often mimicking appendicitis), or the Fitz–Hugh–Curtis syndrome, which is an inflammation of Glisson's capsule of the liver. PID may also be caused by many nonsexually transmitted bacteria that are part of the normal vaginal flora. The proportion of PID caused by *N. gonorrhoeae*, based on the recovery of the organism from laparoscopic specimens, varies from 8 to 70% depending on geographic location. The proportion of women with cervical gonococcal infection who will develop upper tract disease is uncertain. However, one series reported that approximately one-third of women had examination findings suggestive of PID. PID is the most common and costly consequence of gonorrhea, and recurrent episodes of PID are common. Initial PID infections are more likely to be gonococcal or chlamydial, while other bacteria are isolated more frequently from recurrent episodes (*Fig. 6.24*). The consequences of PID include an increased probability of infertility (tubal factor infertility), ectopic pregnancy, and chronic pelvic pain.

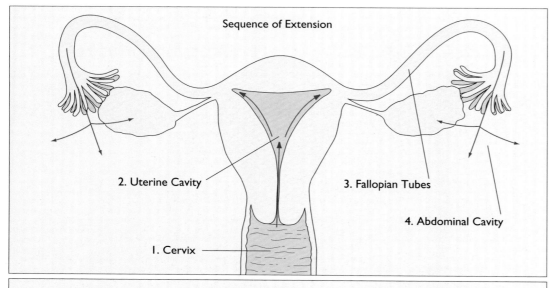

Fig. 6.23 The evolution of gonococcal pelvic inflammatory disease.

Sequence of Extension

2. Uterine Cavity

3. Fallopian Tubes

4. Abdominal Cavity

1. Cervix

Clinical Features

Endocervicitis

May be asymptomatic; vaginal discharge, cervical inflammation, or infection; local tenderness.

Endometritis

Menstrual irregularity.

Endosalpingitis

Constant bilateral lower quadrant abdominal pain aggravated by body motion. Tenderness in one or both adnexal areas. Abscess formation may occur.

Peritonitis

Nausea, emesis, abdominal distention, rigidity, tenderness. Pelvic or abdominal cavity abscess formation may follow.

ETIOLOGIC AGENTS OF PRIMARY AND RECURRENT PELVIC INFLAMMATORY DISEASE

Fig. 6.24 Etiologic agents of primary and recurrent pelvic inflammatory disease.

Neisseria gonorrhoeae	*Bacteroides* spp.
Chlamydia trachomatis	*Peptococcus* spp.
Group B streptococci	*Peptostreptococcus* spp.
Escherichia coli and other enterobacteria	Genital mycoplasmas (?)
Gardnerella vaginalis	*Actinomyces israelii*
Haemophilus spp.	(only with IUD-associated disease)
Fusobacterium spp.	

The clinical diagnosis of PID is imprecise. The disease should be considered in a woman with lower abdominal pain and adnexal tenderness, or midline tenderness indicative of endometritis. Abnormally painful menses and metromenorrhagia are common. PID has been associated with the use of intrauterine contraceptive devices (IUDs). Pelvic actinomycosis, a rare cause of PID, is seen exclusively in women using IUDs. Laparoscopy is the best method for confirming a clinical impression; however, especially in early PID, the inflammation may not have extended to the tubal surface, and the peritoneal mucosa may appear normal despite inflammation within the tubes (*Figs. 6.25* and *6.26*). Endometrial biopsy represents a less invasive alternative to laparoscopic examination. Abnormalities are seen in as many as 90% of endometrial biopsies from women with laparoscopic evidence of salpingitis. Additionally, as many as one-third of women with examination findings suggestive of PID and negative laparoscopic findings will have histopathologic findings that suggest endometritis. Histopathologic findings consistent with endometritis include the presence of plasma cells in stromal tissue and the presence of neutrophils within the epithelium. Misdiagnosis based on clinical criteria alone is common; ectopic pregnancy and acute appendicitis may be mistaken for PID and vice versa (*Figs. 6.27* and *6.28*). In lieu of laparoscopic and endometrial biopsy specimens, endocervical specimens for *N. gonorrhoeae* and *C. trachomatis* must suffice, and are essential. Empiric treatment regimens must be effective against both pathogens, especially since chlamydial disease is associated with a high incidence of tubal scarring and infertility.

LABORATORY TESTS

In usual clinical practice, the laboratory diagnosis of gonorrhea is made presumptively and then confirmed, a process that involves identifying characteristics that distinguish *N. gonorrhoeae* from other *Neisseria* spp. that may be present in the specimen (*Figs. 6.29* and *6.30*). Nonpathogenic *Neisseria* and related spp. are normal flora of the oropharynx and nasopharynx

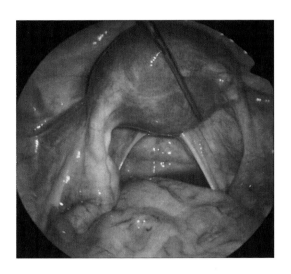

Fig. 6.25 Normal laparoscopic view of the female genital tract: view from above the dome of the uterus.

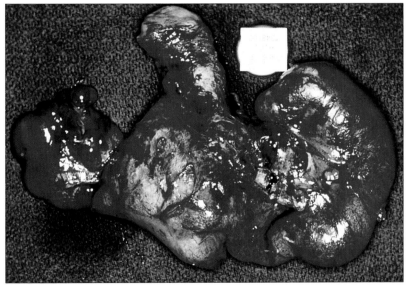

Fig. 6.26 Uterus and fallopian tubes of a patient with advanced recurrent pelvic inflammatory disease, showing so-called 'retort' tubes.

ABDOMINAL PAIN SYNDROMES ERRONEOUSLY DIAGNOSED AS OTHER THAN SALPINGITIS

VISUAL FINDINGS (PREOPERATIVE DIAGNOSIS)	
Ovarian tumor	20
Acute appendicitis	18
Ectopic pregnancy	16
Chronic PID	10
Acute peritonitis	6
Pelvic endometriosis	5
Uterine myoma	5
Uncharacteristic pelvic pain	5
Miscellaneous	6
	91

Modified from Jacobson and Westrom

Fig. 6.27 Abdominal pain syndrome, erroneously clinically diagnosed as other than salpingitis. The correct diagnosis was confirmed by laparoscopy.

ABDOMINAL PAIN SYNDROMES ERRONEOUSLY DIAGNOSED AS SALPINGITIS

VISUAL FINDINGS	
Acute appendicitis	24
Pelvic endometriosis	16
Corpus luteum hematoma	12
Ectopic pregnancy	11
Ovarian tumor	7
Chronic PID	6
Mesenteric lymphadenitis	6
Miscellaneous	16
	98

Modified from Jacobson and Westrom.

Fig. 6.28 Abdominal pain syndrome, erroneously clinically diagnosed as salpingitis. The correct diagnosis was confirmed by laparoscopy.

GROWTH ON SELECTIVE AND NONSELECTIVE MEDIA, REQUIREMENT FOR SUPPLEMENTAL CO₂

Figs. 6.29 and 6.30
Characteristics of human *Neisseria* and related spp. that grow on routine laboratory media selective for the gonococcus. Growth on selective and nonselective media, requirement for supplemental CO_2 (**6.29**). Differential biochemical reactions (**6.30**).

SPECIES	EXTRA CO₂ NEEDED[a]	MTM ML, OR NYC MEDIUM	GROWTH ON CHOCOLATE OR BLOOD AGAR AT 22°C	NUTRIENT AGAR AT 35°C
N. gonorrhoeae	VI	+[b]	–	–
N. meningitidis	I	+	–	+
N. lactamica	D	+	–	+
N. cinerea	D	–[c]	–	+
N. polysaccharea	D	+	–	+
N. flavescens	I	+	–	+
N. sicca	No	–	+	+
N. subflava biovar perflava	No	–[d]	+	+
B. catarrhalis	No	D	+	+
K. denitrificans	I	+	–	–

MTM = modified Thayer-Martin medium; ML = Martin-Lewis medium; NYC = New York City medium; + = Most strains (≥ 90%) positive; – = Most strains (≥ 90%) negative; D = Some strains positive, some strains negative.

[a] Extra CO_2: VI, very important for growth; I, important for growth; No, not needed for growth; D, some strains require extra CO_2.

[b] ≥ 90% of vancomycin-susceptible strains of N. gonorrhoeae may not grow on TM or MTM media.

[c] Some strains of N. cinerea have been isolated on gonococcal selective medium but are colistin-susceptible and will not grow when subcultured on selective media.

[d] Some strains of N. subflava biovar perflava grow on gonococcal selective media in primary culture, are colistin-resistant, and grow on selective media on subculture.

DIFFERENTIAL BIOCHEMICAL REACTIONS

SPECIES	PIGMENT[a]	SUPEROXOL[b]	ACID PRODUCED FROM GLUCOSE	MALTOSE	FRUCTOSE	SUCROSE	LACTOSE (ONPG)	POLYSACCHARIDE FROM 1% SUCROSE[c]	REDUCTION OF NO₃⁻	NO₂⁻[d]	DNase
N. gonorrhoeae	–	+	+	–	–	–	–	–	–	–	–
N. meningitidis	–	–	+	+	–	–	–	–	–	D	–
N. lactamica	–	–	+	+	–	–	+	–	–	D	–
N. cinerea	–	–	–[e]	–	–	–	–	–	–	+	–
N. polysaccharea	–	–	+	+	–	–	–	+	–	D	–
N. flavescens	+	–	–	–	–	–	–	+	–	–	–
N. sicca	–	–	+	+	+	+	–	+	–	+	–
N. subflava biovar perflava	+	–	+	+	+	+	–	+	–	+	–
B. catarrhalis	–	–	–	–	–	–	–	–	+	–	+
K. denitrificans	–	–	+	–	–	–	–	–	+	–	–

ONPG = o-nitrophenyl-β-D-galactopyranoside; DNase = deoxyribonuclease; – = Most strains (≥ 90%) negative; + = Most strains (≥ 90%) positive; D = Some strains positive, some strains negative.

[a] Pigment observed in colonies on nutrient agar. Strains of N. cinerea and N. lactamica are yellow-brown and yellow pigmented when growth is harvested on a cotton applicator or smeared on filter paper.

[b] All Neisseria spp. and B. catarrhalis give a positive catalase test using 3% H_2O_2; N. gonorrhoeae strains give strong reactions with 30% H_2O_2 (superoxol) on chocolatized blood media, whereas other species are usually negative. This test should be used only in conjunction with other tests.

[c] Some strains may be inhibited by 5% sucrose; reactions may be obtained on a starch-free medium containing 1% sucrose. Strains of N. gonorrhoeae and N. meningitidis do not grow on this medium.

[d] Results for tests in 0.1% (w/v) potassium nitrite; N. gonorrhoeae strains and strains of some other species that are negative in 0.1% nitrite can reduce 0.01% (w/v) nitrite.

[e] Some strains of N. cinerea may give a weak reaction in glucose in some rapid tests for the detection of acid from carbohydrates.

and occasionally they are isolated from other sites infected by the gonococcus — for example, the urethra, cervix, and rectum.

PRESUMPTIVE LABORATORY DIAGNOSIS

A provisional diagnosis of gonorrhea may be made from urethral, cervical, and rectal specimens (*Fig. 6.31*) if Gram-negative diplococci are observed intracellularly in polymorphonuclear leukocytes (*Figs. 6.32* and *6.33*). Gram stain is ≥ 95% sensitive in men with symptomatic urethritis. Gram's stain is less sensitive in cervical specimens (50–70%) and is likely to be less (40–60%) in blindly obtained rectal specimens. A presumptive diagnosis of gonorrhea can be made in cervical and rectal specimens if oxidase-positive, Gram-negative diplococci grow on medium selective for the isolation of *N. gonorrhoeae*. Diagnosis of pharyngeal infection cannot be based on the Gram stain or presumptive culture criteria because of the frequent presence of other *Neisseria* and related spp. in the oropharynx.

SPECIMEN COLLECTION AND TRANSPORTATION

Specimens for gonorrhea culture should always be collected before treatment is administered. *N. gonorrhoeae* is most successfully isolated when the specimen is inoculated onto media and incubated at 35–36.5°C in a CO_2-enriched atmosphere immediately after collection. Presence of a CO_2-enriched atmosphere is more important than immediate incubation at 35°C. Thus, streaked plates should be immediately placed in a CO_2 candle-extinction jar held at room temperature until they can be transported to the laboratory incubator. Specimens may be kept at room temperature for up to 5 hours without loss of viability. A candle-extinction jar is easily made from a wide-mouthed screw-cap jar such as a commercial-sized (1 gallon) mayonnaise or relish jar. A damp paper towel is placed on the bottom, and a plain wax candle is lit and placed on the floor of the jar and relit each time a new plate is added to the stack. The cover is then screwed on firmly. This will produce a humid, 3–4% CO_2 atmosphere (*Figs. 6.34* and *6.35*).

PRESUMPTIVE LABORATORY DIAGNOSIS OF
NEISSERIA GONORRHOEAE

Gram-negative diplococci observed intracellularly in PMNs (≥ 95% sensitive in men with symptomatic urethritis)

Gram-negative, oxidase-positive diplococci are isolated on selective media

Fig. 6.31 Presumptive laboratory diagnosis of *N. gonorrhoeae*.

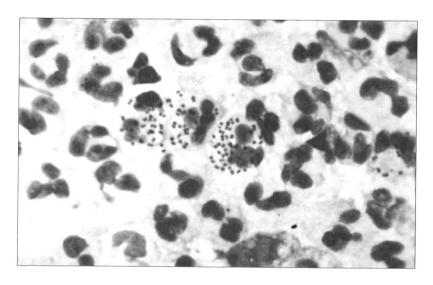

Fig. 6.32 Gram-stained smear of uretheral exudate from a male showing a sheet of neutrophils (PMNs) and many Gram-negative diplococci within PMNs. This finding is sufficient for a presumptive diagnosis of gonorrhea in the male.

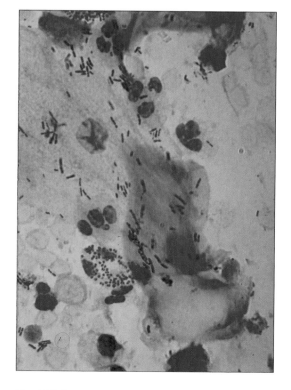

Fig. 6.33 Gram-stained smear of endocervical exudate showing scattered neutrophils and squamous epithelial cells. Gram-negative diplococci are present in one neutrophil. This finding supports a presumptive diagnosis of gonorrhea in the female, but should be confirmed by culture.

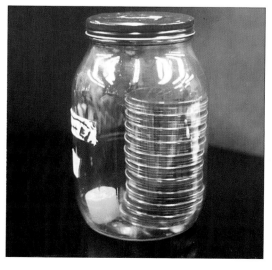

Fig. 6.34 Homemade candle-extinction jar properly filled, with candle on the floor of the jar and cover screwed on tightly.

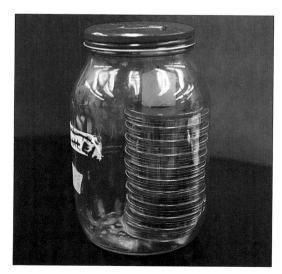

Fig. 6.35 Homemade candle-extinction jar improperly filled. The candle is too close to the lid and will be extinguished before generating the required amount of carbon dioxide.

Specimens for culture may be collected from the urethra, cervix, rectum, and pharynx as well as from the endometrium, fallopian tubes, joint fluid or blood, if PID or DGI is suspected (*Fig. 6.36*). The precise choice of anatomic sites from which to collect specimens is made on the basis of the patient's potential for sexual exposure and presenting symptoms (*Fig. 6.37*). Specimens are collected with cotton, polyester, or calcium alginate swabs. Normally, only urethral specimens are collected from heterosexual men, while urethral, rectal, and pharyngeal specimens are collected from homosexual men. Cervical and rectal specimens are routinely collected from women; specimens may also be collected from the urethra and from Bartholin's and Skene's glands when appropriate. In men, *N. gonorrhoeae* may also be isolated from the culture of urine sediment. Blood cultures should be collected from patients with suspected disseminated infection. In patients with septic arthritis, synovial fluid should be cultured.

If specimens must be transported a significant distance from the clinical facility to the laboratory, they should be inoculated onto an isolation medium (Jembec or Transgrow) and incubated overnight before shipment. The transport medium should be shipped by courier or an express delivery service to ensure delivery of the inoculated medium within 24–48 hours. Transport of specimens in Amies' or Stuart's medium is not advised.

Specimens should be inoculated onto selective media such as Thayer–Martin (TM) medium, modified Thayer–Martin medium (MTM), Martin–Lewis (ML) medium, New York City (NYC) medium, or GC–Lect (GC–L) medium, which are composed of GC base or equivalent media supplemented with growth factors and antimicrobial and antifungal agents; some media contain hemoglobin. If the specimen is obtained from a site that is normally sterile (e.g. blood, synovial fluid, conjunctiva), it may be inoculated on a nonselective medium such as chocolate agar. It should be remembered that other *Neisseria* and related spp. may grow on nonselective media and therefore confirmation procedures should be scrupulously followed.

The specimen should be inoculated over the entire surface of the plate in a 'Z' pattern, followed by streak inoculation of the plate (*Figs. 6.38–6.40*).

This inoculation technique yields isolated colonies that can be more easily processed, particularly in pharyngeal specimens, from which strains of *N. meningitidis*, *N. lactamica*, and *K. denitrificans* may also be isolated.

Inoculated plates should be incubated immediately at 35–36.5°C in a CO_2-enriched, humid atmosphere. Gonococci require CO_2 for primary isolation; the supplemental CO_2 can be provided in a CO_2 incubator, a container with a CO_2-generating tablet, or a candle-extinction jar with white, unscented, nontoxic candles.

GRAM STAIN
A thin smear prepared from the specimen is Gram stained and examined microscopically under an oil-immersion objective ($\times 100$) for intracellular Gram-negative diplococci in polymorphonuclear leukocytes. Smears prepared from suspect colonies should be examined microscopically for the presence of gram-negative diplococci. Cells of *Neisseria* spp. occur as diplococci composed of kidney-shaped cells ($0.8\,\mu m \times 0.6\,\mu m$) with adjacent sides flattened (*see Fig. 6.32*). Thin smears may be stained with a monoclonal FA reagent (*Fig. 6.41*) to confirm the identification of *N. gonorrhoeae*. Cross-reaction with nongonococcal species has not been observed with monoclonal reagents. Occasionally, some gonococcal strains do not react in this test (false negative). FA confirmation with polyvalent antibodies is not recommended because the reagent may react with other *Neisseria* spp. (false positive).

GROWTH CHARACTERISTICS
Plates are examined for growth after incubation for 24 hours; those that show no growth at this time are reincubated for 24–48 hours before being discarded and before a report of negative for *N. gonorrhoeae* is issued. Translucent, nonpigmented-to-brownish colonies measuring 0.5–1.0 mm in diameter on isolation media should be further characterized. Representative colonies are Gram stained and examined for oxidase production. Oxidase is detected either by placing a drop of oxidase reagent (tetramethyl-

SPECIMEN COLLECTION FOR LABORATORY DIAGNOSIS OF GONORRHEA	
SPECIMEN	METHOD OF COLLECTION
Urethral, men	Symptomatic: Express urethral exudate. Asymptomatic: Compress meatus vertically to open the distal urethra, and insert and withdraw a calcium alginate swab to 2 cm with a rotary motion.
Urethral, women	Symptomatic: Massage urethra gently against pubic symphysis. Asymptomatic: Insert and withdraw a calcium alginate swab to 2 cm with a rotary motion.
Endocervical	Insert speculum moistened with warm water (NOT surgical lubricant) into the vagina. Insert a swab 2 to 3 cm into the cervical canal and move in and out with a rotary motion over 10 sec to allow absorption of exudate.
Vaginal	Insert speculum. Rub sterile cotton swab against the posterior vaginal wall and allow swab to absorb specimen. (A swab of the vaginal orifice can be taken if hymen is intact.)
Rectal	Ask patient to spread buttocks and bear down slightly. Insert sterile cotton swab approximately 3 cm into anal canal and rotate to sample crypts just inside the anal ring; allow swab to absorb specimen for 10 sec.
Oropharyngeal	Rub two or three sterile swabs together over the posterior pharynx and tonsillar crypts carefully for 10 sec.

Fig. 6.36 Specimen collection for laboratory diagnosis of gonorrhea.

SPECIMEN COLLECTION SITES	
PATIENT	SITES
Heterosexual men	Urethra Oropharynx
Homosexual men	Urethra Rectum Oropharynx
Women	Cervix Rectum Oropharynx

Fig. 6.37 Sites for usual collection of specimens for the laboratory diagnosis of uncomplicated gonorrhea.

paraphenylenediamine-dihydrochloride) on a few representative colonies or by rubbing representative colonies on filter paper moistened with oxidase reagent with a platinum loop; nichrome loops may react with the oxidase reagent, giving a false-positive reaction. In a positive test, the growth will turn purple within 10 seconds (*Fig. 6.42*). The oxidase reagent should not be placed on all suspect colonies. If few suspect colonies are available, they must be subcultured to chocolate agar immediately after the application of the oxidase reagent because of the toxicity of the reagent to the cells. Thin smears of suspect colonies are Gram stained as described above. If the suspect colonies are oxidase-positive, Gram-negative diplococci, a report of presumptive *N. gonorrhoeae* may be made for cervical, urethral, or rectal specimens. Ideally, all isolates should be confirmed as *N. gonorrhoeae*. Certainly, pharyngeal isolates must be confirmed because other *Neisseria* and related spp. may frequently be isolated on gonococcal selective media (*Figs. 6.43–6.48*).

PRESERVATION

Isolates of *N. gonorrhoeae* must be subcultured every 24–48 hours or suspended in a solution of trypticase soy broth containing 15% glycerol and frozen at −70°C. Strains cannot be stored at −20°C for long periods but can be stored at this temperature for a short time (approximately 2 months).

IDENTIFICATION OF ISOLATES

Traditionally, *Neisseria* and related spp. have been identified by a series of biochemical tests, including acid production from glucose, maltose, sucrose, and lactose; reduction of nitrate; and the production of polysaccharide. Traditional biochemical tests must be incubated for 24–48 hours before results can be interpreted (*Figs. 6.49* and *6.50*). Acid production tests should be incubated at 35–36.5°C without CO_2, which will produce an acid reaction in the media. Rapid tests have been developed that permit identification of strains from the primary isolation plate or within several

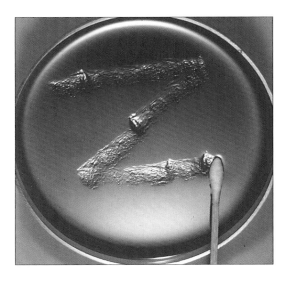

Fig. 6.38 'Z' streak method of inoculation to obtain isolated colonies for the identification of *Neisseria*.

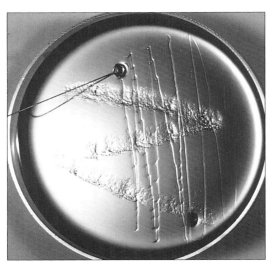

Fig. 6.39 Cross-streaking of 'Z' inoculated plate to ensure separation of colonies.

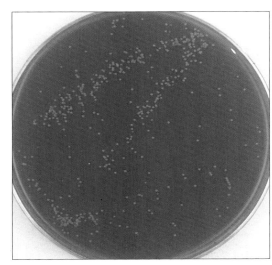

Fig. 6.40 Inoculated plate after 24 hours of incubation.

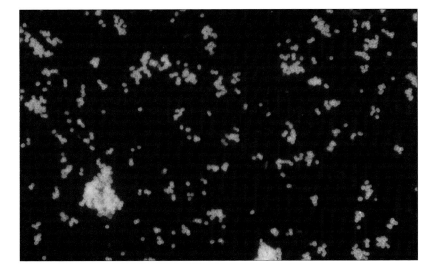

Fig. 6.41 Monoclonal FA stain.

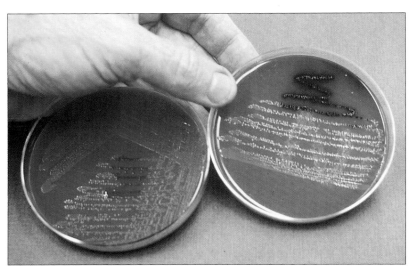

Fig. 6.42 Positive oxidase reaction on culture of *N. gonorrhoeae*.

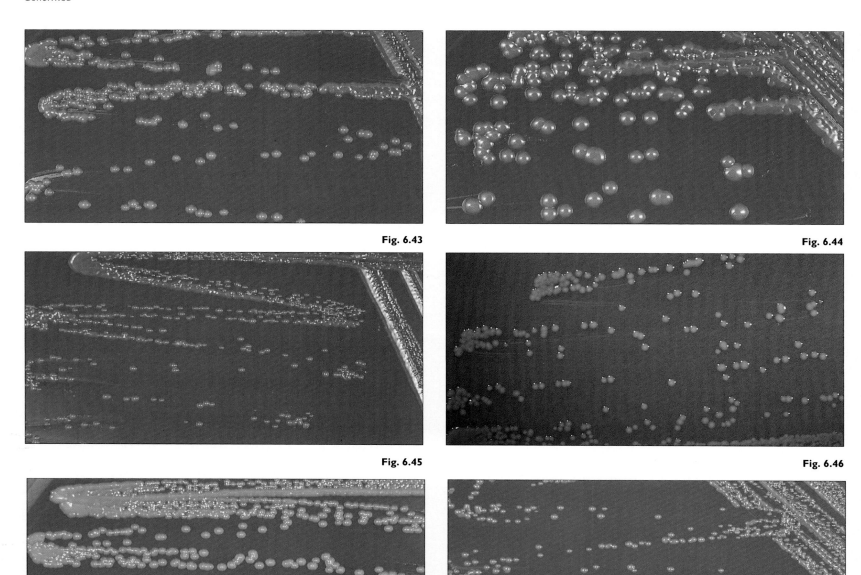

Fig. 6.43

Fig. 6.44

Fig. 6.45

Fig. 6.46

Fig. 6.47

Fig. 6.48

Figs. 6.43–6.48 Typical colonies of *Neisseria* and related spp. (**6.43**) *N. gonorrhoeae*. (**6.44**) *N. meningitidis*. (**6.45**) *N. lactamica*. (**6.46**) *N. cinerea*. (**6.47**) *Branhamella catarrhalis*. (**6.48**) *Kingella denitrificans*.

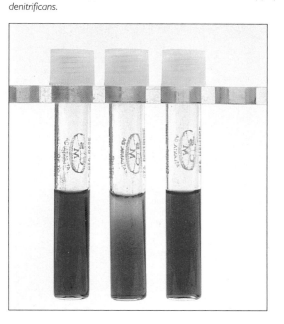

Fig. 6.49 Acid production from carbohydrates in Cystine Trypticase Soy (CTA) medium. Tubes from left to right are CTA base medium containing no carbohydrate, CTA medium containing 1% glucose and CTA medium containing 1% maltose. The organism is *N. gonorrhoeae*.

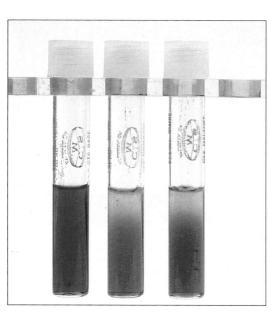

Fig. 6.50 Acid production from carbohydrates in CTA medium (see **6.49** for further details). The organism is *N. meningitidis*.

hours of the isolation of a pure subculture. The rapid confirmation tests may be divided into four categories: carbohydrate, enzyme substrate, serologic, and DNA probe tests.

Rapid Carbohydrate Tests

Rapid carbohydrate tests permit the detection of acid production from glucose, maltose, lactose, and sucrose. Strains of *N. gonorrhoeae* are distinguished by their ability to produce acid only from glucose; most other *Neisseria* spp. produce acid from maltose and thus are easily differentiated from *N. gonorrhoeae*. However, because strains of other *Neisseria* and related spp. may also give strong or weak acid reactions from glucose, additional tests may be required to differentiate between them (*Fig. 6.51*). Strains of several species (maltose-negative *N. meningitidis*, *N. cinerea*, *B. catarrhalis*, and *K. denitrificans*) may be misidentified as *N. gonorrhoeae*. In addition, some strains of *N. gonorrhoeae* produce very weak reactions in glucose tests and may appear to be glucose-negative. Supplemental tests that can be used to distinguish *N. gonorrhoeae* from these species are listed in *Figures. 6.29* and *6.30*.

Enzyme Substrate Tests

Strains of *Neisseria* spp. produce enzymes that may be used to differentiate between them (*Fig. 6.52*). *N. gonorrhoeae* strains produce hydroxyprolyl aminopeptidase, *N. meningitidis* strains produce γ-glutamyl aminopeptidase, and *N. lactamica* strains produce β-galactosidase; strains of *B. catarrhalis* produce none of these enzymes. The use of enzyme substrate tests is limited to the identification of strains isolated on gonococcal selective media because strains of the commensal *Neisseria* spp. may produce hydroxyprolyl aminopeptidase and would be identified as *N. gonorrhoeae* without supplemental tests. In addition, strains of *K. denitrificans* and some strains of *N. subflava* biovar *perflava* and *N. cinerea* have also been isolated on gonococcal selective media and will be misidentified as *N. gonorrhoeae* without additional characterization. Thus using a combination of enzyme substrate and other biochemical tests, strains isolated on selective media can be identified by a process of elimination (*see Figs. 6.29* and *6.30*).

Products that combine acid production, enzyme substrate, and other biochemical tests are also commercially available. These tests provide a more detailed characterization of isolates that will permit the laboratory technician to distinguish *N. gonorrhoeae* from related species. Pure cultures of clinical isolates are required to inoculate all rapid biochemical tests.

Serologic Tests

There are currently no available tests that permit the detection of gonococcal antibodies in serum. Serologic tests for the identification of *N. gonorrhoeae* in primary cultures are commercially available as FA tests (discussed above) or as coagglutination tests. Coagglutination tests consist of cocktails of monoclonal antibodies directed toward gonococcal protein I which have been adsorbed to protein A-producing *Staphylococcus aureus* cells. Suspect colonies are suspended in buffer or saline and heated in a boiling-water bath. A drop of the cooled suspension is mixed with a drop each of the antigonococcal reagents and a negative control. After rotation for 1–2 minutes, the reactions are interpreted. If a suspension gives a positive reaction with the antigonococcal reagent and a negative reaction with the control, the isolate is identified as *N. gonorrhoeae* (*Figs. 6.53–6.55*). Cross-reactions between nongonococcal *Neisseria* and related spp. and the coagglutination reagents have been reported, and some gonococcal strains have not reacted with the reagents.

Nonculture Tests for N. gonorrhoeae

Nonculture tests are available for the detection of gonococcal organisms in patient specimens. Since these tests, unlike culture, do not depend on the presence of viable organisms, they are particularly useful when transport from the clinical facility to the laboratory is difficult. Two nonculture tests are now commercially available in the USA.

Gonococcal antigen is detected by an enzyme-linked immunosorbent assay (Gonozyme; Abbott Laboratories, North Chicago, Illinois). This test has been reported to be as sensitive and specific as the Gram stain in the detection of infection from the male urethra. The test appears less sensitive than culture in detecting endocervical infections. There are no transport dif-

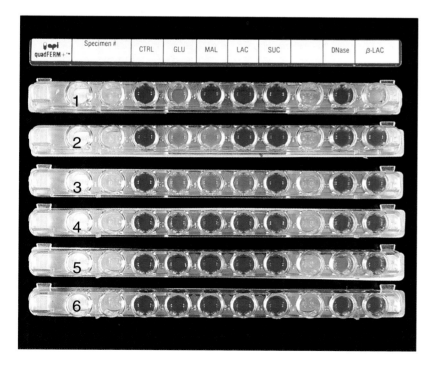

Fig. 6.51 Reactions of *Neisseria* and related spp. in the API Quadferm + rapid carbohydrate test. Tests from left to right are control (no carbohydrate), glucose, maltose, lactose, sucrose, DNase, and β-lactamase. 1. *N. gonorrhoeae* (β-lactamase-positive). 2. *N. meningitidis*. 3. *N. lactamica*. 4. *K. denitrificans*. 5. *B. catarrhalis*. 6. *N. cinerea*.

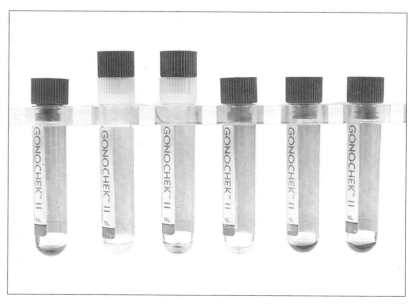

Fig. 6.52 Reactions of *Neisseria* and related spp. in the enzyme substrate test, Gonochek II. From left to right: *N. gonorrhoeae*, *N. meningitidis*, *N. lactamica*, *B. catarrhalis*, *N. cinerea*, and *K. denitrificans*. The production of γ-glutamyl aminopeptidase and β-galactosidase by *N. meningitidis* and *N. lactamica*, respectively, is determined directly without removing the clear inner cap. The ability of strains to produce hydroxyprolylaminopeptidase is determined by exposing the organism suspension to the substrate contained in the red cap. Note that *N. gonorrhoeae*, *N. cinerea*, and *K. denitrificans* give identical reactions in this test, i.e., they produce hydroxyprolylaminopeptidase. Strains of *B. catarrhalis* do not produce any of these enzymes; suspensions will be yellow or colorless after exposure to the substrate contained in the red cap).

ficulties with this test. Because of the possibility of cross-reactions with other *Neisseria* and related species, results should be considered presumptive.

A nucleic acid probe test (PACE; GenProbe, San Diego, California) appears to be quite sensitive and specific in the detection of urethral and endocervical infections in populations with a relatively high prevalence of gonorrhea (see *Fig. 4.78*). Experience with pharyngeal and rectal specimens suggests that the probe test may be less sensitive than culture. Particularly in low-prevalence populations, results of the probe test should be considered presumptive.

PCR and LCR tests for the detection of *N. gonorrhoeae* have been developed (see *Figs. 4.79* and *4.80*). Although these amplification techniques theoretically hold great promise for diagnosis, neither test is yet commercially available.

ANTIMICROBIAL SUSCEPTIBILITY TESTING

Surveillance for antimicrobial resistance in *N. gonorrhoeae* should be an integral part of a routine STD laboratory program. If resources permit, all isolates of *N. gonorrhoeae* should be tested for their susceptibility to clinically important antimicrobial agents. If resources are limited, clinically and epidemiologically important isolates (e.g. isolates from patients with positive test-of-cure culture) should be tested. Clusters of treatment failures may indicate an outbreak of a resistant strain and should be a catalyst for expanded testing.

Fig. 6.53 Reactions of *N. gonorrhoeae*, *N. meningitidis*, and related spp. in the Phadebact coagglutination test: 1. *N. gonorrhoeae*. 2. Negative control. 3. *N. meningitidis*. 4. *N. cinerea*. 5. *N. lactamica*. 6. Negative control.

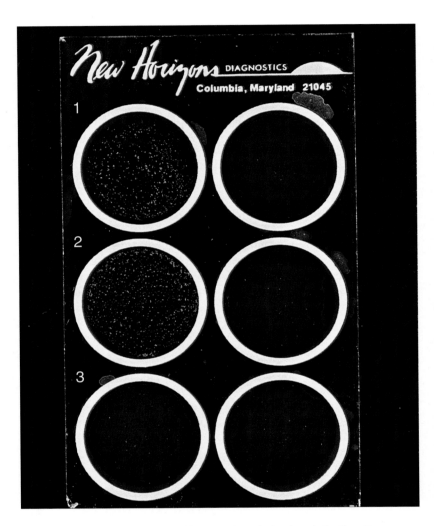

Fig. 6.55 Reactions of *N. gonorrhoeae*, *N. meningitidis*, and related spp. in the GonoGen coagglutination test. From top to bottom, left to right: 1. Positive control and its control (negative) reaction. 2. *N. gonorrhoeae* and its control (negative) reaction. 3. *N. meningitidis* and its control (negative) reaction.

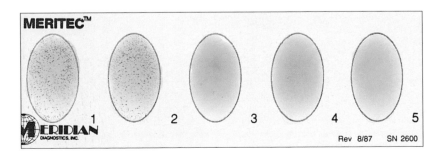

Fig. 6.54 Reactions of *N. gonorrhoeae*, *N. meningitidis*, and related spp. in the Meritec coagglutination test. From left to right: 1. Positive control. 2. *N. gonorrhoeae*. 3. Negative control. 4. *N. meningitidis*. 5. Negative control.

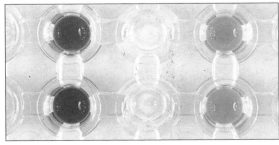

Fig. 6.56 Reactions of β-lactamase-positive (left) and negative (right) strains of *N. gonorrhoeae* in a nitrocefin test.

β-LACTAMASE TESTS

All gonococcal isolates should be tested for β-lactamase, which can be detected in colonies on primary isolation medium or after subculture. Several tests for β-lactamase are available commercially; these include chromogenic cephalosporin (*Fig. 6.56*), acidometric, and iodometric tests. The chromogenic cephalosporin (nitrocefin, PADAC) tests are preferred because the substrates are stable and the reactions are specific and highly sensitive for β-lactamase. The specificity and sensitivity of the acidometric and iodometric tests may be affected by several factors, including incorrect storage of the product, which may result in nonspecific hydrolysis of the substrate. β-lactamase-positive and β-lactamase-negative strains should be included as controls with each batch of clinical isolates.

DETERMINATION OF ANTIMICROBIAL SUSCEPTIBILITY

With the exception of specific β-lactamase tests, resistance in *N. gonorrhoeae* must be detected by measuring the level of susceptibility of strains to an antimicrobial agent. Two methods, the agar-dilution and disk-diffusion procedures, may be used to measure the susceptibilities of isolates.

Agar-Dilution Susceptibility Testing

Agar-dilution susceptibility testing is the reference method for measuring the antimicrobial susceptibilities of strains of *N. gonorrhoeae*. Resistance to antimicrobial agents is measured as the minimal inhibitory concentration (MIC) of the agent that inhibits growth of an isolate. Determination of susceptibilities to relevant antimicrobials, such as broad-spectrum cephalosporins and fluoroquinolones, is recommended. Tests of more traditional antimicrobials, i.e. penicillin and tetracycline, may be included. Susceptibility testing is performed on GC agar base medium containing 1% (vol/vol) IsoVitaleX or an equivalent supplement; antimicrobial agents are incorporated into the base medium in serial twofold dilutions. Isolates to be tested are grown overnight on chocolate agar and suspended in Mueller–Hinton broth to an optical density equivalent to a 0.5 McFarland standard, containing approximately 10^8 colony-forming units (CFU)/ml. The suspensions are diluted 1:10 in Mueller–Hinton broth, and 10^4 CFU/ml are inoculated onto the surface of the antibiotic-containing media and an antibiotic-free control medium with a Steer's replicator or a calibrated loop. Plates are incubated at 35–36°C in a CO_2-enriched atmosphere for 24 hours and then examined for growth. The MIC of the antimicrobial agent for an isolate is the lowest concentration that inhibits its growth.

Disk-Diffusion Susceptibility Testing

Agar-dilution susceptibility testing of *N. gonorrhoeae* isolates is not routinely performed in clinical microbiology laboratories. Instead, disk-diffusion susceptibility testing is most frequently used to measure the antimicrobial resistance of isolates of *N. gonorrhoeae*. The results of disk-diffusion susceptibility testing can be correlated with treatment outcome (*Fig. 6.57*).

ANTIBIOTIC-CONTAINING MEDIA

Medium containing 1.5 μg penicillin/ml has been used to screen for resistant isolates in primary culture. Penicillin-containing media have not been extensively evaluated but have been useful in some geographic areas. The major concern about this method is that it is not standardized. The number of organisms inoculated onto the medium will vary according to their numbers in specimens; urethral specimens from symptomatic men may contain many more organisms than those from women or asymptomatic men. As with the agar-dilution procedure, the result is inoculum-dependent (i.e., the resistance level may be higher if a larger inoculum is used). Whereas a clinical specimen containing many resistant diplococci may yield a positive culture on the penicillin-containing medium, a specimen containing few resistant diplococci may fail to grow on the same medium.

INTERPRETATION OF ANTIMICROBIAL SUSCEPTIBILITY TEST RESULTS

An antimicrobial susceptibility result determined in the laboratory is only a measure of the *in vitro* susceptibility of an isolate. A patient may have a positive test-of-cure culture for a variety of reasons:
- Failure of therapy because of infection with a resistant isolate
- Failure of therapy even when the patient is infected with a strain that is susceptible by *in vitro* measurements
- Reinfection.

Thus, antimicrobial susceptibilities must be used as an adjunct to, but cannot be substituted for, clinical findings.

CORRELATES OF DISK-DIFFUSION SUSCEPTIBILITY RESULTS WITH CLINICAL OUTCOME

SUSCEPTIBLE	Less than 5% likelihood of treatment failure
INTERMEDIATE	Predictable failure rates of 5 to 15% if the patient is treated with the tested antibiotic in the standard dosage (in most cases of intermediate susceptibility, a higher dose or prolonged therapy results in greater than 95% cure rates)
RESISTANT	May be associated with treatment failure rates of greater than 15%

Fig. 6.57 Correlates of disk-diffusion susceptibility results with clinical outcome.

ANTIMICROBIAL THERAPY

In response to the continued emergence of resistant strains in the USA, the 1993 CDC STD Treatment Guidelines recommend treatment of all gonococcal infections presumptively with antibiotic regimens effective against strains resistant to penicillin and/or tetracycline (*Fig. 6.58*). In addition to the four recommended regimens for uncomplicated gonococcal infections, other broad-spectrum cephalosporins such as cefotaxime, cefotetan and cefuroxime axetil, are acceptable alternatives. Spectinomycin, 2 g intramuscularly, is a useful regimen for the treatment of patients who can tolerate neither cephalosporins nor fluoroquinolones. Despite recent reports of fluoroquinolone resistance from Asia, Australia, UK and North America, data are not yet sufficient to modify these recommendations. Treatment recommendations for complicated gonococcal infections (*Fig. 6.59*) are based on expert opinion, not on therapy trials.

Picture credits for this chapter are as follows: Fig. 6.1 Courtesy of GPA, World Health Organization.

RECOMMENDED THERAPY FOR UNCOMPLICATED GONORRHEA

RECOMMENDED THERAPY

Ceftriaxone: 125 mg im in a single dose
or
Cefixime: 400 mg po in a single dose
or
Ciprofloxacin: 500 mg po in a single dose
or
Ofloxacin: 400 mg po in a single dose
plus
A regimen effective against possible co-infection with *C. trachomatis*, such as doxycycline* 100 mg po bid for 7 days.

* For patients in whom tetracyclines are contraindicated (e.g., pregnant women), erythromycin base 500 mg po qid for 7 days may be substituted).

Fig. 6.58 Recommended antimicrobial therapy for uncomplicated gonorrhea.

RECOMMENDED THERAPY FOR PATIENTS WITH COMPLICATED GONOCOCCAL INFECTIONS

SYNDROME	RECOMMENDED THERAPY
Disseminated gonococcal infection	Ceftriaxone*: 1 g, im or iv, every 24 hours All regimens should be continued for 24–48 hours after improvement begins; therapy may then be switched to cefixime 400 mg po bid or ciprofloxacin 500 mg po bid to complete 7 days of therapy
Meningitis/endocarditis	Consultation with an expert is vital. Ceftriaxone 1–2 g iv every 12 hours. Patients with meningitis should be treated for 10–14 days; those with endocarditis should be treated for at least 1 month
Ophthalmia Neonatal	Ceftriaxone: 25–50 mg/kg body weight, im or iv, in a single dose, not to exceed 125 mg
Adult	Ceftriaxone: 1 g im, 1 dose†

*Or cefotaxime 1 g iv every 8 hours, or ceftizoxime 1 g iv every 8 hours, or spectinomycin 2 g im every 12 hours.
†Infected eye should be lavaged with saline solution.

Fig. 6.59 Recommended therapy for patients with complicated gonococcal infections.

BIBLIOGRAPHY

Centers for Disease Control and Prevention: 1993 Sexually Transmitted Diseases Treatment Guidelines. *MMWR* **42**(RR-14):1–101, 1993.

Centers for Disease Control and Prevention: Decreased susceptibility of *Neisseria gonorrhoeae* to fluoroquinolones — Ohio and Hawaii, 1992–1994. *MMWR* **43**:325–327, 1994.

Knapp JS, Rice RJ: *Neisseria* and *Brahamella*. In: Murray PR, Baron EJ, Pfaller MA, Tenover FC, Yolken RH (eds). *Manual of Clinical Microbiology*, 6th ed. Washington, DC, American Society for Microbiology, pp. 324–340, 1994.

Morse SA, Holmes KK: Gonococcal Infections. In: Hoeprich PD, Jordan MC, Ronald AR (eds). *Infectious Diseases*, 5th ed. New York, Harper & Row, pp. 670–685, 1994.

National Committee for Clinical Laboratory Standards: *Approved Standard: Performance Standards for Antimicrobial Disk Susceptibility Tests*, 5th ed. Document M2-A5. National Committee for Clinical Laboratory Standards, Villanova, Pa.

Sarafian SK, Knapp JS: Molecular epidemiology of gonorrhea. *Clin Microbiol Rev* **2**:s49–s55, 1989.

Whittington WL, Knapp JS: Trends in antimicrobial resistance in *Neisseria gonorrhoeae* in the United States. *Sex Transm Dis* **15**:202–210, 1988.

CHAPTER SEVEN

Genital Mycoplasmas

G Cassell, K Waites, and D Taylor-Robinson

INTRODUCTION

Mycoplasmas are the smallest known free-living microorganisms, intermediate in size between bacteria and viruses (*Fig. 7.1*). They are unique among prokaryotes, differing by one or more characteristics from all other major groups of human pathogens and viruses (*Fig. 7.2*). The absence of a cell wall (*Fig. 7.3*) is the single most distinguishing feature of mycoplasmas as a group and is responsible for their inclusion as a separate class, the Mollicutes. Many of the biologic properties of mycoplasmas are due to the absence of a rigid cell wall, including resistance to all β-lactam antibiotics and marked pleomorphism among individual cells. In contrast to L-phase variants of bacteria, mycoplasmas are unable to synthesize cell-wall precursors under any conditions. The mycoplasmal cell membrane contains phospholipids, glycolipids, cholesterol, and various proteins. The extremely small size of the mycoplasmal genome (approximately one-sixth the size of that of *Escherichia coli*) severely limits their biosynthetic capabilities, helps to explain their complex nutritional requirements for cultivation, and necessitates a parasitic or saprophytic existence for most species.

Mycoplasmas usually reside on the mucosal surfaces of the respiratory and urogenital tracts. They are generally limited to the epithelial surface and rarely penetrate the submucosa (*Fig. 7.4*). Most species of mycoplasmas reside

Neisseria (0.6–1.0 μm)	Genital Mycoplasma (0.4–0.5 μm)	Chlamydia (0.25–0.3 μm)	Herpesvirus (0.15–0.2 μm)	Hepatitis B (0.042 μm)

Fig. 7.1 Relative size of mycoplasma in comparison with other sexually transmitted microorganisms. An individual mycoplasmal cell may be as small as 300 nm in diameter.

COMPARISON OF MYCOPLASMAS WITH OTHER MICROBIAL AGENTS

Fig. 7.2 Comparison of mycoplasmas with other microbial agents.

CHARACTERISTIC	MYCOPLASMAS	BACTERIA	CHLAMYDIAE	RICKETTSIAE	VIRUSES
Growth on cell-free media	+	+	–	–	–
Generation of metabolic energy	+	+	–	+	–
Independent protein synthesis	+	+	+	+	–
Contain both DNA and RNA	+	+	+	+	–
Reproduce by fission	+	+	+	+	–
Contain cell wall	–	+	+	+	–
Require sterol for growth	+*	–	–	–	–

* Except for the genus Acholeplasma

Fig. 7.3 Transmission electron micrograph showing mycoplasma between two epithelial cells. Unlike other bacteria, mycoplasmas lack a cell wall.

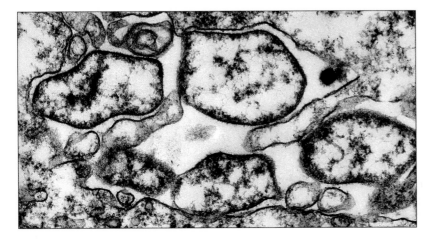

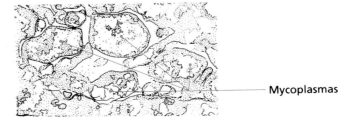

Mycoplasmas

extracellularly, some, like *Mycoplasma fermentans* and *M. penetrans,* can be found intracellularly.

The species of mycoplasmas isolated from the urogenital tract of humans are listed in *Fig. 7.5*. *M. genitalium* (*Fig. 7.6*) occurs infrequently in the lower genital tract of normal males and females. However, several groups of investigators have detected this organism in the urethra of approximately 19–27% of men with NGU and 6–20% of women attending a STD clinic for urethritis or cervicitis. Intraurethral inoculations of this organism into nonhuman primates and the resulting inflammation suggest that it may be a cause of urethritis. Serologic studies in humans and experimental studies

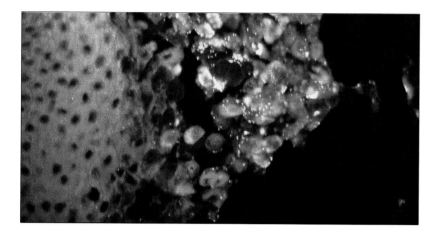

Fig. 7.4 Mycoplasmas attach to epithelial cell surfaces but rarely penetrate the submucosa. Unlike chlamydial organisms, they are extracellular. In this immunofluorescence micrograph, mycoplasmas can be seen attached to the surface of inflammatory cells in the cervix. Note that neither *U. urealyticum* nor *M. hominis* have been shown to be a cause of cervicitis.

MYCOPLASMAS ISOLATED FROM THE GENITOURINARY TRACT OF HUMANS

MYCOPLASMA	KIDNEY	BLADDER URINE	VOIDED URINE	URETHRAL SWAB	SEMINAL FLUID	FALLOPIAN TUBE	CERVIX/ VAGINA	AMNIOTIC FLUID
Mycoplasma hominis	+	+	+	+	+	+	+	+
Ureaplasma urealyticum	+	+	+	+	+	+	+	+
Mycoplasma fermentans			+	+			+	
Mycoplasma penetrans			+					
Mycoplasma primatum				+				
Mycoplasma salivarium	+						+	
Mycoplasma spermatophilum					+			
Mycoplasma genitalium				+				
Acholeplasma laidlawii							+	
Acholeplasma oculi								+

Fig. 7.5 Mycoplasmas isolated from the genitourinary tract of humans.

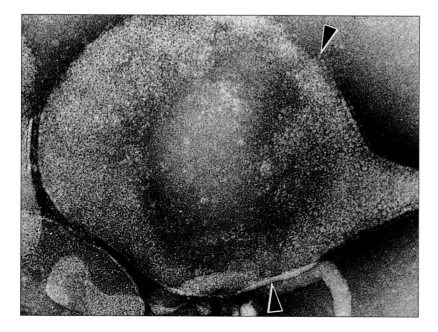

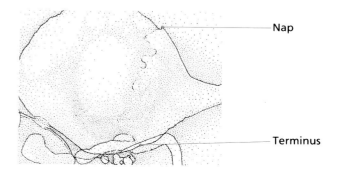

Fig. 7.6 Transmission electron micrograph of *M. genitalium.* Negative staining of an intact mycoplasma cell with ammonium molybdate. The terminus is covered with a nap extending peripherally to the tip.

Nap

Terminus

in nonhuman primates also indicate that *M. genitalium* may be a cause of PID. However, the role of this organism in maternal and fetal infections has not been evaluated. Since *M. genitalium* is a relatively newly described species of mycoplasma and detailed information is lacking concerning its true ecologic niche, more work should be done to evaluate the role of this fastidious mycoplasma in disease during pregnancy and its potential impact upon pregnancy outcome. It is worth bearing in mind that *M. genitalium* has been detected in the respiratory secretions of patients with atypical pneumonia. Thus, future studies in humans should include an assessment of the role of this organism in respiratory disease in infants and children.

M. fermentans has been isolated sporadically from humans for over 40 years. The organism has been recovered from the upper as well as the lower urogenital and respiratory tracts, bone marrow, and supposedly joints. However, little consideration was given to the possibility that *M. fermentans* was a pathogen of humans until its recent detection in patients with AIDS. It has also been implicated in an acute fatal respiratory disease of nonAIDS patients. *M. fermentans* has recently been detected in amniotic fluid collected at the time of cesarean section from four of 232 women with intact membranes. Placental tissues were available for testing from three of these four women and all were positive by PCR. Villitis and chorioamnionitis occurred in two of the four positive cases and no other organisms were detected, suggesting that *M. fermentans* should be investigated further as a cause of maternal and fetal infection. It is therefore also interesting that *M. fermentans* has been detected in the chorionic villi from the placentae of two patients with AIDS. The ecologic niche of *M. fermentans* and its precise incidence in the genital tract of males and females, either those who are asymptomatic or those with AIDS, needs to be established. It was not detected by culture or PCR in the urethral or cervical specimens of 94 males and 87 females, respectively, who lacked symptoms of AIDS but who had cervicitis and/or urethritis.

Ureaplasma urealyticum and *M. hominis* are the mycoplasmal species found most commonly in the genitourinary tract, and are the only two definitively known to cause disease in the genital tract. Thus, the remainder of this chapter will focus on these two organisms.

EPIDEMIOLOGY

The isolation rates of *U. urealyticum* and *M. hominis* in various populations are given in *Figure 7.7*. *U. urealyticum* can be found in the cervix or vagina of 40–80% of sexually mature, asymptomatic women, and *M. hominis* in 20–50%. The incidence of each is somewhat lower in the urethra of normal males. In women, colonization is linked to younger age, lower socioeconomic status,

sexual activity with multiple partners, Black ethnic group, and oral contraceptive use. *U. urealyticum* and *M. hominis* may be transmitted to about 40% of babies born to infected mothers. The colonization of most infants appears to be transient, with a sharp decline in the rate of isolation after 3 months of age. Less than 10% of older children and sexually inexperienced adults are colonized. Colonization after puberty increases with sexual activity.

CLINICAL MANIFESTATIONS

Neither *U. urealyticum* nor *M. hominis* has been shown to cause disease in the lower genital tract of the female. In fact, these organisms are probably commensals in this site. Genitourinary diseases in which they are suspected of having an etiologic role are listed in *Figure 7.8*, and are either diseases of the upper female genitourinary tract or diseases of the male genitourinary tract. Difficulty in accepting these organisms as the cause of disease has usually arisen because either cultural samples cannot be easily obtained from the affected site, or the organisms can be recovered from the affected site in asymptomatic individuals.

Even in diseases in which Koch's postulates have been fulfilled (i.e. *M. hominis* and PID), attempts to link inflammatory lesions of the upper tract with culture isolation from the lower tract have delayed recognition of the etiologic significance of these organisms. Recent carefully controlled clinical studies and experimental infection of laboratory animals have confirmed the disease-producing potential of both *U. urealyticum* and *M. hominis*. A major principle, well illustrated in these studies, is that organisms only reach the upper tract in a subpopulation of individuals infected in the lower genitourinary tract, and that disease then develops in only a few of these individuals. There has been no instance in which the factors predisposing to upper tract colonization or the development of disease have been delineated. In many of the diseases considered, these factors may be more important for the development of lesions than the organism involved. While in some instances, *U. urealyticum* or *M. hominis may* be responsible for directly inducing lesions, they appear primarily to be opportunists. In fact, *U. urealyticum* and *M. hominis* are increasingly being recognized as common causes of extragenital disease in immunocompromised patients and in newborn infants, particularly preterm infants.

URINARY TRACT

Two conditions of the urinary tract, which have been definitively proven to be caused by genital mycoplasmas, are urethritis in males due to *U. urealyticum* and pyelonephritis caused by *M. hominis*. It is possible that some urinary calculi are due to *U. urealyticum* infection.

Fig. 7.7 Epidemiology of *U. urealyticum* and *M. hominis*.

EPIDEMIOLOGY OF *UREAPLASMA UREALYTICUM* AND *MYCOPLASMA HOMINIS*

POPULATION	ISOLATION RATES	
	U. UREALYTICUM	*M. HOMINIS*
Sexually mature, asymptomatic females (cervix or vagina)	40–80%	21–53%
Babies born to infected mothers	ca. 40%	ca. 40%
Older children	< 10%	< 10%
Sexually inexperienced adults	< 10%	< 10%
Normal males	34%	22–54%

Urethritis in Men

Human and animal inoculation studies and the occurrence of urethritis in immunodeficient patients provide indisputable evidence for a causal role for *U. urealyticum* in nonchlamydial NGU, though the exact proportion of cases for which the organism is responsible has not been established (*Fig. 7.9*). Carefully controlled antibiotic and serologic studies also support a causal role. The common occurrence of ureaplasmas in the urethra of asymptomatic men suggests either that only certain biovars or serovars of ureaplasmas are pathogenic or that predisposing factors, such as a lack of mucosal immunity, exist in individuals who do develop disease. There is no evidence supporting a role for *M. hominis* as a cause of urethritis.

Urinary Calculi

Urinary calculi composed of magnesium ammonium phosphate (struvite) and carbonate—apatite account for 20% of all urinary tract stones (*Fig. 7.10*), and may be the most deleterious variety in terms of urologic complications. These

RELATIONSHIP OF *UREAPLASMA UREALYTICUM* AND *MYCOPLASMA HOMINIS* TO DISEASES OF THE GENITOURINARY TRACT OF HUMANS

DISEASE	CAUSATIVE AGENT	
	U. UREALYTICUM	M. HOMINIS
Urethritis of males	+	−
Urethroprostatitis	±	−
Female urethral syndrome	±	−
Pyelonephritis	±	+
Urinary calculi	±	−
Vaginitis	−	−
Cervicitis	−	−
Pelvic inflammatory disease	±	+
Infertility	±	−
Chorioamnionitis	+	±
Spontaneous abortion	±	±
Prematurity/low birth weight	±	−
Intrauterine growth retardation	±	−
Postpartum fever	±	+
Congenital pneumonia	+	+
Pneumonia in newborns	+	+
Meningitis in newborns	+	+
Abscesses in newborns	+	+
Extragenital disease in adults (including septic arthritis)	+	+

− = No association or causal role demonstrated; + = causal role; ± = significant association and/or strong suggestive evidence but causal role not proven.

Fig. 7.8 Relationship of *U. urealyticum* and *M. hominis* to diseases of the genitourinary tract of humans.

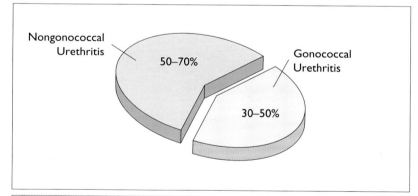

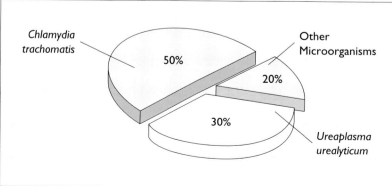

Fig. 7.9 The incidence and causes of nongonococcal urethritis (NGU). (**Top**) Approximate incidence of NGU versus gonococcal urethritis (GU) in the USA. The exact incidence is unknown; however, for the past several years, NGU has outnumbered GU by as much as 2:1. (**Bottom**) Causes of NGU. It is well established that approximately one-half of NGU cases are due to *C. trachomatis*, with the remainder caused by either *U. urealyticum* or other microorganisms whose precise contributions have yet to be identified.

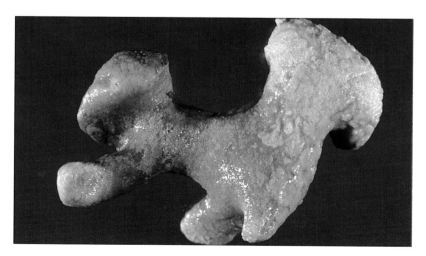

Fig. 7.10 Staghorn renal calculus typically associated with urinary tract infections due to urease-producing bacteria.

so-called infection stones are induced by the enzymatic breakdown of urea by bacterial urease (*Fig. 7.11*). *Proteus* and to a lesser extent *Klebsiella, Pseudomonas, Providencia, Staphylococcus,* and other bacterial species are the usual causes in humans. However, *U. urealyticum* also produces urease and has been demonstrated to induce the crystallization of struvite and calcium phosphates in artificial urine *in vitro* and to produce calculi in animal models. However, there is little evidence that it does so under natural conditions in humans, in the absence of other urease-producing organisms. The major remaining questions concerning the possible role of this organism in urinary calculi are: the frequency with which it reaches the kidney; the predisposing factors that allow this to occur; and the relative frequency of renal calculi which seem to be induced by this organism compared with those induced by other organisms.

Pyelonephritis
Despite the high incidence of *M. hominis* in the lower urogenital tract, this organism has been isolated from the upper urinary tract only in patients with symptoms of acute infection and is often accompanied by a significant antibody response. Overall, *M. hominis* is thought to be involved in 5% of cases of acute pyelonephritis in humans. Predisposing factors, including obstruction or instrumentation of the urinary tract, are found in about 50% of cases in which *M. hominis* is thought to be the etiologic cause.

REPRODUCTIVE TRACT
Pelvic Inflammatory Disease
This disease is an increasingly common disease of multifactorial etiology (*see also Chap. 8*). It can be caused iatrogenically or can occur naturally from infections with various bacteria, the most common of which are *Chlamydia trachomatis* and, to a lesser extent, *Neisseria gonorrhoeae. M. hominis,* but probably not *U. urealyticum,* is also a likely cause of PID, though the exact proportion of cases attributable to it is unknown. *M. hominis* has been isolated in pure cultures from the fallopian tubes of approximately 8% of women with salpingitis diagnosed by laparoscopy, compared with 0% of women without lesions. The organism can also be isolated from the endometrium. In addition, a role for *M. hominis* in cases of PID not associated with either *C. trachomatis* or *N. gonorrhoeae* is supported by significant increases in specific antibody. PID due to *M. hominis* is clinically indistinguishable from similar disease caused by other organisms, and so antimicrobial coverage for *M. hominis* should always be included in the therapy.

While *U. urealyticum* has been isolated directly from affected fallopian tubes, it is found usually in the presence of other known pathogens. Furthermore, the results of serologic studies in humans and those involving animal inoculation and inoculation of fallopian tube organ cultures do not support a causal role.

Prostatitis
A number of studies suggest that the prostate can be infected during the course of an acute ureaplasmal infection of the urethra. Ureaplasmas are isolated more often and in greater numbers from patients with acute prostatitis than from controls. Men with more than 10^4 organisms respond to tetracycline therapy, while those with fewer organisms do not. *U. urealyticum* has not been found in prostatic biopsies from patients with chronic abacterial prostatitis, and *M. hominis* has not been associated with prostatitis of any kind in most studies.

Disorders of Reproduction
Given that *M. hominis* is a cause of salpingitis, it is reasonable to assume that severe tubal infection with this organism may lead to occlusion and infertility. However, this has not been proven. Although the possibility that ureaplasmas may play a role in involuntary infertility in humans was first raised over 20 years ago, the association remains speculative. Prospective studies based on the isolation of *U. urealyticum* and *M. hominis* from the endometrium or placenta, but not studies based only on vaginal–cervical isolation, consistently show an association with spontaneous abortion. Individual case reports indicate that, in some patients, the infection is probably causal.

Chorioamnionitis and Pregnancy Outcome
In a subpopulation of women colonized in the lower genital tract, both *M. hominis* and *U. urealyticum* may colonize the endometrium (*Fig. 7.12*), with or without evidence of inflammation. Attachment of the organisms to sperm (*Fig. 7.13*) has been suggested as one mechanism by which the organisms are introduced into the upper tract. Both organisms can invade the amniotic sac in the first 16–20 weeks of gestation in the presence of intact fetal membranes and in the absence of other microorganisms. Mycoplasmas can be isolated from the endometrium of 20% of unselected individuals with intact fetal membranes at the time of cesarean section and from the placentas of about 10% of unselected individuals with intact membranes and no labor who are undergoing cesarean section. Isolation from fetal membranes increases with the onset of labor, membrane rupture, and the number of vaginal examinations.

The isolation of *M. hominis* from amniotic fluid is virtually always associated with clinical symptoms (maternal fever, uterine tenderness, foul vaginal discharge) and a specific serologic response. *U. urealyticum,* on the other hand, can persist in amniotic fluid for as long as 2 months, in the presence of an intense inflammatory response, without discernible clinical signs or symptoms of amnionitis. A convincing argument that these organisms alone can produce chorioamnionitis is provided by the following (*Figs. 7.15–7.17*):

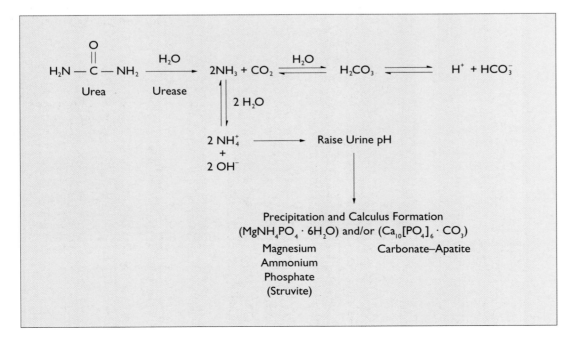

Fig. 7.11 Biochemical reactions leading to the formation of urinary calculi by urease-producing bacteria such as *U. urealyticum.*

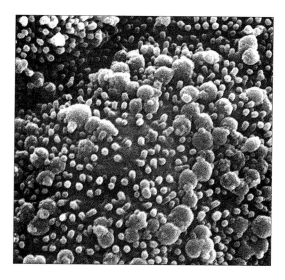

Fig. 7.12 Scanning electron micrograph showing *U. urealyticum* attached to the endometrium. Both *U. urealyticum* and *M. hominis* can be isolated from the endometrium with or without evidence of inflammation. The presence of this organism was demonstrated also by culture of the endometrium and by immunofluorescence.

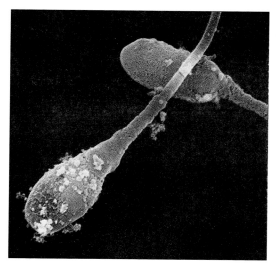

Fig. 7.13 *U. urealyticum* attached to human sperm. These organisms were shown to be ureaplasmas by immunofluorescence and culture.

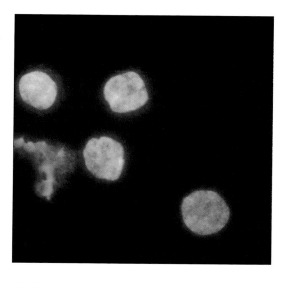

Fig. 7.14 DNA-fluorochrome-stained cytocentrifuged preparation of amniotic fluid collected at 20 weeks' gestation showing amnion cells and the absence of microorganisms. The fluid was shown subsequently to be culturally negative (× 750).

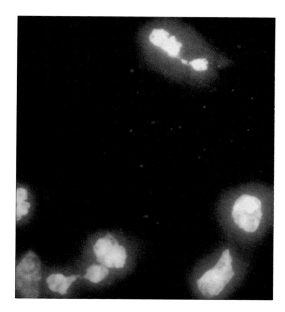

Fig. 7.15 DNA-fluorochrome-stained cytocentrifuged preparation of amniotic fluid collected at 20 weeks' gestation, showing large numbers of *U. urealyticum* (identified by culture) and large numbers of polymorphonuclear leukocytes (× 750). The fluid was culturally negative for other bacteria, viruses, and chlamydiae.

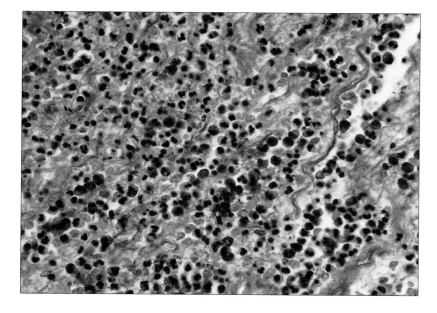

Fig. 7.16 Placenta at 26 weeks' gestation (hematoxylin and eosin × 250). *U. urealyticum* was isolated in pure culture from amniotic fluid 6 weeks prior to delivery. Note the extensive inflammation in the amnion and chorion.

Fig. 7.17 Adjacent section of placenta shown in 7.16 (× 750) stained with rabbit anti-*U. urealyticum* serovar 1 serum and reacted with affinity-purified, fluorescein-labeled, goat anti-rabbit IgG. Ureaplasmas are present in the most intense areas of inflammation. Adjacent sections reacted with normal rabbit serum and conjugate were negative. Brown and Bren-stained adjacent sections of placenta were negative for other bacteria.

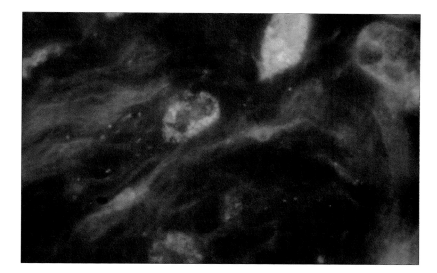

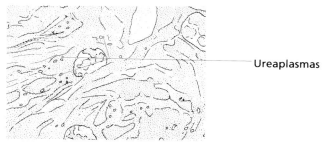

Ureaplasmas

- The demonstration of inflammatory cells and ureaplasmas in amniotic fluid over a 2-month period in the absence of other demonstrable microorganisms
- The direct demonstration of ureaplasmas alone in inflammatory infiltrates in the fetal membranes at the time of premature delivery.

The isolation of U. urealyticum from the placenta is significantly associated with histologic chorioamnionitis and funisitis, stillbirth, and perinatal morbidity and mortality. Individual case reports indicate that, at least sometimes, the infection is causal. Isolation of ureaplasmas from the placenta is inversely related to gestational age and birth weight.

PERIPARTUM INFECTIONS

M. hominis and U. urealyticum are proven causes of postpartum endometritis and are two of the most common causes of postpartum fever. M. hominis and U. urealyticum are both known to cause postabortal fever. These infections are often self-limited and do not require treatment. However, M. hominis septicemia results in a longer hospital stay, and in some cases results in suppurative septic arthritis and postcesarean wound infections.

M. hominis has been isolated from the joints of women who develop acute, suppurative arthritis following childbirth, with the onset of arthritis occurring from 6 hours to 3 weeks after delivery. In most cases, the organism was isolated not only from affected joints but also from blood.

DISEASES OF THE NEWBORN

Respiratory Disease

U. urealyticum and M. hominis are causes of congenital pneumonia and respiratory disease in the newborn (*Fig. 7.18*). In particular, U. urealyticum is a significant cause of respiratory disease in very-low-birth-weight infants. Infants whose birth weights are less than 1,000 g, and in whom ureaplasmas have been isolated from the lower respiratory tract within 24 hours of birth, are twice as likely to develop chronic lung disease and twice as likely to die as are infants of similar birth weights, who are uninfected, or infants weighing more than 1,000 g. Pneumonia and sepsis due to U. urealyticum can be associated with persistent pulmonary hypertension of the newborn. Evidence indicates that many ureaplasmal and M. hominis respiratory infections are acquired *in utero*.

U. urealyticum and M. hominis isolated from tracheal aspirates are likely to be true infections of the lower respiratory tract, since most strains are isolated in pure culture and are often concomitantly isolated from blood. It is not thought that the tracheal isolates are merely due to contamination from the nasopharynx, because of the discrepancy in the isolation rates between the two sites. U. urealyticum has been isolated more often from endotracheal aspirates than from nasopharyngeal swabs. Furthermore, M. hominis has been isolated from as many as 11% of endotracheal aspirates from infants weighing less than 2,500 g with respiratory disease, but rarely from the nasopharynx of these infants. Further evidence that tracheal isolates represent true infection of the lower respiratory tract includes initial isolation from tracheal aspirates in numbers exceeding 10^3 CFUs, and sometimes more than 10^6 CFUs, and repeated isolations of the organisms from tracheal aspirates over several months. The CSF of infants with respiratory disease is often found to be positive for U. urealyticum and M. hominis, again indicating the invasive nature of these organisms in preterm infants.

CNS and Other Systemic Infections

Both U. urealyticum and M. hominis cause meningitis in the newborn. Although their overall prevalence as CNS pathogens has not been thoroughly evaluated, recent evidence suggests that they may be among the most common causes of CSF infections in premature infants within the first few days of life. Congenital infection has been documented in some cases (*Fig. 7.19*).

U. urealyticum in the CSF is significantly associated with severe intraventricular hemorrhage and is often found in the presence of hydrocephalus. Chronic CSF infection of more than one month's duration has been observed with both M. hominis and U. urealyticum. Changes in the CSF may be similar to those seen in bacterial meningitis, namely low glucose, elevated protein, and mononuclear or polymorphonuclear pleocytosis, or there may be no abnormalities detected whatsoever. The range of infection varies from a mild subclinical course with no sequelae to more severe neurologic damage with permanent handicaps.

M. hominis is also a cause of pericardial effusion, adenitis, and subcutaneous abscesses, associated with breaks in the skin due to fetal-monitoring electrodes or forceps wounds.

BACTEREMIA AND OTHER EXTRAGENITAL INFECTIONS

There are numerous individual reports of both M. hominis and U. urealyticum gaining access to the bloodstream. In the case of U. urealyticum, this has been reported in cases of postabortal and postpartum bacteremia, as well as in newborn infants with respiratory distress and/or pneumonia. Bacteremia due to M. hominis has been demonstrated in a variety of conditions following renal transplantation, trauma, and genitourinary manipulations. Wound infections, brain abscesses, and osteomyelitis have also been reported.

The true incidence of extragenital infections caused by either ureaplasmas or M. hominis is unknown as these organisms are not sought routinely. Most reported cases have been discovered by 'accident' due to the occasional

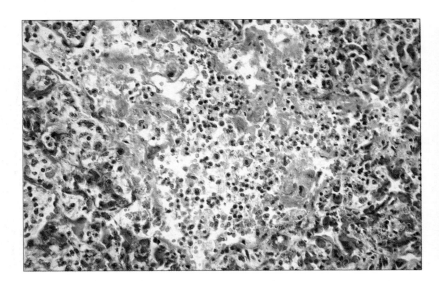

Fig. 7.18 Lung tissue (hematoxylin and eosin × 100) collected at autopsy from a 1-week-old term infant. *U. urealyticum* was isolated in pure culture from blood, tracheal aspirate, and pleural fluid prior to death, and from lung and brain tissue at post mortem. There is a mixed mononuclear and polymorphonuclear cell infiltrate with abundant macrophages, fibrin deposition, and early interstitial fibrosis.

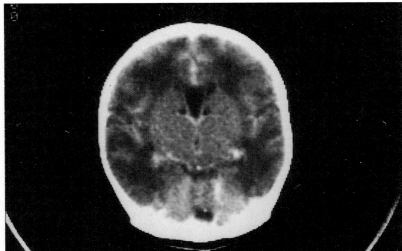

Fig. 7.19 Cranial CT scan of an infant 9 days after birth. *M. hominis* was isolated from the CSF 6 days after birth. There is decreased attenuation, predominantly involving the supratentorial white matter symmetrically, with a few punctate lesions of increased attenuation suggestive of small focal hemorrhage or early calcification. These findings are compatible with diffuse intrauterine infection or a degenerative process.

growth of *M. hominis* on blood agar and in routine blood cultures, or after specific mycoplasmal cultures had been set up following the exclusion of other possible infectious causes.

ARTHRITIS AND OTHER EXTRAGENITAL DISEASE IN IMMUNOCOMPROMISED HOSTS

There is evidence to suggest that mycoplasmas may be responsible for most cases of arthritis in individuals with agammaglobulinemia, since these organisms can be isolated repeatedly from the joints in the absence of any other microbial agent.

In many reported cases, the arthritis was persistent, lasting from several months to over a year. Aggressive, erosive arthritis that progresses in the face of anti-inflammatory therapy and γ-globulin replacement can occur. In some cases involving *U. urealyticum*, the arthritis is associated with subcutaneous abscesses, persistent urethritis, and chronic urethrocystitis/cystitis. Most cases have required aggressive antibiotic therapy, but some of the strains involved are, or have become, resistant to multiple antibiotics.

Septic arthritis, surgical wound infections, septicemia, and peritonitis due to *M. hominis* appear to occur rather frequently in patients following organ transplantation and in other types of patients undergoing immunosuppressive therapy. Sternal wound infections due to *M. hominis* in heart–lung transplant patients seem to be particularly common. Polyarthritis with recovery of both *U. urealyticum* and *M. hominis* has been seen in a kidney allograft patient on an immunosuppressive regimen. However, further evidence that ureaplasmas cause a problem in immunosuppressed patients or in those with AIDS is lacking.

LABORATORY TESTS

Many infections caused by mycoplasmas are discovered accidentally, either by observing the presence of *M. hominis* growing on blood agar, or because of treatment failure with antibiotics directed at common bacterial pathogens but ineffective against mycoplasmas. Unfortunately, a mycoplasmal etiology is often considered only as a last resort.

A mycoplasmal etiology should be considered in diseases in which these organisms have been shown to play a role and when common bacteria have neither been revealed by Gram stain nor isolated. For conditions in which a mycoplasmal etiology has not been proven, it is difficult to justify either examination for the organisms or treatment. In particular, isolation of either *M. hominis* or *U. urealyticum* from the lower female genital tract or urine (other than that collected by catheter or suprapubic aspirations) is not meaningful.

Mycoplasmas are very demanding in terms of laboratory culture requirements. The diagnosis of mycoplasmal infections in general bacteriology laboratories is hampered because the organisms are not visible on Gram stain, reliable culture media specifically designed for mycoplasmal growth have not been available commercially, and the organisms grow poorly or not at all in conventional bacteriologic media. *M. hominis* can be recovered occasionally from blood cultures or other clinical material without special techniques, but this approach is unreliable. Ureaplasmas, *M. genitalium*, *M. fermentans*, and *M. penetrans* are more fastidious than *M. hominis* and cannot be recovered from clinical material unless specific techniques and media are used. If a mycoplasmal infection is suspected, care should be taken to collect a suitable specimen, to ensure that it is transported or stored under conditions known to maintain mycoplasmal viability, and to ensure that its examination is performed by a laboratory experienced in the cultural isolation and identification or detection of mycoplasmas by PCR. Reliable information will be obtained only if these conditions are met.

SPECIMENS FOR CULTURE: ANATOMIC SITES

Liquid specimens, including blood, synovial fluid, CSF, urine, prostatic secretions, sputum, pleural fluid, or tracheal secretions, are acceptable for mycoplasmal culture depending on the nature of the clinical condition. Other suitable specimens include placenta or any tissue collected from a biopsy or at autopsy (brain, lung, liver, kidney) if there is reason to suspect the presence of mycoplasmas.

SPECIMEN COLLECTION AND TRANSPORT

Only calcium alginate-, dacron-, or polyester-tipped swabs should be used, and the swab must always be extracted from the specimen. Blood should be collected free of anticoagulants.

Unlike many bacteria, mycoplasmas, due to their lack of a cell wall, are extremely susceptible to adverse environmental conditions, especially drying, osmotic changes, and toxic metabolites. Particular care must be taken to ensure that specimens are not subjected to extreme environmental fluctuations. No specific transport medium is necessary for tissue or fluid specimens if they can be inoculated directly onto mycoplasmal medium within a reasonable period of time (i.e., no more than 1 hour after collection). However, if specimens are allowed to remain at room temperature and are not inoculated into appropriate transport media, this may result in a significant loss of mycoplasmal viability or overgrowth of bacterial contaminants. When possible, specific mycoplasmal medium such as Shepard's 10 B broth should be provided for direct inoculation of clinical specimens at the time they are collected. If specimens are collected in a facility that does not have immediate access to mycoplasmal broth for transport, satisfactory alternatives include 2SP medium (0.2 M sucrose in 0.02 M phosphate buffer, pH 7.2), trypticase soy broth with 0.5% bovine serum albumin, and commercially available Stuart's medium. Body fluids should be inoculated in an approximately 1:10 ratio (usually 0.1 ml fluid per 0.9 ml broth transport medium). Ideally, some uninoculated material should also be sent to the laboratory. Specimens should be kept refrigerated at 4°C and protected from drying in a sealed container until they can be transported to the laboratory. If transport is not possible within a maximum of 24 hours after collection, the specimen should be stored at −70°C and transported frozen on dry ice. Mycoplasmas are stable for indefinite periods if kept frozen at −70°C in a stable protein-containing supporting medium, such as 10 B broth. Storage at −20°C is less reliable in that a significant gradual loss in titer of organisms may occur.

DETECTION BY CULTIVATION AND POLYMERASE CHAIN REACTION

Although by definition mycoplasmas are free-living (capable of growth on cell-free media), they are fastidious and demanding in their requirements for special media. Various media are available. There are indications that those sold commercially are useful but continued thorough evaluations in a clinical setting are required. In using any medium, but in particular one obtained commercially, it is important to exclude mycoplasmal contamination. Fetal calf serum and horse serum used in most media are occasionally contaminated with mycoplasmas of animal origin.

Mycoplasmas are very sensitive to inhibitors present in some batches of horse serum, yeast extract, and even mycoplasmal media bases, and it is common for the standard medium in a laboratory to be temporarily inadequate for cultivation of mycoplasmas. Without proof of adequacy, negative cultures have little meaning. It is essential that rigorous quality-control procedures are followed, using recent clinical isolates and stock strains (including multiple serotypes, especially with ureaplasmas). A reference mycoplasma laboratory should be consulted before obtaining any specimen if a reliable, experienced laboratory is not locally available.

Clinical specimens for mycoplasmal culture should always be diluted serially in broth to at least 10^{-3} and each dilution inoculated onto agar. Dilution is necessary to overcome potential inhibitory substances or metabolites, including antibiotics, which may be present in the body fluid or tissue, and to facilitate quantitative estimation of the number of organisms present. In theory, greater isolation sensitivity may be obtained by centrifuging urine and performing serial dilutions on an aliquot from the sediment. Tissues should preferably be minced rather than ground for cultivation to circumvent potential growth inhibitors that are more likely to be released with grinding.

Mycoplasmas isolated from the genitourinary tract are very different organisms with their own unique metabolic properties and cultivation requirements. They have different pH ranges for optimal growth, as well as different biochemical substrates from which they derive energy. *U. urealyticum* generates ATP by urea hydrolysis, *M. hominis* metabolizes arginine to ammonia, and *M. genitalium* metabolizes glucose. *M. fermentans* and *M. penetrans* hydrolyze arginine and ferment glucose. No single medium formulation will optimally support the growth of all these organisms. Mycoplasmal growth medium ordinarily contains animal serum, peptones, yeast extract, and metabolic substrates such as glucose, arginine, and urea. Shepard's 10 B broth and A8 agar have been successfully employed for several years for cultivation of both *M. hominis* and *U. urealyticum* (*Fig. 7.20*) . SP-4 broth and agar will support the growth of *M. hominis*, *U. urealyticum*, *M. fermentans*, *M. penetrans*, and *M. genitalium* with appropriate pH and additives (*Fig. 7.21*). Antibiotics, such as penicillin or nystatin, are routinely incorporated into the media to inhibit bacterial and fungal contamination.

Very little information is available concerning the recovery of *M. genitalium*, *M. fermentans*, and *M. penetrans* from clinical material. They are thought to grow best in an atmosphere containing 95% nitrogen and CO_2, but extremely slow multiplication, in particular that of *M. genitalium*, requires that incubation be prolonged over a period of weeks.

M. hominis and *U. urealyticum* are much easier to recover from clinical specimens. Their relatively rapid growth rates make the identification of most positive cultures possible within 2–5 days. Broth cultures may be incubated at 37°C under atmospheric conditions, and agar plates under 5% CO_2 in air or 95% N_2. Ureaplasmas, in particular, are susceptible to a rapid, steep death-phase in culture, which is likely to result from a combination of urea depletion, ammonia production, and elevated pH due to urease activity. The presence of growth in 10 B medium is suggested by an alkaline shift due to the urease activity of ureaplasmas or arginine hydrolysis by *M. hominis*, causing the phenol-red indicator to turn from yellow to pink (*Fig. 7.20*). The presence of growth in SP-4 broth is evident by a red-to-yellow (acidic) shift due to metabolism of glucose, or red to deeper red (alkaline) by arginine hydrolysis (*Fig. 7.21*). Broth cultures showing color changes should be subcultured to agar. This combination of broth-to-agar inoculation technique has been shown to be the most sensitive method for recovery of genital mycoplasmas.

Primers specific for each of the genital mycoplasmas have been identified. Detection by PCR appears to be the method of choice for *M. genitalium* and *M. fermentans* which appear to be more fastidious.

SPECIES IDENTIFICATION

Colonies of *U. urealyticum* can be identified readily on A8 agar by urease production in the presence of $CaCl_2$ indicator (*Figs. 7.22* and *7.23*). *M.*

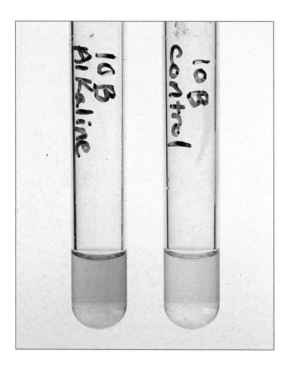

Fig. 7.20 Shepard's 10 B broth. This broth, containing phenol-red pH indicator, is used to cultivate *M. hominis* and *U. urealyticum*. At a pH of 6.0, the broth is yellow. Growth of *U. urealyticum* or *M. hominis* with hydrolysis of urea or arginine, respectively, results in an elevation of the pH and a change in color from yellow to pink without a significant increase in turbidity.

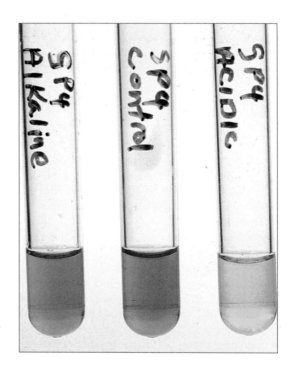

Fig. 7.21 SP-4 broth. This broth may be used for cultivation of *M. hominis*, *U. urealyticum*, *M. fermentans*, *M. penetrans*, or *M. genitalium*. It is normally prepared at a pH of 7.4–7.5. Growth of *M. hominis* with arginine hydrolysis elevates the pH, resulting in a color change from red to deep fuschia, while growth of a glucose-metabolizing mycoplasma, such as *M. genitalium*, results in a decrease in pH due to acidic end-products and a change in color from red to yellow.

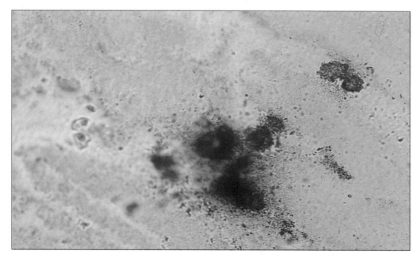

Fig. 7.22 Colonies of *U. urealyticum* growing on A8 agar. The granular brown appearance is due to urease activity in the presence of $CaCl_2$ indicator. The colonies are rather amorphous, as is often the case with ureaplasma colonies produced as a result of an initial isolation attempt from clinical material.

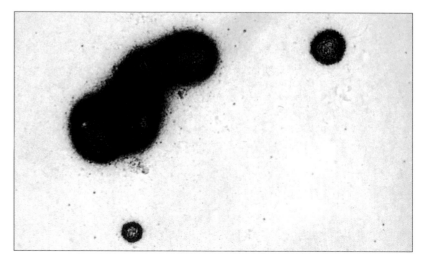

Fig. 7.23 Colonies of *U. urealyticum* growing on A8 agar after several passages on artificial media. Note the characteristics of these discrete colonies compared with those on the initial isolation plate shown in 7.22.

hominis colonies are urease-negative and have a typical 'fried egg' appearance (*Figs. 7.24* and *7.25*). Unlike conventional bacteria, minute mycoplasmal colonies require a stereomicroscope to determine their presence and characterize their morphology.

In addition to *M. hominis*, other mycoplasmal species that may have similar growth requirements may also be present in clinical specimens and be morphologically indistinguishable. There are no biochemical tests that can readily distinguish between the large-colony mycoplasmal species, so serologic or PCR identification methods must be used.

Serologic tests are of two basic types. In the first group, there are procedures using living organisms, in which antiserum inhibits the growth or metabolic functions of the mycoplasma species or type against which it has been prepared. Examples include the growth-inhibition method, metabolism-inhibition method (*Fig. 7.26*), and mycoplasmacidal test. The growth-inhibition method is specific but rather insensitive, making it useful for speciation of mycoplasmas but is of limited, if any, value for antibody measurement. Metabolism-inhibition and mycoplasmacidal tests are sufficiently specific to identify organisms and are also sensitive enough for antibody detection. In a second broad group of serologic methods, organisms are identified by demonstrating the reaction of specific antibody to whole fixed organisms or their antigens. The most widely used of these procedures is colony immunofluorescence.

A problem with any of these techniques is the existence of multiple serotypes of *M. hominis*, *M. fermentans*, and *U. urealyticum*. The many serotypes react specifically with antibody, requiring batteries of antisera if all strains are to be correctly identified.

SEROTYPING

There is some suggestion that certain serotypes of *U. urealyticum* are more likely to be associated with disease, but definitive evidence is lacking. Furthermore, the currently available methods of serotyping are not practical for routine use. However, recent development of PCR technologies allows biotyping and serotyping.

STAINS

Stains that bind to DNA can often aid in detection of mycoplasmas prior to culture results (*see Fig. 7.15*). Extranuclear fluorescence in fluid specimens treated with DNA fluorochrome stains, such as Hoechst 33258, can be used to identify the presence of microorganisms. DNA fluorochrome will stain any prokaryotic DNA present. A Gram stain can be performed to exclude bacteria. Comparison of the specimen with a known positive control will help establish the presence of a mycoplasma, but confirmation with culture is essential for a definitive diagnosis.

Mycoplasmas in exudates can be stained with Giemsa, but most often such preparations are difficult to interpret due to cellular debris and artifacts. Colonies on agar can be more easily visualized by using the Dienes stain (*see Fig. 7.25*).

SEROLOGIC DIAGNOSIS

Almost without exception, patients with invasive *M. hominis* infections seroconvert or show a significant rise in existing antibody. This response can be measured by the metabolism-inhibition assay (*see Fig. 7.26*), enzyme-linked immunosorbent assays, or other serologic procedures. Both acute and

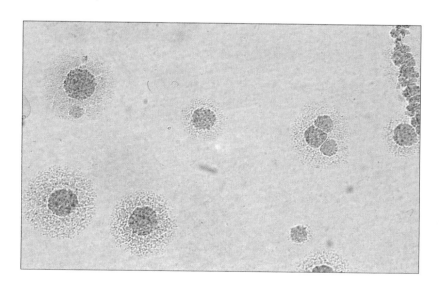

Fig. 7.24 Unstained colonies of *M. hominis* on A8 agar. Mycoplasmal colonies on agar typically exhibit a 'fried egg' appearance due to growth in the agar in the center of the colony. Colonies measure 50–500 µm in diameter. Colonial morphology is dependent to a large extent on local growth conditions and media components.

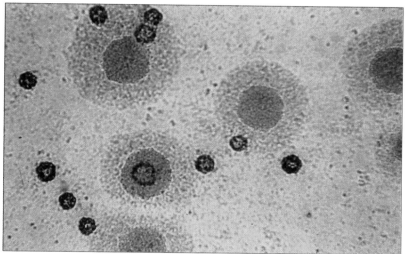

Fig. 7.25 Colonies of *M. hominis* and *U. urealyticum* on A8 agar stained by the Dienes method.

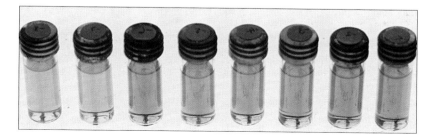

Fig. 7.26 An example of metabolism-inhibition test results. This test is essentially a growth-inhibition technique carried out in liquid medium. Organisms that multiply in liquid medium containing a specific substrate metabolize the substrate, and the products alter the pH of the medium as indicated by a change in color of an appropriate pH indicator. Specific antibody inhibits multiplication of the organisms and therefore indirectly prevents the color change from occurring. The test may be used for determining levels of specific antibody by using a constant number of organisms and multiple dilutions of serum. The titer of the serum is recorded as the highest dilution that prevents the change in color of the medium. In addition, the test can be used for the classification and characterization of clinical isolates by using antisera with known titers.

convalescent sera should be evaluated, with results based on single specimens being difficult or impossible to interpret. Due to the ubiquity of most mycoplasmas in humans, it should be realized that the detection of antibodies alone cannot be considered significant.

The assays mentioned are available for detection of antibodies to *U. urealyticum*. At present, however, the determination of serologic responses is limited to research laboratories. Until more specific information is available about the usefulness of antibody detection, serodiagnosis cannot be recommended for routine diagnostic purposes.

TREATMENT

Some discussion of appropriate chemotherapy is necessary as *M. hominis* and *U. urealyticum* are recognized causes of some genital and extragenital disease entities. Patients should be evaluated for mycoplasmas if they are suspected of having a condition for which mycoplasmas can be etiologically significant (i.e. urethritis in men, PID in women, meningitis in newborns). A positive culture for either *M. hominis* or *U. urealyticum*, particularly in the absence of other microorganisms, is sufficient justification for treatment in most instances. Empiric treatment may be necessary in conditions, such as PID, in which cultures of the affected site may not be readily available, and also because of the general lack of suitable mycoplasmal diagnostic facilities in many areas. However, antimicrobial resistance among clinical isolates of both *M. hominis* and *U. urealyticum* means that chemotherapy without validation by *in vitro* susceptibility testing is risky. The most widely used technique to test the drug susceptibility of mycoplasmas and ureaplasmas is the microtiter broth-dilution method (*Fig. 7.27*).

A summary of the antimicrobial susceptibilities of *U. urealyticum* and *M. hominis* is given in *Figure 7.28*. *M. hominis* and *U. urealyticum* are resistant to sulfonamides, trimethoprim, and all antibiotics that act by inhibiting cell-wall synthesis. Both organisms are often resistant to aminoglycosides and chloramphenicol as well. *M. hominis* is susceptible to clindamycin and resistant to erythromycin, while the reverse is true for ureaplasmas. This differential susceptibility is sometimes helpful in separating mixed cultures so that the additional drug susceptibilities of each mycoplasmal component can be tested. Tetracyclines are the drugs of choice for *M. hominis* and *U. urealyticum* infections if there are no contraindications. However, as many as 40% of clinical isolates of *M. hominis* may be tetracycline resistant. Approximately 80–90% of ureaplasmal strains are sensitive to tetracycline, though the incidence of resistant strains may be increasing. If a mycoplasma is resistant to one drug in the tetracycline group, it is usually resistant to others as well. Erythromycin-resistant strains also occur but high-level resistance is thought

to be uncommon. There may be a correlation between tetracycline resistance and erythromycin resistance. Doxycycline is better absorbed than tetracycline and has a longer half-life.

Standard doses of tetracyclines usually penetrate the meninges and synovial fluid and achieve levels exceeding the MIC for susceptible mycoplasmal or ureaplasmal strains. Clindamycin provides an alternative therapy for *M. hominis* infections not involving the CNS, in which there is a contraindication to using tetracycline, or in cases of tetracycline resistance. In treating conditions known to be sexually transmitted, such as urethritis, the index case as well as all sexual contacts should receive antibiotics to prevent reinfection.

The infant with *M. hominis* meningitis presents a difficult therapeutic situation. Normally, tetracycline therapy is contraindicated in children of less than 8 years of age, but no other currently available drug is approved for use or shown to be effective in this condition. There are precedents for using intravenous tetracycline or doxycycline to treat infants with mycoplasmal or ureaplasmal meningitis, in which the organisms were eradicated.

Erythromycin is the drug of choice for ureaplasmal infections in neonates. Although erythromycin penetrates poorly into the CNS, *U. urealyticum* has been eradicated from CSF with erythromycin in one instance following treatment failure with doxycycline.

The development of resistance in many strains of *U. urealyticum* and *M. hominis* to the aforementioned 'first-line' antibiotics has prompted investigation of many new antimicrobial compounds as they become available.

Clarithromycin and azithromycin have *in vitro* activities against *U. urealyticum* but not *M. hominis*. No published data are available concerning the *in vivo* clinical or microbiologic efficacy of clarithromycin against *U. urealyticum*. However, a single dose of oral azithromycin has been approved for treatment of urethritis due to *Chlamydia trachomatis*. It has been shown to be as clinically effective as doxycycline in patients with urethritis due to *U. urealyticum*, which reflects its *in vitro* activity against this organism.

An advantage of fluoroquinolones is that they are not affected by tetracycline or macrolide resistance in mycoplasmas. Ciprofloxacin is generally less active against *M. hominis* and *U. urealyticum* than ofloxacin. A 7-day course of oral ofloxacin appears to be adequate for treatment of urethritis, but most studies have focused on *C. trachomatis* rather than *U. urealyticum*. Clinical trials of women with uncomplicated PID have shown that monotherapy with ofloxacin is effective, though additional studies with more extensive microbiologic investigations are needed before this drug can be recommended for routine use in PID. Sexual contacts of the index case of urethritis should also receive treatment, just as for any other type of STD.

Guidelines for the duration and routes of drug administration have not been systematically evaluated for either local urogenital or extragenital systemic mycoplasmal or ureaplasmal infections. These should be determined

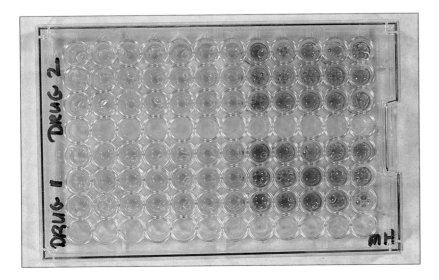

Fig. 7.27 An example of microtiter broth-dilution antibiotic sensitivity test results. This test allows large numbers of isolates to be tested simultaneously against several antibiotics and provides reproducible results. The method depends on the inhibition of mycoplasmal growth by specific dilutions of antibiotic. Growth and inhibition of growth is indicated by the presence and absence, respectively, of a color change in the culture medium containing phenol-red pH indicator.

individually according to the type and location of infection, as well as the age and clinical condition of the patient and specific recommendations of the manufacturer. *Figure 7.29* outlines various oral treatment options. In general, treatment for 10–14 days is recommended. For neonates with meningitis or other systemic infections, parenteral therapy using the same dosage guidelines is advisable, with follow-up cultures to ensure eradication of the organisms. Immunosuppressed persons with systemic mycoplasmal infection, including

the joints and the urinary or respiratory tract, may harbor multiple-resistant strains. Prolonged parenteral therapy, possibly requiring increased dosages, followed by weeks to months of oral therapy may be necessary. This may seem overly aggressive, but previously published cases and personal experience indicate that such infections can be extremely difficult to eradicate. Arthritis due to these organisms can eventually lead to progressive irreversible joint damage if left alone or treated inadequately.

SUSCEPTIBILITIES OF *UREAPLASMA UREALYTICUM* AND *MYCOPLASMA HOMINIS* TO VARIOUS ANTIMICROBIALS

ANTIMICROBIAL	U. UREALYTICUM MIC* (µg/ml)	M. HOMINIS MIC* (µg/ml)
Doxycycline	0.05–1	0.1–0.4
Minocycline	0.03	0.4–0.8
Oxytetracycline	0.4–2	0.5–6.4
Tetracycline	0.05–8	0.2–6.8
Erythromycin	0.1–1.6	> 1000
Clarithromycin	≤ 0.004– > 256	16– > 256
Azithromycin	0.5–4	4–64
Clindamycin	1–50	0.2–1.6
Lincomycin	25– > 500	0.2–1.6
Rosaramicin	0.008–4	< 0.025–0.4
Spiramycin	32	2–16
Chloramphenicol	0.4–3.1	4–25
Gentamicin	3.1–12.5	1.6–12.5
Kanamycin	1.6–12.5	1.6–12.5
Streptomycin	0.4–3.1	4–32
Spectinomycin	16	< 0.3–10
Nitrofurantoin	12.5– > 1000	500
Polymixin	12.5– > 1000	1000
Rifampicin	> 1000	> 100–7100
Vancomycin	500– > 1000	500– > 1000
Penicillin	> 4000	> 1000
Trimethoprim/ sulfamethoxazole	Inactive	Inactive
Ciprofloxacin	0.5– > 64	0.125–4
Lomefloxacin	0.5–16	0.5–8
Ofloxacin	0.2–25	0.125–64

* MIC = minimal inhibitory concentration

Fig. 7.28 Susceptibilities of *U. urealyticum* and *M. hominis* to various antimicrobials.

ORAL TREATMENT OPTIONS FOR MYCOPLASMAL AND UREAPLASMAL INFECTIONS

DRUG	ADULTS	CHILDREN
Tetracycline	250–500 mg qid	25–50 mg/kg/day, divided into 4 equal doses
Doxycycline	Loading doses of 200 mg; then 100 mg/bid	Loading doses of 4 mg/kg, then 2–4 mg/kg/day divided into 1–2 doses
Clindamycin*	150–450 mg qid	10–25 mg/kg/day, divided into 3 to 4 equal doses
Erythromycin**	250–500 mg qid	20–50 mg/kg/day, divided into 4 equal doses
Azithromycin **	1 g single dose	not recommended
Ofloxacin	200–400 mg bid	not recommended

* Effective only for M. hominis

** Effective only for U. urealyticum

Fig. 7.29 Oral treatment options for mycoplasmal and ureaplasmal infections.

BIBLIOGRAPHY

Cassell GH, Baseman JB, Bove J, Lo S-C, Montagnier L, Quackenbush RL, Taylor-Robinson D, Tully JG: The changing role of mycoplasmas in respiratory disease and AIDS. *Clin Infect Dis* **17** (suppl.):S315, 1993.

Cassell GH, Waites KB, Crouse DT: Genital mycoplasmal infections. In: Remington JS, Klein JO (eds): *Infectious Diseases of the Fetus and Newborn Infant*. Philadelphia, W. B. Saunders, pp 619–670, 1994.

Furr PM, Taylor-Robinson D, Webster ADB: Mycoplasmas and ureaplasmas in patients with hypogammaglobulinemia and their role in arthritis: microbiological observations over 20 years. *Ann Rheum Dis* **53**:183–187, 1994.

Krause DC, Taylor-Robinson D: Mycoplasmas which infect humans. In: Maniloff J, McElhaney RN, Finch LR, Baseman JB (eds): *Mycoplasmas. Molecular Biology and Pathogenesis*. Washington DC, American Society for Microbiology Press, pp 417–444, 1992.

Lo S-C: Mycoplasmas and AIDS. In: Maniloff J, McElhaney RN, Finch LR, Baseman JB (eds): *Mycoplasmas. Molecular Biology and Pathogenesis*. Washington DC, American Society for Microbiology Press, pp 525–545, 1992.

Lo S-C, Hayes MM, Wang RY-H, Pierce PF, Kotani H, Shih JW-K: Newly discovered mycoplasma isolated from patients infected with HIV. *Lancet* **338**:1415–1418, 1991.

Shepard MC: Culture media for ureaplasmas. In: Razin S, Tully JG(eds): *Methods in Mycoplasmology*. New York, Academic Press, Vol I, pp 137–146, 1983.

CHAPTER EIGHT

Pelvic Inflammatory Disease

R Rice, D Schwartz, J Knapp, and J Paavonen

INTRODUCTION

Pelvic inflammatory disease (PID) is a serious and costly condition among women of reproductive age. It usually results from infection of the uterus, fallopian tubes, ovaries, and the surrounding structures, and is associated with ascending or contiguous spread of microorganisms from the lower genital tract and cervix (*Fig. 8.1*). Since the 1960s, as the incidence and recognition of certain STDs such as gonorrhea and chlamydial infection have increased, so has the estimated incidence of PID. Despite a continuing decrease in the number of reported cases of gonorrhea in the USA, an increasing proportion of gonococcal infections has been caused by antibiotic-resistant organisms. Likewise, more than four million cases of chlamydial infection are estimated to occur in the USA each year. Efforts to prevent PID and its related complications should therefore be based on strategies which more effectively detect, treat, and reduce the transmission of STDs.

EPIDEMIOLOGY

Globally, PID is an important problem that contributes to considerable morbidity and has significant adverse effects on female reproductive health. At least 20–25% of women who develop PID will experience serious and chronic sequelae such as chronic pelvic pain, ectopic pregnancy, and impaired fertility. In the USA, the estimated direct costs for PID and its sequelae exceeded $2 billion in 1990 (*Fig. 8.2*), while the combined annual direct and indirect costs for PID are projected to exceed $9 billion by the year 2000 (*Fig. 8.3*). Based on estimates from the National Center for Health Statistics (NCHS) at the CDC, approximately 200,000–250,000 women are hospitalized for PID in the USA each year (*Fig. 8.4*), and annually at least one million women seek outpatient care for PID and related complications. Despite an overall trend towards a decline in PID hospitalizations, the number of ambulatory visits to private physicians has remained virtually unchanged (*Fig. 8.5*).

DEFINITION OF PELVIC INFLAMMATORY DISEASE

'Clinical syndrome found in women, resulting from infection of the uterus, fallopian tubes, ovaries, peritoneal surfaces and surrounding anatomic structures, and often associated with ascending or contiguous spread of microorganisms from the lower genital tract and uterine cervix.'

Fig. 8.1 PID is a commonly diagnosed complication of ascending genital tract infection and is frequently associated with pre-existing or concomitant gonococcal or chlamydial infection.

ESTIMATED DIRECT COSTS FOR PID AND ITS ASSOCIATED SEQUELAE (USA, 1990)

CATEGORY OF DISEASE	ESTIMATED DIRECT COSTS ($)
Inpatient PID	1,593,610,000
Outpatient PID	33,951,000
Infertility	187,195,000
Ectopic Pregnancy	361,548,000

Fig. 8.2 The estimated direct costs for PID and associated sequelae, such as ectopic pregnancy and infertility, were estimated to exceed $2 billion in the USA alone in 1990.

Fig. 8.3 The US Public Health Service estimates that total direct and indirect costs for PID will exceed $9 billion by the year 2000.

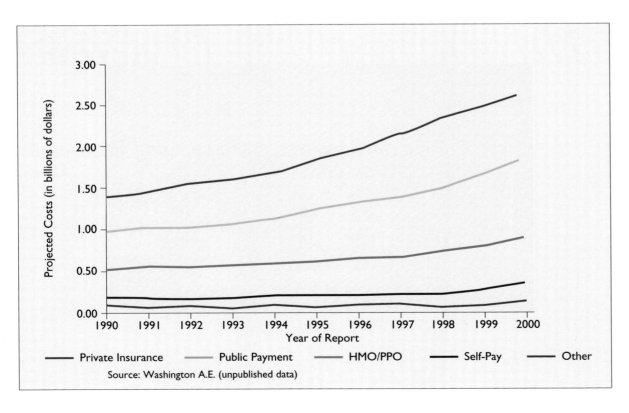

Certain factors may increase a woman's risk for PID. These are young age, socioeconomic status, use of an intrauterine device (IUD), and noncompliance with STD treatment (*Fig. 8.6*). Several authors have reported that the use of oral hormonal contraceptives may decrease the risk for developing acute PID caused by certain organisms; the reasons for this association remain unclear. Other factors, such as douching and smoking, have been cited in selected studies but remain controversial.

MICROBIOLOGY

Traditionally, PID has been characterized as a major complication of genital tract infection caused by the sexually transmitted pathogens, *Neisseria gonorrhoeae* and *Chlamydia trachomatis* (*see Chapters 4* and *6*). However, various studies have demonstrated the recovery of other microorganisms,

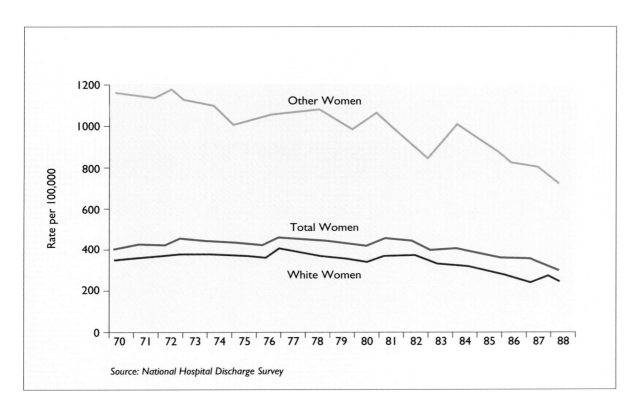

Fig. 8.4 Hospitalizations for PID are almost 250,000 per annum in the USA, though there has been a relative decline in the number of estimated hospitalizations for PID since 1986. This trend may reflect changing sources for PID hospital payments, a changing etiology and clinical severity of disease, or a shift in the utilization of outpatient and alternative health-care providers.

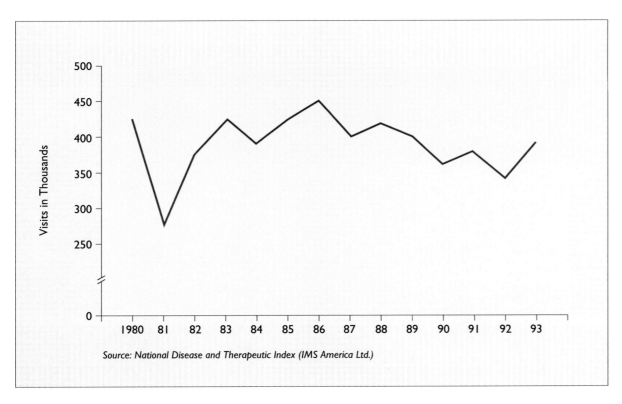

Fig. 8.5 Initial ambulatory visits to private physicians in the USA for PID have remained essentially unchanged over the last several years.

135

particularly anaerobes from the lower genital tract, facultative bacteria, and coliforms. Earlier studies suggested that most cases of PID were the result of a preceding gonococcal infection of the lower genital tract. *Figure 8.7* provides an overview of the isolation of gonococci from women with PID in the preantibiotic and antibiotic eras. In the 1970s and early 1980s, several authors suggested that not all PID was caused by the gonococcus and that other microorganisms including *C. trachomatis* were associated with the development of PID. *Figure 8.8* compares the results of studies on the identification of *C. trachomatis* in acute salpingitis. Recently, more attention has been directed to the microbiology of, and risk factors for, nongonococcal, nonchlamydial PID. In most series, the type of microorganisms (other than *N. gonorrhoeae* and *C. trachomatis*), that have been recovered from upper tract specimens, have been facultative anaerobes representing the endogenous vaginal and perineal microflora. These have included *Gardnerella vaginalis*, *Streptococcus agalactiae*, anerobic streptococci, *Peptostreptococcus* spp., *Fusobacterium* spp., *Bacteroides* spp. (other than *Bacteroides fragilis*), genital mycoplasmas and ureaplasmas, and coliforms (e.g. *Escherichia coli*) (*Fig. 8.9*). As well as these microorganisms, but found less often, are nongenital pathogens, such as *Haemophilus influenzae, H. parainfluenzae,* and *N. meningitidis,* which may be isolated from women with acute PID and salpingitis.

Other less commonly associated microorganisms include *Actinomyces* spp., which are typically linked to IUD usage. In less developed countries or populations with a high prevalence of tuberculosis, PID may be associated with *Mycobacterium tuberculosis*, due to dissemination of the microorganism via the bloodstream rather than via ascending spread from the lower genital tract. In some areas of the world, granulomatous salpingitis may also be caused by organisms such as *Schistosoma* spp.

POTENTIAL RISK FACTORS FOR PID

Demographic and social factors

    Age
    Socioeconomic status
    Marital status

Health behavior, contraception, and other factors*

    Intrauterine device
    Menstrual cycle
    Douching
    Smoking
    Alcohol and illicit drug use
    Treatment noncompliance
    Delayed partner referral

*Data on some factors remain controversial or inconclusive.

Fig. 8.6 Various studies have cited proven or suspected risk factors for the development of PID. Some risk factors, such as douching and smoking, vary and the data remain controversial.

FREQUENCY OF GONOCOCCAL ISOLATION IN SELECTED STUDIES OF PID FROM THE PREANTIBIOTIC AND ANTIBIOTIC ERAS

AUTHOR (YEAR)	NO. OF PID CASES	ISOLATION RATE (%)
Holtz (1930)	1262	33.0
Curtis (1931)	24	66.6
Hundley (1950)	80	41.2
Hedberry (1958)	216	44.0
Falk (1965)	283	41.0
Jacobsen (1969)	563	40.0
Eschenbach (1975)	204	45.0
Thompson (1976)	24	70.8
Soper (1994)	84	61.9

Fig. 8.7 Studies conducted in the preantibiotic and antibiotic eras have demonstrated a wide range of recovery rates for *N. gonorrhoeae* among women with PID.

CHLAMYDIA TRACHOMATIS IN ACUTE SALPINGITIS

STUDY	NUMBER OF PATIENTS	ENDOCERVIX		ISOLATED FROM: PERITONEAL CAVITY		4-FOLD SERUM ANTIBODIES	
Eilard	22	6	(27%)	*2/22	(9%)	5/22	(23%)
Mardh	53	19	(38%)	*6/20	(30%)	—	
Treharne	143	N.S.		N.S.		89/143	(62%)**
Paavonen	228	69	(30%)	—		—	
Eschenbach	100	20	(20%)	†1/54	(2%)	15/74	(20%)
Thompson	30	3	(10%)	*†3/10	(30%)	—	
Sweet	35	2	(6%)	*0/35	(0%)	8/35	(23%)

*Fallopian tubes   ** Had acute phase IgG≥1:64   †Culdocentesis

Fig. 8.8 The recognition of a nongonococcal etiology for PID led to numerous studies that identified *C. trachomatis* as an important etiologic agent for PID and salpingitis in the USA and Scandinavia.

CLINICAL MANIFESTATIONS

The clinical spectrum of PID ranges from endometritis to salpingitis, oophoritis, adnexitis, peritonitis, tubo-ovarian abscess, and perihepatitis. Lower abdominal pain, usually bilateral in nature, is a commonly reported clinical symptom or complaint of women who present with PID. Other common clinical complaints include abnormal and often profuse or grossly purulent vaginal discharge, dysuria, lower back pain, and abnormal vaginal bleeding (*Fig. 8.10*). Women who present with acute PID may also suffer from nausea, vomiting, fever, and prostration. Common findings on pelvic examination may include mucopurulent cervical discharge, uterine or cervical motion tenderness, and bilateral or occasionally unilateral adnexal tenderness or palpable mass. The minimal clinical and additional criteria for the diagnosis of PID are summarized in *Figs. 8.11* and *8.12*. Although clinical findings are highly sensitive for suspected PID, clinical signs and symptoms are at best only 65–70% specific when compared with laparoscopy, which is the 'gold standard' required for confirmatory diagnosis of PID (*Fig. 8.13*).

Clinically, PID must be differentiated from other abdominal and pelvic conditions, including (but not only) life-threatening conditions, such as acute appendicitis and ectopic pregnancy. In a small percentage of women, acute appendicitis or periappendicitis and PID may coexist, thus further complicating diagnosis and the usual management. Laparoscopy is considered the 'gold standard' for confirming a diagnosis of PID because it not only allows direct inspection of the fallopian tubes and surrounding pelvic anatomy (*Fig. 8.14*), but also enables microbiologic sampling of the upper genital tract (e.g. fallopian tube, ovary, and peritoneal fluid) for possible pathogens and other

MICROORGANISMS COMMONLY ISOLATED FROM UPPER GENITAL TRACT SPECIMENS OF WOMEN WITH PID

Sexually transmitted

Chlamydia trachomatis
Neisseria gonorrhoeae
Genital mycoplasmas

Nonsexually transmitted

Bacteroides
   disiens
   intermedius
   melanogenicus
Clostridium spp.
Coliforms
Eubacterium spp.
Fusobacterium spp.
Peptostreptococcus spp.
Prevotella spp.
Propionibacterium spp.
Others

Fig. 8.9 The sexually transmitted microorganisms, *Neisseria gonorrhoeae* and *Chlamydia trachomatis*, are usually associated with the development of PID. However, nonsexually transmitted microorganisms representing vaginal and gut anerobes, facultative bacteria and coliforms have been identified as potential pathogens for PID. Other microorganisms, such as *Haemophilus influenzae* and *H. parainfluenzae*, may be recovered from some cases of PID. Microorganisms that are associated with a granulomatous type of PID, but which are uncommon in North American and European studies of PID, include *Actinomyces* spp., *Mycobacterium tuberculosis*, and *Schistosoma* spp.

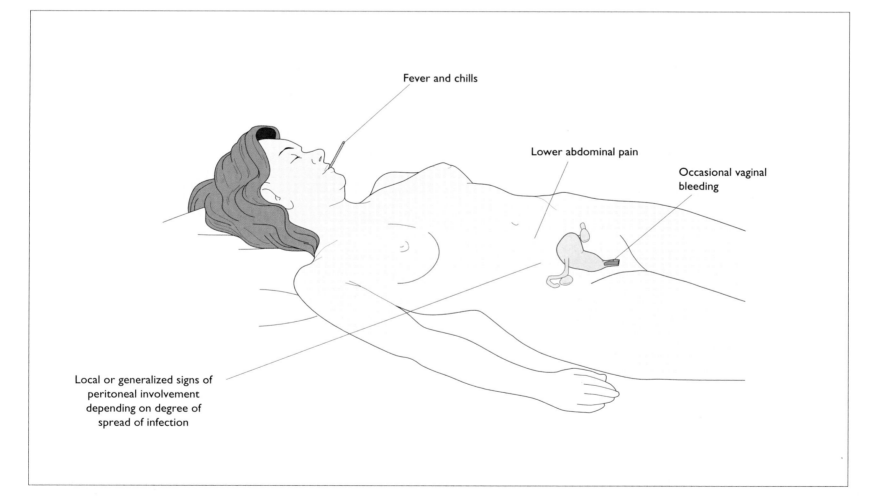

Fever and chills

Lower abdominal pain

Occasional vaginal bleeding

Local or generalized signs of peritoneal involvement depending on degree of spread of infection

Fig. 8.10 Clinical manifestations of acute PID range from lower abdominal pain and pelvic tenderness to fever and severe prostration with peripheral leukocytosis and an elevated erythrocyte sedimentation rate.

etiologic agents, without the risk of contamination of samples by vaginal flora. This contamination was a major problem associated with the older procedure of culdocentesis, which was often used in earlier studies of PID. Laparoscopy may be used to help characterize fallopian-tube inflammation and the severity of salpingitis (*Figs. 8.15* and *8.16*). Studies have demonstrated that the clinical diagnosis of PID may be incorrect in at least 30% of cases when compared with laparoscopic diagnosis. However, the routine use of laparoscopy to confirm a diagnosis of PID is prohibited by cost and availability, especially in the ambulatory or public health clinic setting where PID is often diagnosed. The accuracy of laparoscopy may not be 100% because of expectation bias or because laparoscapy may not detect subtle endosalpingitis. Endometrial biopsy is another diagnostic procedure which may be used in the diagnosis of PID to provide confirmatory histopathologic diagnosis of endometritis. In contrast to laparoscopy, endometrial biopsy can be performed on an outpatient basis and is considerably less invasive. Studies have found at least 90% correlation between the results of endometrial biopsy to confirm endometritis and laparoscopically confirmed salpingitis.

More recently, newer procedures, such as transvaginal sonography and high field magnetic resonance imaging (MRI), have been applied to assist in the diagnosis of PID.

MINIMUM CRITERIA FOR CLINICAL DIAGNOSIS OF PID

Lower abdominal tenderness

Bilateral adnexal tenderness

Cervical motion tenderness

Negative pregnancy test

Fig. 8.11 Minimum criteria required for a clinical diagnosis of PID.

ADDITIONAL CRITERIA USEFUL IN DIAGNOSING PID

ROUTINE

Fever >38.3°C (oral)

Abnormal vaginal discharge

Elevated ESR or CRP

Endocervical evidence of
N. gonorrhoeae or C. trachomatis

EXTENSIVE

Endometrial biopsy

Ultrasound-confirmed
tubo-ovarian abscess

Laparoscopy

Fig. 8.12 Additional criteria or evidence to support or confirm a diagnosis of PID.

CLINICAL DIAGNOSIS OF PID

CLINICAL FINDINGS	SENSITIVITY (%)[*]
Lower abdominal pain	94
Adnexal tenderness	92
Vaginal discharge	55
Pelvic mass	50
Fever (>38°C)	41

Clinical findings 65% specific in 814 cases assessed by laparoscopy.

Fig. 8.13 Clinical signs and symptoms such as lower abdominal pain and tenderness are highly sensitive for PID, but lack specificity. In the best clinical circumstances, when compared to laparoscopy, clinical findings are at best 65–70% specific.

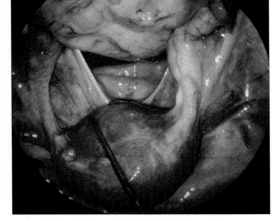

Fig. 8.14 A view through the laparoscope of the female internal pelvic organs and supporting structures (uterus, fallopian tubes, pelvic peritoneum, broad ligament).

SURGICAL EVIDENCE FOR THE DIAGNOSIS OF PID*

Tubal edema
Tubal exudate
Tubal hyperemia

By laparoscopy or laparotomy.

Fig. 8.15 Surgical evidence for salpingitis and PID.

LAPAROSCOPIC CRITERIA OF ACUTE PID

MINIMUM CRITERIA:
Erythema of fallopian tubes
Edema and swelling of fallopian tubes
Seropurulent exudate from fimbriae and/or on serosal surface of fallopian tubes

SCORING:
Mild: minimum criteria; tubes freely movable and patent
Moderate: minimum criteria more marked; tubes not freely movable; patency uncertain
Severe: inflammatory mass

Fig. 8.16 Laparoscopic criteria for scoring the severity of tubal inflammation and salpingitis.

PATHOGENESIS

Anatomically, the female genital tract is composed of the external and internal genitalia (*Fig. 8.17*). Internal genitalia include the vagina, uterus, fallopian tubes, and ovaries. Hormonal changes over the stages of a woman's life influence the mucosal components and cyclical environment of this system and also influence the risk for acquiring certain infections. The cervix, which is the lowest part of the uterus, is probably the most important structural and possibly a functional barrier to infectious agents that may ascend from the lower genital tract and vagina into the uterus. The external mucosal surface of the cervix (ectocervix), extends into the vagina, and consists of stratified, nonkeratinized, and squamous epithelial cells, which undergo cyclical modifications during the normal menstrual cycle in women of reproductive age. However, the endocervix has a mucosal surface consisting of a single stratum of mucous-secreting cuboidal or columnar epithelial cells. It has been hypothesized that cervical mucus may be a natural barrier to the ascending spread of microorganisms, such as *N. gonorrhoeae*, *C. trachomatis*, and endogenous vaginal bacteria into the uterus. The normal fallopian tubal mucosa also consists of ciliated and nonciliated epithelial cells (*Fig. 8.18*).

The mechanisms for the extension of infecting microorganisms into the upper female genital tract may vary according to the organism and continues to be a complex and controversial topic. In the setting of gonococcal PID and salpingitis, it is thought that infection probably extends via a direct canalicular route from the endocervix into the endometrium and subsequently into the fallopian tubes. This causes edema and incites an intense polymorphonuclear leukocyte response. In studies of gonococcal PID, the organism is more frequently recovered during and immediately after the menstrual period. Using *in vitro* organ system models and scanning electron microscopy (*Fig. 8.19*), it has been shown that the gonococcus readily attaches to the microvilli of nonciliated mucosal epithelial cells, enters these epithelial cells, resulting in cell damage and sloughing of ciliated cells (*Fig. 8.20*). Cell damage may be caused by the release of lipopolysaccharide, which may stimulate the production of tumor necrosis factor and other cytokines. Much of the cell damage may be attributed to the acute inflammatory response. Nonhuman primate and other animal models have been developed to study the pathogenesis of chlamydial PID. Experimental chlamydial infection induced in nonhuman primates has been defined as a complex process of immune-mediated responses leading to overt tubal damage. Previous research using scanning electron microscopy has documented the process of chlamydial attachment to nonciliated epithelial cells (*Fig. 8.21*). Intracellular replication of *Chlamydia* results in the release of elementary bodies by rupture of the infected cells (*Fig. 8.22*). Comparable data are not available on the pathogensis of nongonococcal, nonchlamydial PID.

Due to the recognized complexity and polymicrobial nature of PID, the pathogenesis of PID is similarly complex and remains the subject of intense

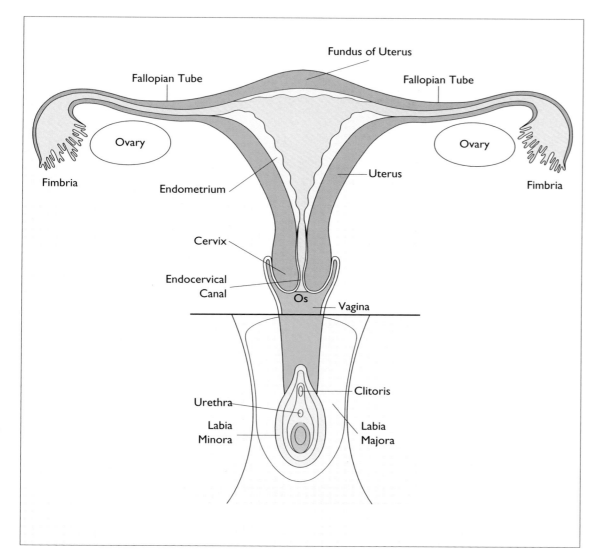

Fig. 8.17 Anatomic depiction of normal internal and external female genitalia.

and continuing investigations. Nonhuman primate and other animal models, e.g., mouse and guinea pig, have been used by various investigators to study the inflammatory response to gonococcal or chlamydial infection in the upper genital tract and fallopian tubes. Serologic studies have shown that a significantly higher proportion of women with tubal occlusion have elevated serum antibodies to *Chlamydia*. PID due to *Chlamydia* may often be subclinical or 'silent' in nature, and thus go undetected and untreated resulting in chronic tubal inflammation and damage. Recent studies have suggested that specific chlamydial antigenic components, such as heat-shock proteins, may play a major role in inducing the inflammatory response in the fallopian tube.

Pathology

Previous studies have estimated that 10–20% of women infected with *N. gonorrhoeae* may develop PID. It is estimated that at least a similar proportion of women with *C. trachomatis* may be at risk of PID. Several studies have suggested that the risk for developing PID may increase at menses, and that hormonal factors may play a role in the pathogenesis of PID by affecting the structural and functional barriers preventing infection of the upper female genital tract. Some investigators have postulated that initial exposure to *N. gonorrhoeae* or *C. trachomatis* increases the risk for developing endometritis

and PID by the ascending spread of these microorganisms, and the concomitant or subsequent ascending infection with nonsexually transmitted endogenous vaginal facultative and anaerobic bacteria, including organisms associated with bacterial vaginosis.

The spectrum of gross and microscopic pathologic changes occurring in the upper genital tract organs as a result of PID are seen in *Figures 8.23–8.32*. *Figure 8.23* illustrates the typical appearance of the endometrium associated with acute gonococcal endometritis, while *Figures 8.24–8.28* illustrate the spectrum of acute salpingitis and pyosalpinx. Acute salpingitis is one of the most severe complications of PID that often results in pyosalpinx or a 'retort tube'. With resolution of acute salpingitis, there may be a series of structural alterations to the tube, termed chronic salpingitis, which are associated with the major complications of PID (*Fig. 8.29*). The mucosal plicae form fibrinous adhesions to one another which progress to bridging between folds (*Fig. 8.30*). Tubo-ovarian adhesions may also form, with occlusion of the tubal ostium, and there may be associated peritoneal inflammation. Eventually, a hydrosalpinx may result (*Figs. 8.31–8.35*). Ovarian involvement in PID is almost always a complication of salpingitis, and typically presents as a unilateral or bilateral tubo-ovarian abscess (*Figs. 8.34–8.37*). Although less common than a tubo-ovarian abscess, an abscess confined to the ovary may also occur. A major complication of PID is tubal

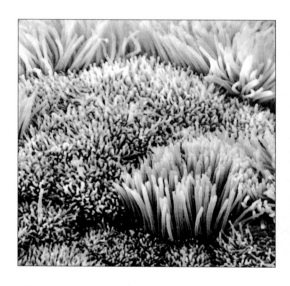

Fig. 8.18 Scanning electron micrograph of cultured human fallopian tube tissue showing both nonciliated cells with microvilli and ciliated cells.

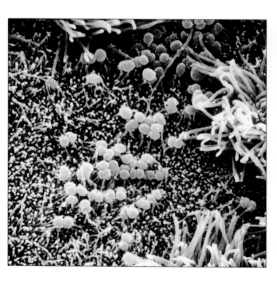

Fig. 8.19 Scanning electron micrograph of gonococci attaching to the microvilli of cultured human fallopian tube tissue. Note that gonococci are only attached to the nonciliated cells.

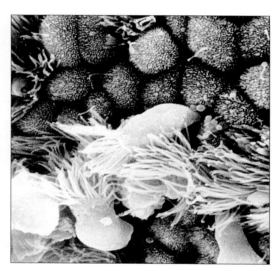

Fig. 8.20 Scanning electron micrograph showing ciliated epithelial cells sloughing from the cultured human fallopian tube mucosa. Some gonococci are still attached to the nonciliated cells, which show some damage as evidenced by their exaggerated borders and abnormal appearance.

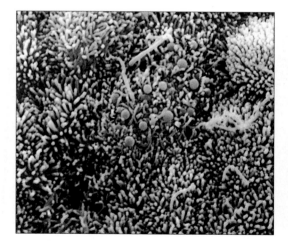

Fig. 8.21 Scanning electron micrograph of chlamydial elementary bodies attaching to the microvilli of nonciliated epithelial cells of the human fallopian tube mucosa

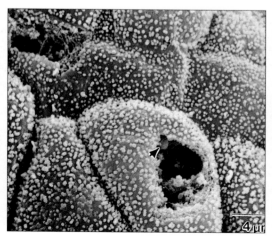

Fig. 8.22 Scanning electron micrograph of a human fallopian tube organ culture infected with *Chlamydia trachomatis*. Note the large hole where the cell has ruptured. The arrow points to an elementary body that remains within the interior of the cell.

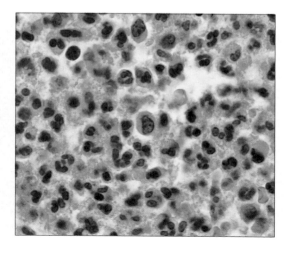

Fig. 8.23 Acute gonococcal endometritis, showing numerous and abundant neutrophils and few plasma cells from endometrial biopsy section (hematoxylin and eosin).

pregnancy. The unruptured fallopian tube is dilated and has a blue discoloration due to hematosalpinx. Almost two-thirds of tubal pregnancies contain an identifiable embryo (*Fig. 8.38*). Continued growth of the conceptus often results in tubal rupture around the eighth week of gestation, resulting in potentially life-threatening hemorrhage. A few tubal pregnancies may proceed to longer gestations (*Fig. 8.39*) and there are rare reports in which the pregnancies have

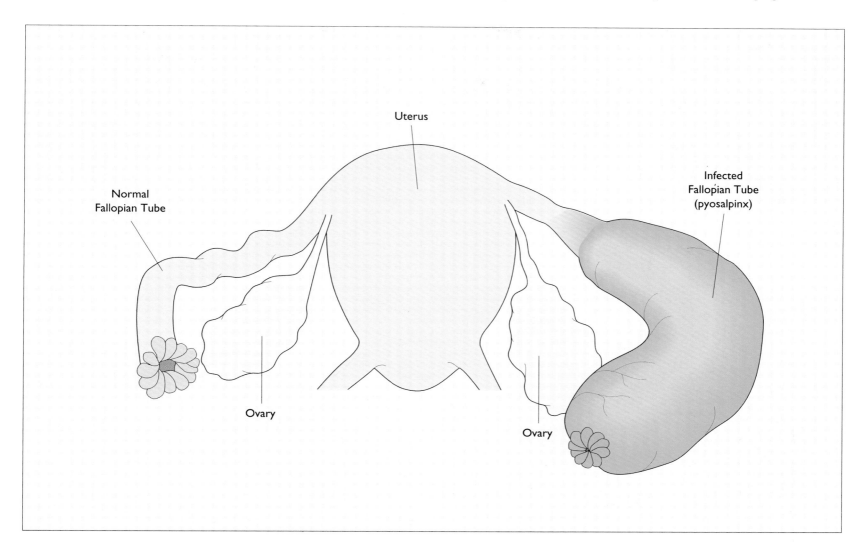

Fig. 8.24 Illustrated drawing of acute salpingitis and pyosalpinx.

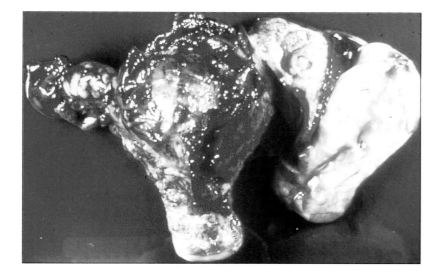

Fig. 8.25 A gross surgical specimen of uterus and infected fallopian tube removed from a patient with salpingitis and ruptured pyosalpinx abscess.

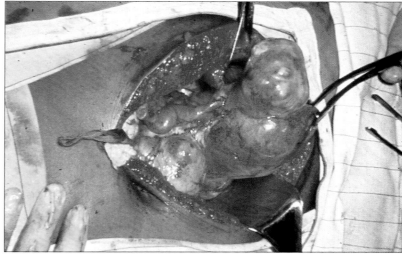

Fig. 8.26 Total abdominal hysterectomy bilateral salpingo-oophorectomy specimen showing unilateral pyosalpinx.

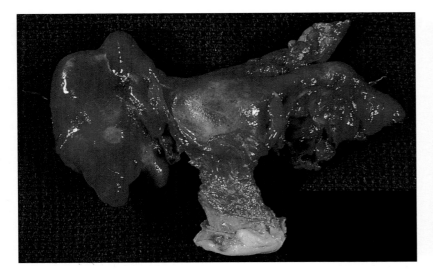

Fig. 8.27 Total abdominal hysterectomy bilateral salpingo-oophorectomy specimen showing unilateral pyosalpinx.

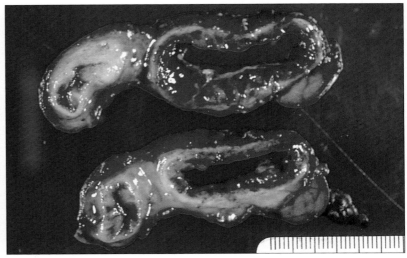

Fig. 8.28 Exudative pyosalpinx from salpingectomy.

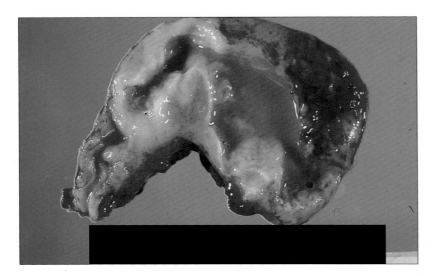

Fig. 8.29 Cross-section of a fallopian tube with chronic salpingitis, showing a thickened wall lined with fibrinohemorrhagic exudate. Salpingitis is the most common infertility problem associated with STDs.

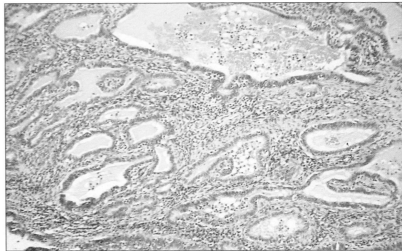

Fig. 8.30 The characteristic microscopic findings of chronic salpingitis are seen here, including thickening and fusion of the plical folds, and plasmacellular infiltration of the lamina propria (hematoxylin and eosin x 100).

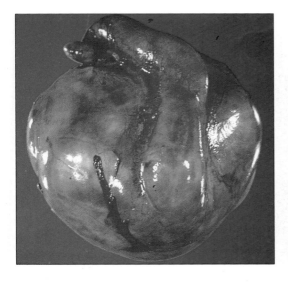

Fig. 8.31 Hydrosalpinx is one of the complications of salpingitis. This case is a typical example of hydrosalpinx, showing a tube, especially the ampullary portion, with dilatation and obliteration of the ostium.

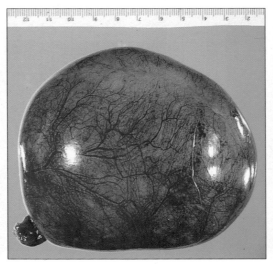

Fig. 8.32 Severe hydrosalpinx. There is marked luminal dilatation, and the wall is thin and translucent.

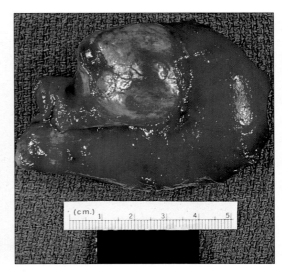

Fig. 8.33 Hydrosalpinx with tubo-ovarian adhesions.

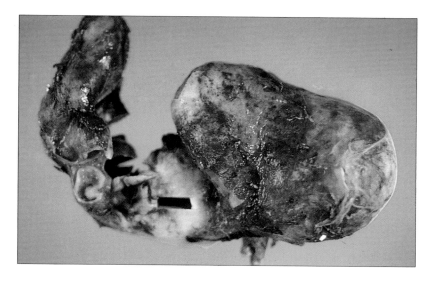

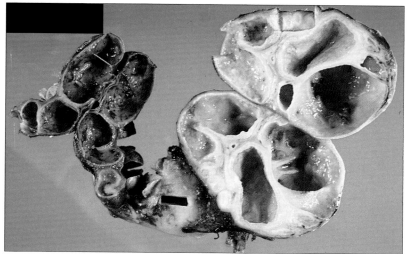

Figs. 8.34 and **8.35** Salpingo-oophorectomy specimen with chronic ovarian abscess and hydrosalpinx, before (**8.34**) and after (**8.35**) opening the specimen. The 'retort' shape of the specimen is typical for this process. The chronicity of the ovarian abscesses is evident from the presence of residual smooth-walled cystic cavities lined by fibrin.

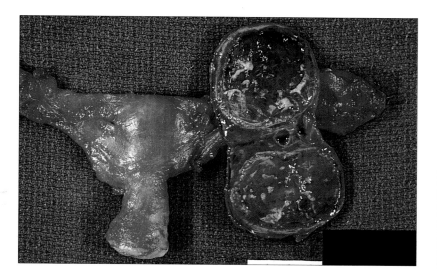

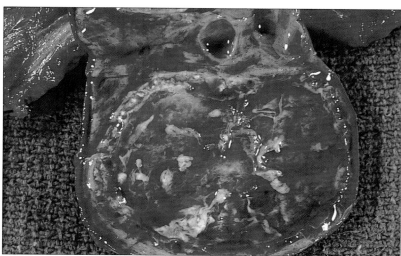

Fig. 8.36 Unilateral tubo-ovarian abscess. The majority of acute and chronic inflammatory lesions of the ovary are infectious, and are a manifestation of PID.

Fig. 8.37 Close-up of abscess in **8.36** showing hemorrhage, fibrin, and suppurative material.

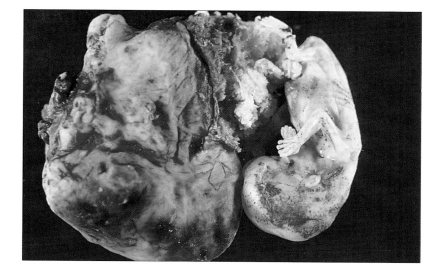

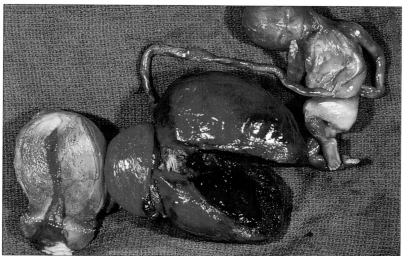

Fig. 8.38 Ectopic pregnancy is a potentially life-threatening complication of PID and salpingitis. In this tubal pregnancy, the placental implantation site into the tube is evident. Among 15–24-year-olds, one in 24 will develop an ectopic pregnancy after her first episode of PID.

Fig. 8.39 This shows an unusually advanced tubal pregnancy which ruptured into the abdominal cavity, associated with hematosalpinx. Damage to the fallopian tube from PID is estimated to confer a 7–10-fold greater risk of ectopic pregnancy.

proceeded to term with a viable fetus. Tuberculosis is the most common etiologic agent of granulomatous salpingitis, and for reasons which are not completely understood the mycobacteria preferentially lodge in the fallopian tube rather than in other parts of the female genital tract. The tube becomes enlarged and nodular, and dense adhesions may form between the tube and ovary (*Fig. 8.40*). The tubal mucosa may appear roughened and micronodular, and microscopically there is granulomatous inflammation, often with multinucleated giant cells (*Fig. 8.41*). Another cause of granulomatous salpingitis is actinomycotic infection. Actinomycotic infections of the fallopian tube are usually associated with the use of an IUD and actinomycosis of the endometrium (*Figs. 8.42* and *8.43*). Similarly to other infections resulting in PID, chronic endometritis may also be present. Grossly, an enlarged fibrous mass involving either the tube and/or the ovary is usually present. The inflammatory mass may contain pus-filled sinus cavities, and have adhesions to other structures in the pelvic cavity. The microscopic finding of actinomycotic grains within the inflamed tube or ovary is diagnostic, but microbiologic culture is necessary to identify precisely the causative species. Other infectious causes of salpingitis include schistosomiasis, which is rare in North America and Europe but is in fact one of the most common causes of granulomatous salpingitis worldwide (*Fig. 8.44*).

LABORATORY STUDIES

The detection of *N. gonorrhoeae* or *C. trachomatis* in genital-tract specimens in the clinical setting of lower abdominal pain, vaginal discharge, and pelvic tenderness is highly suggestive of PID, and the clinician should obtain good biologic specimens to test for these microorganisms. The endocervical Gram-stained smear (*Fig. 8.45*), if positive for typical Gram-negative, intracellular diplococci, may assist in the diagnosis of PID; however, in most clinical situations, the endocervical gram-stained smear is often difficult to interpret and unreliable due to improper specimen collection, contamination with vaginal flora, and under- or overstaining with reagents. Thus, culture of specimens on a solid, selective medium, such as modified Thayer–Martin (MTM), Martin–Lewis (ML), or a similar medium, is the recommended procedure for the isolation and confirmatory identification of *N. gonorrhoeae* from women with suspected genital tract infections. Several nonculture tests, including DNA probes and enzyme immunoassays (EIA) have been developed for the detection of *N. gonorrhoeae* in clinical specimens; however, nonculture results should be considered as presumptive screening tests for gonorrhea (*see Chapter 6*).

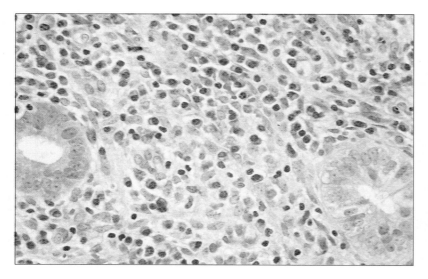

Fig. 8.40 The most common cause of granulomatous salpingitis is *Mycobacterium tuberculosis*. In this case of mycobacterial salpingitis, the tubal lumen is dilated, the mucosal surface is roughened, and the wall is thickened and fibrous. About 10–20% of women who die from tuberculosis have tubal involvement.

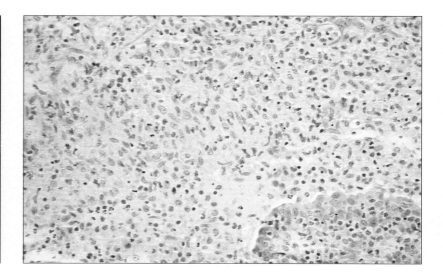

Fig. 8.41 Granulomatous salpingitis from a patient with *M. tuberculosis* infection, showing the replacement of normal tubal architecture by an inflammatory lesion containing mainly histiocytes and lymphocytes (hematoxylin and eosin × 200).

Fig. 8.42 Chronic endometritis in a patient with actinomycotic infection of the endometrium and fallopian tube, associated with an intrauterine device (IUD). Numerous plasma cells infiltrate the stroma (hematoxylin and eosin × 400).

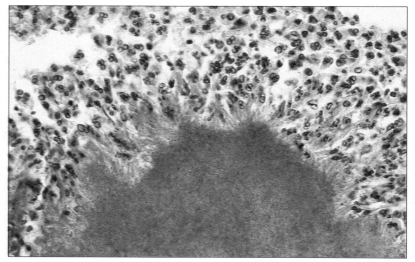

Fig. 8.43 Actinomycotic grain and surrounding acute inflammation from fallopian tube infection. The edge of the grain has radiating eosinophilic material, termed the Splendore–Hoeppli phenomenon (hematoxylin and eosin × 400).

In routine clinical practice, the laboratory diagnosis of *C. trachomatis* (*Fig. 8.46*) continues to be more difficult and costly than for *N. gonorrhoeae*. Cell culture has long been the 'gold standard' for the confirmatory diagnosis of *C. trachomatis*, but is costly and often not available except in academic or reference laboratories. Recently developed diagnostic techniques, such as PCR and LCR, are undergoing extensive evaluation, and in the future may offer reasonable and reliable alternatives to cell culture for confirmatory diagnosis of chlamydial infections. Over the past several years, various nonculture tests including DNA probes, EIA, and direct fluorescent antibody (DFA) tests have been developed for the screening and detection of *Chlamydia* in genital-tract specimens. Although nonculture results for both *C. trachomatis* and *N. gonorrhoeae* may provide valuable clinical information, these results may not be used for medicolegal purposes, such as evidence in cases of rape or sexual assault (*see Chapter 4*).

Other laboratory tests, which are not specific for PID but are often abnormal or elevated in an acute infection or inflammation and which may help in the diagnosis and monitoring of PID, include the erythrocyte sedimentation rate (ESR), quantitative C-reactive protein (CRP), and the total white blood cell (WBC) count. Combining ESR and CRP increases the ability to discriminate severe PID from moderate to mild PID. Serologic tests that detect IgG Antibodies to *C. trachomatis* are generally not diagnostic of, or specific for, PID *per se*, but are at best indicative of a genital tract infection associated with *Chlamydia*.

THERAPY AND MANAGEMENT OF PID

Due to the complex microbiology of PID, a therapeutic approach using broad-spectrum antimicrobial agents is recommended. Problems that often complicate the management of PID include a difficult clinical diagnosis, inaccessibility of clinical sites for culturing, patient compliance in taking prescribed medications, and delayed access to health-care providers skilled and trained in the management of STDs and PID (*Fig. 8.47*). The optimum therapy regimen should include agents known to be active against *N. gonorrhoeae*, *C. trachomatis*, and the broad-spectrum of aerobic and anaerobic bacteria commonly detected in women with PID. The choice of antimicrobial therapy should therefore be guided by knowledge of underlying or presumed etiologic agents, and data on the incidence and

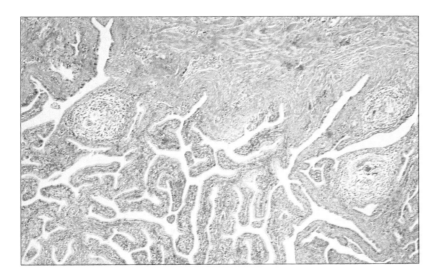

Fig. 8.44 Salpingitis due to *Schistosoma haematobium*. Well-circumscribed granulomas, containing parasite ova, are present within the stroma of several plical folds (hematoxylin and eosin × 40).

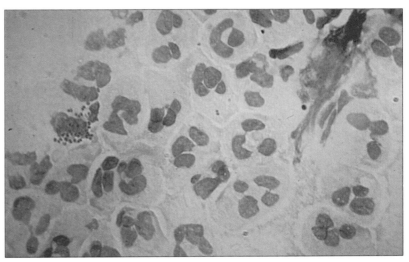

Fig. 8.45 Gram-stained smear of endocervical secretions. Note the polymorphonuclear leukocytes with numerous Gram-negative 'intracellular diplococci'.

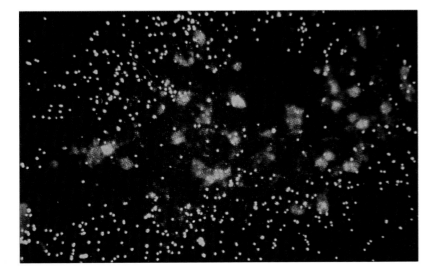

Fig. 8.46 Typical appearance of fluorescein-stained chlamydial inclusions.

PROBLEMS FREQUENTLY ENCOUNTERED WITH PID MANAGEMENT

Difficult clinical diagnosis

Sites of infection inaccessible for routine confirmatory testing

Polymicrobial nature

Optimal antibiotic selection

Poor patient compliance with multiple-day therapy and follow-up

Delayed access to appropriate treatment and prevention services

Lack of partner referral for timely evaluation and treatment

Fig. 8.47 Problems frequently encountered in the management of PID.

prevalence of antimicrobial resistance in confirmed PID pathogens, such as *N. gonorrhoeae*. Recent *in vitro* susceptibility studies of *N. gonorrhoeae* obtained from women with PID in the USA have demonstrated that *in vitro* resistance to penicillin and tetracycline occurs in 20–25% of isolates tested.

The CDC provides recommendations for the outpatient and inpatient therapy and management of PID. For example, recommended outpatient regimens include a single dose of ceftriaxone, 250 mg intramuscularly plus oral doxycycline, 100 mg twice daily for 10–14 days (*Fig. 8.48*). Inpatient therapy regimens recommended by the CDC include cefoxitin (or a comparable cephalosporin) plus doxycycline, or clindamycin plus gentamicin, in appropriate doses (*Fig. 8.49*). Male sex partners should receive prophylactic treatment for gonorrhea and chlamydial infection, and should be counseled on the proper use of condoms to reduce further exposure to and transmission of STDs. PID patients and their sex partners should also receive information and counselling on the prevention of HIV infection as well as STDs, and should be offered confidential HIV testing as an integral part of the management of PID.

The decision to choose outpatient management rather than hospitalization for PID should ideally be based on specific clinical criteria. *Figure. 8.50* provides a summary of previously published and suggested criteria for the hospitalization of women with PID; however, some physicians prefer to hospitalize all women with suspected or proven PID. Regardless of the decision to treat PID on an outpatient or hospital basis, all women with PID should be re-evaluated within 48–72 hours following the initiation of therapy and again following completion of therapy.

Surgical management of PID ranges from laparoscopy, which is primarily used to confirm the diagnosis of salpingitis, to laparotomy that is sometimes used to manage cases of ruptured tubo-ovarian abscess and severe peritonitis. Conservative surgical modalities include procedures, such as irrigation and drainage; more extensive surgical management of PID and its complications ranges from surgical removal of pelvic organs to reconstructive procedures to restore fertility, and is beyond the scope of this chapter. Possible indications for the surgical management of PID are summarized in *Fig. 8.51*.

ACUTE PID OUTPATIENT THERAPY REGIMENS*

Ceftriaxone 250 mg im or cefoxitin (or equivalent cephalosporin) 2 g im with probenecid 1 g po *plus* doxycycline 100 mg po bid for 14 days

or

Ofloxacin 400 mg po bid for 14 days *plus* metronidazole 250 mg po qid for 14 days or doxycycline 100 mg po bid for 14 days

*CDC 1993 STD treatment guidelines

Fig. 8.48 Recommended PID outpatient therapy regimens.

ACUTE PID INPATIENT THERAPY REGIMENS*

Cefoxitin 2 g iv qid or cefotetan (or equivalent cephalosporin) 2 g iv bid plus doxycycline 100 mg po or iv bid

or

Clindamycin 900 mg iv tid plus gentamicin 2 g iv loading dose followed by a maintenance dose 1.5 mg/kg/hr iv. This regimen should be continued for at least 48 hours after demonstrable clinical improvement, then followed with doxycycline 100 mg po bid or clindamycin 400 mg po qid for a total 14-day dosing regimen.

*CDC 1993 STD treatment guidelines

Fig. 8.49 Recommended PID inpatient therapy regimens.

ACUTE PID: INDICATIONS FOR HOSPITALIZATION

Uncertain diagnosis
Surgical emergencies
Suspected pelvic abscess
Severe illness
Pregnancy
Adolescence
Patient noncompliance
Outpatient therapy failure
Inability to arrange interim re-evaluation

Fig. 8.50 Suggested indications for hospitalization for PID.

POTENTIAL INDICATIONS FOR SURGERY IN THE MANAGEMENT OF PID

Failure to improve after adequate therapy
Pelvic abscess refractory to medical therapy
Ruptured abscess and peritonitis
Uncertain diagnosis

Fig. 8.51 Possible reasons or indications for the surgical management of PID.

ACUTE AND CHRONIC COMPLICATIONS OF PID

ACUTE COMPLICATIONS	CHRONIC COMPLICATIONS
Ruptured abscess	Chronic pelvic pain
Pelvic thrombophlebitis	Ectopic pregnancy
Perihepatitis	Infertility
Peritonitis	Menstrual abnormality
Psychosocial problems	Recurrent pelvic infections

Fig. 8.52 Complications of PID.

PID PREVENTION AND TREATMENT STRATEGIES

Emphasize compliance with prescribed medications
Review contraindications and potential side-effects
Schedule follow-up examination
Convey need to abstain from sex until treatment is completed
Emphasize need to refer sex partners for treatment
Provide instruction to reduce 'risky' health behaviors
Develop programs to enhance risk-avoidance skills
Support continuing training and education for providers
Improve access to STD/PID prevention services
Increase access to appropriately trained health-care providers
Support cost-effective STD screening in at-risk groups

Fig. 8.53 Prevention and treatment strategies for PID should include acute-care patient education regarding treatment compliance and partner referral. Prevention should also include the reduction of risky health behaviors including unprotected sexual intercourse and the building of risk-avoidance skills. Health-care providers should receive continuing training and education to enhance their skills in diagnosing and treating PID more effectively in its early stages and to counsel women and their sex partners on STD prevention.

COMPLICATIONS OF PID

Ectopic pregnancy and tubal infertility are the most serious and costly longterm complications and sequelae of PID and salpingitis (*Fig. 8.52*). In the USA, the rate of ectopic pregnancies increased dramatically between 1970 and 1989 (*see Fig. 4.17*); the increase was attributed to the concurrent increase in the number of cases of gonorrhea, STDs, and PID among women of reproductive age. Similar increases in the rate of women diagnosed with infertility were also observed. Studies have shown that the risk for infertility increases with each subsequent episode of PID.

PREVENTION STRATEGIES

Prevention is the most important aspect of PID research and management. Enormous costs could be saved by preventing PID, which as described earlier will cost, both directly and indirectly, more than $9 billion annually in the USA by the year 2000. Reducing the spread and transmission of the sexually transmitted agents, *N. gonorrhoeae* and *C. trachomatis,* is recognized as a critical element in prevention. Since the mid-1980s, the reported incidence of gonorrhea has steadily declined in the USA; however, the prevalence and risk behaviors for exposure to gonorrhea remain unacceptably high among younger, sexually active women and adolescents in certain geographic areas and population subgroups, e.g. inner city, adolescent females. Effective prevention strategies need therefore to target women at highest risk for STD and PID, and to develop innovative approaches to increase access to, and use of, STD screening services, and to provide health education to reduce risk-taking

behaviors (*Fig. 8.53*). Many health-care providers are reluctant to counsel or screen women for STD or to obtain an adequate clinical history for STD.

Ideally, gonococcal and chlamydial vaccines would offer the best preventive strategies, but none are currently available. Previous trials of potential gonococcal vaccines in male volunteers in several settings have failed to demonstrate protection from *N. gonorrhoeae.* Current prevention strategies for PID therefore need to emphasize risk-avoidance skills and the importance of limiting behaviors or sexual practices that increase the likelihood for exposure to *N. gonorrhoeae* and *C. trachomatis.*

However, the prevention of nonsexually transmitted PID is a complex and difficult topic which requires more research and study. More research is needed to define risk factors and direct prevention strategies for nongonococcal, nonchlamydial PID, as well as gonococcal and chlamydial PID.

PID IN HIV-INFECTED WOMEN

Increasing rates of HIV transmission among intravenous drug users and heterosexuals have contributed to a rising incidence of HIV infection and AIDS among women of childbearing age. Attention has therefore been directed towards the clinical spectrum, diagnosis, and management of PID in HIV-infected women. Much of the information on this topic has been derived from retrospective observations, case reports or limited cohort studies of PID in HIV-infected women, which have suggested that PID may be more severe in HIV-infected women. However, the potential for bias in the setting of HIV infection has been raised and case-control studies are in progress to address this issue. Clearly, more data are needed in this important and emerging area of PID prevention and management.

Picture credits for this chapter are as follow: Figs. 8.2 and 8.3 courtesy of AE Washington, MD, University of California, San Francisco; Figs. 8.18–8.22 courtesy of MD Cooper, Southern Illinois University Medical School.

BIBLIOGRAPHY

Centers for Disease Control and Prevention: Pelvic inflammatory disease: guidelines for prevention and management. *MMWR* **40** (RR–5):1–25, 1991.

Centers for Disease Control and Prevention: Sexually transmitted disease surveillance 1992. Public Health Service, Centers for Disease Control, Atlanta, Georgia, 1993.

Cates W, Rolfs RT, Aral SO: Sexually transmitted diseases, pelvic inflammatory disease, and infertility: an epidemiologic update. *Epidemiol Rev* **12**:199–220, 1990.

Eschenbach DA, Buchanan TM, Pollock HM, et al.: Polymicrobial nature of pelvic inflammatory disease. *N Engl J Med* **293**:166–171, 1975.

Eschenbach DA: Acute pelvic inflammatory disease. *Urol Clin North Am* **11**:65–81, 1984.

Eschenbach DA, Hillier S, Critchlow, Stevens C, et al.: Diagnosis and clinical manifestations of bacterial vaginosis. *Am J Obstet Gynecol* **158**:819–828, 1988.

Expert Committee on Pelvic Inflammatory Disease: Pelvic inflammatory disease: research directions in the 1990s. *Sex Transm Dis* **18**:46–64, 1991.

Hager WD, Eschenbach DA, Spence MR, Sweet RL: Criteria for diagnosis and grading of salpingitis. *Obstet Gynecol* **61**:113–114, 1983.

Irwin KL, Rice RJ, Sperling RS, O'Sullivan MJ, Brodman M: Potential for bias in studies of the influence of human immunodeficiency virus infection on the recognition, incidence, clinical course, and microbiology of pelvic inflammatory disease. *Obstet Gynecol* **84**:463–469, 1994.

Jacobsen L, Westrom L: Objectivized diagnosis of acute pelvic inflammatory disease. *Am J Obstet Gynecol* **105**:1088–1098, 1969.

Korn AP, Landers DV, Green JR, Sweet RL: Pelvic inflammatory disease in human immunodeficiency virus-infected women. *Obstet Gynecol* **82**:765–768, 1993.

Mårdh P–A: An overview of infectious agents of salpingitis, their biology and recent advances in methods of detection. *Am J Obstet Gynecol* **138**:933–951, 1980.Mårdh P–A: An overview of titation of damage by pathogenic microorganisms. *Infect Immun* **13**:608, 1976.

Melly MA, et al.: Studies of the toxicity of *Neisseria gonorrhoeae* for human fallopian tube mucosa. *J Infect Dis* **143**:423, 1981.

Miettinen A, Saikku P, Jansson E, Paavonen J: Epidemiologic and clinical characteristics of pelvic inflammatory disease associated with *Mycoplasma hominis*, *Chlamydia trachomatis*, and *Neisseria gonorrhoeae*. *Sex Transm Dis* **1**:24–29, 1986.

Patton DL, Kuo CC, Wang SP, et al.: Distal tubal obstruction induced by repeated *Chlamydia trachomatis* salpingeal infections in pig-tailed macaques. *J Infect Dis* **155**:1292–1299, 1987.

Paavonen J: *Chlamydia trachomatis* in acute salpingitis. *Am J Obstet Gynecol* **138**:957–959, 1980.

Paavonen J, Kiviat N, Brunham R, et al.: Prevalence and manifestations of endometritis among women with cervicitis. *Am J Obstet Gynecol* **152**:280–286, 1985.

Peterson HB, Walker CK, et al.: Pelvic inflammatory disease. Key treatment issues and options. *JAMA* **266**:2605–2611, 1991.

Punnonen R, Terho P, Nikkanen V, Muerman OL: Chlamydial serology in infertile women by immunofluorescence. *Fertil Steril* **31**:656–659, 1979.

Rice PA, Schachter J: Pathogenesis of pelvic inflammatory disease caused by *Chlamydia trachomatis* and *Neisseria gonorrhoeae*: where should research efforts focus? *JAMA* **266**:2587–2593, 1991.

Rolfs RT, Galaid EI, Zaidi AA: Pelvic inflammatory disease: trends in hospitalizations and office visits, 1979–1988. *Am J Obstet Gynecol* **166**:983–990, 1992.

Sellors J, Mahoney J, Goldsmith C, et al.: The accuracy of clinical findings and laparoscopy in pelvic inflammatory disease. *Am J Obstet Gynecol* **164**:113–120, 1991.

Soper DE: Diagnosis and laparoscopic grading of acute salpingitis. *Am J Obstet Gynecol* **164**:1370–1376, 1991.

Soper DE, Brockwell NJ, Dalton HP, Johnson D: Observations concerning the microbial etiology of acute salpingitis. *Am J Obstet Gynecol* **170**:1008–1017, 1994.

Sperling RS, Friedman F, Joyner M, et al.: Seroprevalence of human immunodeficiency virus infection in women admitted to the hospital with pelvic inflammatory disease. *J Reprod Med* **36**:122–124, 1991.

Sweet RL, Draper DL, Hadley WK: Etiology of acute salpingitis: influence of episode, number and duration of symptoms. *Obstet Gynecol* **58**:62–68, 1981.

Washington AE, Katz P: Costs and payment source for pelvic inflammatory disease: trends and projections, 1983–2000. *JAMA* **266**:2565–2569, 1991.

Wasserheit JN, Bell TA, Kiviat NB, et al.: Microbial causes of proven pelvic inflammatory disease and efficacy of clindamycin and tobramycin. *Ann Intern Med* **104**:187–193, 1986.ease and efficacy of clindamycin and tobramycin. *Ann Intern Med* **104**:187–193, 1986.

CHAPTER NINE

Vaginal Infections

S Hillier and R Arko

INTRODUCTION

Vaginal symptoms are extremely common and are the main reason why many women seek health care. During the 1980s, the number of initial visits to physicians for vaginitis due to trichomoniasis remained constant or decreased slightly, while new office visits due to yeast vaginitis and bacterial vaginosis doubled (*Fig. 9.1*). Vaginal symptoms may be caused by vaginal or cervical infections resulting in abnormal discharge, or by noninfectious causes. The most common type of vaginal syndrome is bacterial vaginosis followed by yeast vulvovaginitis. Although trichomoniasis is common in some STD clinics and some prenatal clinics, it is extremely rare in others, and in the USA, is generally agreed to be the least frequent of the three vaginal infections. Desquamative inflammatory vaginitis, caused mainly by group B streptococci, is a recently described cause of infectious vaginitis. Causes of noninfectious vaginitis include a lack of estrogen postpartum or after the menopause, or allergic vaginitis (*Fig. 9.2*).

The vagina is a dynamic ecosystem which is sterile at birth and becomes colonized within a few days with a predominantly Gram-positive flora, consisting of anaerobic bacteria, staphylococci, streptococci, and diphtheroids. The vaginal pH in premenarchal females is near neutral (pH 7.0) until puberty. At puberty, under the influence of estrogen, the vaginal epithelium increases to about 25 cells thick, glycogen levels in the epithelium and vagina increase, the predominant flora changes to lactobacilli, and the vaginal pH decreases to less than 4.5. This low pH is maintained until the menopause, when the vaginal epithelium thins, a mixed flora of anaerobic bacteria, staphylococci, and diphtheroids becomes re-established, and the vaginal pH rises above 6.0.

The normal flora in women of childbearing age is dominated by lactobacilli (*Fig. 9.3*). Nearly 100% of women with normal flora will be colonized by lactobacilli, usually at a concentration of 10 million organisms per gram of vaginal fluid. While staphylococci and diphtheroids are relatively common, they are present at 1,000-fold lower concentrations, approximately 10,000 organisms per gram of vaginal fluid. The anaerobic coccus, *Peptostreptococcus*, is also recovered from nearly all women, but at concentrations similar to that of aerobic cocci. Anaerobic Gram-negative rods, such as *Prevotella bivia*,

Bacteroides ureolyticus, and *Porphyromonas* spp. are found in 30–60% of normal women at concentrations of less than one million per gram. Thus, in the normal woman with adequate levels of estrogen, lactobacilli account for more than 95% of microorganisms present in the vagina (*Fig. 9.4*).

An early hypothesis by Döderlein maintained that the predominant lactic acid-producing lactobacilli in the vagina have a protective function against pathogenic bacteria, and that an abnormal vaginal discharge results from partial replacement of the normal flora by less acidophilic microorganisms. Consistent with this hypothesis, lactobacilli have been shown to have *in vitro* inhibitory effects on other microorganisms. Glycogen is deposited on the vaginal epithelium under the influence of estrogen, and is then metabolized to glucose by the host. The glucose is converted to lactic acid by the lactobacilli, which acidifies the vagina to a level inhospitable to many other species of bacteria.

In addition to lactic acid, lactobacilli produce a number of compounds which inhibit other bacteria, such as hydrogen peroxide (H_2O_2), lactacin, acidolin and others. The H_2O_2 generated may directly inhibit other microorganisms. It may also form, in combination with halide (chloride ion) and myeloperoxidase, the potent halide-H_2O_2-myeloperoxidase microbicidal system (*Fig. 9.5*). Women colonized by H_2O_2-generating lactobacilli are less likely to be colonized by *Gardnerella*, genital mycoplasmas, and anaerobes, and are less likely to have bacterial vaginosis. The lactobacilli are autoinhibited by high levels of H_2O_2, so that the levels of H_2O_2-generating lactobacilli are self-regulated in the vagina.

Lactobacilli vary greatly in size but are generally large, straight, or curved rods (*Fig. 9.4*). They are Gram-positive, but cells from older cultures may stain Gram-negative or Gram-variable. Lactobacilli are facultative or strictly anaerobic and are usually nonmotile. Although they have complex nutritional requirements, they produce lactic acid as the primary end-product of carbohydrate metabolism.

BACTERIAL VAGINOSIS

For many years, *nonspecific vaginitis* was loosely used to refer to vaginal discharges not caused by *Trichomonas vaginalis* or *Candida* spp. In 1955, Gardner

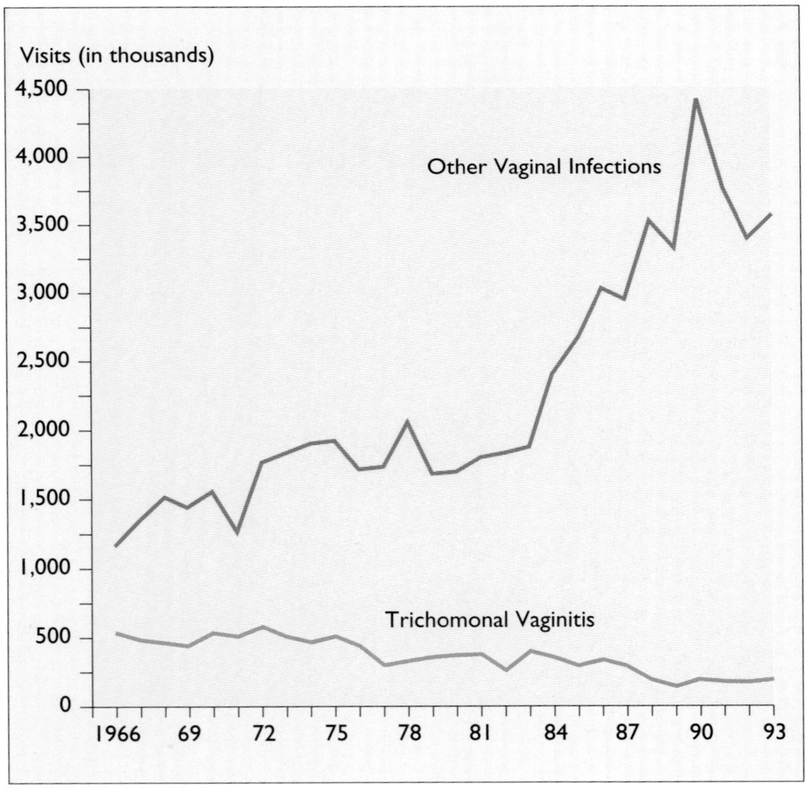

Fig. 9.1 Trichomonal and other vaginal infections, initial visits to physicians' offices, USA, 1966–1993. Source: National Disease and Therapeutic Index (IMS America, LTD).

VAGINAL SYNDROMES AND THEIR ETIOLOGIES

TYPE	ETIOLOGY
Infectious:	
Bacterial vaginosis	Mixed *Gardnerella vaginalis*, anaerobes (*Prevotella, Porphyromonas, Bacteroides, Fusobacterium, Peptostreptococcus, Mobiluncus*), and genital mycoplasmas
Yeast vulvovaginitis	90% *Candida albicans*, 10% other yeasts
Trichomoniasis	*Trichomonas vaginalis*
Desquamative inflammatory vaginitis	Group B streptococci, other unknown causes
Non-infectious:	
Post-partum atrophic vaginitis	Lack of estrogen especially during lactation
Allergic vaginitis	Systemic allergy; passive transfer of IgE in semen; local response to chemical irritants
Atrophic vaginitis	Lack of estrogen during or after menopause

Fig. 9.2 Vaginal syndromes and their etiologies.

and Dukes clinically defined this condition and called it 'Haemophilus vaginalis vaginitis', believing *H. vaginalis* to be the causative organism. This micro-organism has since been renamed *Gardnerella vaginalis*. Today, 'Haemophilus vaginalis' vaginitis' is referred to as *bacterial vaginosis* (or as *anaerobic vaginosis* in Britain), reflecting the lack of inflammation of the vaginal epithelium in this condition. Others use the term *vaginal bacteriosis*, meaning too many

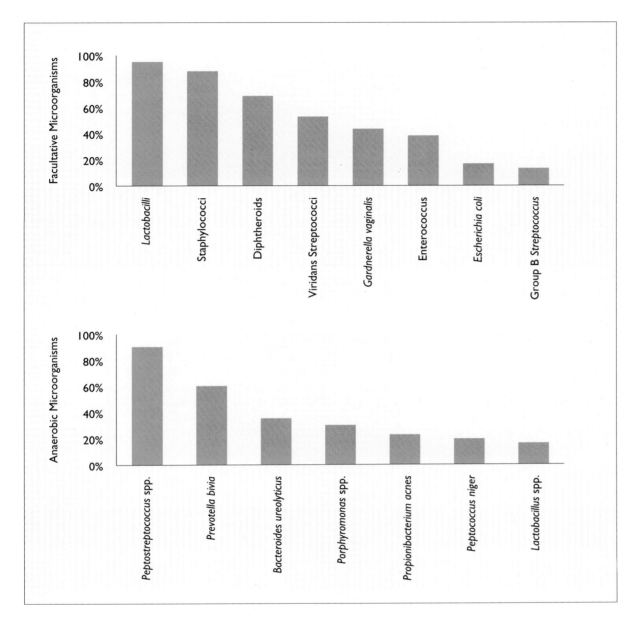

Fig. 9.3 Bacteria in vaginal flora of women without vaginal infections, in order of usual prevalence.

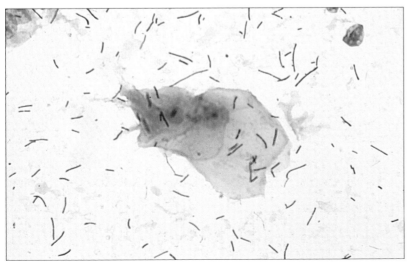

Fig. 9.4 Gram-stained vaginal smear taken from a woman having approximately 10 million (10^7) H_2O_2-producing lactobacilli per gram of vaginal fluid. Note the preponderance of lactobacilli and the lack of other bacterial morphotypes.

bacteria in the vagina. Bacterial vaginosis is thought to be the result of a complex interaction of many species of bacteria. Gardner and Dukes believed the disease was caused by *G. vaginalis* because they identified the organism in women with bacterial vaginosis but not in women without the disease. In retrospect, they seem to have been unable to recover *G. vaginalis* from the latter group because the medium they used was insensitive and because women with bacterial vaginosis have far greater numbers of the organism than do women without the condition. If sensitive culture techniques are used, as many as 50% of asymptomatic women are found to be colonized with *G. vaginalis*.

The involvement of bacterial species other than *G. vaginalis* in bacterial vaginosis was recognized by Pheifer *et al.* in 1978. They recognized that Gram-negative rods (*Prevotella, Porphyromonas, Bacteroides, Fusobacterium*) and *Peptostreptoccus* spp. occur in increased numbers in the vaginal secretions of women with bacterial vaginosis, and found that metronidazole, which is active against anaerobic bacteria, provides effective therapy. Subsequently, *Mobiluncus* spp. have been found to be highly associated with bacterial vaginosis, as has *Mycoplasma hominis*.

The etiologic role of these microorganisms in unclear. However, treatment data suggest that drugs, such as metronidazole or clindamycin which are active against anaerobic bacteria, yield the best clinical response. Other antimicrobial agents, such as sulfa or ampicillin, which are active against *G. vaginalis* but have less activity against anaerobes, are significantly less effective clinically. Although *Mobiluncus* is often resistant to metronidazole, women who have *Mobiluncus* and are treated with this compound have the same rate of cure as women not colonized by *Mobiluncus*. These findings would suggest that anaerobic Gram-negative rods have a more central role in the etiology of bacterial vaginosis than *Gardnerella, Mobiluncus,* or the genital mycoplasmas.

The development of bacterial vaginosis is the result in a shift in the vaginal ecosystem from one predominated by acid-producing lactobacilli to one characterized by a predominance of *Gardnerella* and anerobic bacteria. The triggers thought to cause this shift in the vaginal ecosystem include multiple sexual partners and regular douching (which may kill vaginal lactobacilli). Women who lack lactobacilli which produce H_2O_2 are also more likely to acquire bacterial vaginosis.

G. vaginalis metabolically produces amino acids, which act as substrates for the production of volatile amines (e.g., putrescine) by anaerobic bacteria; these amines are responsible for the unpleasant odor associated with the disease. The amines, in turn, raise the vaginal pH, so favoring the continued growth of *G. vaginalis* over lactobacilli.

EPIDEMIOLOGY

Bacterial vaginosis is the most common of the vaginitides, yet its epidemiology is not well understood. Although the disease is associated with increased numbers of sexual partners, and is rare in women who are not sexually experienced, it is not considered an STD. The treatment of sexual partners is not routinely recommended because no study has documented that treatment of the male sexual partner decreases the recurrence of bacterial vaginosis. Although the use of an IUD and a history of trichomoniasis have been associated with bacterial vaginosis, most affected women have no identifiable risk factors. Without therapy, cases may be self-limited, intermittently recurrent, or chronic.

CLINICAL MANIFESTATIONS

In 1983, an International Working Group on Bacterial Vaginosis formulated clinical criteria for the diagnosis of bacterial vaginosis (*Fig. 9.6*). Many cases are so mild that they are not recognized by patients, and are found only on routine examinations. Some of these women are only apparently asymptomatic, however, and following treatment will notice the disappearance of a previously inapparent vaginal discharge or odor. This finding may be attributable to the fact that many women consider vaginal malodor to be a hygiene problem rather than a symptom resulting from infection.

Women with bacterial vaginosis may complain of increased vaginal discharge or abnormal vaginal odor. In symptomatic women having bacterial vaginosis and without other genital infections, 90% of women will complain of vaginal discharge, over 70% will complain of odor and 45% will complain of vaginal irritation. The discharge, which typically is milky, clings to the vaginal walls (*Fig. 9.7*). The vaginal mucosa and vulva appear normal; this lack of inflammation has led to the use of the term *vaginosis* instead of *vaginitis*. The term *vaginosis* does not denote a lack of polymorphonuclear leukocytes in the vaginal wet mount. More than 30 polymorphonuclear leukocytes per high-powered field will be noted in one-third of women with this syndrome.

Examination of a woman with a complaint of a vaginal discharge or odor should include an evaluation for the clinical criteria of bacterial vaginosis (*Fig. 9.6*). The odor of the vaginal secretions should be tested by smelling

Fig. 9.5 Microbicidal and inhibitory activity of lactobacilli.

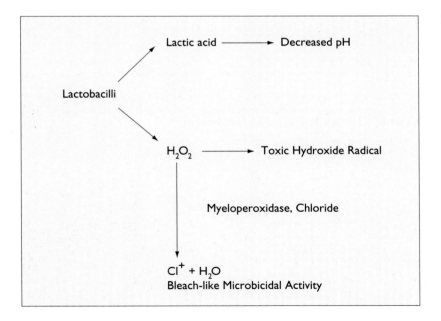

the withdrawn speculum (the 'whiff test'); normal vaginal secretions do not have an unpleasant odor. If this test is negative, a more sensitive procedure for detecting the amines produced is performed by adding a few drops of 10% potassium hydroxide (KOH) to a few drops of vaginal secretions. The mixture should be smelt immediately ('whiffed') for the transient, 'dead fish' odor characteristic of bacterial vaginosis. Potassium hydroxide increases the pH to the point at which the volatilization of polyamines, such as putrescine, cadaverine, and trimethylamine, occurs. Many women first notice vaginal malodor immediately following intercourse, because semen, which has a pH of 8.0, alkalinizes vaginal fluid so releasing the volatile amines.

The pH of vaginal secretions should be determined by using a strip of narrow-range pH paper (about pH 4.0–5.5), which may be applied to the withdrawn speculum or directly pressed against the vaginal wall with a swab (*Figs. 9.8–9.10*). Lastly, a wet mount of vaginal secretions should be done to look for 'clue' cells. These are epithelial cells covered with *G. vaginalis* that Gardner and Dukes called 'clues' to the diagnosis of bacterial vaginosis (*Fig. 9.11*). By comparison, vaginal epithelial cells from women without bacterial vaginosis have clear borders (*Fig. 9.12*).

When examining a woman for bacterial vaginosis, various potential diagnostic pitfalls should be avoided. The clinical or laboratory assessment may be affected by examination during menses, within a day of sexual intercourse, recent douching, or the use of intravaginal products or systemic antimicrobials. Menses, semen, or douching may affect the pH, and a weakly positive whiff test may be produced by menstrual blood or semen. Care should be taken to ensure that the pH paper does not sample either water used to moisten the speculum or cervical secretions, which are relatively alkaline. It is important to exclude trichomoniasis, which may also have an elevated pH and a positive whiff test because of an accompanying overgrowth of anerobes. Lastly, lactobacilli can cling to epithelial cells, so attention should be given to the morphology of organisms seen on clue cells.

LABORATORY TESTS

The Gram stain is the single best laboratory test for diagnosis of bacterial vaginosis. This method is preferable to culture because it has greater specificity and should be available in any laboratory which is licensed to perform moderately complex tasks. To prepare a vaginal smear for a Gram stain, a swab should be used to obtain vaginal fluid and cells from the vaginal wall (not the cervix). This swab should then be rolled across a slide and the material allowed to air-dry. There is no need to heat-fix the smear prior to shipment to the laboratory. Air-dried vaginal smears are stable at room temperature for months.

In the laboratory, the smear should be heat-fixed and Gram-stained. There are two primary methods for diagnosis of bacterial vaginosis from Gram-stained smears. For the Nugent method (*Fig. 9.13*), a score of 0 to 10 is formed, based on the relative quantity of various bacterial morphotypes. Smears having scores of ≥ 7 are considered consistent with bacterial vaginosis.

CLINICAL DIAGNOSTIC CRITERIA FOR BACTERIAL VAGINOSIS

THREE OF THE FOUR FOLLOWING:

- Clue cells (at least 1 in 5 vaginal epithelial cells with edges obscured by bacteria)

- Vaginal pH > 4.5

- Amine odor spontaneously or after addition of 10% KOH to vaginal fluid

- Thin, homogenous discharge

Fig. 9.6 Clinical diagnostic criteria for bacterial vaginosis.

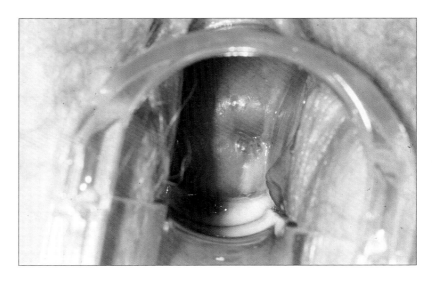

Fig. 9.7 Vaginal examination from a woman with mild bacterial vaginosis. Notice the milky discharge pooling beneath the cervix and the lack of cervical inflammation or vaginal erythema.

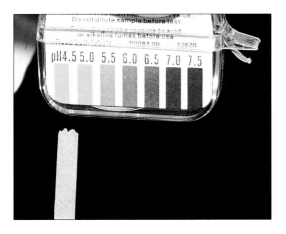 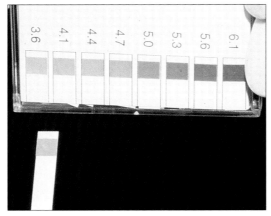 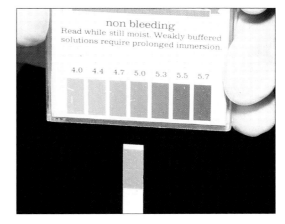

Figs. 9.8–9.10 Measurement of vaginal pH is usually performed using commercially available pH strips. A vaginal pH of more than 4.5 is usually considered abnormal, but pH papers with gradations between pH 4.2 and 5.0 (**9.9** and **9.10**) are usually easier to read than pH paper strips with gradations at each half pH unit (**9.8**).

Scores of 0–3 are categorized as normal, while scores of 4–6 are intermediate. This method has a sensitivity of 85–90% and a specificity of greater than 90%. The advantage of the method is its high reproducibility and intraobserver agreement. Some workers view the requirement for counting and scoring the morphotypes as a disadvantage of this method. Examples of Gram-stained vaginal smears are shown in *Figure 9.14*.

In the more simple Spiegel method, vaginal smears are categorized as bacteria present or absent, based on the relative quantities of *Lactobacillus* and *Gardnerella* morphotypes, not the presence or absence of any other bacterial morphotype. The sensitivity of the Spiegel method has ranged from 62–100%, while specificity has ranged from 73–100% in various studies.

Cultures for *G. vaginalis* should not be used to diagnose bacterial vaginosis because 36–55% of women without bacterial vaginosis will harbor this organism as part of their normal flora. *G. vaginalis* can be recovered at high concentrations – a million organisms per ml of vaginal fluid – even in women lacking clinical signs or symptoms of bacterial vaginosis. Women with bacterial vaginosis generally have 100 million organisms per ml of vaginal discharge (*Fig. 9.15*).

Other laboratory methods for diagnosing bacterial vaginosis include:
- Oligonucleotide probes for high concentrations of *G. vaginalis*
- Tests evaluating various polyamines
- Detection of bacterial enzymes including proline aminopeptidase or sialidase
- Gas-liquid chromatography of vaginal fluid (*Fig. 9.16*).

Although these are presently research techniques, it is likely that one or more of these tests could be adapted for clinic or bedside use.

Bacterial vaginosis is always a mixed infection, including *Gardnerella* and anaerobic Gram-negative rods, such as *Prevotella*, *Porphyromonas*, and *Bacteroides*. *Mycoplasma hominis* is usually present, while *Mobiluncus* is sometimes present. *G. vaginalis* shares many culture and morphologic similarities with *Haemophilus* and *Corynebacterium* spp., although, based on DNA homology studies, *Gardnerella* clearly is a separate genus. Although it is a fastidious, facultative bacterium, it can be grown in an atmosphere of 5–10% CO_2 (candle jar) or in an anaerobic chamber. *G. vaginalis* organisms are Gram-negative or Gram-variable, pleomorphic coccobacilli, or bacilli that average 0.4 mm by 1.5 mm in size (*Fig. 9.17*). In vaginal smears, they are often attached to epithelial cells.

The primary isolation of *G. vaginalis* from specimens containing mixed flora is best performed by using an enriched human or rabbit blood medium containing the selective antibiotics, colistin, and nalidixic acid. The diffuse hemolysis means that cells should be Gram-stained to distinguish Gram-negative *G. vaginalis* from Gram-positive *Lactobacillus* spp. (*Fig. 9.18*).

While anaerobic Gram-negative rods are part of the normal flora of most women, several species are found at higher frequencies in women with bacterial vaginosis (*Fig. 9.19*). These include *Prevotella bivia* (formerly *Bacteroides bivius*), *Prevotella corporis* (formerly one of the *Bacteroides melaninogenicus* group), *Bacteroides ureolyticus*, and *Fusobacterium nucleatum*. Women with

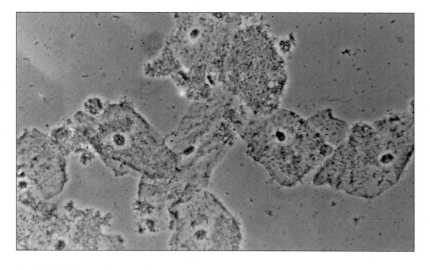

Fig. 9.11 Saline wet mount of vaginal fluid from a woman with bacterial vaginosis. Note that about half of the epithelial cells are clue cells.

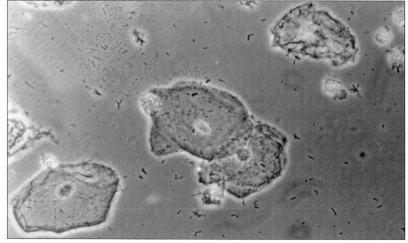

Fig. 9.12 Saline wet mount of vaginal fluid from a normal woman without genital infection. The vaginal epithelial cells are not covered by bacteria. As shown here, some normal vaginal epithelial cells have edges which may be mistaken for clue cells by their irregular appearance. However, true clue cells have edges obscured by bacteria rather than an irregular shape.

Fig. 9.13 Standardized scoring method for evaluation of Gram-stained smears for diagnosis of bacterial vaginosis.

STANDARDIZED SCORING METHOD FOR EVALUATION OF GRAM-STAINED SMEARS FOR DIAGNOSIS OF BACTERIAL VAGINOSIS

BACTERIAL MORPHOTYPE	POINTS* SCORED PER MORPHOTYPE**				
	NONE	1+	2+	3+	4+
Large Gram-positive rod	4	3	2	1	0
Small Gram-negative/variable rod	0	1	2	3	4
Curved Gram-negative/variable rod	0	1	1	2	2

*Score of 0–3 points, normal; 4–6 points, intermediate; 7–10 points, bacterial vaginosis
**1+ < 1/1000× oil immersion field; 2+ 1–5; 3+ 6–30; 4+ >30

clinical signs of bacterial vaginosis have a 100-fold greater concentration of these obligately anaerobic Gram-negative rods compared to women with lactobacilli-predominant microflora. However, it is not practical to perform routine cultures for these fastidious microorganisms. The importance of anaerobes in the etiology of bacterial vaginosis is supported by the increased clinical efficacy of antimicrobials, such as metronidazole and clindamycin, which are effective against anaerobic bacteria. These organisms are easily visualized by Gram stain and their presence in high numbers is a good indicator of bacterial vaginosis.

Mycoplasma hominis, one of the genital mycoplasmas, is found in only 15% of women with a normal vaginal flora, but in over 60% of women with bacterial vaginosis. As these organisms do not have cell walls, they are not visible

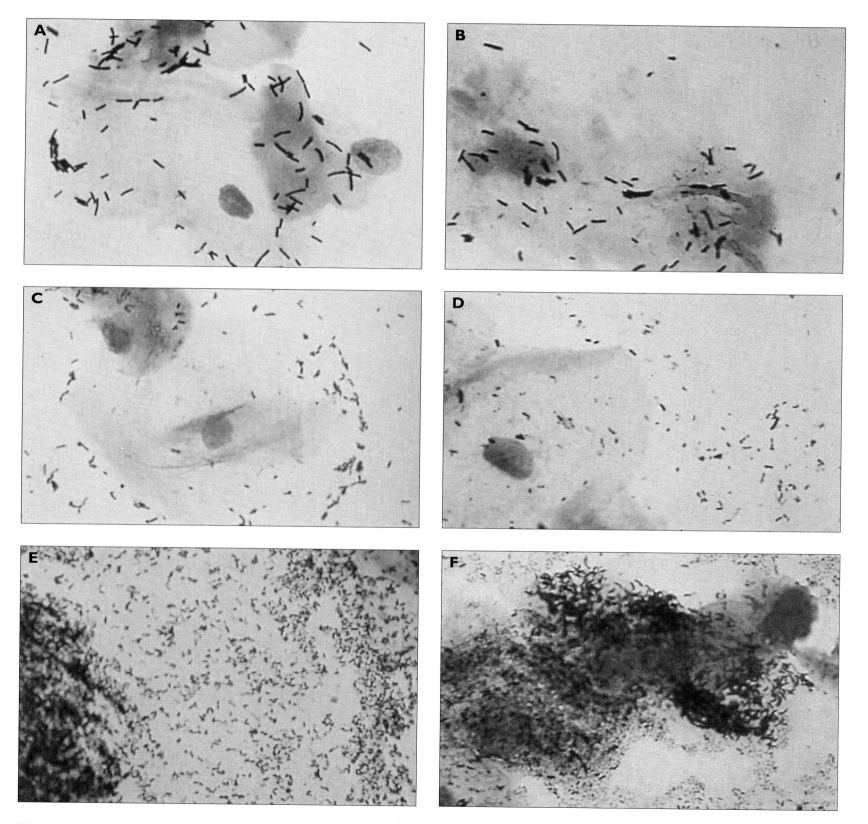

Fig. 9.14 Gram-stained vaginal smears from women with normal vaginal flora (A and B), intermediate vaginal flora (C and D), and bacterial vaginosis (E and F). The scores given to these smears according to the Nugent method are: A = 0; B = 2; C = 4; D = 6; E = 8; and F = 10.

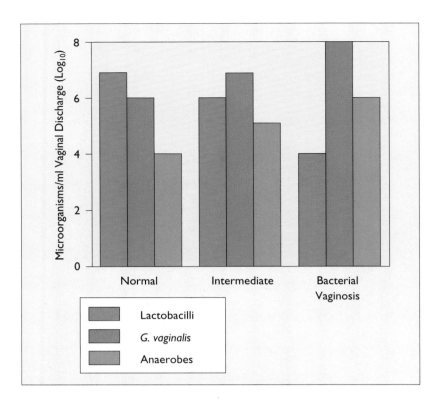

Fig. 9.15 Concentration of lactobacilli, *G. vaginalis*, and anaerobes in vaginal secretions or discharge.

DIAGNOSIS OF BACTERIAL VAGINOSIS BY INDIRECT METHODS		
METHOD	SENSITIVITY (%)	SPECIFICITY (%)
Oligonucleotide probe for *G. vaginalis*	94–95	79–81
Putrescine/cadaverine	87	86
Trimethylamine*	100	100
Succinate/lactate ratio	54–89	80–96
Proline aminopeptidase	74–93	86–93
Sialidase	84	100

Only 10 women included in this study.

Fig. 9.16 Diagnosis of bacterial vaginosis by indirect methods.

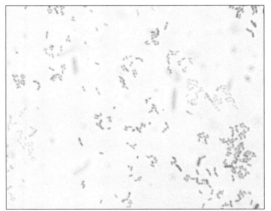

Fig. 9.17 Gram stain of *Gardnerella vaginalis* from 3 day culture showing Gram-negative coccobacilli.

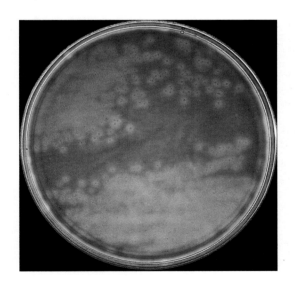

Fig. 9.18 Human blood bilayer plate incubated in an *atmos* phere containing 5% CO_2 for 3 days, showing hemolysis surrounding *G. vaginalis* colonies.

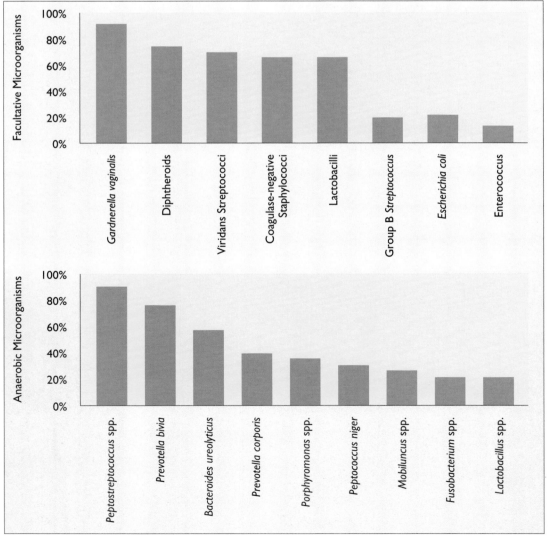

Fig. 9.19 Bacteria found in the vaginal flora of women with bacterial vaginosis, in order of usual prevalence.

by direct stains of vaginal smears (*see Chapter 7*). The role of these organisms in the etiology of bacterial vaginosis is unclear, but they have been shown to be pathogenic in upper genital tract infections.

Mobiluncus ('motile hooks') spp. are a recently 'rediscovered' group of anaerobic bacteria. These curved rods are often observed in vaginal smears from women with bacterial vaginosis (*Fig. 9.20*). Unlike *G. vaginalis*, they are rarely found in vaginal smears from women without bacterial vaginosis. Since culture techniques for *Mobiluncus* spp. are laborious and may be less sensitive than presumptive identification by vaginal smears or other methods, such as DNA probes or fluorescent antibody stains (*Fig. 9.21*), the prevalence of *Mobiluncus* in vaginal secretions is difficult to determine. Consequently, the presence of *Mobiluncus* in the vagina is often based on microscopic results showing organisms with characteristic morphology. Two species, *M. curtisii* (short form) and *M. mulieris* (long form), have been distinguished based on their size and subtle biologic differences (*Figs. 9.22* and *9.23*). Both species are motile, using flagella originating from the concave aspect of the cell, and both have a laminated cell wall consistent with a Gram-positive structure, even though they usually stain as Gram-negative rods.

TREATMENT

The antimicrobial agents that are most effective in treating bacterial vaginosis are those with good activity against anaerobes. Metronidazole or clindamycin, used orally or intravaginally, are the agents which yield the highest cure rates (*Fig. 9.24*). Other antimicrobials (e.g. triple sulfa cream), which have good *in vitro* activity against *G. vaginalis* but not anaerobes, are effective in only 50% of women. Ampicillin and amoxicillin are also only effective in 50% of women, while agents that are effective in cervicitis, including tetracycline, erythromycin, azithromycin, or ofloxacin, have very limited efficacy (less than 30%).

Since bacterial vaginosis is caused by an imbalance in the vaginal ecosystem, some clinicians have used homeopathic remedies such as yogurt, acetic acid gel, lactic acid gel, or hormonal creams. None of these treatments has been proven to be more effective than placebo in carefully controlled trials. It is possible that vaginal recolonization with suitable, human-derived strains of lactobacilli may be a useful adjunct to antimicrobial therapy, but so far no commercially available strain has been proven

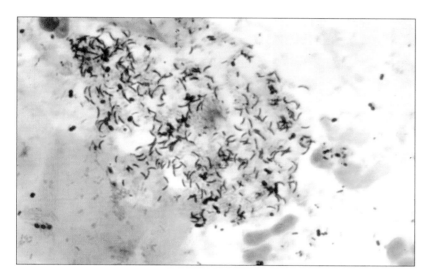

Fig. 9.20 Gram-stained clue cell from a woman with bacterial vaginosis, showing *Mobiluncus curtisii* on the surface.

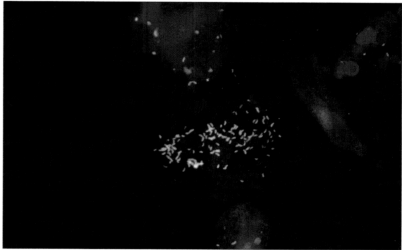

Fig. 9.21 Clue cell from a woman with bacterial vaginosis stained with a fluorescent antibody to *Mobiluncus curtisii*.

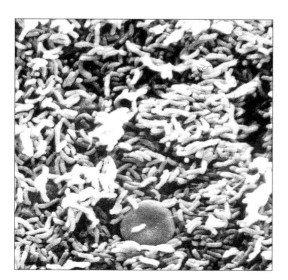

Fig. 9.22 Scanning electron micrograph of *Mobiluncus curtisii*. Notice the red blood cell in the center of the field, with *M. curtisii* on the surface.

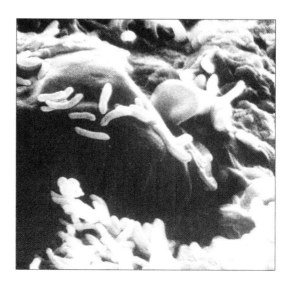

Fig. 9.23 Scanning electron micrograph of *Mobiluncus mulieris*, the longer of the two species of *Mobiluncus*.

to be beneficial. A number of recently published studies have linked bacterial vaginosis to complications of pregnancy, including preterm labor, preterm delivery, and amniotic fluid infection. While concern about the potential teratogenicity and carcinogenicity of metronidazole has limited its use during pregnancy, this drug is generally regarded as safe for use in the second trimester of pregnancy.

TRICHOMONIASIS

INTRODUCTION

Trichomonas vaginalis is a protozoan that infects the genital tract specifically. Although two other species of trichomonads colonize man (*Trichomonas tenax* in the mouth and *Pentatrichomonas hominis* in the large intestine), these organisms do not occur in the vagina. *T. vaginalis* is ovoid, and approximately 10–20 μm wide (about the size of a white blood cell) (*Fig. 9.25*). The organism has four, free, anterior flagella and a fifth flagellum embedded in an undulating membrane that extends around the anterior two-thirds of the cell. The flagella move the protozoan with a jerky movement.

EPIDEMIOLOGY

Women are the main carriers of disease. About one-third of men who are sexual partners of women with *T. vaginalis* have urethral colonization, but men, unlike women, rapidly clear the organism. One study found that 70% of men who had had sex with an infected woman 2 days previously were infected,

with this percentage dropping to 47% by 14 days or longer. Thus, transmission of the disease depends upon relatively frequent intercourse of men with different partners, and/or occasional long-term infections in some men.

In a study of trichomoniasis in over 13,000 women in the second trimester of pregnancy, the prevalence by culture was 13%. Infection by *T. vaginalis* was associated with Black race, being unmarried, a history of gonorrhea, and having multiple sexual partners during pregnancy. The high prevalence of this sexually transmitted pathogen in pregnant women is of concern because of the recent data suggesting that trichomoniasis is linked with an increased risk of low birth weight.

CLINICAL MANIFESTATIONS

As many as one-half of women infected with *T. vaginalis* are asymptomatic. This number depends upon how women are selected for study, how closely the women are questioned for symptoms, and the sensitivity of diagnostic techniques. In symptomatic women, a vaginal discharge is the most common complaint. The discharge usually appears purulent or yellow in color. As in bacterial vaginosis, about 50% of women notice a disagreeable odor, due to the overgrowth of anaerobic microorganisms with resultant amine production. Vulvar itching is also reported by 50% of women with trichomoniasis.

The vaginal mucosa is often erythematous, reflecting the inflammatory nature of the disease process (*Fig. 9.26*). In a few cases, the cervix is inflamed and has punctate hemorrhages (*Fig. 9.27*). Rarely, *T. vaginalis* has been found in the upper genital tract, but the significance of this finding is unknown.

Most men infected with *T. vaginalis* are asymptomatic. About 5–10% of men with nongonococcal urethritis are infected with *T. vaginalis*. The organism has been recovered from semen in association with an inflammatory semen analysis, but whether it is a cause of prostatitis is debatable.

EFFECTIVENESS OF DIFFERENT REGIMENS FOR TREATMENT OF BACTERIAL VAGINOSIS	
AGENT AND REGIMEN	EFFICACY ONE MONTH POST TREATMENT
Metronidazole oral	
500 mg bid for 7 days	78–82%
2 g single dose	72–73%
Intravaginal metronidazole gel	
5 g bid for 5 days	71–73%
Clindamycin oral	
300 mg bid for 7 days	94%
Intravaginal clindamycin cream	
5 g once daily for 7 days	61–85%
Ampicillin	66%
Ofloxacin (300 mg bid for 7 days)	29%
Erythromycin	20%
Tetracycline	20%
Lactate gel	20%
Acetic acid gel	18%
Yogurt	7%
Lactobacilli (10^8 bid for 6 days)	20%
Povidone iodine tablets (200 mg bid for 14 days)	25%

Fig. 9.24 Effectiveness of different regimens for treating bacterial vaginosis.

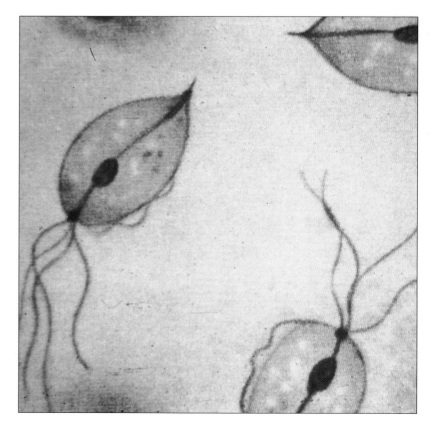

Fig. 9.25 *Trichomonas vaginalis.*

LABORATORY TESTS

A variety of diagnostic techniques for *T. vaginalis* are available but none detect all infected women. The most commonly used and easiest technique is that of a wet mount of vaginal secretions. An aliquot of vaginal secretions, usually obtained with a swab, is mixed with a small amount of saline and examined with light- or phase-contrast microscopy under low power. Trichomonads are about the size of white blood cells and move with a jerky motion. Organisms that are tentatively identified under low power are then examined under high power to confirm their motility and to visualize flagella (*Fig. 9.28*). The sensitivity of the wet mount varies with the concentration of trichomonads in the discharge, the dilution of secretions examined, the experience of the investigator, and the standard to which the wet mount is compared. Sensitivity may be as low as 50%, but most authorities consider it to be about 65–85%.

Culture is the most sensitive means of diagnosis, and a variety of culture media are available. Although *T. vaginalis* can be cultured using solid media, all clinically useful media are liquid. Of the media available in the USA, the best seems to be Diamond's medium or a variant. An aliquot of vaginal secretions is placed into tubes and incubated at 33–37°C. A drop of fluid from the bottom of the tube, where the concentration of trichomonads is greatest, is examined by wet mount daily for 7 days or until positive. If examination cannot be performed daily, then examination at 3–4 days and again at 7 days will detect almost all positive specimens.

Recently, fluorescein-labeled monoclonal antibodies have been used to detect trichomonads on vaginal smears (*Fig. 9.29*). The sensitivity of this procedure exceeds that of the wet mount but appears to be less than that of sensitive culture media. Compared with wet mount, this procedure requires more time, is more expensive, and requires a fluorescence microscope, and thus may be most useful in situations where culture is not available.

The Papanicolaou stain of exfoliated cervical cells may identify trichomonads (*Fig. 9.30*). Cytologic criteria for the diagnosis of trichomoniasis vary, however, from simply visualizing an inflammatory reaction thought to be typical of trichomoniasis to the visualization of flagella arising from a cell. In one study, up to 30% of women with an incidental finding of *Trichomonas* on Papanicolaou smear had negative culture and wet-mount results for this organism.

No widely accepted technique of differentiating strains of *T. vaginalis* exists. Reaction patterns based on panels of monoclonal antibodies and differences between *in vitro* hemolytic activity appear to offer the most promise in differentiating strains when necessary.

TREATMENT

Metronidazole is the only antimicrobial widely recommended to treat trichomoniasis (*Fig. 9.31*). Two regimens are commonly used. A single oral dose of 2 g, which is more than 85% effective, is often used because it can be given as a single dose. Alternatively, 250 mg administered orally three times a day for 7 days is slightly more effective. With both regimens, sexual partners must be simultaneously treated.

Metronidazole-resistant strains of *T. vaginalis* have been reported from at least 26 states. The origin of their resistance is unclear, but many of the resistant strains of *T. vaginalis* appear to be aerotolerant. Organisms which are facultative are generally resistant to metronidazole.

Recurrent trichomoniasis is usually caused by a failure to treat all sexual partners, or by noncompliance of sexual partners with therapy. If a documented case of resistant trichomoniasis is found, concurrent use of oral and intravaginal metronidazole can be used. Intravenous metronidazole therapy has not been found to have a higher efficacy than oral therapy. Unfortunately, intravaginal metronidazole alone cures only half of infected women.

Treatment of trichomoniasis in pregnancy is problematic. Metronidazole may be contraindicated in the first trimester of pregnancy because of the potential carcinogenicity, although human data supporting this is lacking. Metronidazole has a pregnancy B classification, which is the same classification as clotrimazole. Some clinicians have recommended the use of intravaginal clotrimazole for treatment during pregnancy, but this also has a low efficacy.

CANDIDIASIS

INTRODUCTION

Vaginal disease caused by yeasts is common, with most women having at least one symptomatic, vaginal yeast infection during their lifetime. *Candida albicans* causes 90% of vaginal infections (with other *Candida* spp. and *Torulopsis glabrata* causing most of the remainder). Thus, vaginal yeast infections are often referred to as *candidiasis*. However, recovery of the organism from, or identification in, vaginal secretions is not sufficient to diagnose disease, because asymptomatic vaginal colonization occurs in approximately 10–15% of women.

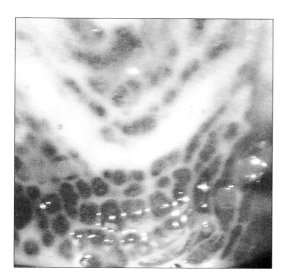

Fig. 9.26 Vaginal erythema and discharge from a patient with trichomoniasis. Note frothiness of discharge.

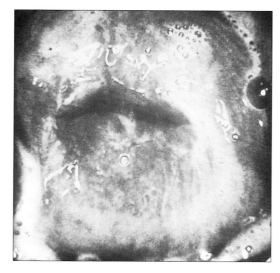

Fig. 9.27 'Strawberry cervix,' seen in about 10% of patients with trichomoniasis. Note frothiness of discharge.

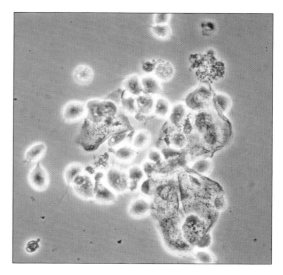

Fig. 9.28 Trichomonads visualized by phase contrast microscopy (× 400).

In 1991, some antifungal agents (clotrimazole and miconazole) became available over the counter. These medications have since become some of the top-selling over-the-counter products in the USA, accounting for over $200 million in annual sales. This figure suggests that 13 million episodes of self-diagnosed and treated episodes of yeast vaginitis occur annually. A clinical examination complicated by large quantities of self-administered vaginal antifungal cream has become a common problem in the past 5 years (*Fig. 9.32*).

CLINICAL MANIFESTATIONS

Candidiasis is a vulvovaginitis whose predominant symptom is prurituis. Typically, the onset is acute and occurs premenstrually. When seen by the clinician, the vulva and vagina may be erythematous and excoriated. Prurituis may occur with a discharge (*Fig. 9.33*), or without one. A curdy white thick discharge may be present in 50% of affected women (*Figs. 9.34* and *9.35*). Symptoms of pruritus should not be used as the sole basis for diagnosis, since other infections may cause vaginal itching.

Many women from whom *Candida* spp. are isolated may not complain of a discharge, and are thus asymptomatic. Nevertheless, women infected with *Candida* spp. are more likely to have a discharge considered to be abnormal by a clinician (and thus have signs of disease) than women not colonized, indicating that the disease is inapparent to some women. The vaginal secretions do not have an offensive odor.

In men, *Candida* spp. may cause balanitis (inflammation of the glans penis) and balanoposthitis (inflammation of the glans penis and prepuce) (*Fig. 9.36*). *Candida* organisms have been recovered from semen and from the urethras of some men with nonspecific urethritis, but the significance of these findings is unclear.

EPIDEMIOLOGY

Although men can be colonized with *Candida* spp., and many male sexual partners of women with candidiasis are transiently colonized, candidiasis is not recognized as an STD. Instead, symptoms occur in women previously

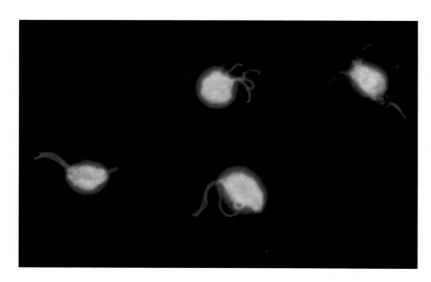

Fig. 9.29 Trichomonads stained with fluorescein-labeled antibody (x 1,000).

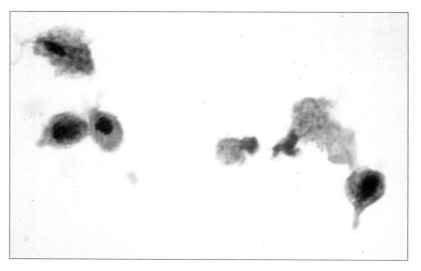

Fig. 9.30 Trichomonads identified by Papanicolaou stain on exfoliated cervical cells.

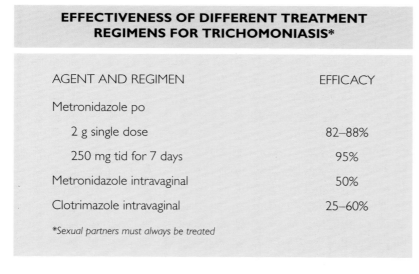

EFFECTIVENESS OF DIFFERENT TREATMENT REGIMENS FOR TRICHOMONIASIS*

AGENT AND REGIMEN	EFFICACY
Metronidazole po	
2 g single dose	82–88%
250 mg tid for 7 days	95%
Metronidazole intravaginal	50%
Clotrimazole intravaginal	25–60%

*Sexual partners must always be treated

Fig. 9.31 Effectiveness of different treatment regimens for trichomoniasis.

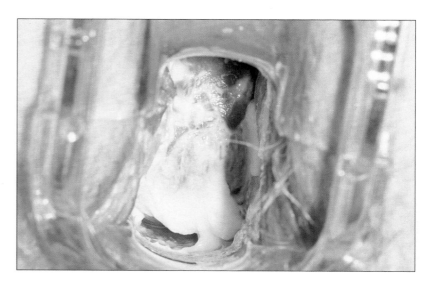

Fig. 9.32 Vaginal examination on a woman who inserted a commercial preparation of vaginal antifungal medication prior to her appointment. Excessive quantities of vaginal cream make evaluation of discharge, vaginal pH, and amine odor difficult. A vaginal Gram stain can usually be successfully performed in these patients if care is taken to sample the vaginal walls.

colonized with *C. albicans*. Although the reasons why symptomatic yeast infections occur are not completely understood, pregnancy, diabetes, use of birth control pills, steroid use, and systemic antimicrobial therapy (which eliminates competing vaginal flora) are recognized predisposing factors to symptomatic infection. Many women who develop yeast vaginitis will have not had any of the recognized risk factors.

LABORATORY TESTS

C. albicans occurs in both yeast and mycelial forms. Yeasts are oval cells about 4–8 mm in diameter (*Fig. 9.37*). In vaginal specimens, yeasts multiply asexually by forming buds (blastoconidia). If the buds keep forming and elongating, and do not detach from one another, they resemble hyphae and are called pseudohyphae (*Fig. 9.38*). The constrictions between buds in the pseudohyphae differentiate them from true hyphae. Hyphae, which form a mycelium when they are abundant and intertwined, are rarely seen in vaginal secretions because they are formed only under poor growth conditions, while the vagina, rich in glycogen and oxygen, provides suitable growth conditions for *Candida* spp.

The diagnosis of candidiasis is most often made by wet-mount microscopy of vaginal fluid; this can be done when the vaginal fluid is examined for clue cells and trichomonads. Estimates of the sensitivity of wet-mount microscopy range from 40–85%; as with trichomoniasis, sensitivity varies with patient selection, observer experience, and sensitivity of the culture media to which wet-mount results are compared. Symptoms appear to be directly correlated to the quantity of yeasts present, and thus if symptomatic women are studied, the wet mount will appear highly sensitive.

The wet-mount specimen is examined for yeasts or pseudohyphae under low-power magnification (× 100), while subsequent high-power examination (× 400) will detail the organism. Debris from epithelial cells or mucus may be mistaken for or may obscure yeasts, but this potential problem can be eliminated by adding a few drops of 10–15% KOH to the wet-mount specimen. The addition of KOH has been shown to improve both sensitivity and specificity.

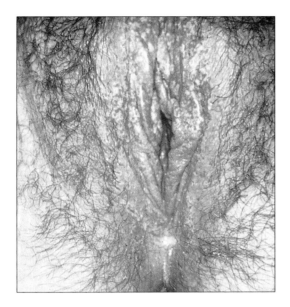

Fig. 9.33 Vulvovaginal candidiasis. Mild discharge and inflammation of the vulva, commonly occurring in vulvovaginal candidiasis.

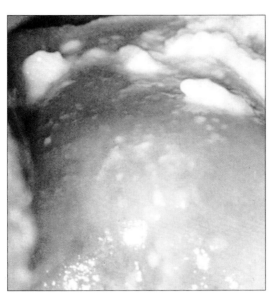

Fig. 9.34 Vaginal candidiasis. Curd-like discharge commonly present in candidiasis.

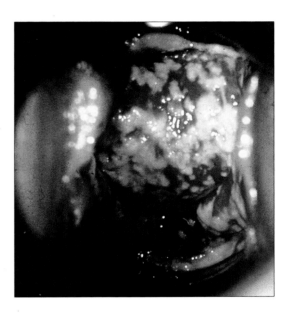

Fig. 9.35 Cervical candidiasis. Clumps of discharge adhering to the cervix.

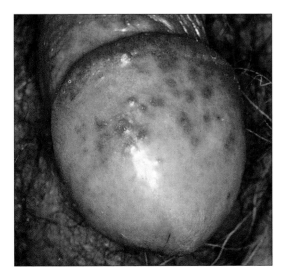

Fig. 9.36 Penile candidal balanitis showing erythematous papules and pustules on the glans penis.

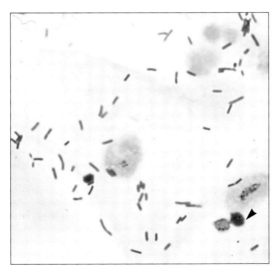

Fig. 9.37 Gram-stained vaginal smear from a woman having a vaginal yeast infection caused by *Candida (Torulopsis) glabrata*, a yeast which does not form hyphae or pseudohyphae. The Gram-positive rods in the background are lactobacilli.

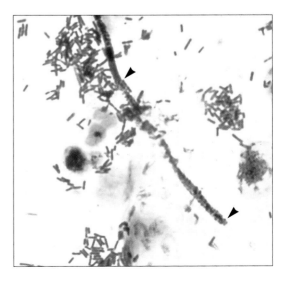

Fig. 9.38 Gram-stained vaginal smear from a woman with vulvovaginal candidiasis. Note the large pseudohyphal element and the abundance of Gram-positive rods resembling lactobacilli.

A Gram stain of vaginal secretions is not as sensitive as wet mount in detecting infection. *Candida* spp. stain intensely Gram-positive (*see Figs. 9.37 and 9.38*). *Candida* spp. may be seen on Papanicolaou-stained samples of exfoliated cervical cells. This method is not sensitive, however, and detects only about 50% of cases of symptomatic women.

Culture is the most sensitive diagnostic test, but should be reserved for those instances in which clinical signs or symptoms of yeast infection are present and the wet mount is negative for hyphae. *Candida* spp. grow on many media, including blood agar. At least two media should be used for greatest yield, one with and one without antimicrobials inhibitory for competing microorganisms. Sabouraud's dextrose, the most widely used medium, supports the growth of all clinically important yeasts. *Candida* spp. will grow at both 25°C and 37°C, so using two temperatures offers no diagnostic advantage. Although *Candida* spp. grow most rapidly at 37°C, more rapidly growing bacteria may obscure fungal colonies at this temperature, and so many authorities prefer to grow *Candida* at 30°C. Pinpoint colonies may be visible at 24 hours but are more apparent at 48–72 hours. Nickerson's agar and its analogs may simplify the identification of *Candida* spp. because the colonies are selectively dark, but this method of identification is not totally reliable. It is important to remember that finding yeast by culture in an asymptomatic woman means only that she harbors this organism as part of her normal flora.

TREATMENT

A number of highly effective oral and intravaginal antifungals are available (*Fig. 9.39*). Nystatin is the least effective with cure rates in the 70–75% range. The remaining antifungals have published efficacies in the 80–88% range. Of the intravaginal imidazoles, clotrimazole and miconazole are available over-the-counter in the USA, while the remainder are available only by prescription. The prescription vaginal products, butoconazole, terconazole, and tioconazole have a greater *in vitro* efficacy against non-*C. albicans* yeasts. However, the clinical significance of this is unclear as the published efficacy for these compounds is similar to that reported for over-the-counter products.

Oral agents which have been used in the USA for treatment of yeast vaginitis include fluconazole, which is supplied as a single 150 mg oral tablet and ketoconazole, which has been used more frequently for women with recurrent infections.

A small subset of women with yeast vulvovaginitis develop recurrent infections, which can cause monthly or even persistent symptoms. Longitudinal data suggest that women are usually persistently infected by the same strain or species of yeast. While some of those women have recognized risk factors for yeast infection, most do not. Risk factors should be considered, but a thorough search for subclinical diabetes mellitus is not warranted.

One approach to the management of recurrent yeast vulvovaginitis is the use of antifungal agents prophylactically prior to or immediately after menses. In placebo-controlled trials, women who use prophylactic antifungals will have fewer episodes of recurrence, but these women will develop increased episodes of yeast vaginitis after stopping prophylactic therapy. Thus, the prophylactic use of antifungals should be viewed as providing suppression rather than cure. Another approach is to prescribe antifungals empirically at the onset of symptoms. Although this approach results in more episodes of yeast vaginitis, the total amount of antifungal used and the total costs for drugs is substantially less.

THERAPIES FOR TREATMENT OF VAGINAL CANDIDIASIS HAVING SIMILAR EFFICACIES

INTRAVAGINAL

Clotrimazole	100 mg vaginal tablet once daily for 7 days
	5 g 1% vaginal cream once daily for 7 days
	500 mg tablet used once
Miconazole	100 mg vaginal suppository once daily for 7 days
	200 mg vaginal suppository once daily for 3 days
	5 g 2% cream once daily for 7 days
Terconazole	80 mg vaginal suppository once daily for 3 days
	5 g 0.4% cream once daily for 7 days
	5 g 0.8% cream once daily for 3 days
Butoconazole	5 g 2% cream once daily for 3 days
Tioconazole	4.6 g 6.5% ointment once

ORAL

Fluconazole	150 mg once
Ketoconazole	400 mg daily for 14 days

Fig. 9.39 Therapies for the treatment of vaginal candidiasis having similar efficacies.

DESQUAMATIVE INFLAMMATORY VAGINITIS

CLINICAL AND LABORATORY FINDINGS
Purulent yellow-green discharge
Vaginal erythema
Vaginal pH > 4.5
Amine odor absent
Increased (3–4+) vaginal PMN's
Parabasal cells and naked nuclei
Gram-positive cocci
Lack of lactobacilli
CHARACTERISTICS OF POPULATION
Usually Caucasian
More frequent post-menopause
Long duration of symptoms
TREATMENT
Primary:
    2% clindamycin vaginal suppositories daily for 14 days
Relapse:
    Oral ampicillin or cephalexin

Fig. 9.40 Desquamative inflammatory vaginitis.

During pregnancy, yeast vaginitis should be treated with one of the pregnancy category A (nystatin) or B (clotrimazole, miconazole) antifungals. Other therapies are not recommended for use during pregnancy, based on animal studies, and have been given a pregnancy category C.

DESQUAMATIVE INFLAMMATORY VAGINITIS

INTRODUCTION

The most recently described cause of infectious vaginitis is desquamative inflammatory vaginitis. It is considered a type of infectious vaginitis because it has been associated with group B streptococci and it responds to therapy with antimicrobial agents effective against this microorganism. As this syndrome has been described very recently, and occurs rarely in comparison to other types of infectious vaginitis, comparatively little is known about this syndrome.

EPIDEMIOLOGY

Desquamative inflammatory vaginitis occurs more frequently in perimenopausal or postmenopausal women than in women of reproductive age.

This syndrome has been documented much more frequently in Caucasian than in African-American women, even when the study population has a majority of African-American women (*Fig. 9.40*).

CLINICAL FEATURES

Women with desquamative inflammatory vaginitis often present with complaints of vaginal irritation lasting months or even years. On examination, these women will have profound vaginal erythema (*Fig. 9.41*). While the vaginal pH will usually be greater than 4.5, amine odor is almost universally absent, indicating a lack of anaerobic microorganisms. A purulent yellow-green discharge may be present.

Diagnosis is made on the basis of elevated pH and a lack of amine odor coupled with the microscopic evaluation of vaginal fluid. The wet-mount examination is characterized by the presence of parabasal cells and naked nuclei, suggesting severe desquamation of the vaginal epithelium. A Gram-stained vaginal smear usually shows the presence of many polymorphonuclear leukocytes, the absence of lactobacilli, and the presence of abundant Gram-positive cocci (*Fig. 9.42*).

Treatment with 2% clindamycin, as an intravaginal cream or suppository, used once daily for 2 weeks will treat most cases effectively. In the case of relapse, oral cephalexin or ampicillin is recommended. In some cases, a culture for β-hemolytic streptococci can be obtained to monitor the response to therapy.

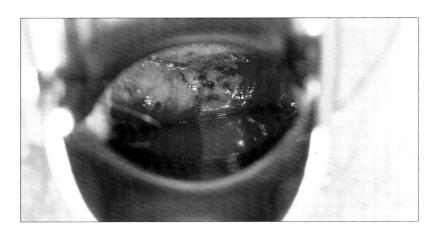

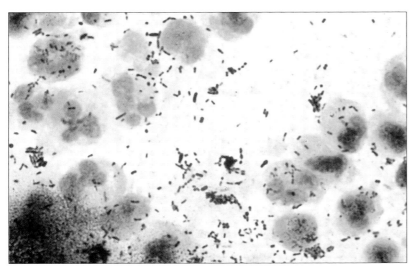

Fig. 9.41 Desquamative inflammatory vaginitis. Areas of intense vaginal erythema from group B streptococci in this case of desquamative inflammatory vaginitis.

Fig. 9.42 Gram-stained vaginal smear from a woman with desquamative inflammatory vaginitis caused by group B streptococci. Notice the presence of many polymorphonuclear leukocytes and Gram-positive cocci, and the lack of gram-positive rods resembling lactobacilli.

CONCLUSIONS

Vaginal infections are common in women, and lead them to seek medical care or to pursue self-diagnosis and treatment. A careful examination of the vaginal fluid, measurement of vaginal pH, evaluation of vaginal odor after addition of 10% KOH, and an assessment of vaginal discharge are essential components of office diagnosis. Cultures are not useful at all in the diagnosis of bacterial vaginosis. They are only occasionally indicated for yeast vaginitis, but are vastly superior to wet mount for *Trichomonas*. Several different treatment options are available for these infections, but additional care should be taken when choosing a therapy for use during pregnancy.

Picture credits for this chapter are as follows: Fig. 9.13 Nugent RP Krohn MA, Hillier SL: Reliability of diagnosing bacterial vaginosis is improved by a standardized method of Gram stain interpretation. J Clin Microbiol **29**:297–301, 1991; by permission of the American Soceity for Microbiology;

Figs. 9.33, 9.35, and 9.36 courtesy of Bingham JS: Pocket picture Guide Series. Sexually transmitted diseases. London, Gower Medical Publishing Ltd., 1984.

BIBLIOGRAPHY

Amsel, R, Totten PA, Spiegel CA, Chen KCS, Eschenbach DA, Holmes KK: Nonspecific vaginitis: diagnostic criteria and microbial and epidemiologic associations. *Am J Med* **74**:14–22, 1983.

Boeke AJP, Dekker JH, van Eijk JTM, Kostense PJ, Bezemer PD: Effect of lactic acid suppositories compared with oral metronidazole and placebo in bacterial vaginosis: a randomised clinical trial. *Genitourin Med* **69**:388–392, 1993.

Bump RC, Zuspan FP, Buesching WJ, III, Ayers LW, Stephens T: The prevalence, six-month persistence and predictive values of laboratory indicators of bacterial vaginosis (nonspecific vaginitis) in asymptomatic women. *Am J Obstet Gynecol* **150**:917–924, 1984.

Chaltopadhyay B: The role of *Gardnerella vaginalis* in 'non-specific' vaginitis. *J Infect Dis* **9**:113, 1984.

Chen KCS, Amsel R, Eschenbach DA, Holmes KK: Biochemical diagnosis of vaginitis: determination of diamines in vaginal fluid. *J Infect Dis* **145**:337–345, 1982.

Covino JM, Black JR, Cummings M, Zwicki B, McCormack WM: Comparative evaluation of ofloxacin and metronidazole in the treatment of bacterial vaginosis. *Sex Transm Dis* **20(3)**:262–264, 1993.

Eschenbach DA, Hillier SL, Critchlow CW, Stevens CE, Koutsky LA, DeRouen T, Holmes KK: Diagnosis and clinical features associated with bacterial vaginosis. *Am J Obstet Gynecol* **158**:819–828, 1988.

Gardner HL, Dukes CD: *Haemophilus vaginalis* vaginitis. *Ann NY Acad Sci* **83**:280, 1959.

Glupczynski Y, Labbe M, Crockaert F, Pepersack F, Van Der Auwera P, Yourassowsky E: Isolation of *Mobiluncus* in four cases of extragenital infections in adult women. *Eur J Clin Microbiol* **3**:433–435, 1984.

Gravett MG, Nelson HP, DeRouen T, Critchlow CW, Eschenbach DA, Holmes KK: Independent association of bacterial vaginosis and *Chlamydia trachomatis* infection with adverse pregnancy outcome. *JAMA* **256**:1899–1903, 1986.

Greenwood JR: Current taxonomic status of *Gardnerella vaginalis*. *Scand J Inf Dis* **40**(suppl.):11, 1983.

Hillier SL, Krohn MA, Rabe LK, Klebanoff SJ, Eschenbach DA: The normal vaginal flora, H_2O_2-producing lactobacilli, and bacterial vaginosis in pregnant women. *Clin Infect Dis* **16**(suppl. 4):S273–281, 1993.

Hillier SL, Krohn MA, Watts DH, Wölner–Hanssen P, Eschenbach DA: Microbiological efficacy of intravaginal clindamycin cream for the treatment of bacterial vaginosis. *Obstet Gynecol* **76**:407–413, 1990.

Krieger JN, Tam MR, Stevens CE, et al.: Diagnosis of trichomoniasis. Comparison of conventional wet-mount examination with cytologic studies, cultures, and monoclonal antibody staining of direct specimens. *JAMA* **259**:1223–1227, 1988.

Lebherz TB, Ford LC: *Candida albicans* vaginitis: The problem is diagnosis, the enigma is treatment. *Chemotherapy* **28**(suppl. 1):73, 1982.

Livengood CH, III, Thomason JL, Hill GB: Bacterial vaginosis: treatment with topical intravaginal clindamycin phosphate. *Obstet Gynecol* **76**:118–23, 1990.

Lossick JG: The diagnosis of vaginal trichomoniasis. *JAMA* **259**:1230, 1988.

Mårdh PA, Taylor–Robinson D (eds): *Bacterial Vaginosis*. Almquist and Wiksell International, Stockholm, 1988.

Norrod PE, Morse SA: Presence of hydrogen peroxide in media used for cultivation of *Neisseria gonorrhoeae*. *J Clin Microbiol* **15**:103, 1982.

Nugent RP, Krohn MA, Hillier SL: Reliability of diagnosing bacterial vaginosis is improved by a standardized method of Gram stain interpretation. *J Clin Microbiol* **29**:297–301, 1991.

O'Connor MI, Sobel JD: Epidemiology of recurrent vulvovaginal candidiasis: identification and strain differentiation of *Candida albicans*. *J Infect Dis* **154**:358–362, 1986.

Pheifer TA, Forsyth PA, Durfee MA, et al.: Nonspecific vaginitis: role of *Haemophilus vaginalis* and treatment with metronidazole. *N Engl J Med* **198**:1429–1434, 1978.

Roberts MC, Hillier SL, Schoenknecht F, Holmes KK: Comparison of Gram stain, DNA probe and culture for the identification of species of *Mobiluncus* in female genital specimens. *J Infect Dis* **152**:74–77, 1985.

Schmitt C, Sobel JD, Meriwether C: Bacterial vaginosis: treatment with clindamycin cream versus oral metronidazole. *Obstet Gynecol* **79**:1020–1023, 1992.

Sobel JD: Vulvovaginal candidiasis — what we do and do not know. *Ann Intern Med* **101**:390, 1984.

Sobel JD: Desquamative inflammatory vaginitis: a new subgroup of purulent vaginitis responsive to topical 2% clindamycin therapy. *Am J Obstet Gynecol* **171**:1215, 1994.

Spiegel CA, Amsel R, Eschenbach DA, Schoenknecht F, Holmes KK: Anaerobic bacteria in nonspecific vaginitis. *N Engl J Med* **303**:601–607, 1980.

Spiegel CA, Amsel R, Holmes KK: Diagnosis of bacterial vaginosis by direct Gram stain of vaginal fluid. *J Clin Microbiol* **18**:170–177, 1983.

Spiegel CA, Eschenbach DA, Amsel R, Holmes KK: Curved anaerobic bacteria in nonspecific vaginosis and their response to antibiotic therapy. *J Infect Dis* **148**:817–822, 1983.

Spiegel CA, Roberts M: *Mobiluncus* gen. nov., *Mobiluncus curtisii* subsp. *curtisii* sp. nov., *Mobiluncus curtisii* subsp. *holmesii* subsp. nov., and *Mobiluncus mulieris* sp. nov., curved rods from the human vagina. *Int J Syst Bacteriol* **34**:177–184, 1984.

Thomason JL, Schreckenberger PC, Spellacy WN, et al.: Clinical and microbiological characterization of patients with nonspecific vaginosis associated with motile, curved anaerobic rods. *J Infect Dis* **149**:801–809, 1984.

Totten PA, Amsel R, Hale J, Piot P, Holmes KK: Selective differential human blood bilayer media for isolation of *Gardnerella* (*Haemophilus*) *vaginalis*. *J Clin Microbiol* **15**:141–147, 1982.

Ventkataramani TK, Rathbun HK: *Corynebacterium vaginale* (*Haemophilus vaginalis*) bacteremia: clinical study of 29 cases. *John Hopkins Med J* **139**:93, 1976.

Wathne B, Holst E, Hovelius B, Mårdh PA: Erythromycin versus metronidazole in the treatment of bacterial vaginosis. *Acta Obstet Gynecol Scand* **72**:470–474, 1993.

Weston TET, Nicol CS: Natural history of trichomonal infection in males. *Br J Vener Dis* **39**:251–257, 1963.

Wilson A, Ackers JP. Urine culture for the detection of *Trichomonas vaginalis* in men. *Br J Vener Dis* **56**:46, 1980.

CHAPTER TEN

Human Immunodeficiency Virus and the Acquired Immunodeficiency Syndrome

D Spach and P Keen

INTRODUCTION

Throughout the world, the spread of human immunodeficiency virus (HIV) continues at an alarming rate. This pandemic has created a dramatic, often devastating, impact on many countries. Although much has been learned about this disease, researchers do not predict a cure in the immediate future, and an increasing number of HIV-infected individuals is expected.

CLASSIFICATION

In the spring of 1981, the CDC received many reports from New York and California that described previously healthy gay males with *Pneumocystis carinii* pneumonia (PCP) and Kaposi's sarcoma. Initially, no apparent cause was discovered for the immunosuppression of these individuals and the CDC termed the disorder, the acquired immunodeficiency syndrome (AIDS). Soon afterwards, the CDC also formulated a definition of an AIDS case: 'any disease, such as PCP or Kaposi's sarcoma, that predicts a defect in cell-mediated immunity in a person who has no documented cause for the immunodeficiency'. Investigators subsequently identified HIV as the causative agent for AIDS and the CDC revised the surveillance definition to include a positive serologic test for HIV antibody. In 1987, they further revised the AIDS case definition to include a presumptive diagnosis of several conditions, namely PCP, Kaposi's sarcoma, esophageal candidiasis, and toxoplasmosis of the brain. They also added encephalopathy and wasting syndrome to the list of AIDS-defining conditions. In 1993, the CDC expanded the AIDS case definition to include patients with CD4 counts of less than 200 cells/mm^3 (or a CD4 of less than 14%). They also added three new clinical conditions – recurrent bacterial pneumonia, pulmonary tuberculosis, and invasive cervical cancer. This most recent classification system categorizes patients both on the basis of their CD4 cell count and their clinical condition (*Fig. 10.1*).

EPIDEMIOLOGY

WORLDWIDE
Globally, an estimated 14 million people are infected with HIV (*Fig. 10.2*). By the year 2000, projections estimate that between 38 million and 108 million people will be HIV-infected (*Fig. 10.3*). To date, 80% of AIDS cases have occurred among individuals living in developing countries, usually in regions with limited resources for treatment and prevention. Africa continues to have the largest population of HIV-infected individuals, with infection rates now exceeding 10% of the general population in some regions of this continent. Projections indicate that a dramatic increase in the number of AIDS cases will occur in southeast Asia, southern Asia, and India. In areas of the world other than the USA or Europe, heterosexual transmission of HIV predominates, with male to female ratios of approximately 1:1. In contrast, male homosexuality and injection-drug use account for most cases in the USA and Europe.

In almost all regions of the world, HIV-1 continues to predominate as the virus responsible for causing AIDS. HIV-2, which can also cause AIDS, predominantly occurs in West Africa (*Fig. 10.4*). Although HIV-1 and HIV-2 have similar gene products and similar modes of transmission, HIV-2 appears to have less potential for infection and causes slower clinical progression. Up to April 1992, there were fewer than 40 cases of HIV-2 infection in the USA, with all cases identified among individuals who had previously lived in West Africa or had sexual partners from that region.

USA
In the USA, an estimated 1 million people are infected with HIV, and as of 1995, approximately 350,000 AIDS-related cumulative deaths will have occurred. Although every state has reported cases of AIDS (*Figs. 10.5* and *10.6*), most have come from large urban areas, particularly New York City, San Francisco, Los Angeles, Miami, and Houston. Recent trends show that the number of AIDS cases from nonmetropolitan areas is increasing at a faster rate than in urban areas. Overall, the incidence of AIDS continues to increase on an annual basis (*Fig. 10.7*).

The major HIV transmission categories include men who have sex with men, injection-drug users, heterosexuals, and hemophiliacs (*Fig. 10.8*). Most AIDS cases have occurred among men who have sex with men, but in recent years, AIDS cases attributable to heterosexual contact have shown the largest proportional increase (*Fig. 10.9*). The growth in AIDS cases in the heterosexual category has been caused by the rapid increase in cases among heterosexual females (*Fig. 10.10*). The use of non-intravenous drugs, including cocaine and alcohol, has probably been a major factor in this increase, through the exchange of sex for drugs and due to disinhibition leading to unprotected sex. Overall, AIDS cases among adult females have increased from 3% in the early years of the epidemic to 13% in 1992.

Although the number of adolescents with AIDS remains relatively small, this number has sharply risen in recent years. Moreover, most individuals who develop AIDS in their early 20s probably acquired HIV in their early to mid-teenage years. Males, ethnic minorities, and racial minorities are disproportionately affected among adolescents with AIDS. Approximately 5,228 AIDS cases have been reported in children under 13 years of age, with most of these cases resulting from perinatal transmission. Sexual abuse may play a role in some pediatric cases with no identifiable risk factor (*Fig. 10.11*).

African-Americans and Hispanics are disproportionately represented in the total number of AIDS cases: each group makes up only approximately 10% of the US population, but comprises 36% and 18%, respectively, of reported AIDS cases in 1993 (*Fig. 10.12*). These observed racial differences are most notable among female and pediatric cases.

Modes of Transmission
The transmission of HIV occurs via three major routes:
- Sexual contact that exchanges body fluids (semen or vaginal fluid)
- Exchange of blood (injection-drug use, transfusion of blood products, and percutaneous needlestick injuries)
- Perinatal exchange of fluids between mother and child (transplacental, vaginally at the time of birth, and via breast milk).

There is no evidence to suggest that HIV infection is spread by nonsexual close contact, by the airborne route, by insect bites, by water, or by food handlers. In most regions of the world, the transmission of HIV predominantly occurs via sexual contact. Thus, educational programs that promote 'safe sex' among both heterosexuals and homosexuals remain the most effective means of preventing the spread of HIV. Other preventive measures include needle-exchange programs and screening blood products for HIV antibody.

In health-care settings, reports of HIV transmission have occurred among individuals stuck with needles containing HIV-infected blood, or when infected blood has entered the worker's bloodstream though openings in the skin or mucus membranes. No transmission from airborne droplets, environmental surfaces, or exposure to blood of intact skin have been reported. Following an accidental percutaneous needlestick injury, the estimated risk of acquiring HIV infection is approximately 0.3%, much less than the risk of acquiring hepatitis B after a similar exposure. HIV is susceptible to common disinfectants such as alcohol, phenol, formalin, sodium hypochlorite (household bleach), and glutaraldehyde. Customary dishwashing and laundering procedures are considered sufficient to provide adequate decontamination of food-service items and linens.

PATHOGENESIS

Many research laboratories have confirmed that HIV, a member of the lentivirus subfamily of human retroviruses, is indeed the cause of AIDS. HIV, like all human retroviruses, contains reverse transcriptase, an enzyme that permits transcription of viral RNA into DNA. This process also allows for incorporation of the newly formed DNA into the host cellular genome. Structurally, HIV consists of three major components:

- A host-derived outer lipid bilayer studded with knob-like outer projections
- A cone-shaped viral core that contains RNA
- A matrix sandwiched between the outer lipid bilayer and the viral core (*Figs. 10.13* and *10.14*).

The HIV RNA genome consists of nine viral genes, each one of which encodes a viral protein with a unique function (Fig. 10.15). Three of the proteins (gag, env, and pol) are produced as precursor proteins and are subsequently cleaved into smaller proteins. HIV predominantly binds to cells

1993 CDC REVISED CLASSIFICATION SYSTEM FOR HIV INFECTION AND EXPANDED AIDS SURVEILLANCE CASE DEFINITION FOR ADOLESCENTS AND ADULTS*

Fig. 10.1 1993 CDC revised classification system for HIV infection and expanded AIDS surveillance case definition for adolescents and adults.

CLINICAL CATEGORIES

CD4$^+$ T-CELL CATEGORIES	(A) ASYMPTOMATIC, 1° HIV, OR PGL	(B) SYMPTOMATIC, NOT A OR C CONDITIONS	(C) AIDS-INDICATOR CONDITIONS
(1) ≥ 500 cells/mm^3	A1	B1	C1
(2) 200–499 cells/mm^3	A2	B2	C2
(3) < 200 cells/mm^3	A3	B3	C3

*shaded areas indicate AIDS-defining categories

B CONDITIONS (listed in alphabetical order): bacillary angiomatosis; bacterial endocarditis, meningitis, or sepsis; candidiasis (oral); candidiasis (persistent vulvovaginal); cervical dysplasia or carcinoma in situ; constitutional illness (persistent unexplained fever or diarrhea or weight loss or disabling weakness); herpes zoster (multidermatomal); listeriosis; myelopathy; nocardiosis; hairy leukoplakia (oral); pelvic inflammatory disease (particularly if complicated by tubo-ovarian abscess); peripheral neuropathy; thrombocytopenia.

C CONDITIONS

Bacterial Infections
    Mycobacterium avium complex
    Mycobacterium kansasii (disseminated or extrapulmonary)
    Mycobacterium tuberculosis
    Mycobacterium of other or unidentified species (disseminated or extrapulmonary)
    Salmonella (recurrent septicemia)

Fungal Infections
    Candidiasis (bronchial, esophageal, trachea, or pulmonary)
    Coccidioidomycosis (disseminated or extrapulmonary)
    Cryptococcosis (extrapulmonary)
    Histoplasmosis (disseminated or extrapulmonary)
    Pneumocystis carinii pneumonia

Protozoan Infections
    Cryptosporidiosis (intestinal, for longer than 1 month)
    Isosporiasis (intestinal, for longer than 1 month)
    Toxoplasmosis (brain)

Viral Infections
    Cytomegalovirus (other than liver, spleen, or nodes)
    Herpes simplex (chronic ulcers >1 month duration or esophagitis or bronchitis or pneumonitis)

Malignancies
    Cervical cancer (invasive)
    Kaposi's sarcoma
    Lymphoma (Burkitt's, immunoblastic, or primary of brain)

Other
    Encephalopathy (HIV-related)
    Progressive multifocal leukoencephalopathy
    Pneumonia (2 or more episodes in 1-year period)
    Wasting syndrome (greater than 10% weight loss or fever and chronic weakness lasting longer than 30 days in absence of a concurrent illness that could explain this finding)

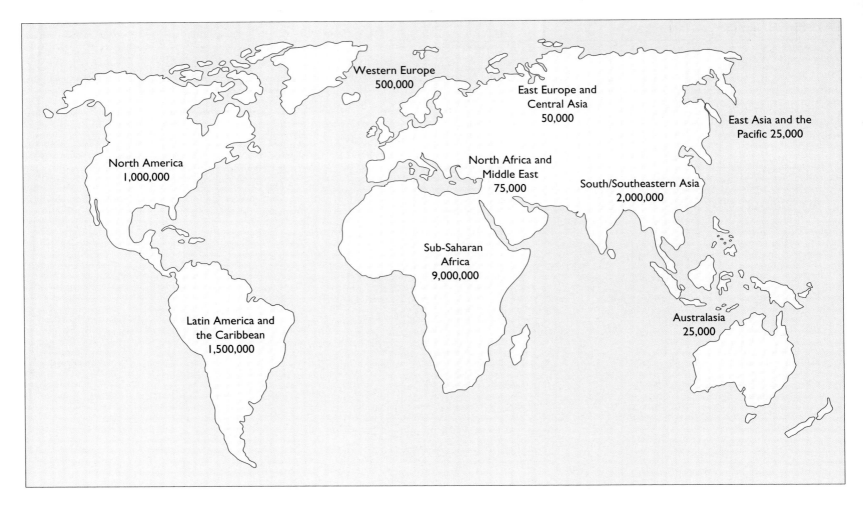

Fig. 10.2 Estimated global prevalence of HIV infection, 1994. (Source: World Health Organization.)

Fig. 10.3 Global projections of HIV infections, 1992 (Source: World Health Organization).

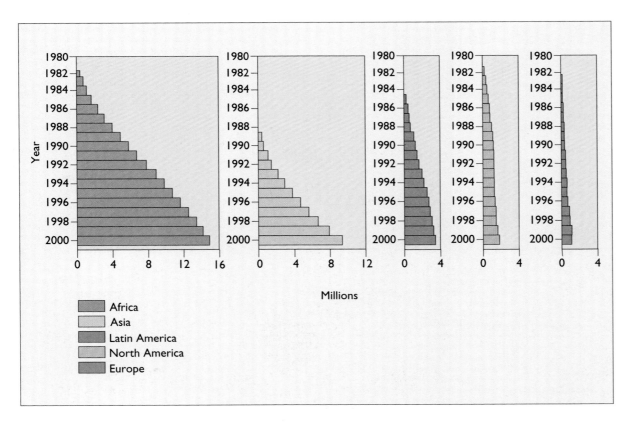

with the CD4 protein on the cell surface, namely CD4+ (T4) lymphocytes, monocytes, and microglial cells. Once HIV binds to the CD4 protein, complex conformational changes occur that lead to fusion of the viral and host membranes (*Fig. 10.16*). Following this process, the viral core enters the cell, the viral reverse transcriptase converts the single-stranded viral RNA into viral DNA, and the viral DNA integrates into the host DNA. This integrated DNA is referred to as the provirus and can remain latent or can reactivate intermittently. During the reactivation process, the host cell transcribes proviral DNA into viral messenger RNA, followed by translation of viral mRNA into viral proteins. These proteins are then cleaved and assembled into an incomplete virion that eventually buds from the cell (*Fig. 10.17*). During the budding process, the incomplete virion becomes coated with host membrane components, thus forming a complete HIV virion.

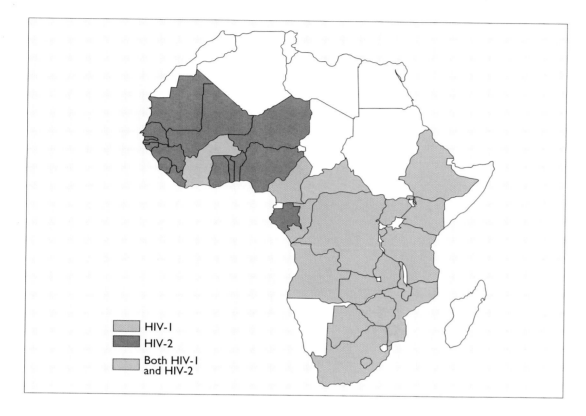

Fig. 10.4 HIV infection in Africa. The highest incidences of HIV-1 and HIV-2 infection and AIDS have been reported from central and southern Africa, as shown within the outlined areas.

HIV-1

HIV-2

Both HIV-1 and HIV-2

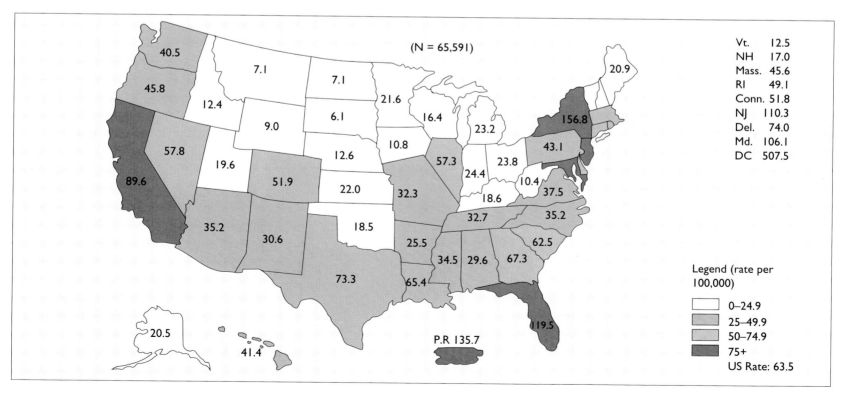

Fig. 10.5 Male adult/adolescent AIDS annual rates per 100,000 population for cases reported in the USA, 1994.

Although the binding of HIV to CD4[+] 'helper' lymphocytes probably plays a critical step in the immunopathogenesis of HIV infection, the exact mechanism whereby HIV gradually depletes these CD4[+] cells remains unknown. Presumably, CD4[+] cells are destroyed by a combination of direct cellular HIV infection and by indirect immunologic processes. The CD4[+] cell counts decrease by an average of 50–80 cells/mm^3 per year, and this CD4[+] cell depletion has a profound adverse effect on the immune system — most notably, a severely diminished response to a wide array of infectious pathogens and malignant tumors (*Fig. 10.18*). Clinically, CD4[+] cell count measurements are currently the most widely used marker to gauge

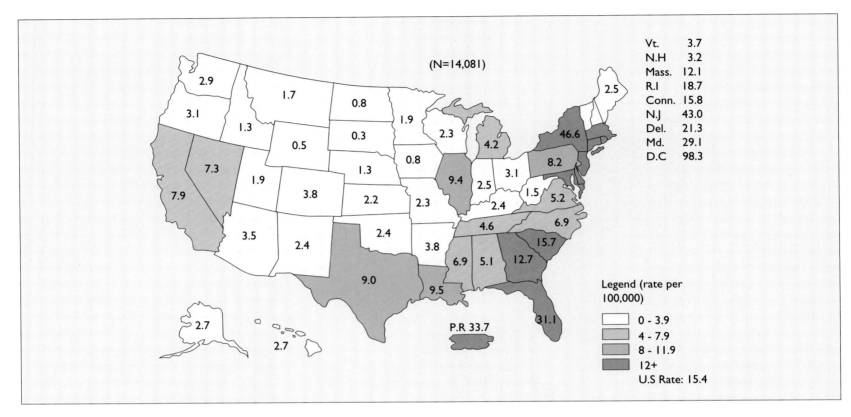

Fig. 10.6 Female adult/adolescent AIDS annual rates per 100,000 population, for cases reported in the USA, 1994.

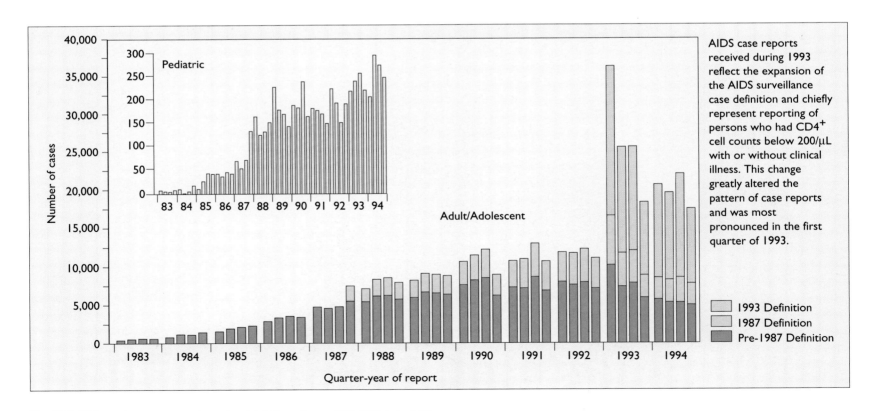

Fig. 10.7 AIDS cases by quarter-year of report and definition category, 1983–1994, in the USA.

the overall immunocompetence of an HIV-infected individual. HIV also has profound effects on other cells of the T-cell branch of the immune system, particularly CD8$^+$ (T8) cells. The normal ratio of CD4$^+$ to CD8$^+$ cells is approximately 2:1, but with HIV infection, this ratio gradually decreases, firstly as a result of increases in CD8$^+$ cells, and then mainly because of the profound decrease in CD4$^+$ cells.

SEROLOGIC TESTING

Serologic testing is the most common laboratory method used to detect HIV infection. The enzyme-linked immunosorbent assay (ELISA or EIA), which usually becomes positive within 3 months after infection (and

Fig. 10.8 Adult/adolescent AIDS cases by exposure category reported through 1994, USA.

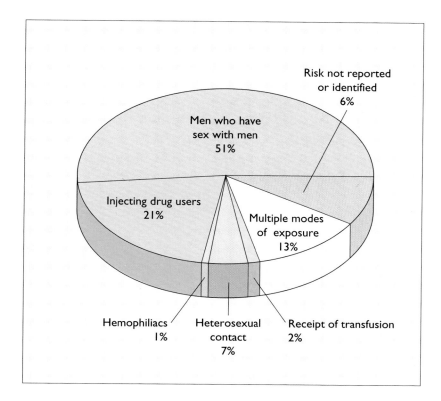

Fig. 10.9 Heterosexual AIDS cases in the USA.

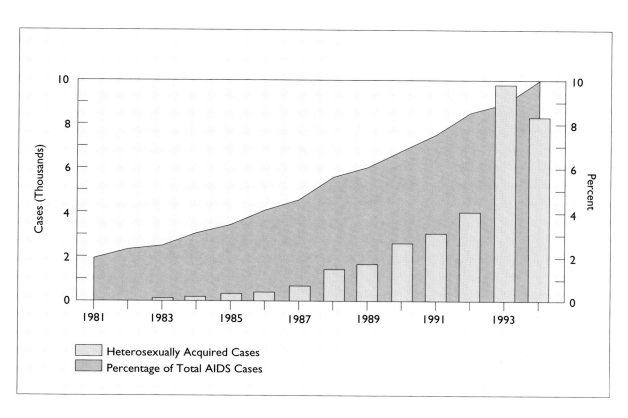

almost always by 6 months), remains the most commonly used serologic test (*Fig. 10.19*). The sensitivity of the commercially available ELISA test kits ranges from 93.4–99.6%, with a specificity ranging from 99.2–99.8%. Nevertheless, in a population with a low prevalence of infection, even a

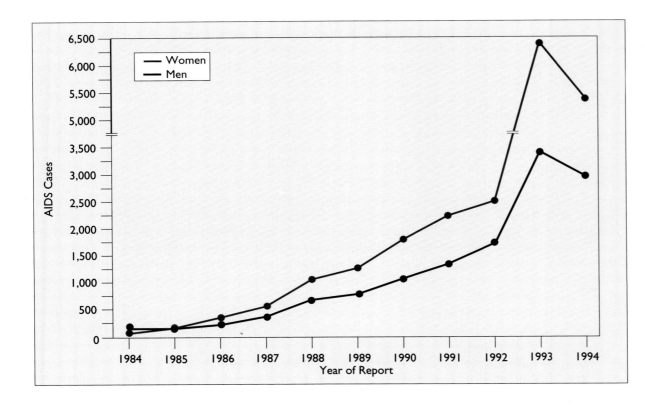

Fig. 10.10 Number of AIDS cases due to heterosexual contact by gender, 1984–1994, in the USA.

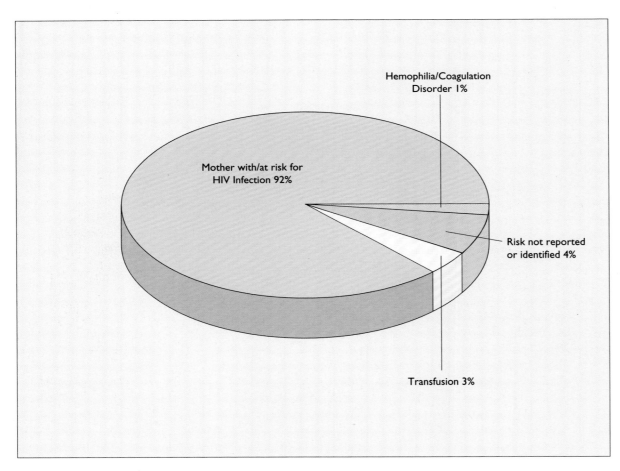

Fig. 10.11 Pediatric cases of AIDS by exposure category reported in 1994, USA.

specificity of 99.8% does not provide 100% predictive value for a positive test, and thus false-positive results may occur. For this reason, the Western Blot test, which has a significantly greater specificity than the ELISA, is used as a confirmatory test (*Fig. 10.20*).

The Western blot can determine which specific proteins (antibody bands) are present; those that are considered specific for HIV-1 include core (p17, p24, p55), polymerase (p31, p51, p66), and envelope (gp41, gp120/160) proteins. The CDC has defined a positive Western blot as the presence of at least two of the following antibody bands: p24, gp41, or gp120/160. A negative result is defined as the presence of no specific antibody bands for HIV-1. Individuals with one or more HIV-1-specific proteins, but who do not meet CDC criteria, are considered to have an indeterminate Western blot. Current widely used HIV-1-specific Western blots can detect HIV-2 with a sensitivity of approximately 80%.

Other methods used to detect HIV infection include HIV culture, direct detection of HIV antigens, and PCR testing. Current HIV culture techniques are cumbersome, time consuming, of low sensitivity, and generally available only at research facilities. As a diagnostic test, the HIV p24 antigen test is mainly used to diagnose patients with acute HIV infection who are in a 'window period' and have not yet developed antibodies to HIV. All individuals who undergo any type of HIV testing should receive pretest and post-test counseling.

ANTI-HIV THERAPY

There are many points in the life cycle of HIV that could theoretically be targets for therapeutic intervention (*Figs. 10.16* and *10.21*). However, to date, the most widely used compounds are those that inhibit the enzyme reverse transcriptase. The first drug specifically approved for use in the treatment of patients with AIDS and ARC was zidovudine, formally known as azidothymidine, or AZT. Zidovudine is a thymidine analog (*Fig. 10.22*), which will prevent viral DNA chain synthesis (*Fig. 10.23*) once it has been incorporated into the viral DNA. Common adverse effects caused by zidovudine include leukopenia, anemia, headache, and nausea. Less commonly, zidovudine may cause myopathy by inhibiting mitochondrial DNA polymerase. Two additional antiretroviral compounds are now widely used: didanosine (formerly dideoxyinosine, or ddI) and zalcitabine (formerly dideoxycytidine, or ddC). The major adverse effects observed with didanosine have been peripheral neuropathy and pancreatitis. With zalcitabine, the major adverse effects consist of peripheral neuropathy and oral stomatitis. A fourth antiretroviral medication, stavudine (D4T), has recently been approved for use; its major adverse affect is also peripheral neuropathy. The recommendations for proper use of antiretroviral drugs are controversial and a detailed discussion is beyond the scope of this chapter; a summary of recent

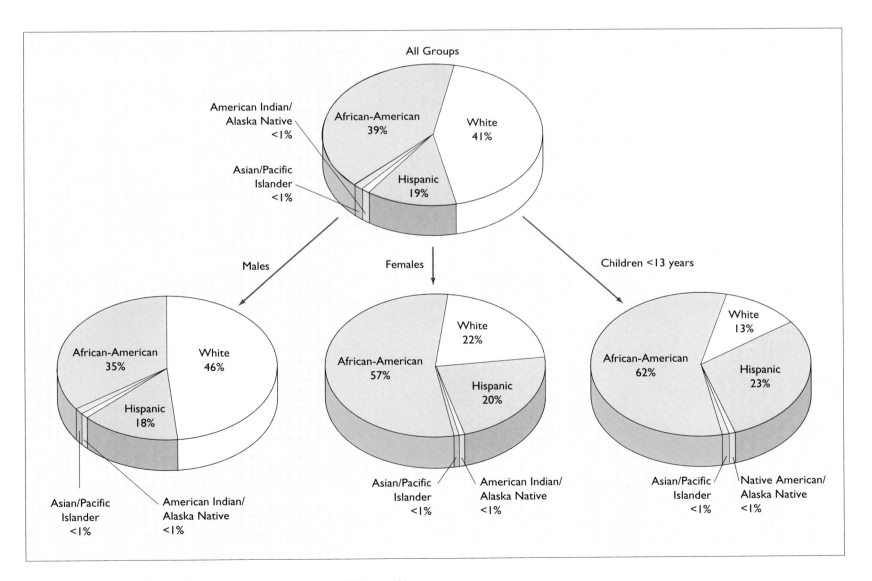

Fig. 10.12 Percentage of AIDS cases by race or ethnic group reported in 1994 in the USA.

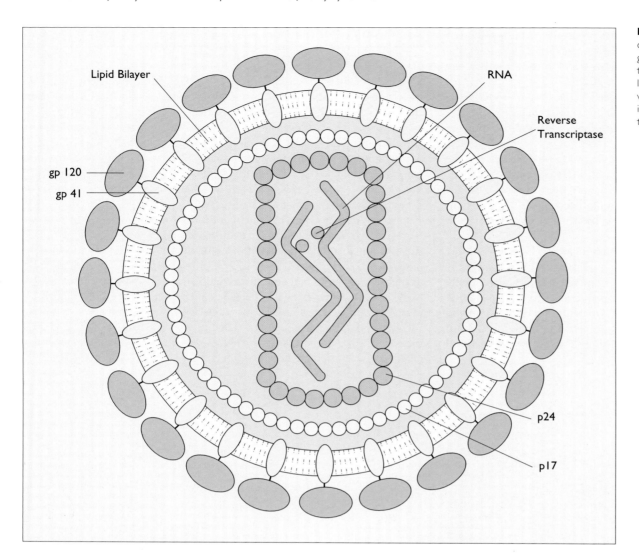

Lipid Bilayer

gp 120

gp 41

RNA

Reverse
Transcriptase

p24

p17

Fig. 10.13 The HIV virion. The retrovirus consists of an outer lipid bilayer studded with glycoprotein molecules, each of which consists of two subunits, gpl 20 and gp41. The membrane lipids are derived from the host cell. The major viral core proteins are p24 and p17. The RNA is in the core along with the enzyme reverse transcriptase.

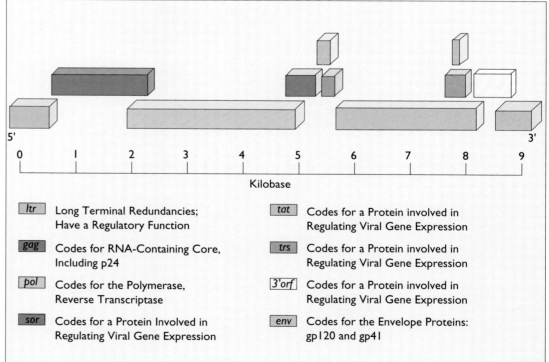

| | 5' | 0 | 1 | 2 | 3 | 4 | 5 | 6 | 7 | 8 | 9 | 3' |

Kilobase

ltr	Long Terminal Redundancies; Have a Regulatory Function
gag	Codes for RNA-Containing Core, Including p24
pol	Codes for the Polymerase, Reverse Transcriptase
sor	Codes for a Protein Involved in Regulating Viral Gene Expression

tat	Codes for a Protein involved in Regulating Viral Gene Expression
trs	Codes for a Protein involved in Regulating Viral Gene Expression
3'orf	Codes for a Protein involved in Regulating Viral Gene Expression
env	Codes for the Envelope Proteins: gp120 and gp41

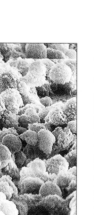

Fig. 10.14 Scanning electron micrograph (low magnification) of a population of HIV-infected lymphocytes.

Fig. 10.15 The HIV provirus. Organization of the HIV genome. At each end, there are DNA segments called long terminal redundancies (ltr), which have a regulatory function. There are at least seven genes: *gag* codes for the RNA-containing core, *pol* for reverse transcriptase, and *env* for the envelope proteins, while four others (*tat, trs, sor,* and *3'orf*) encode small proteins that regulate gene expression.

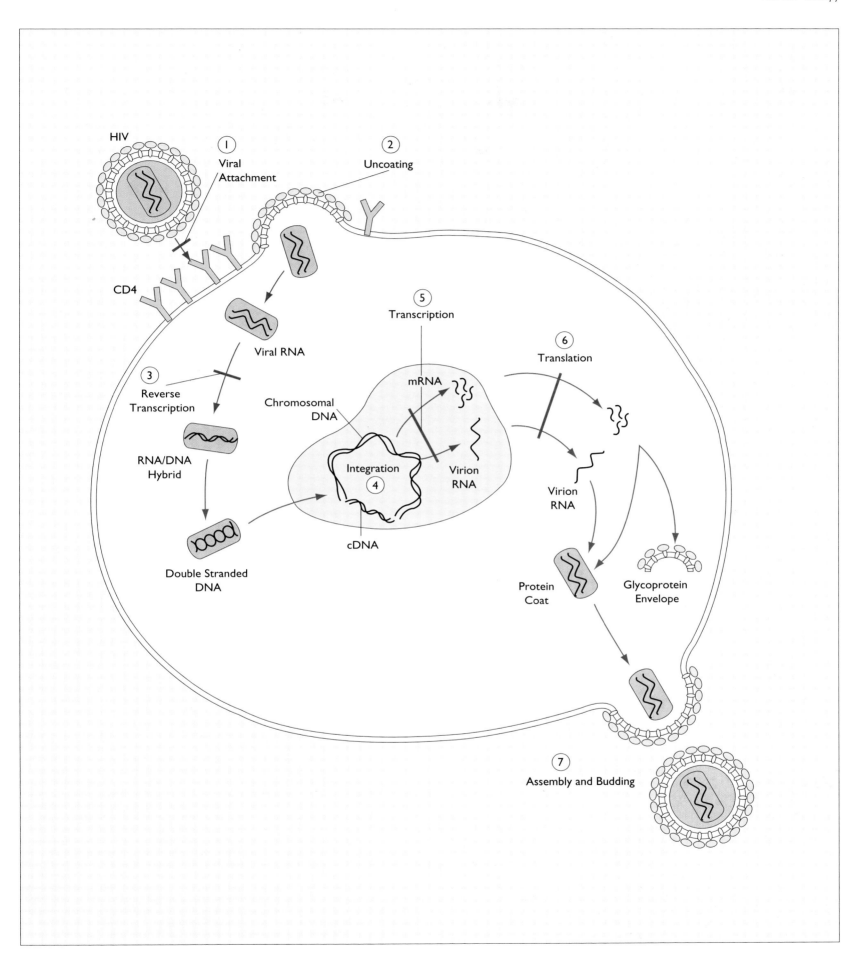

Fig. 10.16 The life cycle of HIV.

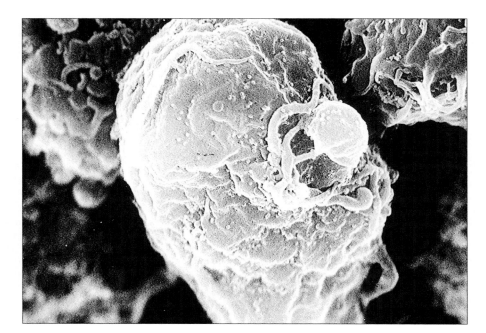

Fig. 10.17 Scanning electron micrograph of HIV-infected CD4+ lymphocyte showing virus budding from the plasma membrane.

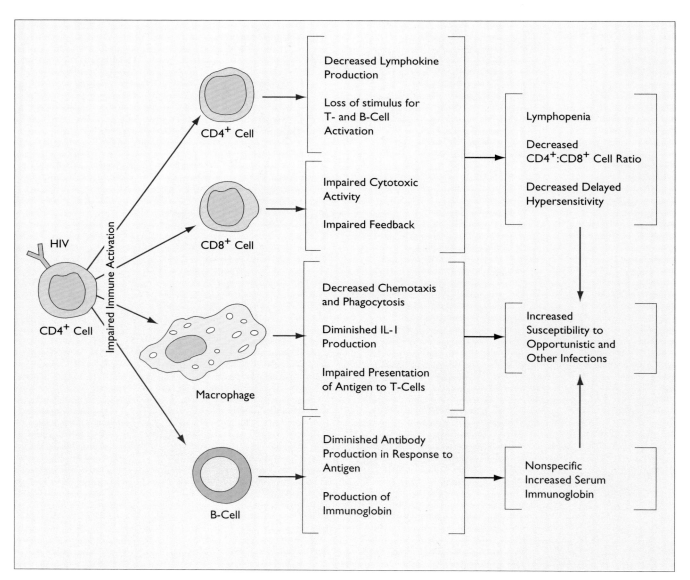

Fig. 10.18 The effect of HIV infection on the immune system.

guidelines (prior to approval of stavudine) is shown in *Figure 10.24*. Among the other potential therapeutic drugs, the protease inhibitors appear to be the most promising, and there are many studies being carried out at present to determine the effectiveness and toxicity of these agents.

CLINICAL MANIFESTATIONS

Patients with HIV infection can develop a wide array of clinical disorders as a result of the virus-induced immunosuppression. Following the acute HIV illness, cutaneous and oral disorders are predominant in patients with early-stage (CD4+ cell counts > 500 cells/mm³) and middle-stage HIV disease (CD4+ cell

counts between 200 and 500 cells/mm³). Subsequently, with late-stage HIV infection (CD4+ counts < 200 cells/mm³), patients often develop opportunistic infections and/or malignancies that most commonly involve the pulmonary and gastrointestinal systems and CNS. Patients often present with multiple clinical problems, especially those with late-stage disease.

Acute HIV Infection

Following acquisition of HIV, an estimated 30–50% of persons will develop a clinical illness associated with this acute infection, typically 2–4 weeks after becoming infected with HIV. The clinical symptoms and signs are most often described as a mononucleosis-like illness characterized by fever, rash (*Fig. 10.25*), sore throat, and lymphadenopathy. Other associated symptoms and signs include myalgias, headache, mucosal ulcerations (oral,

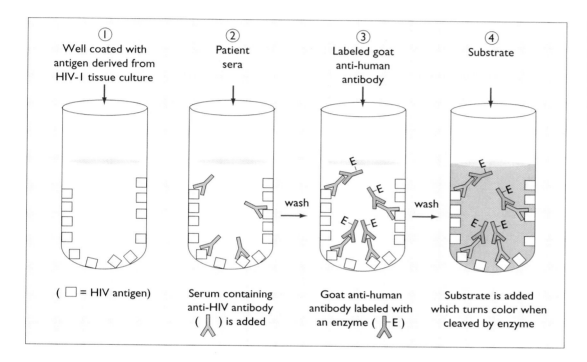

Fig. 10.19 HIV-1 ELISA. First, a microwell plate is coated with antigens derived from an HIV-1 tissue culture. Second, the patient's serum is added to the microwell plate. Third, goat-antihuman antibody that has been labeled with an enzyme binds to the patient's anti-HIV antibody. Finally, substrate is added which, when cleaved by the conjugated enzyme, produces a colored product that can be measured photometrically.

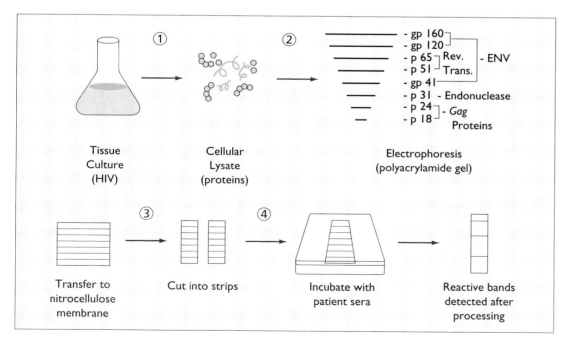

Fig. 10.20 HIV-1 Western blot. First, a cellular lysate is made from HIV-infected tissue culture. Second, the lysate (proteins and glycoproteins) is separated by polyacrylamide gel electrophoresis. Third, the separated proteins and glycoproteins are transferred onto a nitrocellulose membrane which is then cut into strips. Fourth, a strip is incubated with a patient's serum. Anti-HIV antibodies in the patient's serum, which have bound to specific HIV-associated proteins, are detected following incubation with an enzyme-labeled anti-human antibody and substrate.

vaginal, penile), facial palsy, and hepatosplenomegaly. Generally, this acute illness lasts 1–2 weeks. During this time, CD4⁺ cell counts often fall transiently, followed by a brisk increase in CD8⁺ cell counts. Presumably the marked CD8 response plays an important role in the initial control of the acute HIV infection. The diagnosis of acute HIV infection is usually confirmed by obtaining a positive p24 antigen test in the setting of a negative HIV antibody test.

Dermatologic

A wide range of dermatologic disorders of varying etiologies occurs in HIV-infected individuals, including bacterial, fungal, viral, and noninfectious disorders. Common noninfectious disorders include xerosis and eosinophilic folliculitis. Patients with xerosis develop dry rough skin with a predilection for the anterior tibial areas, dorsal surface of the hands, and the forearms (*Fig. 10.26*). Kaposi's sarcoma, recently shown to be caused

STAGES IN THE REPLICATIVE CYCLE OF A PATHOGENIC HUMAN RETROVIRUS THAT MAY BE TARGETS FOR THERAPEUTIC INTERVENTION	
STAGE	**POTENTIAL INTERVENTION**
Binding to target cells	Antibodies to the virus or cell receptor
Early entry into target cell	Drugs that block fusion or interfere with retroviral uncoating
Transcription of RNA to DNA by reverse transcriptase	Reverse transcriptase inhibitors
Degradation of viral RNA in an RNA–DNA hybrid	Inhibitors of RNase H activity
Integration of DNA into host genome	Drugs that inhibit *pol* gene-mediated 'integrase' function
Expression of viral genes	'Anti-sense' constructs; inhibitors of the *tatIII* protein or *art/trs* protein
Viral component production and assembly	Myristylation, glycosylation, and protease inhibitors or modifiers
Budding of virus	Interferons

Fig. 10.21 Stages in the replicative cycle of a pathogenic human retrovirus that may be targets for therapeutic intervention.

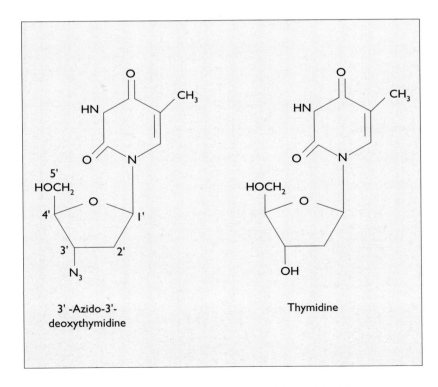

Fig. 10.22 Structures of zidovudine (3'-azido-3'-deoxythymidine) and thymidine.

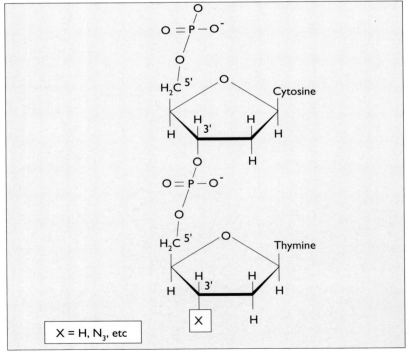

Fig. 10.23 Possible mechanism of activity against HIV of 2',3'-dideoxynucleosides as triphosphate products. When the 3'-carbon of the deoxyribose is modified by certain substitutions (shown by X) that replace the normal 3'-OH, it is not possible to form the 5' —> 3' phosphodiester linkages that are necessary for DNA elongation in the replication of the virus from an RNA form to a DNA form.

by infection with a novel herpes virus, often presents as an asymptomatic reddish-purple papule or nodule and may appear anywhere on the skin (*Figs. 10.27–10.32*). In addition, Kaposi's sarcoma can develop in other organ systems, such as the lungs or gastrointestinal tract. The clinical diag-

ANTIRETROVIRAL THERAPY FOR HIV-INFECTED ADULTS: RECOMMENDATIONS FROM 1993 NIAID STATE-OF-THE-ART CONFERENCE

Clinical Status	CD4+ Range, Cell Count × 10⁹/L	Recommendation
No Previous Antiretroviral Therapy		
Asymptomatic	> 0.50	No therapy
Asymptomatic	0.20–0.50	Zidovudine or no therapy
Symptomatic	0.20–0.50	Zidovudine
Asymptomatic	< 0.20	Zidovudine
Symptomatic	< 0.20	Zidovudine
Previous Antiretroviral Therapy		
Stable	≥ 0.30	Continue zidovudine
Stable	< 0.30	Continue zidovudine or change to didanosine
Progressing	0.05–0.50	Change to didanosine or zalcitabine
Progressing	< 0.50	Change to didanosine or zalcitabine
Intolerant to Zidovudine		
Stable or progressing	< 0.05	Change to didanosine or zalcitabine

NIAID = National Institute of Allergy and Infectious Diseases.

Sande MA et al. Antiretroviral therapy for adult HIV-infected patients: recommendations from a state-of-the-art conference. JAMA 1993; 270: 2583–9.

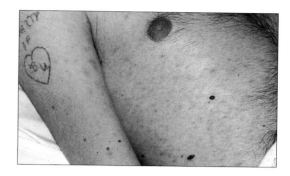

Fig. 10.24 Recommendations for antiretroviral therapy for HIV-infected adults.

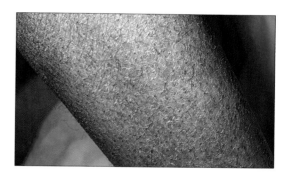

Fig. 10.25 Cutaneous maculopapular eruption associated with acute HIV infection.

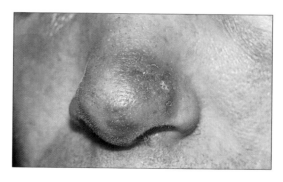

Fig. 10.26 Dry scaling skin showing the typical appearance of xerosis.

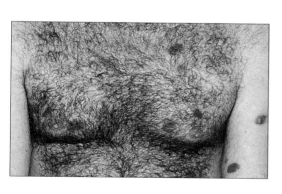

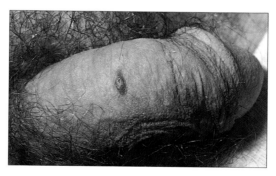

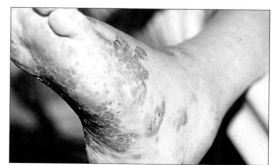

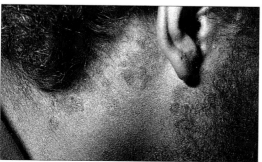

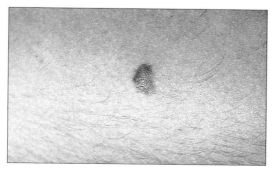

Figs. 10.27–10.32 Multiple locations and variable appearances of biopsy-proven Kaposi's sarcoma lesions.

nosis of Kaposi's sarcoma can be confirmed from the characteristic histology of a biopsy of a lesion (*Figs. 10.33–10.36*).

Eosinophilic folliculitis typically presents as pruritic perifollicular papules located on the face, scalp, trunk, and upper extremities; the diagnosis is confimed by biopsy. Staphylococcal folliculitis is the most common cutaneous bacterial infection in HIV-infected patients and may occur in any hair-bearing area, particularly on the trunk and face. This type of folliculitis may be difficult to distinguish from noninfectious eosinophilic folliculitis. The diagnosis is most often based on the patient's response to antistaphylococcal antimicrobial therapy. Another less common cutaneous disorder, cutaneous bacillary angiomatosis, is caused by a bacterium belonging to the genus *Bartonella* (formerly *Rochalimaea*) and can present as dermal or subcutaneous lesions (*Fig. 10.37*). Although some investigators have isolated the causative organism from skin lesions, the diagnosis is most often made from a Warthin–Starry silver stain on a biopsy sample (*Fig. 10.38*).

Seborrheic dermatitis, a common and early manifestation of HIV infection, is believed to result from the host response to a fungal (*Pitysporum*) infection (*Fig. 10.39*). The diagnosis is based on the clinical appearance of this disorder. Other fungal infections, such as cryptococcosis and histoplasmosis, may cause multiple cutaneous lesions when they disseminate (*Fig. 10.40*). In addition, disseminated infection with *Penicillium marneffei* manifesting as multiple cutaneous lesions has been recently reported to occur frequently in areas of Southeast Asia, such as northern Thailand (*Figs. 10.41* and *10.42*).

Molluscum contagiosum, which is caused by a pox virus, typically presents as umbilicated papular lesions, most commonly on the face (*Fig. 10.43*) and genital tract (*Fig. 10.44*). In contrast with immunocompetent individuals who usually show spontaneous resolution of these lesions, patients with HIV infection usually have progressively enlarging and spreading lesions that do not spontaneously resolve (*Fig. 10.45*). Often confused with molluscum contagiosum, HPV-related warts develop as thick, hyperkeratotic papular growths most often seen on the hands (*Fig. 10.46*), feet, vulva, or penis, or in the perianal region. The diagnosis of molluscum and warts is almost always based on the clinical appearance of the lesions. Herpes zoster virus infection can develop at any stage of a patient's HIV disease, and, in some instances, it may be their first HIV-related manifestation. Patients typically develop painful grouped vesicles along a dermatomal distribution (*Figs. 10.47* and *10.48*). Although the clinical presentation is often similar to that in the immunocompetent patient, the duration of disease may be longer and the risk of dissemination higher. The diagnosis is often made on clinical grounds alone, but can be confirmed using fluorescent antibody and culture tests (scrape the base of the lesion to obtain cells) (*see Chapter 11*). HIV-infect-

ed patients with mucocutaneous HSV infections often present with painful and ulcerative lesions, rather than vesicular lesions (*Fig. 10.49*). These lesions can be chronic and are most often located on the face, penis, or vulva, or in the perianal region. The diagnosis is made similarly to that of herpes zoster.

Most HIV-infected patients who become infested with scabies usually present with multiple pruritic papules, which are typically located on the hands (particularly on the wrist and between fingers), along the belt line, and, in males, on the glans penis (*Fig. 10.50*). An unusual variant of scabies called Norwegian crusted scabies can develop in late-stage AIDS patients and is characterized by nonpruritic hyperkeratotic plaques and an extraordinarily large number of mites (*Fig. 10.51*). With any type of scabies, the diagnosis is made by scraping a skin lesion and identifying mites under the microscope (*Fig. 10.52*) (*see also Chapter 15*). A summary of the common dermatologic disorders and their treatment is shown in *Figure 10.53*.

Oral

Oral candidiasis, which is caused by the yeast *Candida albicans*, occurs very commonly among HIV-infected individuals, especially those with CD4+ cell counts of less than 300 cells/mm³. Oral candidiasis can appear in three different forms:
- Pseudomembranous (thrush)
- Atrophic (erythematous) candidiasis
- Angular cheilitis (*Figs. 10.54–10.56*).

Symptoms associated with candidiasis often depend on the degree of candidiasis and may include pain or alterations in taste. Although most experienced clinicians diagnose oral candidiasis on the basis of the clinical appearance of this disorder, a KOH wet mount or Gram stain of a scraping can confirm the diagnosis.

Oral hairy leukoplakia, another common oral disorder, occurs as a result of Epstein–Barr virus-induced epithelial thickening of the tongue. Often confused with candidiasis, oral hairy leukoplakia generally develops on the side of the tongue and is not removed by scraping (*Fig. 10.57*). The diagnosis is made on the clinical appearance of the lesion. This disorder rarely causes symptoms and rarely requires treatment.

Patients with early-stage HIV disease who develop oral HSV infection typically present with symptoms similar to those seen in immunocompetent individuals, namely vesicular lesions on the lips or pharynx, which resolve in 5–7 days. Individuals with advanced HIV disease, however, generally develop nonhealing ulcerative lesions that may involve the tongue, gums, pharynx, or palate (*Fig. 10.58*). The diagnosis is made by either fluorescent antibody testing or by viral culture on a sample obtained from scraping the base of the lesion.

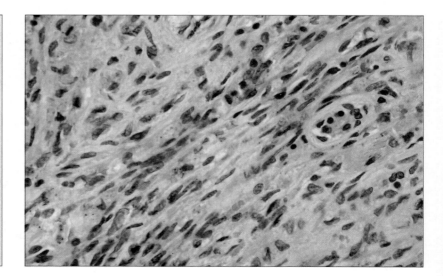

Fig. 10.33 Histology of Kaposi's sarcoma. Low-power photomicrograph of cutaneous Kaposi's sarcoma. The neoplasm is poorly circumscribed and diffusely involves the reticular dermis. Both the vascular and spindle-cell features are readily apparent. Very early lesions often contain a chronic inflammatory infiltrate, demonstrate little cytologic atypia, and strongly resemble benign reactive granulation tissue, making the diagnosis exceedingly difficult if not impossible at that stage (hematoxylin and eosin × 40).

Fig. 10.34 Kaposi's sarcoma. The spindle-cell neoplastic component predominates in this photomicrograph. Occasional extravasated erythrocytes are present (hematoxylin and eosin × 400).

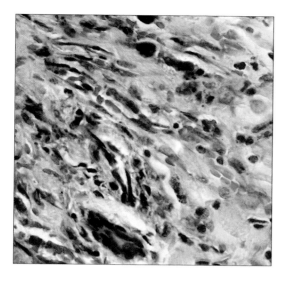

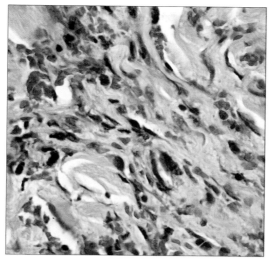

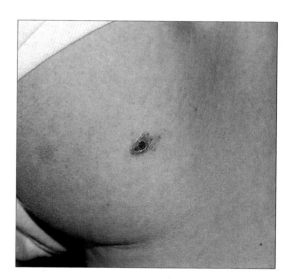

Figs. 10.35 and 10.36 Kaposi's sarcoma. Neoplastic vessels, multiple abnormal slit-like vascular spaces, marked cytologic atypia, extravasated erythrocytes, and a small amount of brownish granular hemosiderin pigment can be seen. These features are characteristic of this sarcoma of endothelial cell origin (hematoxylin and eosin × 400).

Fig. 10.37 Subcutaneous bacillary angiomatosis lesion that has eroded the skin surface.

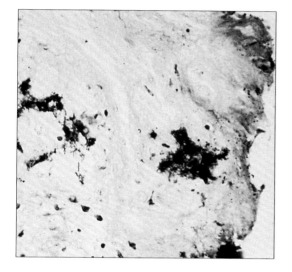

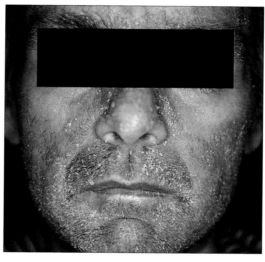

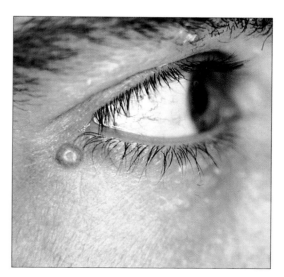

Fig. 10.38 Warthin–Starry stain of a skin biopsy taken from a patient with bacillary angiomatosis showing multiple clumps of organisms.

Fig. 10.39 Typical seborrheic dermatitis showing erythema and scaling of the nasolabial folds, facial creases, and eyebrows.

Fig. 10.40 Skin lesion of a patient with disseminated cryptococcal infection.

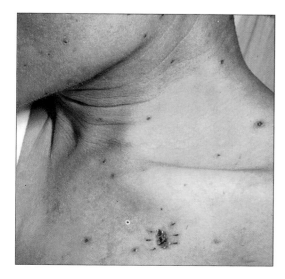

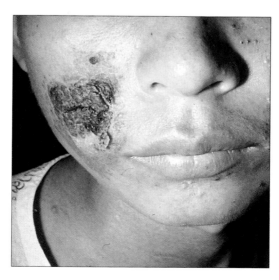

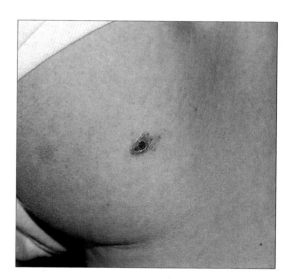

Fig. 10.41 Multiple cutaneous lesions caused by disseminated *Penicillium marneffei* in an HIV-infected patient from Thailand.

Fig. 10.42 Facial lesions caused by disseminated *Penicillium marneffei* in an HIV-infected patient from Thailand.

Fig. 10.43 Typical umbilicated molluscum contagiosum lesion.

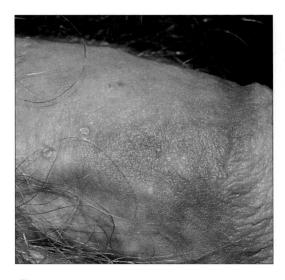

Fig. 10.44 Penile molluscum contagiosum.

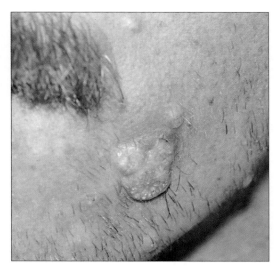

Fig. 10.45 Large molluscum contagiosum lesion.

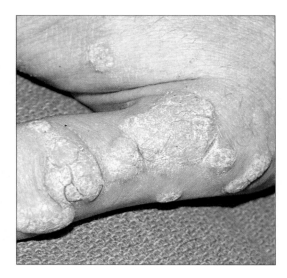

Fig. 10.46 Extensive hyperkeratotic warts located on a patient's hands.

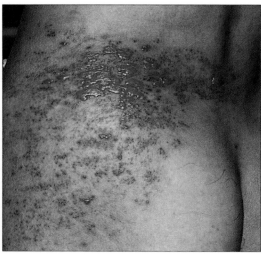

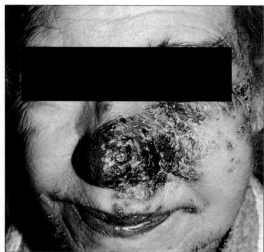

Figs. 10.47 and 10.48 Typical grouped vesicular lesions of herpes zoster in dermatomal distribution.

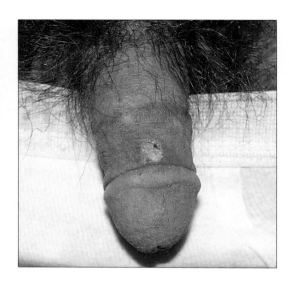

Fig. 10.49 Chronic ulcerative painful herpes simplex lesion.

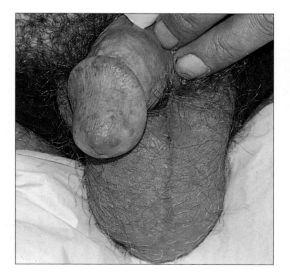

Fig. 10.50 Scabies lesions on the glans penis.

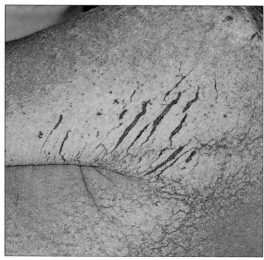

Fig. 10.51 Thick hyperkeratotic lesions of Norwegian crusted scabies.

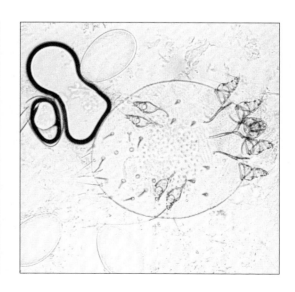

Fig. 10.52 Typical appearance of scabies mite (× 200).

TREATMENT OF COMMON DERMATOLOGIC DISORDERS

CONDITION	TREATMENT
Xerosis	Mild: emollients (e.g., eucerin cream) Severe: add mild topical steroid
Kaposi's sarcoma	Liquid nitrogen Intralesional vinblastine Intralesional interferon-α
Eosinophilic pustular folliculitis	Antihistamines Topical steroids Ultraviolet light therapy 3–5 × /week
Bacterial folliculitis	Antibiotics (dicloxacillin or cephalexin); prolonged therapy often needed
Bacillary angiomatosis	Erythromycin 500 mg po qid for 2–3 months
Seborrheic dermatitis	Mild: 2% ketoconazole cream bid Moderate–Severe: 2% ketoconazole cream bid plus 1% hydrocortisone bid Refractory: ketoconazole 200 mg po qid
Molluscum contagiosum	Liquid nitrogen Retin-A
Warts	Liquid nitrogen Podophyllin Podophylox
Herpes zoster	Acyclovir 800 mg bid for 7–10 days
Herpes simplex	Acyclovir 400 mg tid for 7–10 days
Scabies	Permethrin (5% cream) Lindane (1% lotion)

Fig. 10.53 Treatment of common dermatologic disorders.

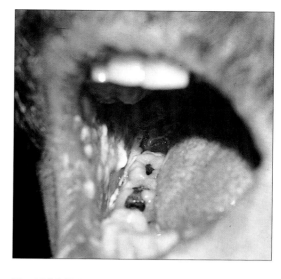

Fig. 10.54 Clinical presentation of oral candidiasis. Pseudomembranous candidiasis with thick plaque-like lesions on the buccal mucosa.

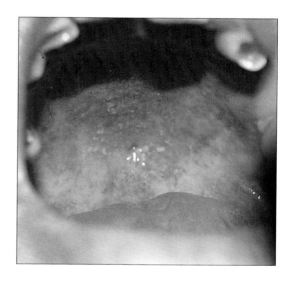

Fig. 10.55 Clinical presentation of oral candidiasis. Erythematous candidiasis showing reddened upper palate.

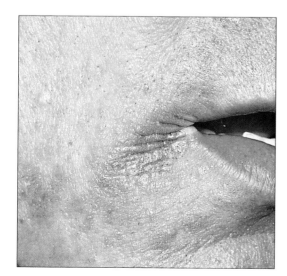

Fig. 10.56 Clinical presentation of oral candidiasis. Angular cheilitis with fissuring at the corners of the mouth.

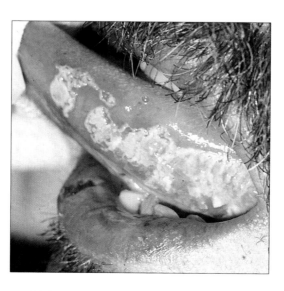

Fig. 10.57 Fine, reticulate, white plaques characteristic of oral hairy leukoplakia in a patient with AIDS.

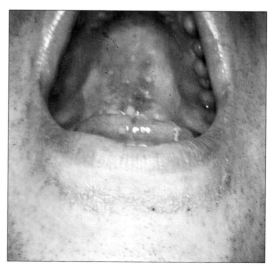

Fig. 10.58 Vesicles of herpes simplex infection on the palate of a patient with AIDS.

Less frequently, patients may develop other oral disorders, such as recurrent aphthae, gingivitis, or Kaposi's sarcoma (*Fig. 10.59*). A summary of the common oral disorders and their treatment is shown in *Figure 10.60*.

Pulmonary

Streptococcus pneumoniae is the most common bacterial cause of severe pneumonia among HIV-infected individuals, occurring 10 times as often as in the general population. Patients who develop pneumococcal pneumonia usually do so before they develop AIDS and most have clinical signs and symptoms similar to those in HIV-negative individuals. In general, the onset of disease is abrupt and often includes high fever, pleuritic chest pain, and sputum production. Chest radiographs show segmental, lobar, or multilobar consolidation in approximately 75% of patients (*Fig. 10.61*). The major distinctive feature of pneumococcal pneumonia in HIV-infected patients is the 20-fold (or higher) incidence of pneumococcal bacteremia. Although HIV-infected patients usually respond well to typical treatment regimens, such as penicillin, they do have a higher relapse rate. As 85% of the infections involve strains contained in the 23-valent pneumococcal polysaccharide vaccine, patients should receive pneumococcal vaccination, preferably early in the course of their HIV disease. Although other bacteria, such as *Haemophilus influenzae*, can cause pneumonia, they occur much less often than pneumococcal pneumonia.

P. carinii pneumonia has remained the most common AIDS-defining opportunistic infection, despite its marked decrease as a result of effective prophylaxis. Early in the course of PCP, patients usually have nonspecific systemic symptoms, such as fever, night sweats, malaise, and weight loss. Typically, patients then develop a nonproductive cough followed by dyspnea. The physical examination is generally unhelpful, but on occasion may reveal dry sounding rales on chest auscultation. Patients with PCP usually have CD4$^+$ counts of less than 200 cells/mm^3. The chest radiograph most often shows diffuse or perihilar interstitial infiltrates (*Fig. 10.62*). Less characteristic findings include upper-lobe infiltrates, lobar consolidation, and cystic changes (*Figs. 10.63* and *10.64*). In addition, up to 20% of patients with PCP may present with a normal chest radiograph.

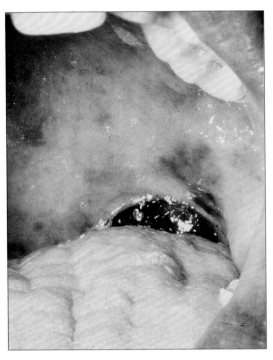

Fig. 10.59 Violaceous Kaposi's sarcoma lesion located in the posterior pharynx.

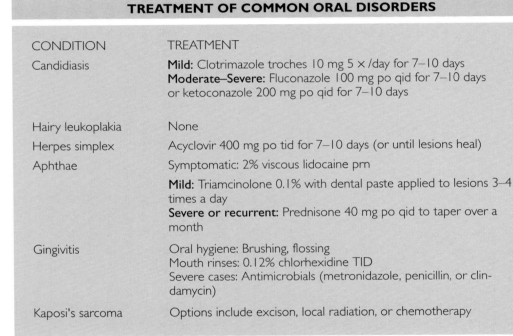

TREATMENT OF COMMON ORAL DISORDERS

CONDITION	TREATMENT
Candidiasis	**Mild:** Clotrimazole troches 10 mg 5 × /day for 7–10 days **Moderate–Severe:** Fluconazole 100 mg po qid for 7–10 days or ketoconazole 200 mg po qid for 7–10 days
Hairy leukoplakia	None
Herpes simplex	Acyclovir 400 mg po tid for 7–10 days (or until lesions heal)
Aphthae	Symptomatic: 2% viscous lidocaine prn
	Mild: Triamcinolone 0.1% with dental paste applied to lesions 3–4 times a day **Severe or recurrent:** Prednisone 40 mg po qid to taper over a month
Gingivitis	Oral hygiene: Brushing, flossing Mouth rinses: 0.12% chlorhexidine TID Severe cases: Antimicrobials (metronidazole, penicillin, or clindamycin)
Kaposi's sarcoma	Options include excison, local radiation, or chemotherapy

Fig. 10.60 Treatment of common oral disorders.

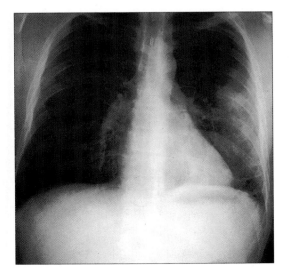

Fig. 10.61 Lobar pneumonia in a patient with pneumococcal pneumonia.

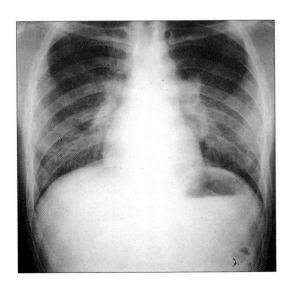

Fig. 10.62 Characteristic diffuse interstitial perihilar infiltrates in a patient with *Pneumocystis carinii* pneumonia.

The approach to the evaluation of the patient with suspected PCP depends on the index of suspicion for PCP and the clinical stability of the patient. An approach to a stable patient with suspected PCP is presented in *Figure 10.65*. A definitive diagnosis can be made using Papanicolaou smears, silver stains, or monoclonal antibody tests on material obtained from an induced sputum, bronchoalveolar lavage, or rarely, transbronchial biopsy (*Figs.10.66–10.70*). Although the diagnostic yield of induced sputum is significantly less than with bronchoalveolar lavage, it is often performed first because it is a noninvasive test. Those patients with negative results from induced sputum should proceed to bronchoscopy. As bronchoalveolar lavage is diagnostic in more than 90% of PCP cases, transbronchial biopsy is rarely necessary. Although effective treatment for PCP has made a significant impact on the survival of HIV-infected patients with PCP, fatalities still occur (*Fig. 10.71*). Patients with CD4+ counts less than 200 cells/mm³ or a history of PCP should be given prophylactic therapy.

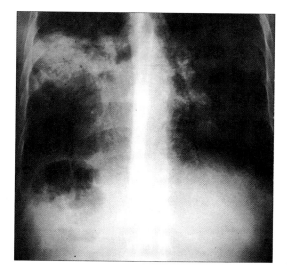
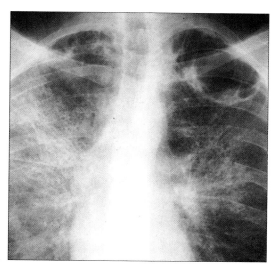

Figs. 10.63 and 10.64 *Pneumocystis carinii* pneumonia.(**10.63**) Chest x-ray shows consolidation changes in right lung, which is a less typical finding than the characteristic interstitial infiltrate.(**10.64**) Cystic changes in left upper lobe.

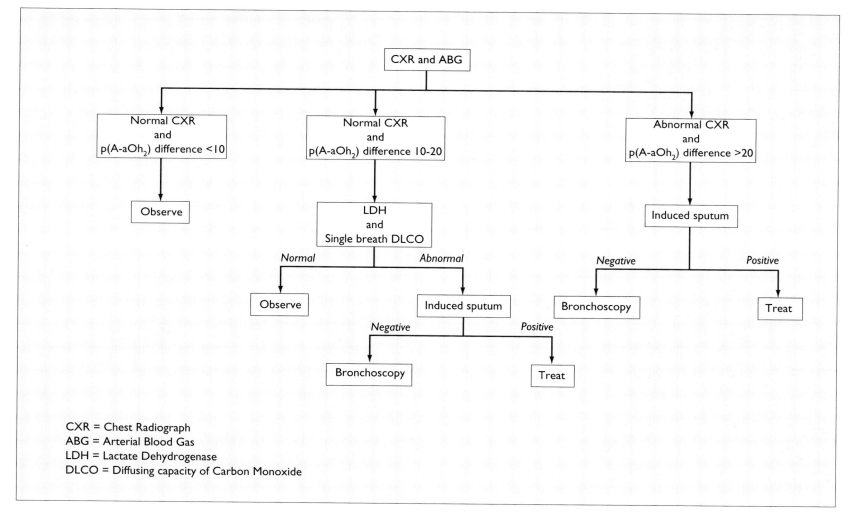

CXR = Chest Radiograph
ABG = Arterial Blood Gas
LDH = Lactate Dehydrogenase
DLCO = Diffusing capacity of Carbon Monoxide

Fig. 10.65 Approach to stable patient with suspected *Pneumocystis carinii* pneumonia.

In recent years, the incidence of *Mycobacterium tuberculosis* infection in the USA has increased (*Fig. 10.72*), predominantly as a result of the increased number of cases among HIV-infected individuals. Tuberculosis can occur at any stage of HIV disease. In general, tuberculosis in patients with early-stage HIV has a different presentation than in patients with AIDS. Patients with early HIV present in a similar way to HIV-negative individuals. Thus, the purified protein derivative (PPD) test is usually positive, chest radiographs show upper-lobe involvement (frequently with cavitation) (*Fig. 10.73*), and extrapulmonary disease infrequently occurs. In contrast, patients with AIDS often have an atypical presentation, characterized by a negative PPD, diffuse infiltrates on chest radiographs (often involving the lower and middle lobes), and rarely extrapulmonary disease. Regardless of the stage of HIV disease, the diagnosis of tuberculosis pneumonia is based on the isolation of *M. tuberculosis* from material from the respiratory tract (usually sputum); in addition, one can immediately suspect tuberculosis if characteristic 'red snappers' are present on an acid-fast stain of this material (*Fig. 10.74*). Patients at all stages of HIV disease generally respond to standard antituberculosis therapy, assuming the causative strains are not drug resistant. Among the HIV-infected population, multiresistant tuberculosis has increased at an alarming rate: treatment in this situation remains problematic. All HIV-infected patients should undergo PPD testing.

There are other less common processes that may involve the lung. For example, although HIV-infected patients with *Mycobacterium avium* complex (MAC) infection generally present with disseminated disease, occasionally they may present with focal pulmonary disease. In addition, isolation of MAC from the respiratory tract has a good predictive value for the development of MAC bacteremia, even among patients without pulmonary symptoms. Obtaining respiratory cultures for screening purposes, however, is not recommended, mainly because of their low sensitivity. Most patients who develop disease caused by MAC have CD4+ cell counts of less than 75 cells/mm³.

Previously, cytomegalovirus (CMV) was believed to play a major role in causing pulmonary disease in HIV-infected patients. At present, most authorities believe that CMV rarely causes clinically significant pulmonary disease, despite its frequent isolation from the respiratory tract. Moreover, the isolation of CMV from the respiratory tract is not a good predictor for the development of CMV-induced disease of the retina or gastrointestinal tract.

Among HIV-infected individuals, infection with *Cryptococcus neoformans* most commonly involves the CNS, but because the lungs serve as the portal of entry for this organism, patients may develop pulmonary cryptococcosis. When pulmonary cryptococcosis does occur, approximately 70% of patients have evidence of disseminated infection, with positive cultures from either blood or CSF. Patients who develop pulmonary cryptococcosis usually present with nonspecific symptoms, such as fever, cough, dyspnea, headache, and weight loss. Chest radiography most often shows either focal or diffuse interstitial infiltrates, but less commonly, focal or nodular patterns, pleural effusions, or lymphadenopathy are apparent (*Figs. 10.75* and *10.76*). The diagnosis depends on identifying cryptococcal organism from fluid or tissue specimens. In addition, tests for serum cryptococcal antigen are

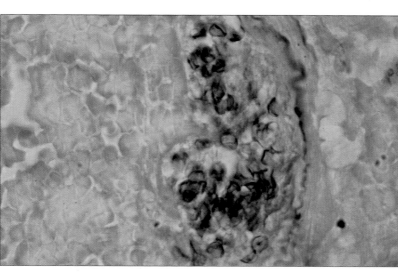
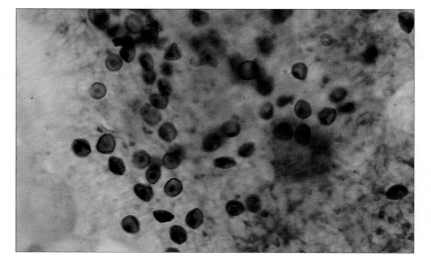
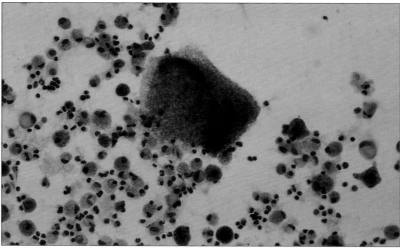
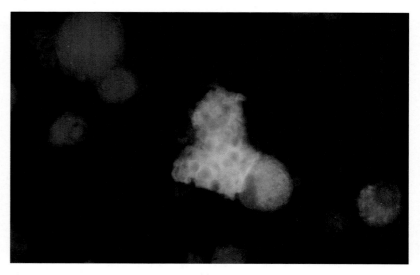

Figs. 10.66–10.69 *Pneumocystis carinii* pneumonia bronchoalveolar lavage, cytospin preparations. (**10.66**) Mass of *Pneumocystis* organisms having a 'dirty' green-brown appearance with Papanicolaou stain (× 250). Individual cysts are not readily discernible. Note adjacent large pigmented alveolar macrophages. (**10.67**) Morphology of individual *Pneumocystis carinii* cysts with Gomori methanamine silver (GMS) stain, which stains cyst walls. The cysts are often round to ovoid, but helmet-, comma-, or sickle-shaped forms are also common. Note the characteristic central 'dot' seen in many as well as occasional transverse grooves (× 1,000). (**10.68**) Transbronchial lung biopsy of PCP. The morphology of the cysts in tissue sections may appear somewhat more distorted than in smear preparations (GMS × 1,000). (**10.69**) Indirect immunofluorescent stain using monoclonal antibody specific for *P. carinii*. Organisms appear green and are clustered; alveolar macrophages are red × 400).

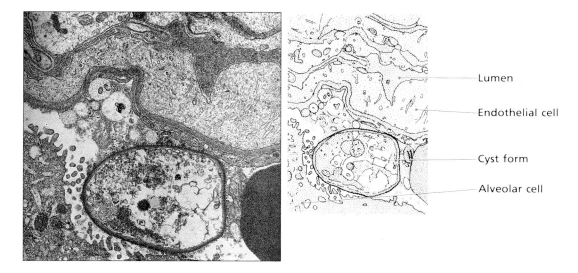

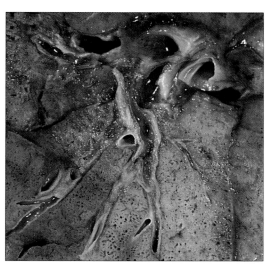

Fig. 10.70 An electron micrograph of the cyst form of *Pneumocystis carinii* in the lung.

Fig. 10.71 Autopsy lung tissue from an AIDS patient with diffuse *Pneumocystis* pneumonitis. Diffuse consolidation is present with patchy areas of induration and mucous plugging of bronchioles.

Fig. 10.72 Incidence of tuberculosis in the USA, 1980–1992.

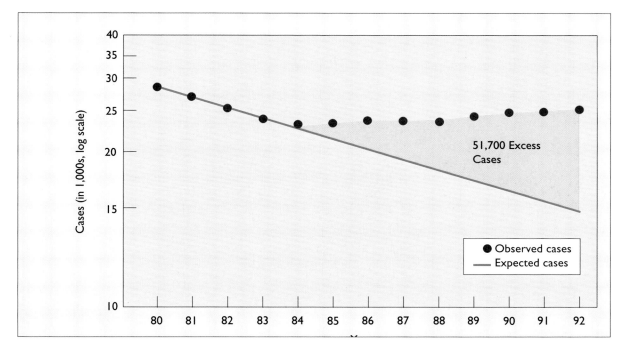

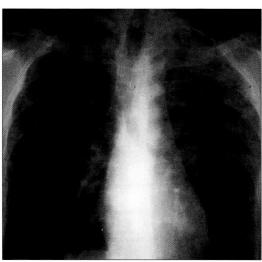

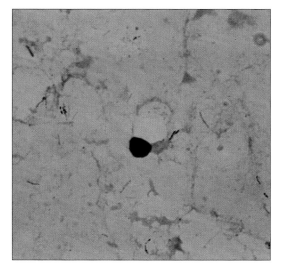

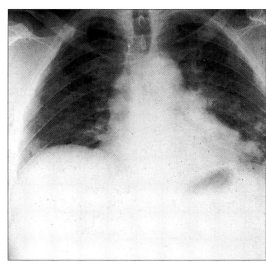

Fig. 10.73 Chest radiograph showing left upper lobe infiltrate due to *Mycobacterium tuberculosis* in an HIV-infected patient.

Fig. 10.74 Sputum. Numerous acid-fast bacilli are present in the background, several of which demonstrate the typical beaded morphology (Kinyoun stain × 1,000).

Fig. 10.75 Chest radiograph showing a nodular pulmonary infiltrate due to *Cryptococcus neoformans* (see also **10.76**).

usually positive. *Histoplasma capsulatum* is a rare cause of pulmonary disease, except among patients from highly endemic areas located in the midwestern USA. Almost all HIV-infected patients who develop histoplasmosis present with disseminated disease. Approximately 5% of patients, however, will develop focal pulmonary disease (*Fig. 10.77*).

Kaposi's sarcoma is a common serious pulmonary disorder among HIV-infected patients. Pulmonary Kaposi's sarcoma causes symptoms that include dyspnea, cough, and on occasion, hemoptysis. Although most patients have concomitant cutaneous involvement, some may have isolated pulmonary disease. Chest radiographic appearances include diffuse reticular-nodular lesions with irregular borders, mediastinal enlargement, and less often, pleural effusion (*Figs. 10.78* and *10.79*). The diagnosis is made by viewing endobronchial lesions during bronchoscopy, or by histologic examination of a transbronchial or open-lung biopsy specimen. If untreated, patients with pulmonary Kaposi's sarcoma usually experience a rapidly progressive deterioration. Even with therapy, the prognosis remains poor. A summary of the common pulmonary disorders and their treatment is shown in *Figure 10.80*.

Gastrointestinal
Two major types of gastrointestinal manifestations predominate in HIV-infected patients:
* Esophagitis
* Diarrhea.

The major causes of esophagitis include *Candida* (*Fig. 10.81*), CMV (*Figs. 10.82* and *10.83*), HSV (*Fig. 10.84*), and acid reflux. These disorders, except for acid reflux, most commonly occur in patients with CD4$^+$ counts less than 100 cells/mm^3. Occasionally, esophageal Kaposi's sarcoma may mimic these disorders. In general, regardless of the cause of the esophagitis, patients present with odynophagia and retrosternal chest pain. As candidal esophagitis is the most common of these disorders, most authorities recommend treating the patient empirically for candidal esophagitis, and if the condition does not improve within 3–5 days, proceeding to upper endoscopy with biopsy (*Fig. 10.85*). The treatment of common esophageal disorders is shown in *Figure 10.86*.

Among HIV-infected patients, diarrhea is a common cause of morbidity. The differential diagnosis is extensive and the more common causes of diarrhea are listed in *Fig. 10.87*. The diagnosis of the offending pathogen generally requires a stepwise approach (*Fig. 10.88*). The most common HIV-associated bacterial enteric pathogens, *Salmonella* spp., *Shigella* spp., and *Campylobacter* spp., occur more frequently among HIV-infected patients than in the general population. These infections usually cause diarrhea and fever and patients often have cultures that are positive from both stool and blood. As HIV-infected patients frequently receive antimicrobials, *Clostridium difficile* infection may develop and cause diarrhea.

The parasite *Cryptosporidium parvum*, a coccidian protozoan, causes severe, watery, cholera-like diarrhea with cramps, and sometimes nausea and vomiting. Its life cycle

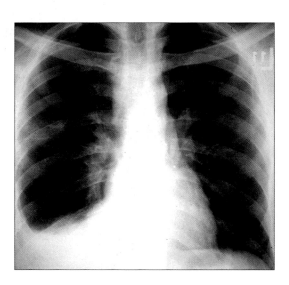

Fig. 10.76 Chest radiograph showing a right pleural effusion, which on culture grew *Cryptococcus neoformans*. This patient also had disseminated cryptococcal infection with positive blood cultures.

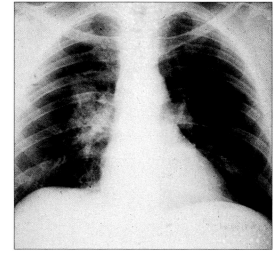

Fig. 10.77 Chest radiograph showing pulmonary histoplasmosis. The diagnosis is made by bronchoscopy and biopsy.

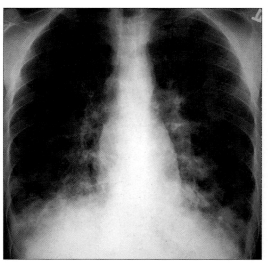

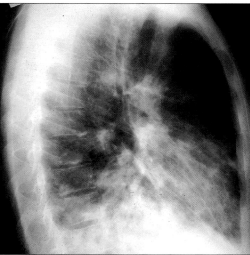

Figs. 10.78 and 10.79 Chest radiograph showing Kaposi's sarcoma of the lung. The bilateral interstitial and nodular infiltrates were proven by transbronchial biopsy to be Kaposi's sarcoma. (**10.78**) PA view. (**10.79**) Lateral view.

TREATMENT OF COMMON PULMONARY DISORDERS

CONDITION	TREATMENT
Pneumococcal pneumonia	Penicillin: 500,000 U iv q 4h
PCP (Treatment)*	TMP/SMZ: 15–20 mg/kg (TMP)/day po or iv in 3–4 divided doses or TMP/Dapsone: TMP 15–20 mg/kg/day in 3–4 divided doses plus dapsone 100 mg po qid or Pentamidine: 4 mg/kg iv qid or Clindamycin/Primaquine: clindamycin 600 mg po tid plus primaquine 30 mg po qid or Atovaquone: 750 mg po bid
PCP (Prophylaxis)	TMP/SMZ: 160/800 mg po qid or Dapsone: 100 mg po qid or Aerosolized pentamidine: 300 mg q month
Tuberculosis	Isoniazid: 300 mg po qid for 9 months plus Rifampin: 600 mg po qid for 9 months plus Pyrazinamide: 20 mg/kg po qid for 2 months plus Ethambutol: 20 mg/kg po qid (discontinue if isolate not drug-resistant)
MAC pneumonia	Clarithromycin: 500 mg po bid plus Ethambutol: 15 mg/kg po qid
Cryptococcal pneumonia	(Initial) Amphotericin B: 0.7 mg/kg iv qid (Maintenance) Fluconazole: 200 mg po qid
Kaposis sarcoma	Systemic chemotherapy

*Patients with marked hypoxia (pO$_2$< 70) should receive adjunctive corticosteroid therapy.

Fig. 10.80 Treatment of common pulmonary disorders.

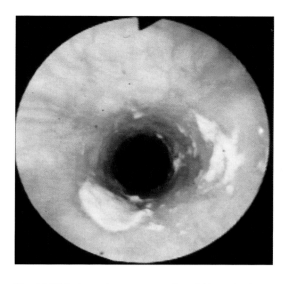

Fig. 10.81 Endoscopic appearance of candidal esophagitis.

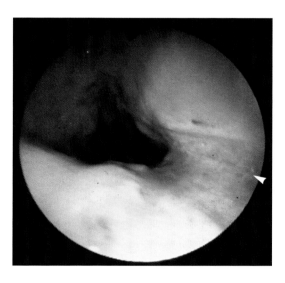

Fig. 10.82 Endoscopic view showing large ulcerated esophageal lesion (arrow) caused by cytomegalovirus.

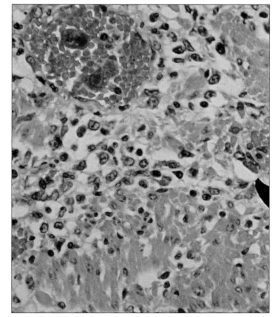
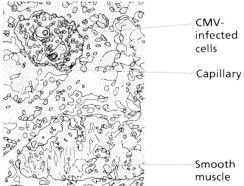

CMV-infected cells

Capillary

Smooth muscle

Fig. 10.83 Typical intranuclear and intracytoplasmic inclusions are seen within two cytomegalovirus-infected endothelial cells that have desquamated into the lumen of a capillary in this esophageal tissue (hematoxylin and eosin × 400).

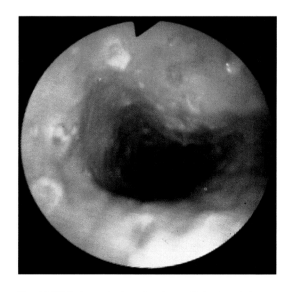

Fig. 10.84 Endoscopic view showing multiple ulcerated esophageal lesions caused by herpes simplex infection.

is shown in *Figure 10.89*. Among HIV-infected patients with CD4⁺ cell counts greater than 200 cells/mm³, cryptosporidiosis usually causes a self-limiting diarrheal illness, similar to the illness that occurs in normal hosts. In contrast, patients with CD4⁺ cell counts of less than 200 cells/mm³ typically develop unremitting diarrhea associated with weight loss and generalized wasting. In one study, cryptosporidia were found in 21% of patients with AIDS and diarrhea. A diagnosis can be made by finding oocysts in the stool using a modified acid-fast stain (*Fig. 10.90*). Although the diagnosis can also be made by small-bowel biopsy (*Figs. 10.91* and *10.92*), this test is usually not required. In addition to causing intestinal disease, cryptosporidia can cause biliary tract disease.

Microsporidiosis, which is caused by a number of closely related coccidian protozoan parasites, has recently been described as a probable cause of diarrhea among HIV-infected individuals. Not all patients with microspor-

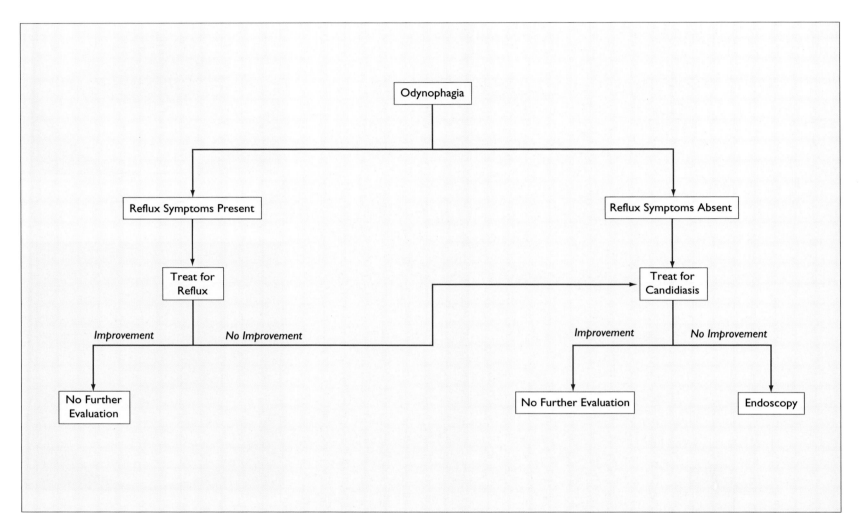

Fig. 10.85 Evaluation of odynophagia.

Fig. 10.86 Treatment of common esophageal disorders.

TREATMENT OF COMMON ESOPHAGEAL DISORDERS

CONDITION	TREATMENT
Candida esophagitis	Fluconazole: 200 mg po qid for 3 days then 10 mg po qid for 21 days
Cytomegalovirus esophagitis	Ganciclovir: 5 mg/kg iv bid for 2–4 weeks then 6 mg/kg iv qid Foscarnet: 60 mg/kg iv tid for 2–4 weeks then 100 mg/kg iv qid
Herpes esophagitis	Acyclovir: 400 mg po tid (may require larger doses or iv dosing)
Kaposi's sarcoma	Systemic chemotherapy

CAUSES OF DIARRHEA IN PATIENTS WITH HIV INFECTION

Fig. 10.87 Common causes of diarrhea in HIV-infected patients.

BACTERIAL	VIRAL	PARASITIC	NEOPLASTIC
Salmonella spp.	Cytomegalovirus	*Cryptosporidium parvum*	Kaposi's sarcoma
Shigella spp.	HIV	*Entamoeba histolytica*	Lymphoma
Campylobacter spp.		*Giardia lamblia*	
Mycobacterium avium-complex		*Isospora belli*	
Clostridium difficile			

EVALUATION OF DIARRHEA IN HIV INFECTED PATIENTS

Fig. 10.88 Evaluation of diarrhea in HIV-infected patients.

INITIAL STUDIES

Stool culture (for *Salmonella*, *Shigella*, and *Campylobacter*)

Modified acid-fast stain (for *Cryptosporidium* and *Isospora*)

Microscopic evaluation of stool for ova and parasites × 3

Evaluation of stool for *Clostridium difficile* toxin (if patient has been taking antibiotics recently)

IF INITIAL STUDIES ARE NONDIAGNOSTIC CONSIDER THE FOLLOWING

Weber Stain (for Microsporidia)

Sigmoidoscopy with biopsy

Upper endoscopy with duodenal drainage or small bowel biopsy

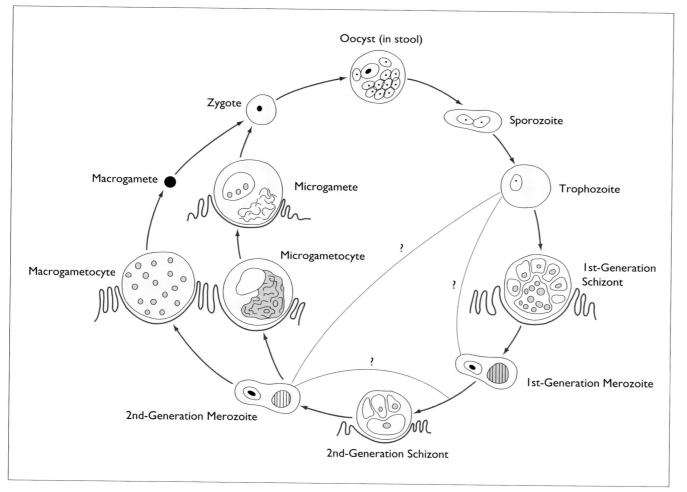

Fig. 10.89 Life cycle of *Cryptosporidium parvum*.

idiosis manifest symptoms and its exact role in causing diarrhea remains poorly defined. The diagnosis is made using a modified trichrome stain (Weber stain) or using the fluorochrome, calcofluor white (*Figs. 10.93* and *10.94*).

Another coccidian protozoan parasite, *Isospora belli*, can cause a diarrheal illness similar to cryptosporidiosis. Isosporiasis is most frequently seen in the tropics, particularly in Haiti. Iodine-stained wet mounts and modified acid-fast stool smears may reveal oocysts that are significantly larger than the cryptosporidial oocysts (*Fig. 10.95*).

Giardia lamblia is a common pathogen among HIV patients. It causes problems ranging from asymptomatic infection to profuse watery diarrhea, abdominal cramps, bloating, nausea, and severe malabsorption. Direct stool examination may reveal trophozoites or cysts (*Fig. 10.96*). Other tests used to diagnose giardiasis include stool antigen and upper endoscopy with duodenal biopsy (*Figs. 10.97* and *10.98*).

Amebiasis, which is caused by *Entamoeba histolytica*, may manifest as proctocolitis with diarrhea, tenesmus, cramps, abdominal pain, and rectal discharge. Amebic colitis may also resemble ulcerative colitis (*Fig. 10.99*). For HIV-infected patients, this disorder is found predominantly among homo-sexual men. When the diagnosis is suspected, multiple stool samples for ova and parasites should be collected (*Figs. 10.100* and *10.101*), and if negative, the diagnosis can usually be made with bowel biopsy.

CMV infection may cause disease ranging from diarrhea to intestinal perforation. Barium studies are often abnormal. As serologic evidence of prior CMV infection is almost universal in this patient population, measurement of CMV antibody titer is generally not helpful. Appearance at endoscopy is variable, showing either normal mucosa or discrete lesions. The diagnosis is made histologically by observing cytoplasmic inclusion bodies in biopsied samples (*Fig. 10.102*).

Mycobacterium avium complex (MAC) is another important cause of gastrointestinal symptoms. Manifestations include abdominal pain, diarrhea, anemia, and weight loss. Abdominal computerized tomographic (CT) scans may show associated enlarged retroperitoneal lymph nodes. Diagnosis of intestinal MAC can be made from stool culture, or in some cases, by bowel biopsy (*Figs. 10.103–10.107*). Isolation of MAC from stool culture suggests that the patient will progress to develop disseminated MAC disease. Although MAC can be found in biopsies from liver, bone marrow or lymph nodes, disseminated disease is reliably diagnosed with blood cultures.

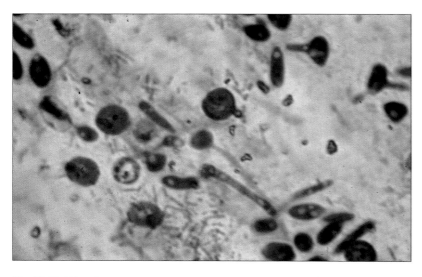

Fig. 10.90 Although cryptosporidia are occasionally identified in unstained and iodine-stained concentrated wet mounts, they are best identified by performing a modifed acid-fast stain on smears. Oocysts appear as circular red bodies 4–6 µm in diameter. Sporozoites can occasionally be seen within oocysts. (Modified acid-fast stain × 1,000).

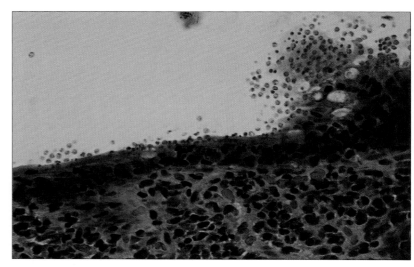

Fig. 10.91 Innumerable cryptosporidia seen infecting the mucosal brush border in this duodenal biopsy. The organisms appear as small, 4–6 µm, round basophilic bodies, adherent to the mucosal surface on routine hematoxylin-and-eosin stained histologic sections (× 40).

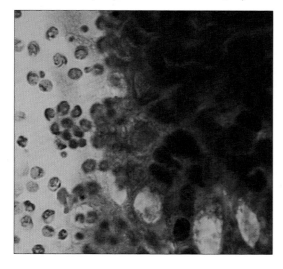

Fig. 10.92 Higher magnification of the section shown in **10.91** demonstrates numerous cryptosporidia adherent to the brush border of duodenal mucosa. In histologic sections, the organisms are not acid-fast perhaps because the organisms seen infecting the brush border of small bowel mucosa represent a different stage in the life cycle of cryptosporidia than is passed in stool (hematoxylin and eosin × 400).

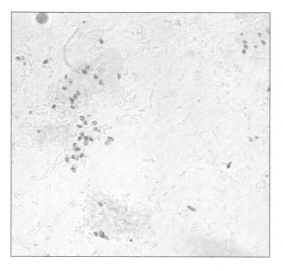

Fig. 10.93 Stool sample showing red-stained microsporidia (modified trichrome stain [Weber stain] × 400).

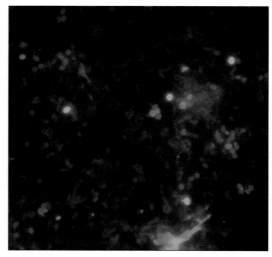

Fig. 10.94 Stool specimen stained with the fluorochrome calcofluor white showing brightly staining scattered microsporidia organisms that are few in number; abundant, less intense staining bacteria are present as background material (× 400).

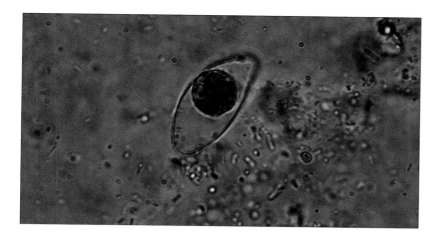

Fig. 10.95 Iodine-stained wet mount of fecal concentrate demonstrating the coccidian protozoa *Isospora belli*. Seen in this photomicrograph is an immature oocyst (approximately 25–30 μm) with a single central granular zygote (× 1,000). Similar to *Cryptosporidia, Isospora* are best identified with a modified acid-fast stain.

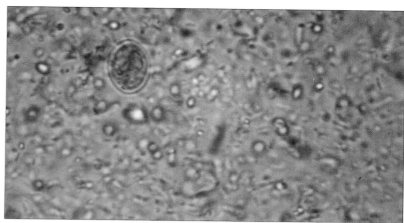

Fig. 10.96 Cyst of *Giardia lamblia* showing ovoid shape, prominent cyst wall, granular cytoplasm, and at least two nuclei.

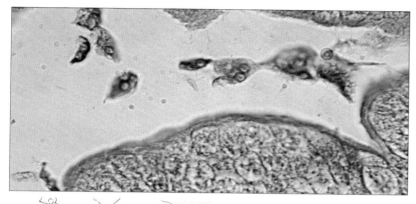

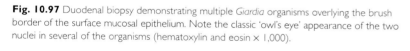

Giardia with "owl's eye" appearance of nuclei

Fig. 10.97 Duodenal biopsy demonstrating multiple *Giardia* organisms overlying the brush border of the surface mucosal epithelium. Note the classic 'owl's eye' appearance of the two nuclei in several of the organisms (hematoxylin and eosin × 1,000).

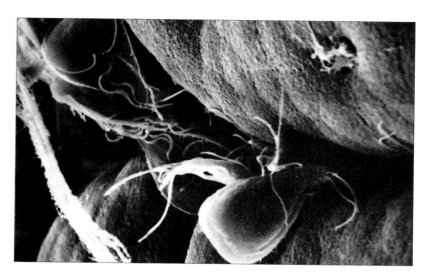

Fig. 10.98 Scanning electron micrograph of *Giardia* trophozoites in a crevice of a human jejunal villus (× 1,550).

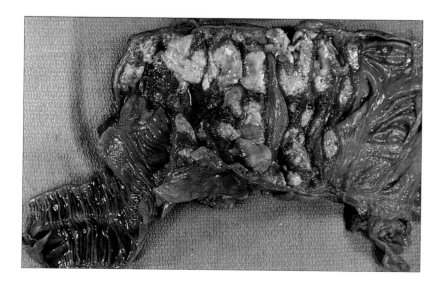

Fig. 10.99 Markedly dilated segment of proximal large bowel demonstrating numerous ulcers (whitish-green mucosal defects) secondary to *Entamoeba histolytica* infection.

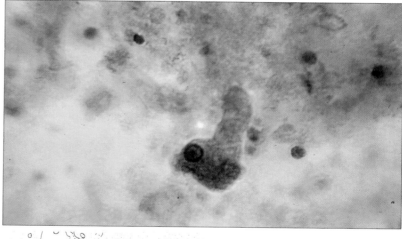

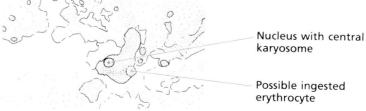

Nucleus with central karyosome

Possible ingested erythrocyte

Fig. 10.100 *Entamoeba histolytica* trophozoite. Note the single nucleus with evenly distributed peripheral chromatin, a central karyosome, and granular cytoplasm with a suggestion of an ingested erythrocyte within the peripheral cytoplasm (Trichome stain × 1,000).

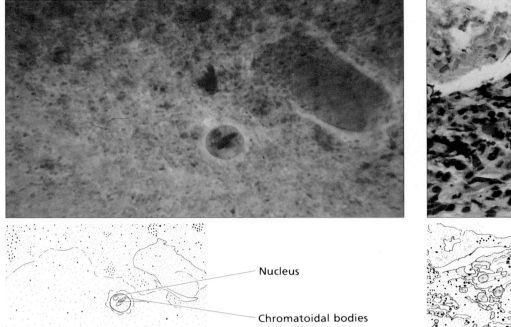

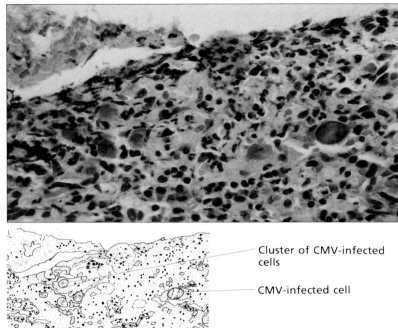

Fig. 10.101 *Entamoeba histolytica* cyst. Spherical cyst with only visible nucleus (immature cyst) and several cytoplasmic chromatoidal bodies (iodine wet mount × 400).

Fig. 10.102 Numerous cytomegalovirus-infected cells are present within the lamina propria of this colon biopsy. Kaposi's sarcoma was also present in several other of the tissue fragments from this biopsy. The neoplasm, however, is not present in this photomicrograph (hematoxylin and eosin × 400).

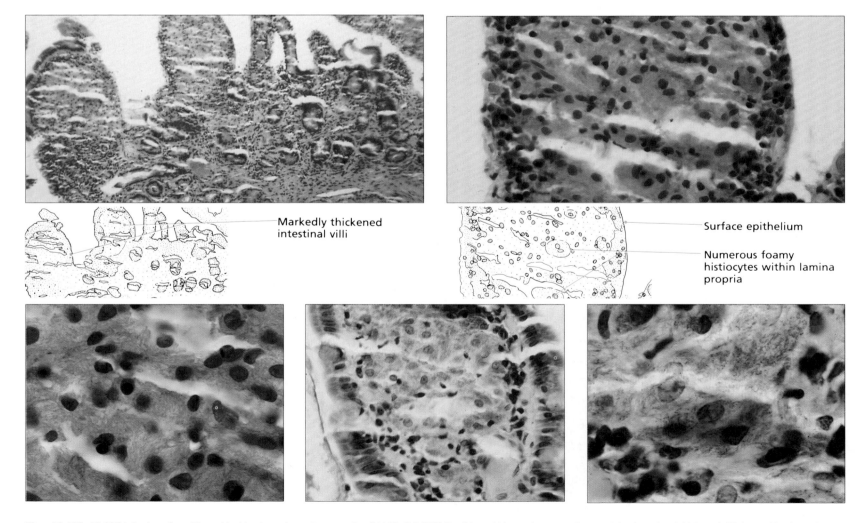

Figs. 10.103–10.107 Infection of small bowel by *Mycobacterium avium*-complex (MAC). (**10.103**) Small bowel biopsy demonstrating several enlarged and thickened villi due to *Mycobacterium avium*-complex infection (hematoxylin and eosin × 100). (**10.104**) Higher magnification of a thickened intestinal villus demonstrating prominent expansion of the lamina propria by numerous histiocytes having pale, eosinophilic cytoplasm (hematoxylin and eosin × 400). (**10.105**) High magnification of foamy histiocytes. This appearance is due to the presence of large numbers of intracytoplasmic mycobacteria. However, the appearance with routine hematoxylin-and-eosin stained sections is essentially identical to that seen in Whipple's disease, and an acid-fast stain is necessary to confirm the presence of mycobacteria (hematoxylin and eosin × 1,000). (**10.106**) The cytoplasm of the histiocytes appears red due to the large numbers of intracytoplasmic mycobacteria stained with this acid-fast stain (Ziehl-Neelson stain × 400). (**10.107**) Numerous acid-fast bacilli filling the cytoplasm of histiocytes (Ziehl-Neelson stain × 1,000).

Among the tumors of the gastrointestinal tract described in patients with AIDS, the most common is Kaposi's sarcoma. Lesions can develop in the stomach, small bowel, large bowel, and the anorectal area. These lesions are usually asymptomatic, but in some instances, they can bleed, obstruct the bowel lumen, or cause perforation. As superficial biopsy will not detect these submucosal tumors, biopsies are sometimes falsely negative. The treatment of common intestinal disorders is shown in *Figure 10.108*; as noted some of these disorders are more responsive to therapy than others.

In addition to developing esophagitis and diarrhea, homosexual HIV-infected males can develop proctitis (*Fig. 10.109*) and perianal lesions such

TREATMENT OF COMMON INTESTINAL DISORDERS

CONDITION	TREATMENT	RESPONSE
Salmonellosis	Ciprofloxacin: 500 mg po bid for 21 days	Good
Campylobacter	Ciprofloxacin: 500 mg po bid for 14 days	Good
Shigellosis	Ciprofloxacin: 500 mg po bid for 14 days	Good
Clostridium difficile	Metronidazole: 500 mg for 10 days	Good
	or	
	Vancomycin: 125 mg po qid for 10 days	Good
Cryptosporidiosis	Paromomycin: 500 mg po tid for 30 days, then 500 mg po bid	Fair
	or	
	Azithromycin: 500 mg po bid for 30 days, then 500 mg po qid	Fair
Microsporidiosis	Albendazole: 400 mg po bid for 4 weeks	Fair
	or	
	Atovaqone 750 mg po tid	Fair
Amebiasis	Metronidazole: 750 mg po tid for 10 days, followed by either Paromomycin: 500 mg po tid for 7 days	Good
	or	
	Iodoquinol: 650 mg po tid for 20 days	
Isosporiasis	TMP/SMZ: 1 DS po qid for 10 days, then 1 DS po bid for 20 days	Good
Giardiasis	Metronidazole: 500 mg po tid for 10 days	Good
Cytomegalovirus (enteritis, colitis)	Ganciclovir: 5 mg/kg iv bid for 2–4 weeks	Fair
	or	
	Foscarnet: 90 mg/kg iv bid for 2–4 weeks	Fair
MAC enteritis	Clarithromycin: 500 mg po qid plus Ethambutol: 15 mg/kg po qid plus Clofazimine: 100–200 mg po qid	Good
Kaposi's sarcoma	Systemic chemotherapy	Fair

Fig. 10.108 Treatment of common intestinal disorders.

CAUSES OF PROCTITIS IN HOMOSEXUAL MEN

DISEASE	SIGNS AND SYMPTOMS	DIAGNOSIS
Herpes simplex	Atypical and ulcerative lesions, pain	Tzanck prep (or Wright's stain) of base of lesion Viral FA, culture
Syphilis	Atypical and multiple chancres	Rapid Plasma Reagin (RPR)/ Venereal Disease Research Laboratory (VDRL) tests, darkfield microscopy, FA
Gonorrhea	Rectal discharge, pain	Gram stain and culture
Chlamydia trachomatis	Rectal discharge, fistula, pain	*Chlamydia* cultures, rapid diagnostic tests

FA – fluorescent antibody

Fig. 10.109 Causes of proctitis in homosexual men.

as perianal warts (*Fig. 10.110*), HSV infection (*Fig. 10.111*), Kaposi's sarcoma, and anal carcinoma.

Neurologic

HIV-infected patients often develop neurologic problems, especially as their immune suppression progresses and they develop AIDS (*Fig. 10.112*). Any patient with AIDS, who presents with a new neurologic complaint or a new abnormal neurologic finding, should be given a complete neurologic examination as part of their clinical evaluation. If either meningitis, encephalopathy, or a brain mass lesion is suspected, further evaluation should be performed as outlined in *Fig. 10.113*.

Cryptococcal meningitis is the most common opportunistic CNS infection in patients with AIDS, occurring in approximately 7% of AIDS patients. This infection, which is caused by the fungus *C. neoformans*, usually involves patients who have CD4+ cell counts of less than 100 cells/mm^3. Typically, it manifests as a subacute-to-chronic illness characterized by fever, headache, malaise, and less frequently, altered mental status, photophobia, or neck stiffness. Patients with altered mental status have a poor prognosis. The diagnosis of cryptococcal meningitis can be confirmed from CSF with one or more of three available tests: India ink, cryptococcal antigen, or culture. Of these three, India ink (*Figs. 10.114* and *10.115*) is the most rapid, but has a significantly lower sensitivity than the cryptococcal antigen test. For the initial

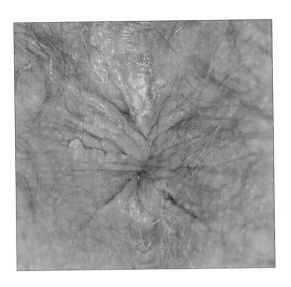

Fig. 10.110 Raised, irregular perianal warts.

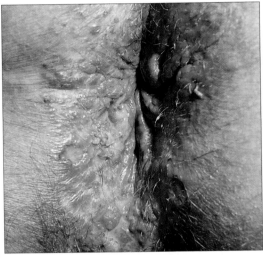

Fig. 10.111 Perinanal vesicular and ulcerative lesions of herpes simplex infection.

COMMON NEUROLOGIC PROBLEMS IN PATIENTS WITH AIDS

Cryptococcal meningitis

Toxoplasmosis

Primary CNS lymphoma

Progressive multifocal leukoencephalopathy

Cytomegalovirus encephalitis

Neurosyphilis

Peripheral neuropathy or myelopathy

HIV-associated dementia

Fig. 10.112 Common neurologic problems in patients with AIDS.

Fig. 10.114 Irregular violet-staining budding yeast with prominent clear-to-slightly opaque capsule typical of *Cryptococcus* present in a CSF cytology specimen. A darkly staining, poorly preserved small lymphocyte is also present (cytospin preparation, Wright's stain × 1,000).

EVALUATION OF NEUROLOGIC PROBLEMS IN PATIENTS WITH AIDS

CT scan with contrast (and/or MRI)

Lumbar puncture (if no mass effect on CT scan) with CSF sent for:

    Gram stain

    Cell count

    Glucose

    Protein

    India ink stain

    Cryptococcal antigen

    Venereal Disease Research Laboratory (VDRL) Slide Test

    Cytology

    Culture—routine, acid-fast, and fungal (viral, if available)

Fig. 10.113 Evaluation of neurologic problems in patients with AIDS.

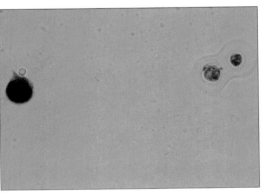

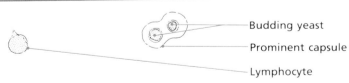

— Budding yeast

— Prominent capsule

— Lymphocyte

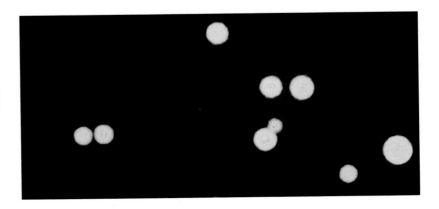

Fig. 10.115 India-ink preparation of CSF specimen demonstrating numerous yeasts, some of which are budding. These are seen as clear spaces against the dark background. This appearance is largely due to displacement of the ink by large amounts of capsular material and is characteristic of *Cryptococcus* (× 400).

diagnosis, one should consider any detectable cryptococcal antigen titer on a CSF specimen as reliable evidence of cryptococcal meningitis. Patients with treated cryptococcal meningitis, however, frequently maintain a positive CSF titer without evidence of persistent CNS infection. Cultures, which generally take at least several days to turn positive, are predominantly used to confirm the initial diagnosis and to follow treatment responses. Patients with cryptococcal meningitis also have positive serum cryptococcal antigen titers more than 95% of the time. As the organism may also invade brain tissue, one may occasionally find evidence of cryptococcosis on brain biopsy or autopsy specimens (*Fig. 10.116*).

Toxoplasma encephalitis, which is caused by the protozoan parasite *Toxoplasma gondii*, is the most common cause of focal CNS mass lesions in patients with AIDS. In almost all cases, *Toxoplasma* encephalitis is due to the reactivation of latent infection in patients who have CD4⁺ cell counts of less than 200 cells/mm³. The clinical presentation is characterized by fever, headache, mental status changes, and less often seizures. If the patient has serologic evidence of previous infection with *T. gondii*, and if CT scans show multiple ring-enhancing lesions (*Fig. 10.117*), a presumptive diagnosis of toxoplasmosis can be made and empiric therapy started without the need for

a brain biopsy. If patients do not respond to anti-toxoplasmosis therapy within 14 days, or if they deteriorate despite therapy, a brain biopsy is generally indicated (*Figs. 10.118* and *10.119*). In addition, brain biopsy may be indicated for patients who have a negative serology for *T. gondii*, or who have a solitary brain lesion seen by magnetic resonance imaging (MRI). Spinal fluid examination is nonspecific and may be normal. In addition, serology to determine acute rises in IgM titers is not helpful.

Patients who develop CNS lymphoma present with symptoms and signs that are similar to those seen in patients with *Toxoplasma* encephalitis. This tumor is usually induced by Epstein–Barr virus and occurs in patients with advanced HIV disease. The diagnosis is initially suggested by a patient who has only one or two lesions present on CT (or MRI) scanning and a negative *Toxoplasma* serology. The likelihood that a lesion is lymphoma is also markedly increased by a failure to respond to anti-toxoplasmosis therapy. *Figures 10.120* and *10.121* show a CT scan and MRI scan of a large lymphoma. To confirm the diagnosis of lymphoma, biopsy is required.

Progressive multifocal leukoencephalopathy (PML) is a rare, progressive, demyelinating disease caused by a papovavirus known as JC virus. This disorder results from reactivation of the JC virus, which typically occurs when

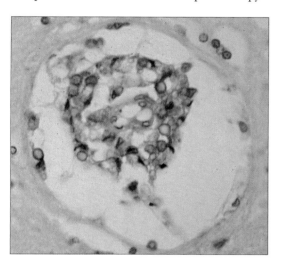

Fig. 10.116 Cryptococcal organisms present within a perivascular space in autopsy brain tissue from a patient with AIDS. A mucicarmine stain was used, which stains the polysaccharide capsule of *Cryptococcus* red and is specific for encapsulated forms of *Cryptococcus*. Other yeast will not stain with mucicarmine (× 400).

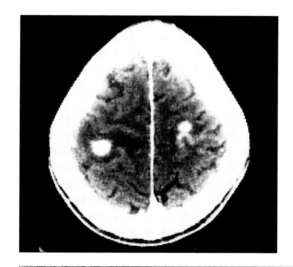

Fig. 10.117 CT scan with contrast of the brain in a patient with AIDS showing two enhancing lesions compatible with CNS toxoplasmosis.

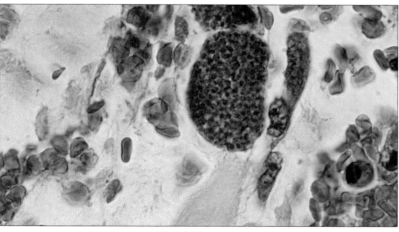
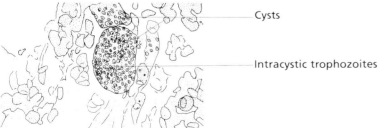

Cysts

Intracystic trophozoites

Fig. 10.118 Brain biopsy showing extracellular *Toxoplasma* cysts containing large numbers of trophozoites.

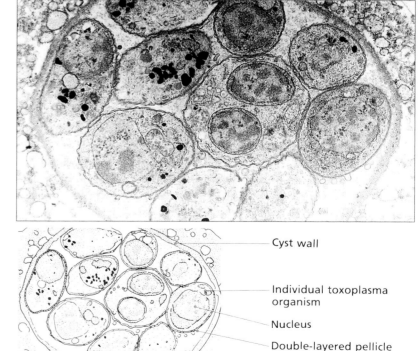

Cyst wall

Individual toxoplasma organism

Nucleus

Double-layered pellicle

Fig. 10.119 Transmission electron photomicrograph of an intracellular *Toxoplasma* cyst containing portions of 10 intracystic organisms. The cyst wall appears slightly more dense peripherally, and is less dense, granular, and slightly irregular internally. The wall of the individual organism is composed of a double-layered pellicle. Nuclei can be seen within some of the organisms, as well as a variety of cytoplasmic organelles, including dense bodies, endoplasmic reticulum, and finely granular material.

a patient's CD4+ cell count decreases to less than 100 cells/mm³. Signs and symptoms are often nonspecific and include headache, behavioral changes, mental impairment, dementia, visual-field deficits, ataxia, limb weakness, and dysarthria. The diagnosis can be strongly suggested by the characteristic appearance of white-matter lesions on a CT scan (*Fig. 10.122*) or MRI scan (*Fig. 10.123*). The MRI scan generally shows more numerous and extensive lesions than a CT scan, and in some instances, the MRI scan is strongly positive when the CT scan does not show any evidence of PML. Although a brain biopsy can confirm the diagnosis, this is rarely indicated.

Patients with early neurosyphilis (meningeal or meningovascular) present with headaches, photophobia, cranial nerve involvement, or stroke, typically within 10 years after the patient has developed secondary syphilis. The diagnosis is suspected in patients with positive serologic tests and confirmed with CSF studies. Late neurosyphilis (paresis and tabes dorsalis) rarely occurs among HIV-infected patients, or in any other patients, in the present-day antibiotic era.

HIV itself may cause significant neurologic disease, including aseptic meningitis, peripheral neuropathy, and HIV-associated dementia. The most common of these, HIV-associated dementia, usually presents with mental slowing, impaired memory, decreased concentration, and the loss of fine motor skills. In most circumstances, the diagnosis is made clinically. A brain CT scan may show atrophy and dilated ventricles; a brain biopsy, when performed, may show evidence of direct HIV invasion of the CNS (*Fig. 10.124*). The treatment of common neurologic disorders is shown in *Figure 10.125*.

Ophthalmic

An array of ocular manifestations can develop in HIV-infected patients (*Fig. 10.126*). Cotton-wool spots, which are believed to result from direct retinal microvascular HIV infection, are common in HIV-infected patients (*Fig. 10.127*). Although these lesions do not usually cause symptoms, they can be confused with CMV retinitis, which is the most common serious ocular finding among HIV-infected patients. CMV retinitis results from reactivation of CMV in patients who almost always have CD4+ cell counts of less than 100 cells/mm³. Most patients complain of seeing floaters or flashing lights and some notice a visual-field deficit. The diagnosis is made by fundoscopy (*Figs. 10.128* and *10.129*) and biopsy is not required. Other retinal lesions, such as those caused by *T. gondii* (*Fig. 10.130*) or *P. carinii*, can occur, but are much less common than CMV retinitis or cotton-wool spots. Reiter's syndrome has

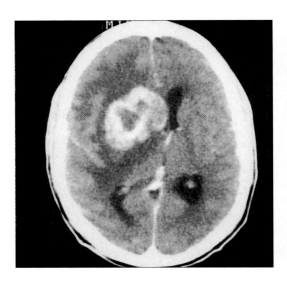

Fig. 10.120 CT scan with contrast showing a large lesion impinging on the ventricle with shift of midline structures. Biopsy of this lesion revealed lymphoma.

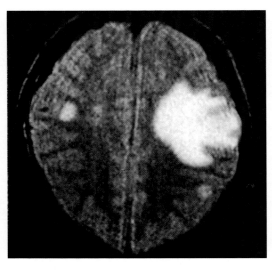

Fig. 10.121 MRI scan showing a large lesion, which on biopsy showed lymphoma.

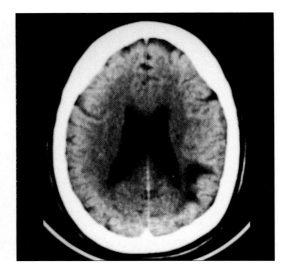

Fig. 10.122 CT scan showing markedly dilated ventricles. A brain biopsy revealed progressive multifocal leukoencephalopathy.

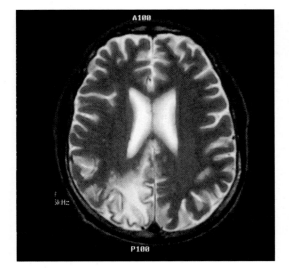

Fig. 10.123 MRI scan of patient with progressive multifocal leukoencephalopathy showing extensive white matter disease.

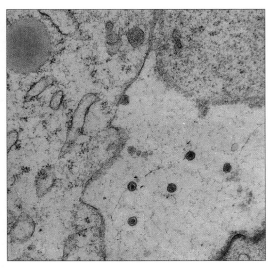

Fig. 10.124 HIV virions in extracellular space of brain tissue of a patient with HIV-associated dementia.

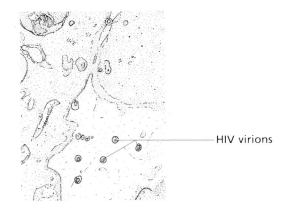

HIV virions

TREATMENT OF COMMON NEUROLOGIC DISORDERS

CONDITION	TREATMENT
Cryptococcal meningitis	(Initial) Amphotericin B: 0.7 mg/kg iv qid (Maintenance) Fluconazole: 200 mg po qid
Toxoplasma encephalitis	(Initial) Pyrimethamine: 100 mg po once then 75 mg po qid plus Sulfadiazine: 1.5 g po qid (or clindamycin: 600 mg po qid) (Maintenance) Pyrimethamine: 50 mg po qid plus Sulfadiazine: 1.0 g po tid
CNS Lymphoma	Radiation therapy
PML	Zidovudine: 1,000–1,500 mg/day in 5 divided doses ?Interferon-α ?Intravenous ARA-C ?Intrathecal ARA-C
Neurosyphilis	Penicillin G: 2–4 million units iv every 4 hours for 14 days
HIV-associated dementia	Zidovudine: 1,000–1,500 mg/day in 5 divided doses

Fig. 10.125 Treatment of common neurologic disorders in HIV-infected patients.

OCULAR FINDINGS IN HIV-INFECTED PATIENTS

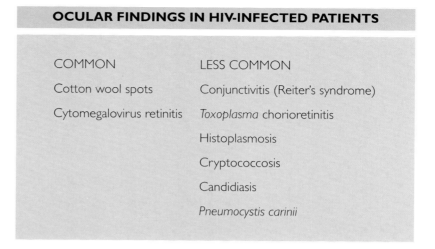

COMMON	LESS COMMON
Cotton wool spots	Conjunctivitis (Reiter's syndrome)
Cytomegalovirus retinitis	*Toxoplasma* chorioretinitis
	Histoplasmosis
	Cryptococcosis
	Candidiasis
	Pneumocystis carinii

Fig. 10.126 Ocular findings in HIV-infected patients.

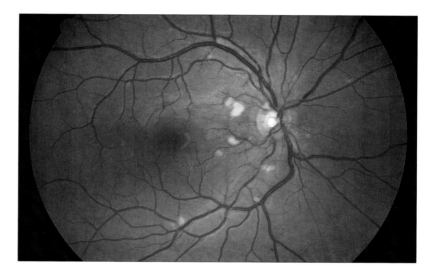

Fig. 10.127 Cotton-wool spots in an HIV-infected patient.

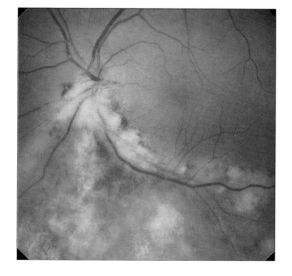
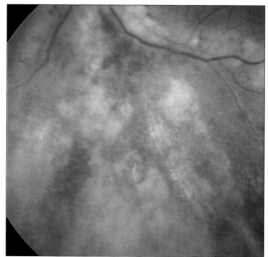

Figs. 10.128 and 10.129 Cytomegalovirus retinitis. Note the typical retinal swelling, hemorrhage and necrosis.

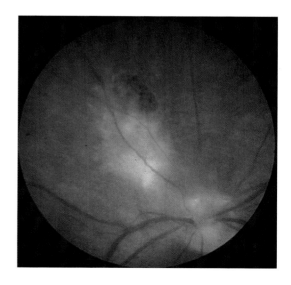

Fig. 10.130 Reactivation of ocular *Toxoplasma* chorioretinitis in an area of previous scarring.

occurred with increased frequency among HIV-infected patients and patients may develop conjunctivitis as part of the constellation of findings (*Fig. 10.131*). The treatment of common ocular disorders is summarized in *Fig. 10.132*.

Hematologic/oncologic

There are many lymphohematologic disorders in patients with AIDS (*Fig. 10.133*). Lymphadenopathy frequently develops in HIV-infected patients and may result from one of three major causes:

- HIV-related
- Non-Hodgkin's (or Hodgkin's) lymphoma
- Opportunistic infections.

Early in the course of their HIV illness, patients may develop significant HIV-related lymphadenopathy. In some cases, the node will show hyperplasia, and with progressive immunosuppression the node architecture may change (*Figs. 10.134–10.136*). Recent studies have suggested that these nodes harbor abundant quantities of HIV. Malignant lymphoma frequently causes a patient to develop fever, weight loss, and enlarged lymph nodes (*Fig. 10.137*). The diagnosis requires a node biopsy (*Figs. 10.138–10.140*). Enlarged lymph nodes may also result from infection with opportunistic pathogens, such as *M. avium* complex (*Figs. 10.141–10.143*), *M. tuberculosis*, and disseminated histoplasmosis (*Figs. 10.144* and *10.145*).

Hematologic abnormalities (anemia, neutropenia, and thrombocytopenia) can result from either HIV-related effects, opportunistic infections, or from medications used to treat HIV-related opportunistic infections. As there may be many possible causes for a hematologic disorder, the exact cause may be difficult to identify. In some instances, bone-marrow examination with

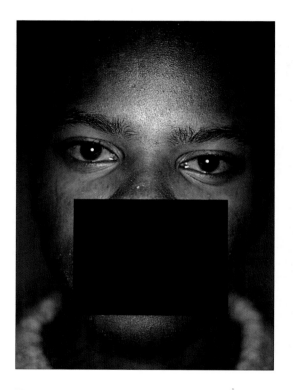

Fig. 10.131 Conjunctivitis of Reiter's syndrome. The patient complained of tearing, itching, and redness of the eyes. In addition, he had arthritis and urethritis.

TREATMENT OF COMMON OCULAR DISORDERS

CONDITION	TREATMENT
Cytomegalovirus retinitis	Ganciclovir: 5 mg/kg iv bid for 2–3 weeks then 6 mg/kg iv qid Foscarnet: 60 mg/kg iv tid for 2–3 weeks then 100–120 mg/kg iv qid
HIV retinopathy	None

Fig. 10.132. Treatment of common ocular disorders.

TUMORS IN HIV-INFECTED PATIENTS

Kaposi's sarcoma	Central nervous system lymphoma
Small bowel lymphoma	Squamous cell carcinoma of the rectum
Non-Hodgkin's lymphoma (small noncleaved lymphoma – either Burkitt or non-Burkitt type – and immunoblastic sarcoma)	Cloacogenic carcinoma of the rectum
	Hodgkin's lymphoma

Fig. 10.133 Tumors in HIV-infected patients.

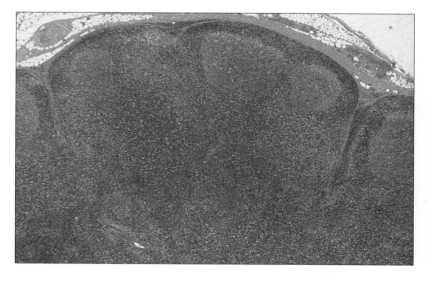

Fig. 10.134 Low-power photomicrograph of a lymph node biopsy demonstrating prominent follicular hyperplasia with multiple large and somewhat irregular follicles that are occasionally confluent. Focal effacement of the mantle zone of small lymphocytes surrounding the germinal centers can be seen. In addition, there is paracortical hyperplasia and irregular sheets of pale histiocyte or epithelioid cells (hematoxylin and eosin × 40).

Fig. 10.135 Prominent effacement of the normal lymph node architecture. There are scattered 'burnt-out' germinal centers and vascularity is prominent (hematoxylin and eosin × 40).

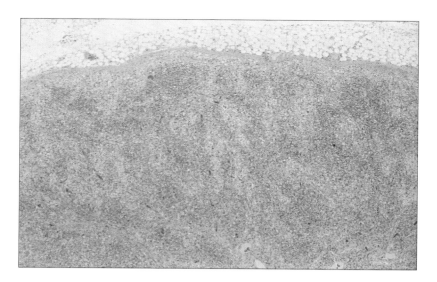

Fig. 10.136 Severe lymph node effacement. The node has a pale quality due to the complete loss of follicles and marked lymphoid depletion (hematoxylin and eosin × 40).

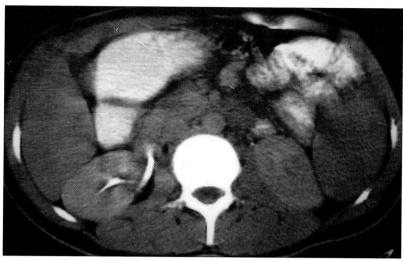

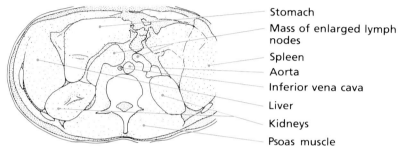

Stomach
Mass of enlarged lymph nodes
Spleen
Aorta
Inferior vena cava
Liver
Kidneys
Psoas muscle

Fig. 10.137 Abdominal CT scan showing retroperitoneal lymphoadenopathy in a patient with AIDS.

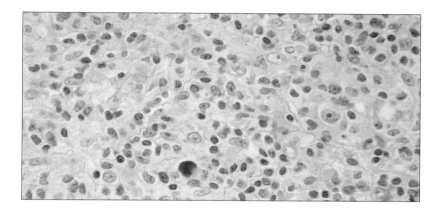

Fig. 10.138 Hodgkin's lymphoma, mixed cellularity type, retroperitoneal lymph nodes. Note the effacement of the normal nodal architecture (absence of typical germinal centers and other normal landmarks), numerous larger histiocytic cells, scattered large atypical mononuclear cells with prominent nucleoli, few lymphocytes, and plasma cells and a large cell with a darkly staining pyknotic nucleus and eosinophilic cytoplasm (the so-called 'mummified cell' of Hodgkin's lymphoma) (hematoxylin and eosin × 250).

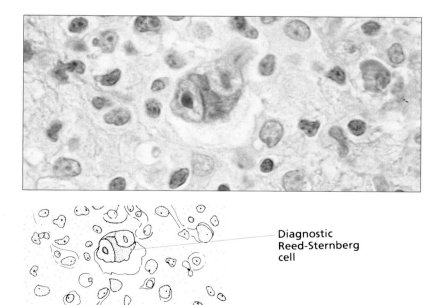

Diagnostic
Reed-Sternberg
cell

Fig. 10.139 Hodgkin's lymphoma, mixed cellularity type. Note the Reed-Sternberg cell (binucleated cell with large eosinophilic nucleoli) requisite for a diagnosis of Hodgkin's disease (hematoxylin and eosin × 1,000).

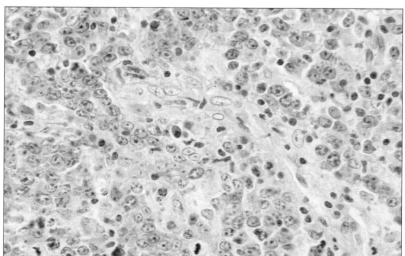

Fig. 10.140 Malignant non-Hodgkin's lymphoma, diffuse, large-cell type (histiocytic lymphoma, Rappaport classification), retroperitoneal lymph node. This is from the same patient as in **10.138** and **10.139**, who was found to have both Hodgkin's and non-Hodgkin's lymphomas in separate retroperitoneal lymph nodes at laparotomy. Lymph node is effaced by large neoplastic lymphoid cells, some with prominent nucleoli (hematoxylin and eosin × 400).

aspirate, biopsy, and culture may be a valuable diagnostic tool. *Figures 10.146* and *10.147* show bone marrow invaded by *H. capsulatum* and *C. neoformans*, respectively. In some instances, the peripheral blood smear has revealed a diagnosis of disseminated histoplasmosis (*Fig. 10.148*).

Women and HIV

Although there has only been limited research on how gender affects the clinical course of HIV infection, available data suggest that women and men have similar early HIV-related symptoms, laboratory findings, and

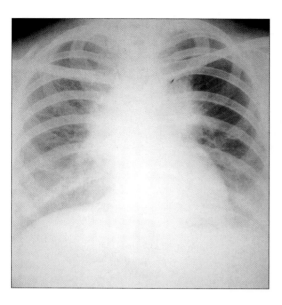

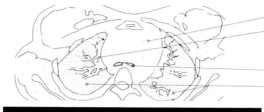

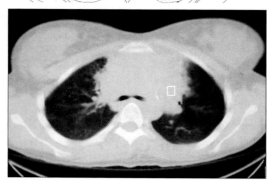

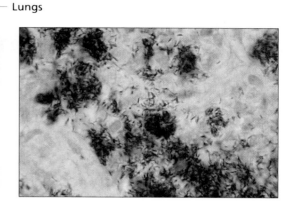

Figs. 10.141–10.143 Lymphadenopathy caused by *Mycobacterium avium*-complex. (**10.141** and **10.142**) Chest radiograph and CT scan showing mediastinal widening due to lymphadenopathy. (**10.143**) Large numbers of acid-fast bacilli are present predominantly within an intracellular location in histiocytes in this lymph node section. Although the pattern of large numbers of acid-fast bacilli completely filling and obscuring the cytoplasm is typical of *Mycobacterium avium*-complex, it is not possible to speciate mycobacteria on a morphologic basis, and culture with identification is necessary (Ziehl–Neelson stain × 1,000).

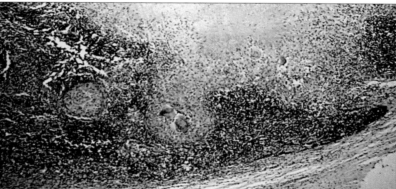

Fig. 10.144 Lymph node showing caseating granulomatous inflammation in an AIDS patient with disseminated histoplasmosis. *Histoplasma* organisms were identified in tissue sections with fungal stains as well as in cultures from lymph node tissue (hematoxylin and eosin × 100).

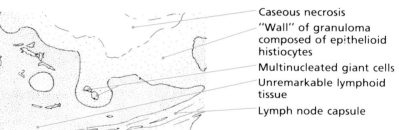

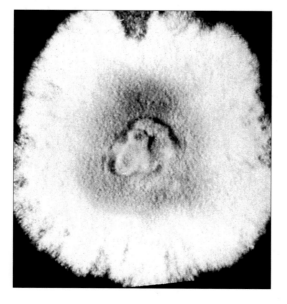

Fig. 10.145 Colony of *Histoplasma capsulatum* on Sabouraud's agar cultured from the lymph node of the patient in **10.144**. Note the white, fluffy, cottony aerial mycelium. With aging, the colony may turn gray–brown, as seen centrally in this colony.

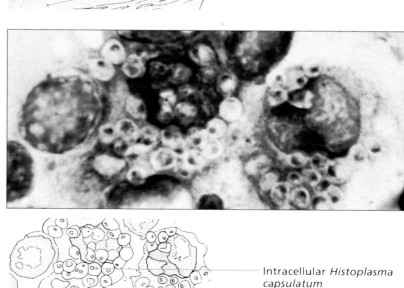

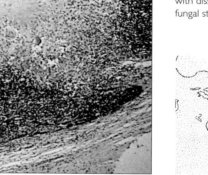

Fig. 10.146 *Histoplasma capsulatum* within the cytoplasm of several macrophages in this marrow aspirate smear (Wright's stain × 1,000).

survival. Patterns of opportunistic infection also appear similar, with two exceptions: women may develop esophageal candidiasis more frequently and Kaposi's sarcoma less frequently. In most areas of the world, clear epidemiologic differences exist. In particular, women in the pandemic tend to be younger, more socioeconomically disadvantaged, and more often of African and Hispanic ethnicity. Many HIV-infected women have children, and are more likely to be single head-of-households and live with other HIV-positive family members. These socioeconomic differences

may decrease access to health care and may lead to increases in morbidity and mortality.

HIV infection may affect many reproductive health concerns, with specific issues developing at different stages of the HIV illness (*Fig. 10.149*). The frequency, severity, and treatment response of many gynecologic problems may be linked to the extent of immunosuppression. Whatever the stage of HIV infection, however, early detection, intervention, and aggressive treatment of gynecologic problems are warranted in HIV-infected women.

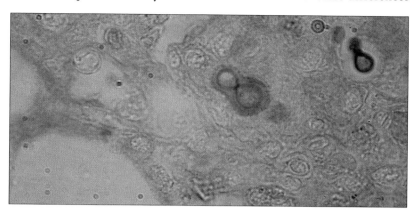

Fig. 10.147 *Cryptococcus neoformans* in bone-marrow biopsy. Two yeast are seen demonstrating narrow based budding. In this Alcian blue/periodic-acid Schiff (PAS) stained section, the cell wall stains faintly pink with PAS, which is typical of fungi. The Alcian blue component stains the polysaccharide capsule light blue and can be used as an equally effective alternative to mucicarmine stain to demonstrate the capsule of *Cryptococcus neoformans* (Alcian blue/PAS × 1,000).

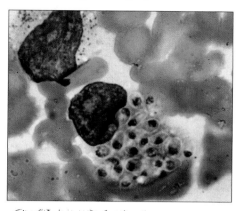

Fig. 10.148 Numerous intracellular *Histoplasma* organisms can be seen within the hematopoietic cells in the center of the photomicrograph. The yeast, which measures 2–5 µm, are usually seen within macrophages, giant cells, or neutrophils. However, they can also be found extracellularly (Wright's stain × 1,000).

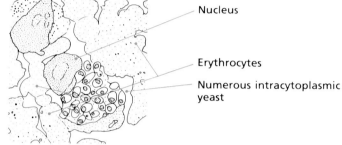

Nucleus

Erythrocytes

Numerous intracytoplasmic yeast

REPRODUCTIVE CONCERNS AND RELATIONSHIP TO STAGES OF HIV INFECTION

STAGE OF HIV INFECTION

INFECTION: SEROCONVERSION	SYMPTOM-FREE	EARLY SYMPTOMS	DISCRETE ILLNESS: CASCADE OF ILLNESS: ENDSTAGE
HIV serologic tests initially negative, so sex partner(s) and offspring may be placed at risk	May be tested as part of routine prenatal screening	Aggressive, recurrent vulvo-vaginal candidiasis; other aggressive STDs should prompt HIV evaluation	Assist with arranging child care
	Offer anticipatory guidance on future pregnancy planning		Pregnancy may result in prematurity, low birth weight, premature rupture of membranes, other complications
	Pap smear every 6 months, aggressive management of abnormal findings	Pregnancy likely to be uncomplicated by HIV	
	Offer personalized, explicit safer-sex skill building	Pap smear every 6 months, aggressive management of abnormal findings	Pap smear every 6 months, aggressive management of abnormal findings
	Pregnancy likely to be uncomplicated by HIV	Aggressive management of gynecologic infections	Aggressive management of gynecologic infections
		Assess contraception, safer sex status	Assess contraception, safer sex status
			Manage opportunistic infections and malignancies

Source: Modified from McKusick (1992). In Contraceptive Technology, 16th ed.

Fig. 10.149 Reproductive concerns and relationship to stages of HIV infection.

Increased rates of HPV and cervical dysplasia may occur more often among HIV-infected women when compared with HIV-seronegative women (*Figs. 10.150 and 10.151*). Moreover, invasive cervical carcinoma has recently been added to the list of AIDS-defining conditions. In order to detect early cervical abnormalities, Papanicolaou smears are recommended at 6-month intervals, with follow-up colposcopy and biopsy if the Papanicolaou smear is abnormal (*Figs. 10.152 and 10.153*). Genital warts, or condylomata acuminata, are also caused by HPV and have been linked to cervical dysplasia. Warts may also develop into extensive refractory lesions. Condylomata on the cervix are usually asymptomatic, requiring colposcopy to visualize them.

Pelvic inflammatory disease may be more common and requires more extensive treatment among HIV-infected women. Clinically, it may appear less severe on physical examination, but may have a more aggressive course. Vulvovaginal candidiasis can be an early manifestation of HIV disease. It is not known whether women with recurrent vulvovaginal candidiasis have an increased risk of developing esophageal candidiasis. Although increased rates of genital HSV infection have not been reported among HIV-positive women, lesions are often slower to heal.

The effect of HIV on the course of pregnancy remains unknown. The offspring of HIV-infected women may become infected *in utero*, at the time of delivery, or through breastfeeding. Estimates of HIV transmission rates range from 13–30%, with higher rates observed among women in developing countries. A recent study has suggested that zidovudine may markedly diminish the risk of maternal-to-fetal HIV transmission.

Miscellaneous Clinical Manifestations

Over the years, it has become clear that, although HIV has a predilection for certain organs, HIV can adversely affect any organ system of the human body. Organ systems that less frequently develop clinically significant problems include the renal, endocrine, and cardiac systems. A variety of renal lesions in patients with HIV infection has been described, consisting of both glomerular and tubular changes. AIDS-associated nephropathy, which consists of nephrotic-range proteinuria and focal and segmental glomerulosclerosis, usually results in end-stage renal disease. Other HIV-related renal abnormalities include other glomerular morphologic changes as well as nonspecific lesions such as acute tubular necrosis, nephrocalcinosis, and interstitial nephritis.

Numerous reports have described adrenal insufficiency in HIV-infected patients, predominantly those with AIDS. The most frequent cause has been CMV infection of the adrenal gland, but other microorganisms, including *M. tuberculosis* and *H. capsulatum,* can also cause adrenal insufficiency.

The clinical spectrum of cardiac disorders in HIV-related disease includes HIV-induced myocarditis, congestive cardiomyopathy (presumed to be of viral origin), nonbacterial thrombotic endocarditis, Kaposi's sarcoma of the myocardium, and non-Hodgkin's lymphoma of the pericardium.

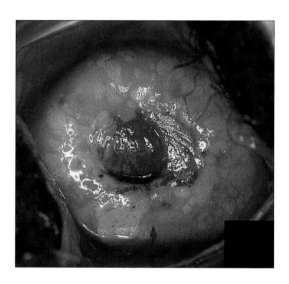

Fig. 10.150 Cervicitis, with cervical condylomata acuminata. Viewed through colposcope.

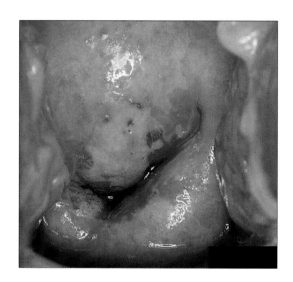

Fig. 10.151 Cervicitis in an HIV-infected woman, later found to have a high-grade squamous intraepithelial lesion (SIL) on cervical biopsy.

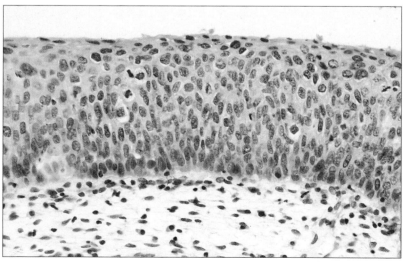

Fig. 10.152 Histopathology slide consistent with high-grade SIL. Koliocytotic changes present which are consistent with HPV.

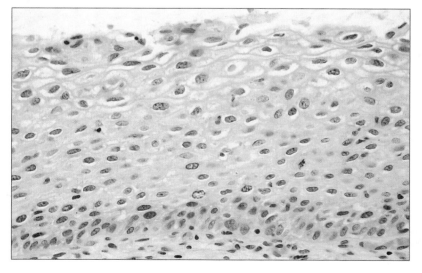

Fig. 10.153 Histopathology slide showing low-grade SIL. Koliocytotic changes present which are consistent with HPV.

BIBLIOGRAPHY

Barnes PF, Bloch AB, Davidson PT: Tuberculosis in patients with HIV infection. *N Engl J Med* **324**:1644–1650, 1991.

Berger TG, Greene I: Bacterial, viral, fungal, and parasitic infections in HIV disease and AIDS. *Dermatol Clin* **9**:465–492, 1991.

Centers for Disease Control and Prevention: 1993 revised classification system for HIV infection and expanded surveillance case definition for AIDS among adults and adolescents. *MMWR* **41**(no. RR–17), 1992.

Centers for Disease Control and Prevention: Update – Acquired immunodeficiency syndrome — United States, 1992. *MMWR* **42**:547–557, 1993.

Chaisson RE, Griffin DE: Progressive multifocal leukoencephalopathy in AIDS. *JAMA* **264**:79–82, 1990.

Cohen PR, Beltrani VP, Grossman ME: Disseminated herpes zoster in patients with human immunodeficiency virus infection. *Am J Med* **84**:1076–1080,1988.

Consensus statement on the use of corticosteroids as adjunctive therapy for *Pneumocystis* pneumonia in the acquired immune deficiency syndrome. *N Engl J Med* **323**:1500–1504, 1990.

Cotton D: AIDS in women. In: S, Broder, T. Merigan, Bolognest, D (eds). *Textbook of AIDS Medicine*. Baltimore, MD, Williams & Wilkins, Section IV, Ch. 11, 161–168, 1994.

Donabedian H, Khazan U: Norwegian scabies in a patient with AIDS. *Clin Infect Dis* **14**:162–164,1992.

Eeftinck Schattenkerk JKM, van Gool T, van Ketel RJ, et al.: Clinical significance of small-intestinal microsporidiosis in HIV-infected individuals. *Lancet* **337**:895–898, 1991.

Ellerbrock TV, Bush TJ, Chamberland ME, Oxtoby MJ: Epidemiology of women with AIDS in the United States, 1981–1990. *JAMA* **265**:2971–2975, 1991.

El–Sadr W, Oleske JM, Agins BD, et al.: Evaluation and management of early HIV infection. Clinical practice guideline no 7. AHCPR publication no. 94–0572. Rockville, Md, Agency for Health Care and Policy and Research, Public Health Services, US Department of Health and Human Services, January 1994.

Feingold AR, Vermund SH, Burk RD, et al.: Cervical cytologic abnormalities and papillomavirus in women infected with human immunodeficiency virus. *J Acquir Immune Defic Syndr* **3**:896–903, 1990.

Flanigan T, Whalen C, Turner J, Soave R, Toerner J, Havlir D, Kotler D: Cryptosporidium infection and CD4 counts. *Ann Intern Med* **116**:840–842, 1992.

Gerberding JL, Henderson DK: Management of occupational exposure to bloodborne pathogens: hepatitis B virus, hepatitis C virus, and human immunodeficiency virus. *Clin Infect Dis* **14**:1179–1185, 1992.

Greenspan D, Greenspan JS: Oral manifestations of HIV infection. *Dermatol Clin North Am* **9**:517–522,1991.

Guest F: HIV and AIDS. In: *Contraceptive Technology*, 16th ed. New York, Irvinton Publishers, pp 51–75, 1993.

Hirsch MS, D'Aquila RT: Therapy for human immunodeficiency virus infection. *N Engl J Med* **328**:1686–1695, 1993.

Horsburgh CR, Jason J, Longini IM, et al.: Duration of human immunodeficiency virus infection before detection of antibody. *Lancet* **ii**:637–639, 1989.

Horsburgh CR: *Mycobacterium avium* complex infection in the acquired immunodeficiency syndrome. *N Engl J Med* **324**:1332–1338, 1991.

Jacobson MA, Mills J: Serious cytomegalovirus disease in the acquired immunodeficiency syndrome. Clinical findings, diagnosis, and treatment. *Ann Intern Med* **108**:585–594,1988.

Katz MH, Greenspan D, Westerhouse J, et al.: Progression to AIDS in HIV-infected homosexual and bisexual men with hairy leukoplakia and oral candidiasis. *AIDS* **6**:95–100, 1992.

Kessler HA, Blaaauw B, Spear J, Paul DA, Falk LA, Landay A: Diagnosis of human immunodeficiency virus infection in seronegative homosexuals with an acute viral syndrome. *JAMA* **258**:1196–1199,1987.

Kinloch-de Löes S, de Saussure P, Saurat J–H, Stalder H, Hirschel B, Perrin LH: Symptomatic primary infection due to human immunodeficiency virus type 1: review of 31 cases. *Clin Infect Dis* **17**:59–65,1993.

Koehler JE, Tappero JW: Bacillary angiomatosis and bacillary peliosis in patients infected with human immunodeficiency virus. *Clin Infect Dis* **17**:612–624,1993.

Krown SE, Myskowski PL, Paredes J: Kaposi's sarcoma. *Med Clin North Am* **76**:235–252,1992.

Laine L, Dretler RH, Conteas CN, et al.: Fluconazole compared with ketoconazole for the treatment of candida esophagitis: a randomized trial. *Ann Intern Med* **117**:655–660,1992.

Levine AM: Acquired immunodeficiency syndrome-related lymphoma. *Blood* **80**:8–20,1992.

Luft BJ, Remington JS: Toxoplasmic encephalitis in AIDS. *Clin Infect Dis* **15**:211–222,1992.

Markovitz DM: Infection with human immunodeficiency virus type 2. *Ann Intern Med* **118**:211–218,1993.

Masur H, and the Public Health Service Task Force on Prophylaxis and Therapy for *Mycobacterium avium* complex. Recommendations on prophylaxis and therapy for disseminated *Mycobacterium avium* complex diseases in patients infected with the human immunodeficiency virus. *N Engl J Med* **329**:898–904, 1993.

Masur H: Prevention and treatment of *Pneumocystis carinii* pneumonia. *N Engl J Med* **327**:1853–1860,1993.

Minkhoff HL, Dehovitz JA: Care of women infected with the human immunodeficiency virus. *JAMA* **266**:2253–2258, 1991.

Pantaleo G, Graziosi C, Fauci AS: The immunopathogenesis of human immunodeficiency virus infection. *N Engl J Med* **328**:327–335,1993.

Peterson C: Cryptosporidiosis in patients with the human immunodeficiency virus. *Clin Infect Dis* **15**:903–909, 1992.

Powderly WG: Cryptococcal meningitis and AIDS. *Clin Infect Dis* **17**:837–842, 1993.

Rabeneck L, Gyorkey F, Genta RM, Gyorkey P, Foote LW, Risser JM: The role of *Microsporidia* in the pathogenesis of HIV-related chronic diarrhea. *Ann Intern Med* **119**:895–899,1993.

Sande MA, Carpenter CJ, Cobbs CG, Holmes KK: Antiretroviral therapy for adult HIV-infected patients: recommendations from a state-of-the-art conference. *JAMA* **270**:2583–2589, 1993.

Sloand EM, Piyy E, Chiarello RJ, Nemo GJ: HIV testing: state of the art. *JAMA* **266**:2861–2866, 1991.

Stein DS, Korvick JA, Vermund SH: CD4+ lymphocyte cell enumeration for prediction of clinical course of human immunodeficiency virus disease: a review. *J Infect Dis* **165**:352–363, 1992.

Weiss RA: How does HIV cause AIDS? *Science* **260**:1273–1279, 1993.

Wheat LJ, Connolly-Springfield PA, Baker RL, et al.: Disseminated histoplasmosis in the acquired immunodeficiency syndrome: clinical findings, diagnosis and treatment, and review of the literature. *Medicine* (Baltimore) **69**:361–374, 1990.

Wilcox CM, Diel DL, Cello JP, Margaretten W, Jacobson MA: Cytomegalovirus esophagitis in patients with AIDS. *Ann Intern Med* **113**:589–593, 1990.

Wofsy C: Therapeutic issues in women with HIV disease. In: M. Sande, P. Volberding (eds): *The Medical Management of AIDS*, 3rd ed. Philadelphia, PA, WB Saunders, 1992.

Zalla MJ, Su WPD, Fransway AF: Dermatologic manifestations of human immunodeficiency virus infection. *Mayo Clin Proc* **67**:1089–1108, 1992.

CHAPTER ELEVEN

Genital Herpes

A Moreland, S Shafran, J Bryan, and P Pellett

INTRODUCTION

Genital herpes is a common, often painful disease that has serious consequences for certain populations. Medical research in this century has significantly expanded our knowledge of the infection and its treatment. Prior to the 19th century, the term *herpes* (Greek for 'to creep') was used in medical literature for a variety of skin eruptions. Gradually, the meaning of the term narrowed to mean primarily the classic appearance of grouped vesicles on an erythematous base. A viral etiology was eventually suggested by transmission experiments in the early 1900s, and was confirmed and classified in relation to other viral diseases by the 1950s.

Genital herpes infections are caused by the herpes simplex virus (HSV), a large (150–200 nm) virus consisting of approximately 152,000 base pairs of double-stranded DNA encapsulated in a proteinaceous capsid, which is itself surrounded by a less well-defined structure, known as the tegument. The virus is contained in a host cell-derived lipid bilayer, studded with virus-specified glycoproteins and integral membrane proteins (*Figs. 11.1* and *11.2*). Two types of HSV exist: HSV type 1 (HSV-1) and HSV type 2 (HSV-2). These constitute two of the eight known human herpesviruses (*Fig. 11.3*). The nucleotide sequences of HSV-1 and HSV-2 are approximately 50% identical and their encoded proteins are even more closely related. There are no genes unique to either virus. HSV-1 is responsible for more than 90% of orolabial herpes and herpes keratitis, while HSV-2 is responsible for approximately 90% of genital herpes. The infection is characterized by viral shedding from affected skin or mucous membranes and the production of several types of specific humoral antibodies. The neutralizing antibodies, which are produced early in the course of infection and persist for variable lengths of time, do not prevent recurrence of the active phase of the disease, perhaps because extracellular virus is inactivated by these antibodies while intracellular viral replication and direct cell-to-cell transfer of new infectious virus still occur. The exact role of humoral antibodies in reactivation of the infection is not fully understood; however, antibodies appear to attenuate the severity of the disease since recurrences generally are less severe than the primary infection. Cell-mediated immune responses undoubtedly play an important role in the manifestation of herpes infections as evidenced by severe, prolonged, and frequently recurring infections in patients who have impaired cell-mediated immunity.

EPIDEMIOLOGY

Accurate data regarding the incidence and prevalence of genital herpes are not available, though several estimates have been made. Studies in several Western countries have found a wide range of HSV-2 seroprevalence, which varies according to the population studied from less than 10% in some groups of young women to over 75% in groups of female prostitutes. A national

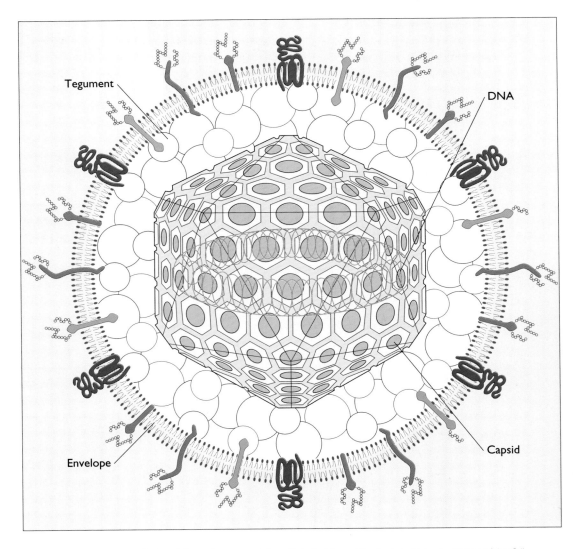

Fig. 11.1 Herpesvirus morphology. Schematic representation. (Adapted from Alberts et al., *Molecular Biology of the Cell*, Garland Press, NY, 1989.)

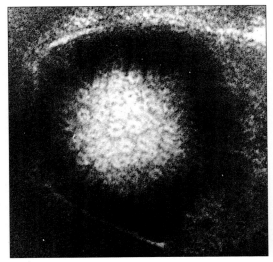

Fig. 11.2 Herpesvirus morphology. Electron micrograph.

study in the USA found a seroprevalence of 16% in adults of 15 years of age or older, with 13% of whites and 41% of blacks being positive (*Fig. 11.4*). Fewer than 40% of HSV-2 seropositive women report having experienced clinical symptoms, and as many as 5% of these women may be shedding virus at any given time. These data suggest that asymptomatic genital herpes is more prevalent than symptomatic cases.

Fig. 11.3 Human herpesviruses.

HUMAN HERPESVIRUSES

VIRUS	PRINCIPAL DISEASES
Herpes simplex virus type 1 (HSV-1)	Skin and mucosal vesicles and ulcers, especially oral
Herpes simplex virus type 2 (HSV-2)	Skin and mucosal vesicles and ulcers, especially genital
Varicella-zoster virus (VZV)	Chickenpox, shingles
Epstein–Barr virus (EBV)	Infectious mononucleosis
Cytomegalovirus (CMV)	Serious disease in immunosuppressed patients and congenital infection
Human herpesvirus 6 (HHV-6)	Roseola infantum, non-rash febrile illness in young children, and possibly pneumonia in immunosuppressed patients
Human herpesvirus 7 (HHV-7)	Some cases of roseola infantum
Human herpesvirus 8 (HHV-8)	Associated with Kaposi's sarcoma and some lymphomas

Fig. 11.4 Prevalence of HSV-2 antibody in the USA in 1978, according to age, race, and sex.

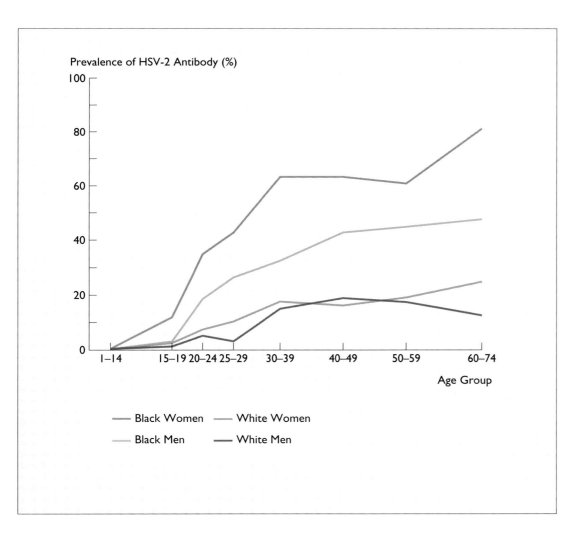

Genital herpes accounted for 2% of visits to STD clinics in the UK in 1979 and 4% of visits to an STD clinic in Seattle in 1980. There is a widely held belief that the prevalence of genital herpes increased dramatically in the 1960s and 1970s. Data supporting this view were analyzed by the CDC and are shown in *Figure. 11.5*.

In developed countries, symptomatic genital herpes, like NGU, is more prevalent among economically advantaged individuals. This contrasts with gonorrhea, which is more prevalent in the economically disadvantaged.

Spread of HSV infection occurs when viral particles enter the skin or mucous membranes through traumatic microscopic openings or fissures. Friction to genital mucosal surfaces often occurs during intercourse, resulting in a favorable environment for passage of virus into keratinocytes. Once inside a keratinocyte, the virus replicates inside the cell's nucleus, and thence spreads to surrounding cells (*Figs. 11.6* and *11.7*). The infected epidermal cells are destroyed, resulting in damage to the involved skin (and may even damage dermis). The virus then enters the peripheral sensory or autonomic nerve endings, and ascends to sensory or autonomic root ganglia, where it becomes latent. Subsequently, viral reactivation may occur, causing the virus to descend along the involved nerve root back to, or very close to, the original site of infection on the skin or mucous membrane. Clinically, this is called a 'recurrence'. Recurrences may be either symptomatic or asymptomatic. Transmission of the infection can occur readily by contact with open vesicles, but can also occur in persons who are asymptomatically shedding the virus. In fact, transmission occurs most commonly from partners asymptomatically shedding virus, rather than from partners with active lesions. This observation is not surprising, as individuals are less likely to be sexually active

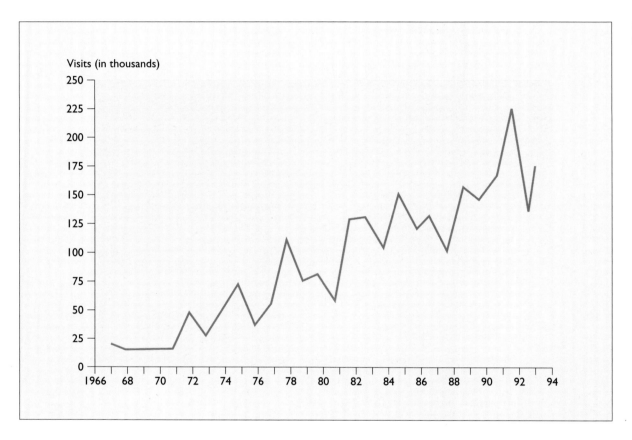

Fig. 11.5 Genital HSV infections: initial visits to physicians' offices, USA, 1966–1993.

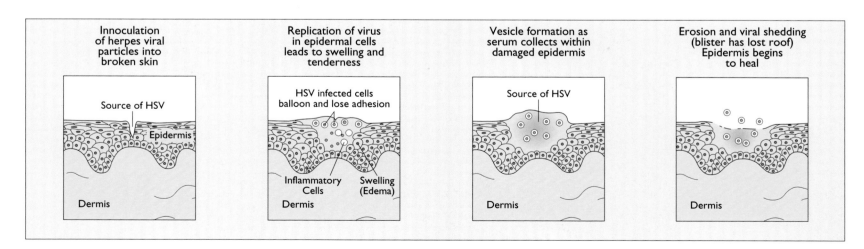

Fig. 11.6 Infection with HSV.

while active herpetic lesions are present. The prominence of asymptomatic viral shedding in the transmission of genital herpes underscores the need for consistent, safer sexual practices. The older recommendation that unprotected sexual activity is safe in the absence of symptoms and signs of genital herpes is clearly incorrect.

Association with Cervical Neoplasia

Since 1969, many studies have shown an association between genital herpes and cervical carcinoma in women. Both conditions appear to be STDs and therefore patients have common risk factors. More recently, however, a much stronger association between cervical cancer and HPV has been demonstrated. Although HSV is not causally associated with cervical cancer, HSV-2 genetic material is occasionally found in neoplastic tissues and some epidemiologic studies have found that concomitant infection with HSV and HPV increases the risk of cervical cancer.

CLINICAL MANIFESTATIONS

Types of Genital Herpes

There are four types of genital herpes (*Figs. 11.8* and *11.9*):
- First-episode primary
- First-episode nonprimary
- Recurrent
- Asymptomatic.

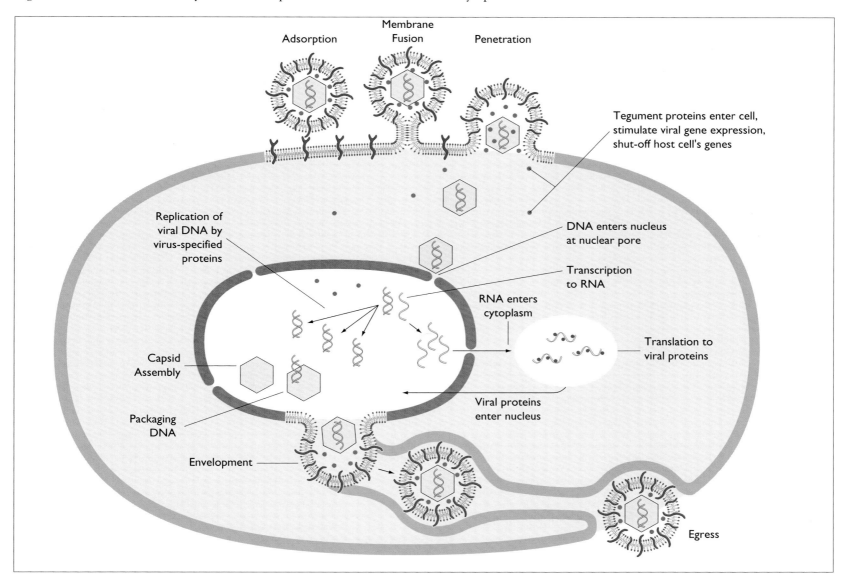

Fig. 11.7 HSV replication cycle. (Modified from Alberts et al, *Molecular Biology of the Cell*. Garland Press, NY, 1989.)

TYPES OF GENITAL HERPES	

First episode genital herpes
  Primary
  Nonprimary
	Recurrent genital herpes
	Asymptomatic genital
	herpes

Fig. 11.8 Types of genital herpes.

First-episode primary genital herpes is a true primary infection. The affected individual has no history of previous genital herpetic lesions and is seronegative for HSV antibodies. In general, this type of genital herpes is the most severe clinically.

First-episode nonprimary genital herpes refers to the first recognized episode of genital herpes in individuals whose sera contain HSV antibodies. In general, first-episode nonprimary genital herpes is less severe than first-episode primary genital herpes, but more severe than recurrent disease. Pre-existing antibody is thought to attenuate the severity of

disease. The distinction between first-episode primary and first-episode nonprimary genital herpes cannot be made clinically in any one individual. The prior acquisition of oral herpes has an ameliorating effect on primary genital herpes infections.

Recurrent genital herpes refers to repeated episodes of genital herpes in the same individual. The recurrence rate for genital infections is higher with HSV-2 than with HSV-1. A comparison of the mean duration of symptoms and signs in patients with first-episode primary, first-episode nonprimary, and recurrent genital herpes is shown in *Figure. 11.10*.

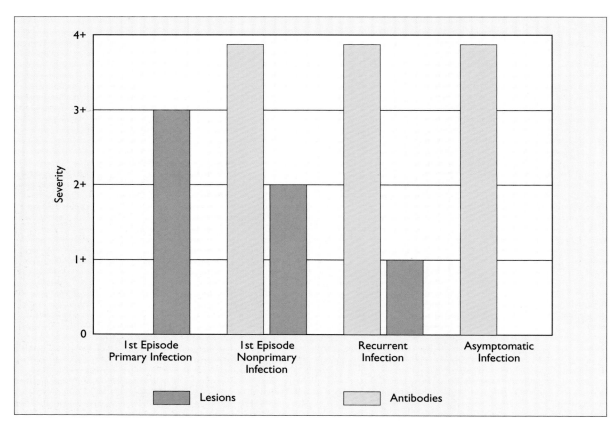

Fig. 11.9 Clinical severity and antibody response in genital herpes.

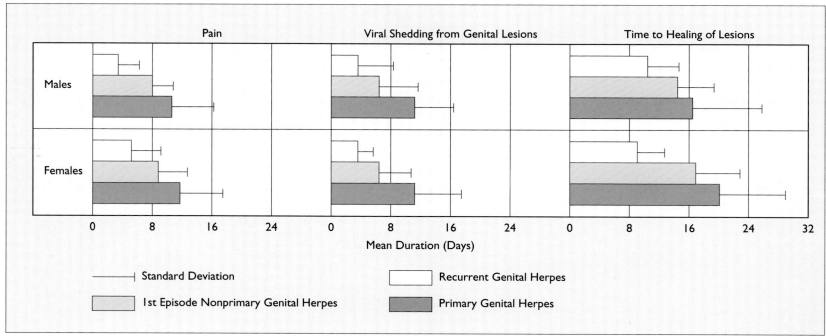

Fig. 11.10 Comparison of symptoms and signs in different types of genital herpes.

Asymptomatic genital herpes refers to episodes in which individuals shed HSV at genital sites in the absence of symptoms. Some of these individuals have genital lesions that they do not notice, but many do not know they have genital herpes. While the quantity of virus shed by these individuals is much less than is found in clinical lesions, asymptomatic shedders can transmit infection and thus are important epidemiologically.

Primary Genital Infection

After intimate contact with an infected person and an incubation period of approximately 1 week (2–12 days), painful, grouped, discrete vesicles appear (*Fig. 11.11*). The vesicles usually evolve into pustules, which then erode, creating an ulcer. The remaining grayish plaques crust before healing takes place (*Fig. 11.12*). This process takes 15–20 days before re-epithelialization occurs. The lesions shed infectious particles of virus for at least 10–12 days, and new lesions may appear until the 10th day. Typical lesions in men occur on the glans penis, coronal sulcus, urethra (*Fig. 11.13*), shaft of the penis, or perianal region. Less frequently, lesions occur on the scrotum, mons area, thighs, or buttocks. In women, lesions usually occur around the introitus, the urethral meatus, or the labia (*Figs. 11.14* and *11.15*), but can also occur in extragenital sites, such as the perineal or perianal regions or on the thighs and buttocks. Cervicitis is common, occurring in 70–90% of women with the first episode of genital herpes; cervical infection may occur in the absence of vulvar disease. Cervicitis occurs less often in recurrent genital herpes. The appearance of the cervix is usually normal, though it may have ulcerations and appear red and friable (*Figs. 11.16* and *11.17*).

Due to individual differences in immunity, environmental factors, or other skin diseases, the presentation of primary genital herpes may be unusual or may differ significantly from this classical picture. Immunosuppression resulting from either medications or disease (*Fig. 11.18*) is sometimes a contributory factor in more severe or prolonged infections. Chronic tinea cruris is characterized by scaling, vesicles or pustules, excoriations, and erosions in the folds of the groin. Exposure of this skin to fresh genital herpes lesions may lead to a superinfection with herpes (*Fig. 11.19*). Chronic eczema may also render the skin susceptible to HSV infection (eczema herpeticum) (*Figs. 11.20* and *11.21*), which can involve the genitals.

Associated genitourinary symptoms in primary genital herpes include dysuria in most cases in both women and men. Vaginal discharge, urethral discharge, and inguinal adenopathy are not uncommon. Pain often occurs

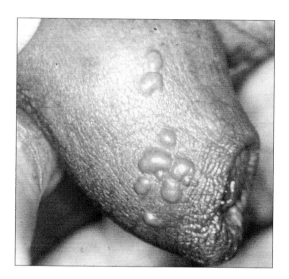

Fig. 11.11 Early lesions of primary genital herpes. Clear, grouped vesicles appear on an erythematous base. Some vesicles are discrete and some coalesce, which frequently results in a scalloped border.

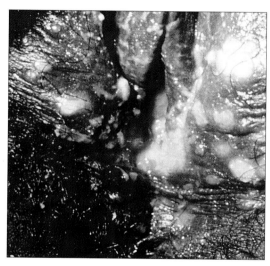

Fig. 11.12 Vulvar herpes of several days' duration. Several stages in the natural evolution of the eruption are apparent here: clear vesicles, pustules, and grayish exudate cover plaques where the roofs of blisters have eroded.

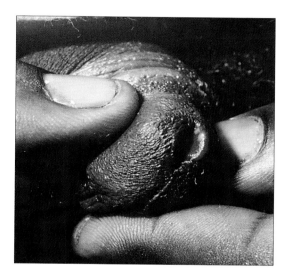

Fig. 11.13 Herpes erosion in the urethral meatus. Dysuria resulted from this erythematous and painful erosion. Urethral involvement is less common than lesions on the shaft or the foreskin of the penis.

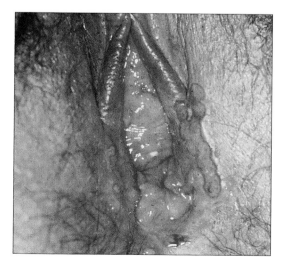

Fig. 11.14 Primary vulvar herpes. The linear appearance of these painful herpetic erosions on the labia is a result of coalescence of several closely grouped vesicles, which have subsequently shed the vesicle roof.

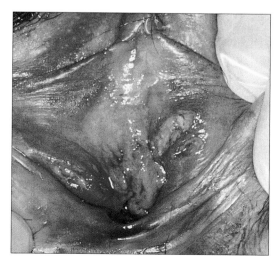

Fig. 11.15 Primary vulvar herpes. These painful ulcers were present on the vulva of the patient in **11.16**.

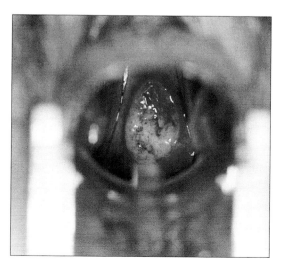

Fig. 11.16 Herpetic cervicitis. Erosive cervicitis was present in this case of primary herpes presenting with vulvar ulcers (see **11.15**).

in men and women with primary symptomatic genital herpes infections. Pain is usually present for at least 1 week, but may sometimes persist for 2 weeks.

In addition, patients with primary genital herpes often have other associated systemic symptoms, including headache, fever, malaise, and myalgia. These symptoms appear more common in women than in men. Pharyngitis, aseptic meningitis, transverse myelitis, and radiculitis are also associated with genital herpes infections in some patients. Neurologic complications occur in about 13–35% of patients. Complaints of a stiff neck, headache, or photophobia ordinarily occur about 3–12 days after the onset of genital lesions. Sacral radiculitis may result in urinary retention. Serious neurologic sequelae are rare, but have been reported. Herpetic autoinoculation of extragenital sites — most often the fingers — is another complication of genital herpes, which probably occurs during primary infection. Such infections are more common in women (*Fig. 11.22*).

Recurrent Genital Herpes
Recurrent genital herpes may vary in individual patients from completely asymptomatic episodes of viral shedding to mild episodes (*Figs. 11.23* and

11.24) or may cause severe discomfort (*Figs. 11.25* and *11.26*). Although the recurrence rate is highly variable in any one individual, most individuals experience 5–8 recurrences per year. In the most cases, however, the symptoms and signs are milder and of shorter duration than in primary infection, and often a prodrome of itching (*Fig. 11.27*), burning, or tingling occurs at the affected site a few hours to a day before the lesions appear. Dysuria is less common and viral shedding is shorter, lasting only about 4 days. The duration of lesions is approximately 10 days to re-epithelialization in recurrent herpes. In immunocompromised patients, recurrences may be atypical in appearance or have a prolonged duration (*Fig. 11.28*). Some individuals experience 'trigger factors', which seem to precipitate a recurrence. Commonly noted trigger factors include stress, fatigue, and menses. Erythema multiforme occasionally occurs with recurrences and may become more troublesome than the herpetic lesions (*see Figs. 1.72–1.74*).

Nearly half of all individuals with recurrent genital herpes with lesions will also experience some prodromes without lesions, in which a typical herpetic prodrome is not followed by the development of lesions. Prodromes without lesions are also known as 'false' prodromes or 'aborted' prodromes,

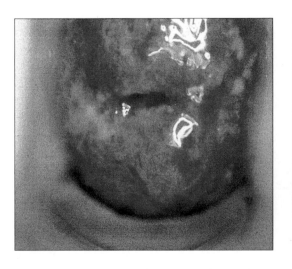

Fig. 11.17 Herpetic cervicitis. Erythema, purulent exudate, and erosions were present on the cervix of this patient with genital herpes.

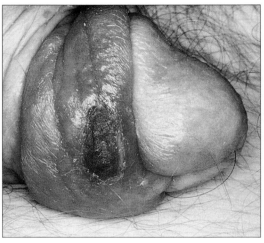

Fig. 11.18 Herpes in a patient with leukemia in whom edema is notable around a large herpetic erosion on the penis. The duration of the lesions was much longer than in healthy individuals.

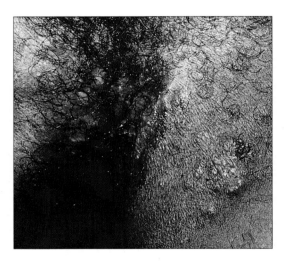

Fig. 11.19 Primary herpes arising in chronic tinea cruris infection. Hyperpigmentation and scaling in inguinal folds are signs of a chronic dermatitis. Tzanck smears from moist erosions and vesicles in the inguinal fold and at the border on the thigh showed characteristic multinucleated giant cells.

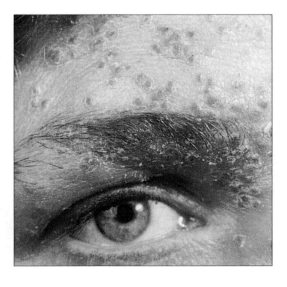

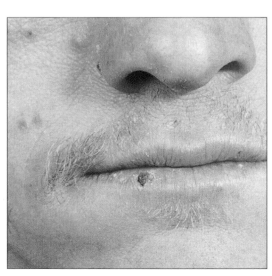

Figs. 11.20 and 11.21 Eczema herpeticum. Generalized herpes simplex (**11.20**) in this case started with an oral lesion (**11.21**) in a patient with atopic dermatitis. Genital eruptions may also be the source of a generalized infection in predisposed individuals.

and are probably due to better immunologic control than is present when lesions develop. It is possible that virus shedding is increased following these 'false' prodrome episodes.

Genital Herpes and Pregnancy

The manifestations of genital herpes do not differ between pregnant and nonpregnant women. Nevertheless, the consequences of maternal genital herpes infection can be very severe for the fetus. Maternal–fetal transmission almost always occurs during parturition, but rarely can occur *in utero*. The rate of transmission depends primarily on whether the mother is experiencing primary or recurrent infection. In primary maternal infection, the rate of fetal transmission is about 50%, compared to less than 8% in recurrent maternal disease. The major reason for the marked discrepancy in the rate of fetal transmission between primary and recurrent maternal infection is the transmission of maternal HSV antibodies to the fetus in recurrent disease. This helps to prevent or attenuate fetal infection. In addition, primary genital herpes is associated with larger quantities of virus and a much greater likelihood of cervicitis. Despite the lower fetal transmission rate of recurrent herpes, transmission at this stage is epidemiologically

significant since recurrent maternal infection is much more prevalent than primary infection.

Pregnant women with a history of genital herpes should be examined very carefully for genital lesions under good light early in labor. If any lesions are detected, the infant should probably be delivered by cesarean section, preferably before the amniotic membrane has ruptured, to prevent direct exposure of the infant to maternal virus. A small percentage of transmission occurs *in utero* and will not be prevented by cesarean delivery.

Neonatal Infection

Unfortunately, 50–60% of infants with neonatal HSV infection are born to mothers with no history of genital herpes. Thus, no matter how carefully women with a history of genital herpes are monitored, there will still be many babies with neonatal herpes infection.

Neonatal HSV infection (*Figs. 11.29* and *11.30*) is very serious. It is associated with prematurity, but is seldom clinically manifested at birth. Clinical disease usually manifests at 3–30 days of age, with 71% of cases presenting with localized infections of the skin, eye, and mouth. Three out of four of these cases will progress to disseminated or CNS involvement. Involvement

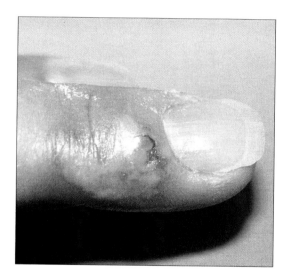

Fig. 11.22 Autoinoculation. Commonly called a herpetic whitlow, these herpes blisters are extremely painful and can be recurrent, but heal spontaneously.

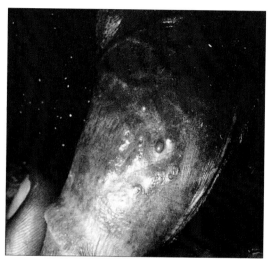

Fig. 11.23 Recurrent genital herpes. Many vesicles have eroded and are healing quickly in this mildly symptomatic case.

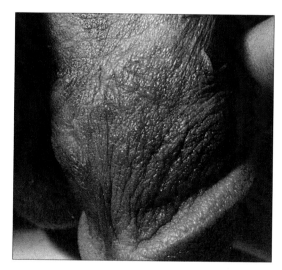

Fig. 11.24 Recurrent genital herpes. Erythema, groups of vesicles, erosions, and edema seen on the shaft of the penis.

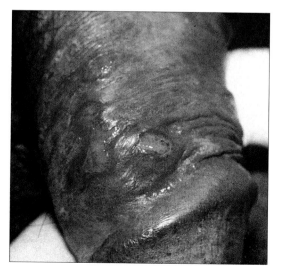

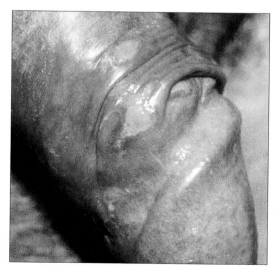

Figs. 11.25 and 11.26 Recurrent penile herpes. These discrete and confluent well-demarcated shallow ulcerations on the shaft of the penis were extremely painful in this 32-year-old diabetic patient.

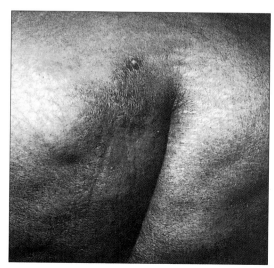

Fig. 11.27 Extragenital HSV of the buttocks. Pruritus and irritation were the first symptoms in this recurrent episode. (The black circle is the site chosen for biopsy.)

of the CNS is associated with considerable morbidity and mortality. The diagnosis of neonatal herpes is particularly challenging when mucocutaneous lesions are absent, as it may resemble bacterial sepsis or other congenital infections (e.g. rubella or toxoplasmosis). Neonatal herpes infection should be diagnosed as early as possible since treatment with either acyclovir or vidarabine reduces both morbidity and mortality.

Any vesicle, bulla, or erosion on the skin of a neonate should be cultured for herpes as well as routine bacterial cultures. Rapid information can be obtained by a Tzanck smear (*see* Cytopathology on page 218), electron microscopy, or direct immunofluorescence, but results should be confirmed by viral culture. Confirmed and highly suspected cases should be treated as soon as possible with intravenous acyclovir or vidarabine. (*See Chapter 14, Perinatal STDs.*)

Differential Diagnosis

When painful grouped vesicles with an erythematous base appear on the genital skin, the diagnosis is almost certainly herpes, but other STDs besides herpes can cause erosions that may be painful. Of these, chancroid (*Figs. 11.31* and *11.32*) most closely resembles herpes in the clinical presentation, frequently with multiple, painful erosions that develop an exudate similar to that seen in the postvesicular stages of genital herpes (*see Chapter 3, Chancroid*).

Syphilis also causes erosions on the genitals (*Figs. 11.33* and *11.34*), but a primary chancre of syphilis that is not secondarily infected with bacteria is usually solitary and not painful. In primary syphilis, dark-field examination of lesion exudate is usually positive if the area has not been recently treated with topical agents and the patient has not been taking oral antibiotics. In adults, secondary syphilis is rarely erosive, but never vesicular. Serologic tests are invariably positive in secondary syphilis and should be done in any erosive genital lesions since STDs often coexist in such patients (*see Chapter 2, Syphilis*).

Traumatic genital ulcers are painful but are not usually multiple or grouped. They have angular borders rather than the scalloped edges seen in herpes erosions (*see Chapter. 1, Genital Dermatoses*).

Contact dermatitis of the genitals is usually itchy and results in vesicles, crusting, and erosions. Secondary infection may result in tenderness. As contact with the offending allergen may occur as much as 2 weeks before the dermatitis appears, diagnosis may be difficult. Vesicles and erosions should be sampled for cytology (Tzanck smears), and viral cultures or antigen detection should be done to rule out herpes before the patient is treated for contact dermatitis (*see Chapter 1, Genital Dermatoses*). Other bullous or erosive diseases, such as impetigo, pemphigus, pemphigoid, Hailey–Hailey disease (benign familial pemphigus) (*Fig. 11.35*), Darier's disease, Behçet's

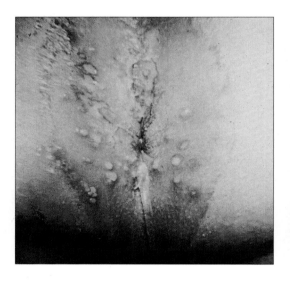

Fig. 11.28 Chronic perianal herpes in an AIDS patient. This infection was very difficult to control even with acyclovir therapy.

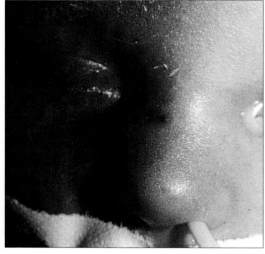

Fig. 11.29 Neonatal herpes. The crusted areas on the bridge of the nose were the only visible cutaneous lesions in this neonate with herpes who developed encephalitis and died.

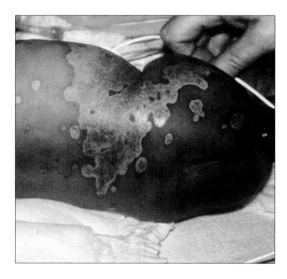

Fig. 11.30 Neonatal herpes. Extensive erosions in another case of neonatal herpes.

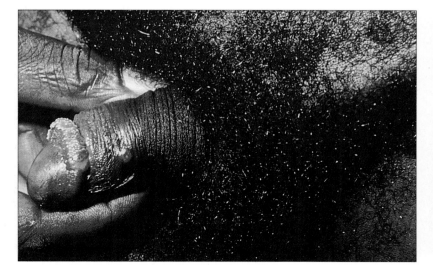

Fig. 11.31 Chancroid. The multiple erosions, like those of herpes, are painful, but blisters are not seen and the lymphadenopathy is more prominent than in comparable herpes eruptions.

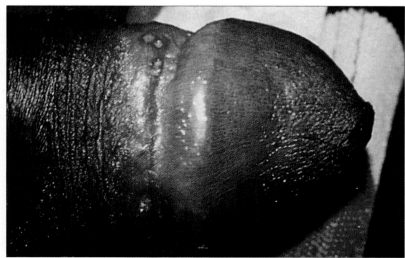

Fig. 11.32 Chancroid. Grouped ulcers resembling genital herpes; however, *Haemophilus ducreyi* was isolated by culture from these lesions.

disease, and Crohn's disease, may either resemble herpes because of bullae or erosions, or may become secondarily infected with the virus. Clinical history and diagnostic tests, including Tzanck smears, Gram stains, and cultures, usually clarify the problem, but biopsies may occasionally be necessary.

LABORATORY TESTS

The most commonly used specific and clinically useful techniques in the diagnosis of genital herpes are the direct examination of clinical materials for viral nucleic acid sequences or viral antigens and the isolation and identification of viruses from clinical specimens.

Direct Examination of Clinical Specimens

Direct examination of clinical specimens permits the most rapid recognition and identification of HSV. Direct methods include histopathology, cytopathology, electron microscopy, immunofluorescence (FA) and immunoenzyme (IE) techniques, enzyme immunoassay (EIA), and nucleic acid probes (NAPs), and the polymerase chain reaction (PCR). Histopathology and cytopathology permit the identification of nuclear–cytoplasmic inclusions and other cellular alterations by light microscopy, while electron microscopy permits the direct ultrastructural visualization of viral particles. With FA, IE, and EIA, the specimen is incubated with an antibody specific for the virus (viral antigen), which will then be identified and examined for the presence of specific fluorescence (FA) or color development (IE, EIA). NAPs use segments of RNA or DNA to detect and identify viral pathogens; PCR amplifies a specific nucleic acid sequence which can then be detected by using a NAP or EIA.

Histopathology

Early HSV infections are characterized by intracellular edema, suprabasal intraepidermal vesicles (*Fig. 11.36*), ballooning degeneration, and homogenization and margination of nuclear chromatin. Intranuclear inclusions and multinucleated giant cells are seen at the periphery of the lesions (*Fig. 11.37*). In later ulcerative stages, keratinocyte necrosis and lysis predominate. Inflammatory cells, such as polymorphonuclear leukocytes and lymphocytes, appear within the vesicle and dermis. As the lesion progresses, the epidermis sloughs, and the remaining erosion re-epithelializes as it heals. Cervical HSV infections are characterized by multinucleated giant cells and intranuclear 'ground-glass' viral inclusions visualized on Papanicolaou smears.

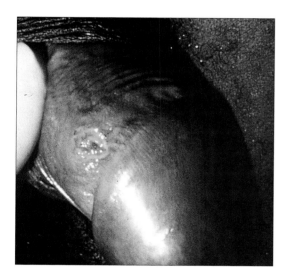

Fig. 11.33 This small primary chancre of syphilis resembles a herpetic erosion.

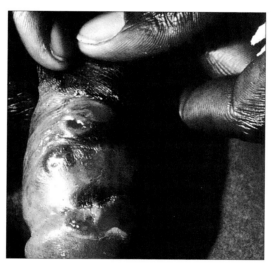

Fig. 11.34 These multiple primary penile syphilitic chancres mimic penile herpes.

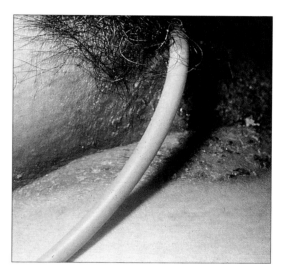

Fig. 11.35 Benign familial pemphigus (Hailey–Hailey disease). Multiple fragile vesicles and bullae are seen at the edge of these characteristic erosive plaques. The clinical history and biopsies are diagnostic.

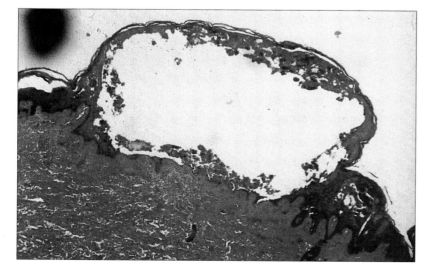

Fig. 11.36 Intraepidermal vesicle of HSV infection.

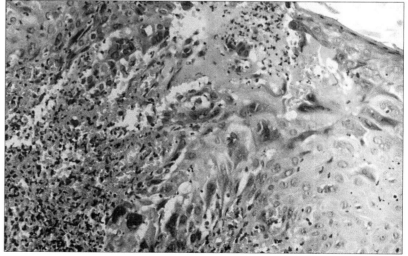

Fig. 11.37 Periphery of HSV erosion showing single and multinucleated epithelial cells with 'ground-glass' nuclei.

Biopsies are not usually performed, but will show changes similar to those described above.

Cytopathology

Cytopathology is useful in identifying HSV infections because characteristic cytopathic effects occur in infected cells. Specimens from vesicular skin and mucosal lesions may be obtained by scraping the edge of the 'unroofed' lesion with a sterile swab or scalpel blade and fixing the prepared slide in 95% ethanol, Zenker's solution, or Bouin's solution (Tzanck smear), and staining with Giemsa or methylene blue stain. HSV-infected cells usually exhibit a combination of virus-induced and degenerative changes. The virus predominantly infects immature epithelial cells. Early manifestations of infection include:

- Nuclear hypertrophy
- Disappearance of nucleoli
- Progressive increase in deoxyribonuclear protein (DRNP), which imparts a distinct, homogeneous, 'ground-glass' appearance to the nucleus
- Displacement of the nuclear chromatin to the periphery, where it adheres and imparts a 'thicker' appearance to the nuclear membrane (*Fig. 11.38*).
- Multinucleated giant cells, produced by the fusion of cytoplasmic membranes of individual infected cells, are often observed. The nuclei vary in size and shape and usually mold against one another (*Fig. 11.39*).

Later in the course of HSV infection, the DRNP condenses, moves to the center of the nucleus, and forms a single, coarsely granular, acidophilic, intranuclear inclusion surrounded by a prominent halo (Fig. 11.40). Degenerative changes (not HSV-specific) also occur in infected cells, including increased cytoplasmic and nuclear vacuolization, loss of normal cell shape, and in later stages of infection, breakage of cytoplasmic and nuclear membranes. Cytologic changes alone cannot serve to differentiate primary HSV infections from recurrent HSV and, similarly, do not distinguish HSV-2 infections from those due to HSV-1. Reliable discrimination of HSV from varicella–zoster virus infections cannot be made on the basis of histology alone.

Electron Microscopy

Electron microscopy is the most applicable method for investigating viral infections, in which the concentration of viral particles in the clinical specimen is greater than 10^6–10^7 particles/ml. To permit the detection and definitive identification of virus morphology, the specimen must also be free of background debris. The types of specimens examined usually include biopsies or fluid and scrapings from vesicles.

Following appropriate preparation, clinical specimens are negatively stained with 2–4% phosphotungstic acid and are examined directly for the presence of virus (*Fig. 11.41*). Enhancement techniques can be used to increase the sensitivity of electron microscopy when examining clinical specimens with virus titers lower than 10^6 particles/ml. Pseudoreplica and agar gel diffusion, which can be used to concentrate and purify clinical specimens, are useful procedures for identifying HSV in vesicle or body fluids. Since all viruses in the herpes group have an identical ultrastructural morphologic appearance, the technique of immune electron microscopy must be used for specific identification. This technique provides direct observation of the interaction of the virus with homologous antibody (*Fig. 11.42*).

Immunofluorescence Methods

These techniques are time-honored, reliable methods for the diagnosis of HSV. They can be used to detect viral antigens in clinical specimens (*Fig. 11.43*) or to confirm the presence of HSV in cell cultures inoculated with clinical materials (*Fig. 11.44*). Clinical specimens or viral cultures can be evaluated for HSV by either direct (DFA) or indirect (IFA) methods. With DFA staining, fluorescein isothiocyanate (FITC)-labeled HSV-specific immunoglobulin (anti-HSV) binds directly to HSV-infected cells present in the specimen (*Figs. 11.45–11.47*). With IFA staining, the anti-HSV is not FITC-labeled (*Fig. 11.48*), and a FITC-labeled antispecies immunoglobulin is used to detect the anti-HSV bound to the HSV-infected cells. Although IFA methods are more sensitive than DFA methods, DFA has several advantages over IFA, including greater specificity, cleaner background (less nonspecific fluorescence), fewer necessary manipulations and reagents, and less time required for incubation (one step instead of two). DFA permits detection of viral antigens only, whereas IFA can be used to detect either antibodies to HSV or HSV antigens. Most commercially available reagents for HSV detection are monoclonal antibody products intended for use with DFA methodology (*Fig. 11.45*). Some of these products are also licensed for use in 'typing' HSV present in clinical specimens, though this procedure is not always necessary. Specimens that can be used for FA diagnosis include frozen sections of tissue, impression smears, lesion scrapings, or resuspended cells from centrifuged sediment. After preparation, the slides are air-dried completely and fixed (usually in acetone or methanol) prior to staining with anti-HSV. If needed, slides can be stored for long periods of time at −70°C.

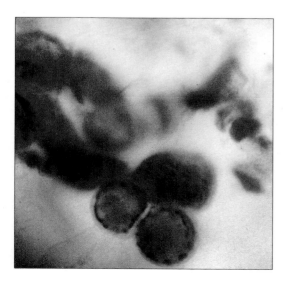

Fig. 11.38 HSV-infected cells in a cytology specimen exhibiting homogeneous, 'ground-glass'-appearing nuclei and peripheral chromatin margination imparting an irregular and more distinct appearance to the nuclear membrane.

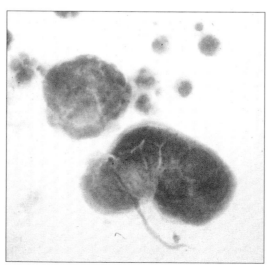

Fig. 11.39 Multinucleated giant HSV-infected cell showing variation in nuclear size and shape and the molding of individual nuclei against one another.

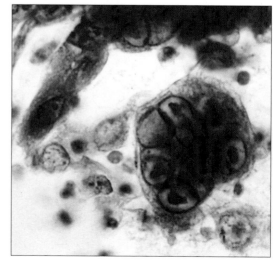

Fig. 11.40 Multinucleated giant HSV-infected cell with prominent intranuclear inclusions surrounded by distinct haloes.

Strict criteria and appropriate positive and negative controls must be used when interpreting FA results. Fluorescence must be bright apple-green in color (with FITC conjugates), and appropriate in cellular location. To diagnose HSV infection, nuclear fluorescence must be observed; cytoplasmic fluorescence may also occur. False-positive fluorescence can be encountered with leukocytes, mucus, and yeasts; leukocytes possess immunoglobulin Fc receptors that can nonspecifically bind conjugates (*Fig. 11.49*). False-negative tests can occur when an insufficient number of viral particles (antigens) are present or when reagents do not perform optimally.

Immunoenzyme Methods

These methods are now being widely used instead of FA procedures to examine smears taken from clinical lesions for the presence of HSV. The general principles of specimen handling and preparation are similar. However, the ability to identify a colored final reaction product using an ordinary bright-field microscope has great advantages for diagnostic histopathology and cytology. The enzyme, which is attached to the specific antibody to be used, substitutes for the FITC used as the detector system in FA methodology. The enzyme, when reacted with its specific chromogenic substrate, yields a colored product. Enzyme-conjugate methods are generally more sensitive than fluorochrome-conjugate ones because the former produce a higher signal, the intensity of which is determined by the length of the enzyme reaction time. New designs in methodology and the introduction of monoclonal antibodies and the avidin–biotin amplification system have greatly increased the sensitivity and specificity of these immunocytochemical methods. These procedures are easy to perform, do not require a fluorescence microscope, and constitute a permanent record since the color of the chromogenic product remains stable for indefinite periods.

Enzyme Immunoassays (Solid Phase)

Enzyme immunoassays, including the enzyme-linked immunoabsorbent assay (ELISA or EIA), also detects viral antigens by using the action of an enzyme on its specific substrate as an indicator. However, EIA methods detect viral antigens present in solutions, which are usually contained in a small cylindrical tube or in microtiter plate wells. Appropriate specimens for detecting HSV antigens by EIA are swabs of vesicular fluid or genital tract lesions. Several EIA systems currently are available for detec-

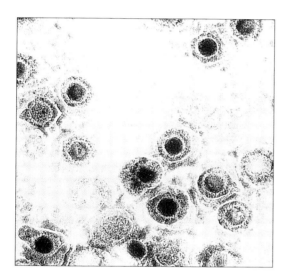

Fig. 11.41 HSV particles detected by direct electron microscopy. Defective or damaged particles have dark centers due to the penetration of phosphotungstic acid stain into the viral nucleocapsid.

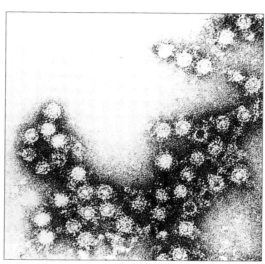

Fig. 11.42 Immune electron microscopy of coxsackie B4 viral particles. An aggregate is formed of individual particles linked together by specific antibody (anti-coxsackie B4).

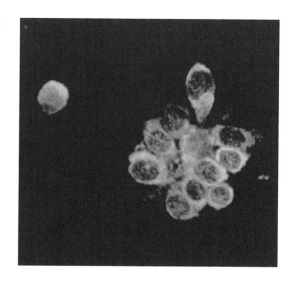

Fig. 11.43 Direct fluorescent antibody test of HSV-infected cell obtained from scraping an ulcerated genital lesion.

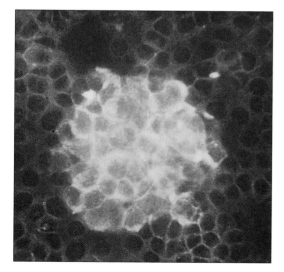

Fig. 11.44 Fluorescent antibody test of HSV-infected cells in a cell culture monolayer previously inoculated with a clinical specimen from a genital lesion.

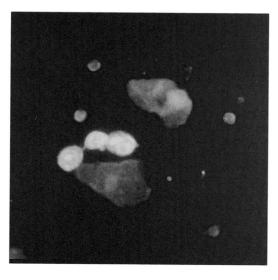

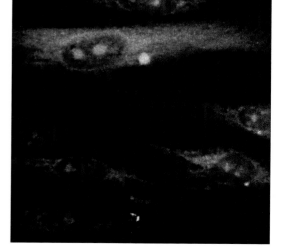

Figs. 11.45 and 11.46 Direct fluorescent antibody test. (**11.45**) Positive result for HSV-2 with monoclonal antibody. (**11.46**) Negative result for HSV-2 with monoclonal antibody.

tion of HSV. A commercially available EIA (Herpchek, Dupont) has a sensitivity that compares well with virus culture methods and also provides the results more quickly.

Nucleic Acid Probes

Nucleic acid probes (*Fig. 11.50*) are discrete segments of single-stranded RNA or DNA that can bind noncovalently (hybridize) with their specific complementary strand of nucleic acid. Hybridization can occur between complementary DNA strands (DNA–DNA duplex), complementary RNA strands (RNA–RNA duplex), or complementary RNA and DNA strands (RNA–DNA hybrid). NAP technology can detect and identify viral pathogens in only a few hours. The probe is mixed with the clinical specimen under proper conditions so that denaturation (separation of double-stranded DNA) can occur. If the specimen contains a nucleic-acid segment complementary to the probe's labeled nucleic-acid sequence, hybridization will take place and a double-stranded structure containing the probe will be formed. The labeled probe (i.e. labelled with a radioactive tag or enzyme label) can then be treated to allow visualization. Biotin–avidin labeling is often used to increase the sensitivity of the reaction. At present, most materials to be tested, such as clinical specimens or viral isolates, need to be affixed

to a solid matrix (usually some type of filter or glass microscope slide). However, newer techniques and probes being developed will not require a solid matrix for testing. NAPs are presently available commercially for use in detecting HSV-1 and HSV-2 DNA sequences.

Polymerase Chain Reaction

This biochemical process can detect a single target DNA molecule within a complex mixture of nontarget DNA, for example, a single viral genome in a milieu of thousands of uninfected cell genomes. This is accomplished by amplifying the target DNA by using specific DNA primers and a thermostable DNA polymerase in a series of iterated reactions, the number of amplified segments (amplimers) increasing by a factor of approximately two at each step. From a single template molecule, $2^{(n-1)}$ amplimers may be obtained after n amplification cycles. Thus, after 30 cycles, more than 500 million amplimer molecules can be generated from a single target. There is an obvious analogy between the biochemical amplification involved and the amplification of viral material that occurs in cell culture, but PCR has the advantages of being able to amplify material that might not be viable in culture and of taking only several hours from the time that the sample is processed to results being generated (*see Fig. 4.79*). The clinical relevance of quantitative PCR is an area of active research.

The appropriate choice of primer sequences and conditions for amplification enables high specificity. This can be further enhanced by an amplimer detection system, which depends on the hybridization of a detection probe with sequences internal to the amplified segment. Although radioactive detection systems are commonly used, there are now nonradioactive EIA-based detection systems, which are compatible with standard EIA plate formats and suitable for clinical laboratory use.

The exquisite sensitivity of PCR is its potential Achilles' heel. A single stray target molecule can lead to a false-positive result, and thus scrupulous attention must be paid to sample acquisition, storage, shipping, and processing procedures. The amplification products themselves are substrates for the amplification reaction, requiring the physical partitioning of sample-preparation areas from areas where amplification products are processed for detection.

PCR assays have been developed for HSV-1 and HSV-2, although none are licensed for clinical use. The greatest clinical value of these assays is the rapid detection of HSV in CSF in the diagnosis of herpes encephalitis. PCR has been of epidemiologic use in demonstrating that HSV is asymptomatically shed even more frequently than indicated by culture-based methods.

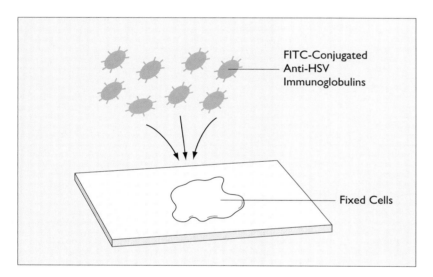

Fig. 11.47 The direct immunofluorescence test.

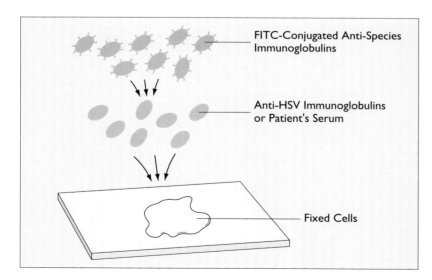

Fig. 11.48 The indirect immunofluoresence test.

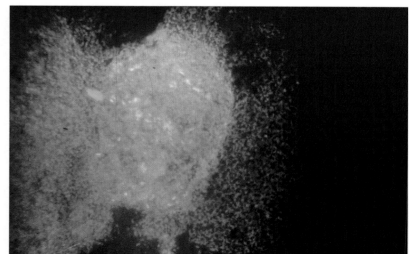

Fig. 11.49 Nonspecific fluorescent antibody test due to binding of labeled antibody via the Fc portion of the molecule to leukocyte Fc receptors.

Identification of Viruses from Clinical Specimens

Virus Isolation

In general, virus isolation takes longer than direct methods to detect viruses in clinical specimens. Yet isolation is a more sensitive technique (except, perhaps, for PCR) because clinical specimens usually contain only small numbers of viral particles and amplification in host systems is necessary for detection. Moreover, virus isolation has the added advantage of permitting recovery of additional viral agents (other than the one primarily being considered) from clinical specimens. Host systems for isolating HSV from clinical specimens include cell cultures and embryonated chickens' eggs. Most diagnostic virology laboratories use cell monolayers in HSV isolation.

The likelihood of recovery of HSV in culture relates to the clinical phase of the lesion; the yield is generally higher from vesicular (94%) than from pustular (87%), ulcerated (70%), or crusted (27%) lesions. HSV-1 and HSV-2 replicate well in many primary or established cell lines of human or primate origin. However, Vero cells (a continuous African monkey kidney cell line) and human diploid lines (such as foreskin fibroblasts or embryonic lung fibroblasts) (*Fig. 11.51*) are especially recommended.

When a specimen contains a high titer of HSV particles, a cytopathic effect (CPE) may be detected as early as 24 hours after inoculation. In most cases, visible CPE usually develops within 2–4 days. HSV-infected cells in the monolayer develop a cytoplasmic granularity and become enlarged, ballooned, and eventually round and refractile or glassy (*Fig. 11.52*). Individual lesions grow in size as cell-to-adjacent-cell spread of virus occurs. Eventually, the entire monolayer becomes infected. Multinucleated giant cells are usually identified. If typing of the HSV isolates is desired, isolates of HSV-1 may be distinguished from isolates of HSV-2 by a variety of procedures, most commonly IFA or EIA.

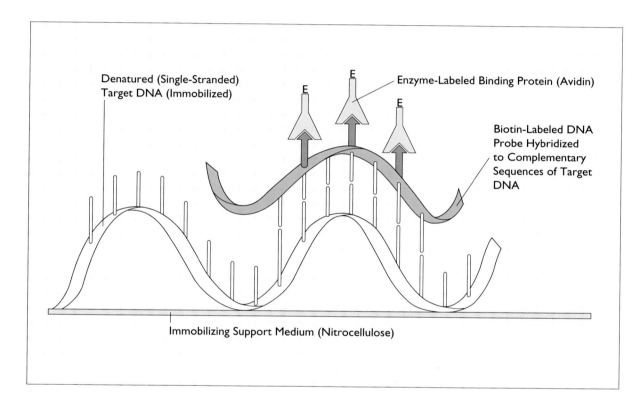

Fig. 11.50 Nucleic acid probe. DNA probes bind to viral DNA to form a visible reaction product indicating the presence of HSV-DNA sequences in clinical specimens or viral isolates.

Fig. 11.51 Uninoculated human diploid fibroblast monolayer.

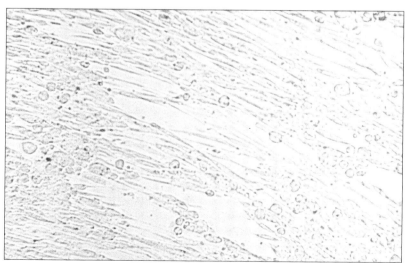

Fig. 11.52 Human diploid fibroblasts infected with HSV and showing cytopathic effects. There is extensive cell rounding, and many degenerated cells have fallen off the glass surface.

The rapid detection of HSV in cell culture is possible as early as 16 hours following inoculation, and before the development of visible CPE which usually requires 2–4 days. This is accomplished using coverslip monolayers in shell vials (*Fig. 11.53*). Key elements in this procedure are the centrifugation of the specimen onto the monolayer and the use of monoclonal antibodies specifically directed against HSV early antigens, which are expressed on cell membranes within a few hours following HSV attachment and penetration. Positive reactions may be visualized using a fluorochrome-labeled antibody or by immunoenzymatic reactions that generate a visible color. This technique has the advantages of:

- Increased sensitivity (due to host amplification of the number of virus particles) compared with rapid methods performed directly on clinical specimens
- A reduction in the time required to detect viral agents in cell culture (16–24 hours) compared with conventional methods (2–4 days).

Serology

A variety of serologic techniques have been developed to detect HSV antibodies. In individuals presenting with a first episode of genital herpes, serologic studies can differentiate between primary and nonprimary infection, but such knowledge will have no effect on management. In recurrent genital herpes, less than 10% of individuals will develop a significant rise in antibody titer. Serology is therefore not recommended in the diagnosis of genital herpes. The combined seroprevalence of HSV-1 and HSV-2 is nearly 100% in most populations.

Accurate assays for HSV type-specific serology are not available commercially. The only truly type-specific HSV serologic assays are based on HSV glycoprotein G (gG). As mentioned earlier, HSV-1 and HSV-2 are very similar genetically, with virtually every gene present in HSV-1 virus having a closely related counterpart in HSV-2. This is the basis for their strong antigenic cross reactivity. The only exception is the gene that encodes gG of HSV-1 (gG-1), which is nearly 1,500 base pairs shorter than the gene encoding HSV-2 gG (gG-2). This difference is sufficient for there to be no detected antigenic cross reactivity between these proteins in humans. True type-specific assays based on gG-1 and gG-2 have been developed (*Fig. 11.54*), but are only available in a very few clinical laboratories.

TREATMENT

Perhaps the most important aspect in the management of genital herpes is educating patients regarding their condition. This includes advising patients to abstain from sexual contact if prodromal symptoms or lesions are present, as well as informing them that transmission may occur via asymptomatic shedding, and that, in fact, asymptomatic shedding is the most common means of transmission. Some patients will require extensive counseling. Women should be advised to inform their obstetric-care provider(s) of their condition if they are pregnant.

As of 1994, acyclovir is the only licensed drug approved for the treatment of genital herpes (*Fig. 11.55*). Famciclovir, the oral prodrug of penciclovir, currently licensed for the treatment of herpes zoster, and valaciclovir, the valine ester of acyclovir, have both been effective in treating genital herpes and will probably be approved for genital herpes in the near future. At the present time, treatment guidelines for both famciclovir and valaciclovir are not available. Acyclovir is an acyclic derivative of the nucleoside guanosine. Acyclovir is actually a 'prodrug', which must be phosphorylated by a virus-specified enzyme, thymidine kinase, to acyclovir monophosphate. Cellular enzymes further phosphorylate the compound into the active drug, acyclovir

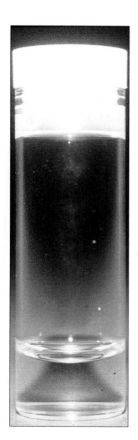

Fig. 11.53 One-dram shell vial containing cell media and coverslip with cell monolayer.

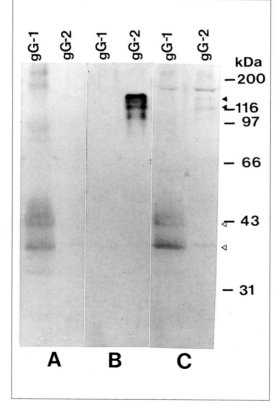

Fig. 11.54 HSV-type-specific serologic assay based on baculovirus expressed gG-1 and gG-2. The serum specimen in Panel A is HSV-1-specific and reacts only with gG-1 (open triangles), the HSV-2-specific specimen in Panel B reacts only with gG-2 (closed triangles), and the dual positive specimen in panel C reacts with both molecules.

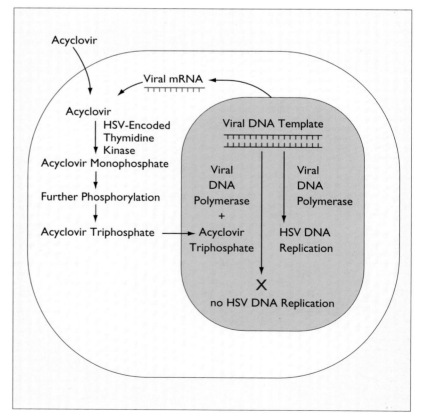

Fig. 11.55 Mechanism of action of acyclovir in infected cell.

triphosphate, which is a potent inhibitor of viral DNA polymerase. Additionally, some acyclovir triphosphate is incorporated into new viral DNA and functions as a DNA-chain terminator. Many individuals with genital herpes do not require acyclovir because:

- Lesions will heal spontaneously
- Acyclovir is expensive
- The benefits of acyclovir are modest, except in immunosuppressed patients.

Acyclovir is contraindicated in pregnancy because there is insufficient data on its safety. Presently, acyclovir should be used in pregnancy only for severe maternal disease. When acyclovir is used in pregnancy, intentionally or otherwise, its use and the outcome of the pregnancy should be reported to the International Acyclovir in Pregnancy Registry, which is collecting data on the safety of acyclovir in pregnancy. The experience with 312 pregnancies in the first 6 years of the registry has not indicated an increase in birth defects as compared with the general population. Recommendations regarding treatment of genital herpes are discussed below and summarized in *Fig. 11.56*.

Acyclovir resistance in HSV is rare, but can occur, particularly in individuals with advanced HIV disease who have had significant prior acyclovir treatment. In most cases, acyclovir resistance is due to mutant strains of HSV which are deficient in thymidine kinase. The treatment of choice for acyclovir-resistant HSV infection is foscarnet, which must be given intravenously. The usual dosage is 60 mg/kg every 8 hours in individuals with normal renal function.

First-Episode Genital Herpes

Individuals with severe first-episode HSV infection occasionally require hospitalization, particularly when serious neurologic complications occur. This small subset of individuals should be treated with intravenous acyclovir, 5 mg/kg over 60 minutes every 8 hours for 5 days. In addition to supportive care, which often includes analgesics, some women need urinary catheterization either for urinary retention or because voiding is extremely painful due to spillage of urine onto herpetic lesions (external dysuria). Most other individuals with first-episode genital herpes should be treated with oral acyclovir, 200 mg 5 times daily for 10 days. Occasional individuals with first-episode genital herpes do not require acyclovir therapy. These include pregnant women, individuals with mild manifestations, and individuals presenting later in their course with most or all lesions in the crust stage.

The benefit of acyclovir therapy in first-episode genital herpes is greater in primary than in nonprimary infection, but such a distinction is available only retrospectively. Acyclovir treatment of first-episode genital herpes has no effect on the subsequent recurrence pattern.

Recurrent Genital Herpes

Four strategies can be used in the treatment of recurrent genital herpes:

- No specific therapy
- Episodic oral acyclovir
- Chronic suppressive oral acyclovir
- Episodic suppressive oral acyclovir.

No antiviral therapy is required for many individuals with recurrent genital herpes, particularly those with mild and/or infrequent episodes.

Oral acyclovir, 200 mg 5 times daily for 5 days, may be given for each episode. Such episodic therapy will accelerate healing by about one day with little pain reduction, and is particularly suited for individuals with infrequent severe episodes, particularly with a long prodrome.

Chronic suppressive oral acyclovir is highly effective, suppressing about 90% of recurrences. Many individuals will respond to 200 mg twice daily, but the dose frequency may need to be increased to three or four times daily in a few patients. Suppressive therapy is safe and effective for at least a year at a time. Chronic suppressive therapy is particularly suited to individuals with

Fig. 11.56 Treatment of genital herpes.

TREATMENT OF GENITAL HERPES

PRESENTATION	TREATMENT
First episode	
Severe, requiring hospitalization	Acyclovir 5 mg/kg iv over 60 min tid for 5 days
Presentation when lesions are already crusted	No antiviral treatment
All others	Acyclovir 200 mg po 5 times daily for 10 days
Recurrent episodes	
Infrequent and/or mild	No antiviral treatment
Infrequent and moderate–severe	Episodal acyclovir 200 mg po 5 times daily for 5 days, or acyclovir 400 mg PO TID for 5 days, or acyclovir 800 mg po bid for 5 days
Frequent	Chronic suppressive acyclovir PO 200–400 mg 2–4 times/day
Pregnant women	Acyclovir is contraindicated in pregnancy, but may be considered for severe neurologic complications of primary disease

frequent recurrences (more than six episodes per year). It is recommended that a temporary 'drug holiday' be given after a year of continuous therapy to re-evaluate the natural frequency of recurrence. In some individuals, the frequency of recurrence will diminish sufficiently so that chronic prophylaxis is no longer required.

To date, some individuals have been treated safely and effectively with chronic suppressive acyclovir therapy for over 6 years, except for brief drug holidays. Despite the widespread use of acyclovir for many years, the development of acyclovir resistance has been remarkably rare and largely restricted

to immunosuppressed individuals. Recently, a recombinant glycoprotein-based HSV-2 vaccine was shown to decrease the frequency of recurrence of clinical episodes in individuals with frequently recurring genital herpes. This vaccine and others remain under clinical investigation.

Topical Acyclovir

Topical acyclovir is ineffective in recurrent genital herpes and shows only trivial benefit in primary genital herpes. It is less effective than oral acyclovir, and its use is not recommended.

Picture credits for this chapter are as follows: Fig. 11.2 courtesy of McKendrick GDW, Sutherland S: An Introduction to Herpes Infections. London, Gower Medical Publishing Ltd, 1983; Fig. 11.4 adapted with permission from Johnson et al: A seroepidemiologic survey of the prevalence of herpes simplex virus type 2 infection in the United States. *N Engl J Med* **312**:7,1989; Fig. 11.6 courtesy of Milton Tam, MD; Figs. 11.14 to 11.17 courtesy of Barbara Romanowski, MD; Fig. 11.20 and 11.21

courtesy of David Mandeville and Peter Lane, MD; Figs. 11.29 and 11.30 courtesy of Mary Spraker, MD; Fig. 11.54 adapted with permission from Sánchez-Martínez D, Pellett PE: Expression of HSV-1 and HSV-2 glycoprotein G in insect cells by using a novel baculovirus expression vector. *Virology* **182**:229, 1991; Fig. 11.55 adapted from Mertz GJ, Corey L: Genital herpes simplex virus infections in adults. Urol Clin N Am 11:107: 1983.

BIBLIOGRAPHY

Andrews EB, Yankaskas BC, Cordero JF, Schoeffler K, Hampp S, and the Acyclovir in Pregnancy Registry Advisory Committee. Acyclovir and Pregnancy Registry: six years' experience. *Obstet Gynecol* **79**:7–13, 1992.

Arvin AM, Prober CG: Analysis of the epidemiology and pathogenesis of herpes simplex virus (HSV) infections in pregnant women and infants using the HSV-2 glycoprotein G antibody assay. *Infect Agents Dis* **2**:375, 1994.

Ashley RL: Genital herpes infections. *Clinics Lab Med* **9**:405, 1989.

Ashley R, Cent A, Maggs V, et al.: Inability of enzyme immunoassays to discriminate between infections with herpes simplex virus types 1 and 2. *Ann Intern Med* **115**:520, 1991.

Bryan JA: Laboratory diagnosis of viral infections. In: Conn RB (ed): *Current Diagnosis*, 7th ed. Philadelphia, WB Saunders, pp 174–182, 1985.

CDC. Genital herpes infection – United States, 1966–1979. *MMWR* **31**:137, 1982.

Coen DM: The implications of resistance to antiviral agents for herpesvirus drug targets and drug therapy. *Antiviral Res* **15**:287, 1991.

Cone RW, Hobson AC, Palmer J, et al.: Extended duration of herpes simplex virus DNA in genital lesions detected by the polymerase chain reaction. *J Inf Dis* **164**:757, 1991.

Fife KH, Crumpacker CS, Mertz GJ, Hill EL, Boone GS, and the Acyclovir Study Group. Recurrence and resistance patterns of herpes simplex virus following cessation of ≥6 years of chronic suppression with acyclovir. *J Infect Dis* **169**:1338–41, 1994.

Gill MJ, Arlette J, Buchan K: Herpes simplex virus infection of the hand: a profile of 79 cases. *Am J Med* **84**:89, 1988.

Guinan ME, Wolinsky SM, Reichman RC: Epidemiology of genital herpes simplex infections. *Epidemiol Rev* **7**:127, 1985.

Johnson RE, Nahmias AJ, Magder LS, et al.: A seroepidemiologic survey of the prevalence of herpes simplex virus type 2 infection in the United States. *N Engl J Med* **321**:7, 1989.

Koutsky LA, Stevens CE, Holmes KK, et al.: Underdiagnosis of genital herpes by current clinical and viral-isolation procedures. *New Engl J Med* **326**:1533, 1992.

Lafferty WE, Coombs RW, Benedetti J, et al.: Recurrences after oral and genital herpes simplex virus infections: influence of site of infection and viral type. *N Engl J Med* **316**:1444, 1987.

Mertz GJ, Benedetti J, Ashley R, et al.: Risk factors for the sexual transmission of genital herpes. *Ann Intern Med* **116**:197, 1992.

Nahmias AJ, Lee FK, Beckman-Nahmias S: Sero-epidemiological and sociological patterns of herpes simplex virus infections in the world. *Scand J Infect Dis* **69**(suppl.):19, 1990.

Prober CG, Corey L, Brown ZA, et al.: The management of pregnancies complicated by genital infections with herpes simplex virus. *Clin Infect Dis* **15**:1031, 1992.

Prober CG, Sullender WM, Yasukawa LL, et al.: Low risk of herpes simplex virus infections in neonates exposed to the virus at the time of vaginal delivery to mothers with recurrent genital herpes virus infections. *N Engl J Med* **316**:240, 1987.

Rooney JF, Felser JM, Ostrove JM, Strauss SE: Acquisition of genital herpes from an asymptomatic sexual partner. *N Engl J Med* **314**:1561, 1986.

Sacks SL: Frequency and duration of patient-observed recurrent genital herpes simplex virus infection: characterization of the nonlesional prodrome. *J Infect Dis* **150**:873, 1984.

Sacks SL: The role of oral acyclovir in the management of genital herpes simplex. *Can Med Assoc J* **136**:701, 1987.

Safrin S, Crumpacker C, Chatis P, et al.: Controlled trial comparing foscarnet with vidarabine for acyclovir-resistant mucocutaneous herpes simplex in the acquired immunodeficiency syndrome. *N Engl J Med* **325**:551–555, 1991.

Sánchez-Martínez D, Pellett PE: Expression of HSV-1 and HSV-2 glycoprotein G in insect cells by using a novel baculovirus expression vector. *Virology* **182**:229, 1991.

Sánchez-Martínez D, Schmid DS, Whittington W, Brown D, Reeves WC, Chatterjee S, Whitley RJ, Pellett PE: Evaluation of a test based on baculovirus-expressed glycoprotein G for detection of herpes simplex virus type-specific antibodies. *J Inf Dis* **164**:1196, 1991.

Stavraky KM, Rawls WE, Chiavetta J, et al.: Sexual and economic factors affecting the risk of past infections with herpes simplex virus type 2. *Am J Epidemiol* **118**:109, 1983.

Stone KM, Whittington WL: Treatment of genital herpes. *Rev Infect Dis* **12** (suppl. 6): S610, 1990.

Straus SE (moderator): Herpes simplex virus infection: biology, treatment, and prevention. *Ann Intern Med* **103**:404, 1985.

Straus SE, Corey L, Burke RL et al.: Placebo-controlled trial of vaccination with recombinant glycoprotein D of herpes simplex virus type 2 for immunotherapy of genital herpes. *Lancet* **343**:1460–1463, 1994.

Straus SE, Croen KD, Sawyer MH, et al.: Acyclovir suppression of frequently recurring genital herpes: efficacy and diminishing need during successive years of treatment. *JAMA* **260**:2227, 1988.

Whitley RJ, Gnann JW: The epidemiology and clinical manifestations of herpes simplex virus infections. In: Roizman B, Whitley RJ, Lopez C (eds): *Human Herpesvirus Infections*. New York, Raven Press, pp 69–105, 1993.

Whitley RJ, Gnann JW: Antiviral therapy. In: Roizman B, Whitley RJ, Lopez C (eds): *Human Herpevirus Infections*. New York, Raven Press, pp 329–348, 1993.

CHAPTER TWELVE

Genital Human Papillomavirus Infections

A Moreland, B Majmudar, and S Vernon

INTRODUCTION

Infection of the human genital tract with the human papillomavirus (HPV) is one of the most common viral STDs. Genital warts (venereal warts, condylomata acuminata, fig warts) have long been recognized, but until recently were considered trivial, and sexual transmission was even questioned by some. Current understanding of this infection requires recognition that condylomata acuminata are only the most obvious manifestation of HPV infections of the anogenital region. A large body of evidence now supports the concept that subclinical HPV infections are much more common than was previously recognized. Additionally, the current diagnosis and management of HPV infections needs to take into account that some HPV types are often associated with squamous atypia and less frequently with invasive carcinoma of the anogenital tract.

The HPV is a 55 nm DNA virus that belongs to the papovavirus family (*Fig. 12.1*). It infects the skin and mucous membranes and replicates in the nuclei of infected epithelial cells. Late viral gene expression, capsid protein synthesis, viral DNA replication and virion assembly occur almost exclusively in terminally differentiated epithelial cells. To date, the HPV group consists of 70 distinct types; 34 of these 70 types have been associated with anogenital lesions. A subset of the genital HPV types are most often detected in genital lesions (*Fig. 12.2*).

HPV cannot be grown routinely in tissue culture. Inoculation experiments at the turn of the century and electron microscopy evidence from 30 years ago offered the first direct and reproducible evidence of the viral etiology of condylomata. Recently, the localization of HPV DNA by in situ hybridization and molecular hybridization techniques has been used to confirm the presence of virus in tissues.

EPIDEMIOLOGY

Although cases of genital warts are not routinely reported, several limited surveys have suggested that prevalence has increased in recent years, and that genital papillomavirus is now the third most common STD (*Fig. 12.3*). The incidence of genital warts has also increased during the past 20 years. Genital warts are now the most common viral STD, with only the incidence of trichomoniasis, gonorrhea, and *Chlamydia* exceeding that of genital warts. However, new visits to private physicians' offices (*Fig. 12.4*) for genital warts outnumber those for gonorrhea and genital herpes.

Genital warts account for approximately 5% of all STD clinic visits in the USA. In some clinics, cases of genital warts outnumber those of gonorrhea. The risk factors for genital warts or subclinical HPV infection have not been well studied, but probably differ from those for gonorrhea. Genital warts are most commonly seen in persons aged 20–24 years. The use of oral contraceptives and cigarette smoking may also be associated risk factors.

Cervical HPV infection is almost always asymptomatic and is much more common than clinically apparent genital warts. Many women with genital warts have coexistent cervical infection. In the USA and Canada, 0.5–3% of routinely screened Papanicolaou smears show evidence of HPV infection, with prevalence generally decreasing with age. However, prevalence is much higher in the few STD clinic populations that have been studied; approximately 10% of women have cytologic evidence of HPV infection. If a battery of diagnostic tests for HPV infection (colposcopy or cervicography, DNA hybridization, and PCR) is used in addition to cytology, this prevalence increases to 25–50%. Latent or subclinical genital HPV infection appears to be much more common than clinical wart disease, but has been studied less extensively than cervical infection.

Although genital warts were recognized as an STD in ancient times, the medical community has accepted this mode of transmission only in the last 20–25 years. Congenital transmission from mother to baby, causing juvenile laryngeal papillomatosis and oral and skin condylomata, is discussed in *Chapter 14*.

The interval between exposure and detection of genital warts is 3–8 months. Penile lesions have been found in up to 70% of male partners of women with CIN. The additional percentage of partners who will become subclinically infected is unknown (*Fig. 12.5*).

Natural History and Association with Cancer

The natural history of genital warts and subclinical HPV infections has not been well established. Warts may persist or recur despite treatment, may regress spontaneously, or rarely, may undergo malignant transformation. Cervical HPV infection appears to have a similar spectrum of behavior, though the subsequent development of malignant precursors is not unusual. In one study, up to 40% of women developed CIN within 24 months of HPV types 16 or 18 being first detected. This work has been supported by numerous smaller studies suggesting that the type of HPV is important in the development of neoplasia.

The epidemiology of cervical and other genital cancers is consistent with a sexually transmissible infectious etiology, and HPV meets several criteria for oncogenicity. Although mounting evidence suggests a strong association between HPV and genital dysplasia and cancer, a causal role has not been

Fig. 12.1 Electron micrograph of HPV (negative stain, phosphotungstic acid). The HPV has an icosahedral capsid 55 nm in diameter.

MOST FREQUENT CLINICAL MANIFESTATIONS OF COMMON HPV TYPES

HPV TYPE	GENITAL LESIONS
6, 11	Anogenital condylomata
16, 18, 31, 42	Bowenoid papulosis, vulvar intraepithelial neoplasia, Bowen's disease
6, 11, 16, 18, 31, 33, 35	Cervical intraepithelial neoplasia, dysplasias of genital mucosa
16, 18, 31, 33, 35	Invasive cancer

Fig. 12.2 HPV types frequently associated with genital lesions.

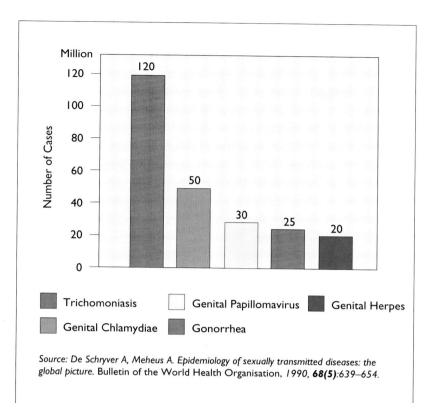

Fig. 12.3 Annual worldwide total of sexually transmitted infections, 1990.

Source: De Schryver A, Meheus A. *Epidemiology of sexually transmitted diseases: the global picture.* Bulletin of the World Health Organisation, *1990,* **68(5)**:639–654.

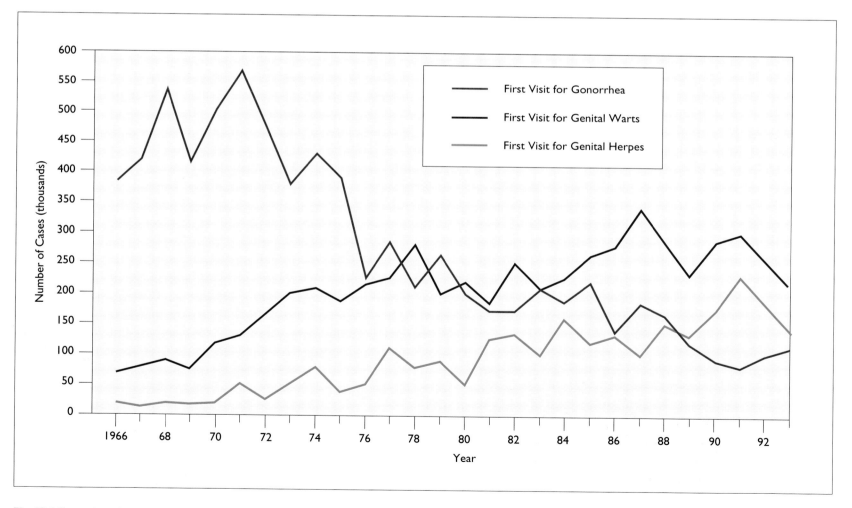

Fig. 12.4 Comparison of visits to private physicians for genital warts, genital herpes, and gonorrhea. (Source: CDC and National Disease and Therapeutic Index, IMS America, Ltd.)

established (*Fig. 12.6*). Papillomaviruses are known to produce tumors in animals, and certain types are capable of transforming normal cells to neoplastic cells *in vitro*. The integration of HPV DNA into the genome of the host cell is usually observed in invasive carcinomas and cervical carcinoma cell lines, whereas in benign and premalignant lesions HPV DNA is usually extrachromosomal. Certain types of HPV DNA (especially types 16, 18 and 31) have been found in all types of genital cancers and cancer precursors. However, many clinically and microscopically normal tissues harbour HPV DNA. Epidemiologic studies show that women with cytologic evidence of HPV have an increased risk of cervical dysplasia and cancer. Prospective studies are needed to show whether HPV infection actually precedes the development of dysplasia or cancer, and to investigate the role of HPV infection as a cofactor rather than the sole etiologic agent.

CLINICAL MANIFESTATIONS

The spectrum of HPV-associated conditions found in the anogenital region ranges from the typical papillomas of condylomata acuminata seen on the external genitalia, perineum, and vaginal, cervical, perianal, and urethral mucosa to clinically inapparent infection of the same areas. Additionally, HPV has been found in vulvar, vaginal, and penile carcinoma *in situ* or intraepithelial neoplasia, including bowenoid papulosis, CIN, and invasive carcinoma of the the genital tract.

Condylomata Acuminata

These papillomatous, pedunculated or sessile growths occur anywhere on the vulvar, penile, scrotal, perineal, or perianal skin, or in the urethra (*Fig. 12.7*). They may be smooth or may have fingerlike projections that cause them to have a rough surface — hence the term *condylomata acuminata* (*condylomata*, knuckles; *acuminata*, pointed) (*Fig. 12.8*). Single lesions usually range from 1 to 4 mm in diameter and from 2 to 15 mm in height. Multiple papules may become confluent, plaquelike, or multilobed masses (*Fig. 12.9*). Condylomata are usually flesh-colored, but may be hyperpigmented or erythematous (*Fig. 12.10*). Penile or vulvar intraepithelial neoplasia (PIN or VIN), also called bowenoid papulosis, occurs more frequently in hyperpigmented lesions and may be interspersed within groups of condylomata (*Figs. 12.11* and *12.12*). HPV 16 is more often associated with PIN or VIN than are HPV 6 or 11. Progression to invasive

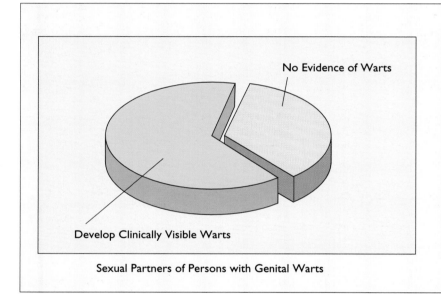

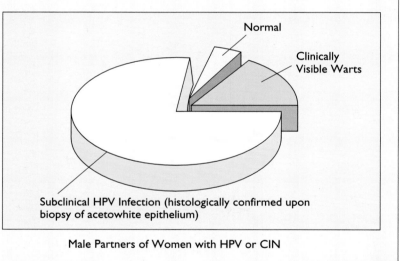

Fig. 12.5 Transmission of HPV infection. Although only two-thirds of sexual partners of patients with genital warts develop genital warts within 3 months, many more may be infected subclinically. Limited studies suggest as many as 90% of partners are infected, yet only a small fraction have clinically apparent warts.

EVIDENCE LINKING HPV WITH CIN AND CERVICAL CANCER

Epidemiology suggests a sexually transmissable infectious etiology of CIN and cervical cancer

40 to 95% of cases of CIN contain HPV DNA

25 to 50% of CIN is associated with HPV types 16 or 18

80 to 90% of cases of invasive cancer contain HPV DNA

Cervical HPV increases risk of CIN and cervical cancer

Fig. 12.6 Evidence linking HPV with CIN and cervical cancer.

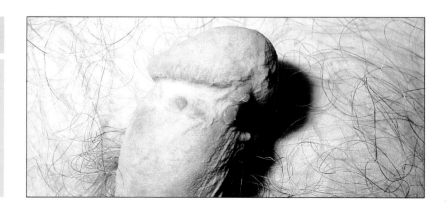

Fig. 12.7 Condylomata acuminata — penile. Asymptomatic, flesh-colored papules are present on the shaft of the penis.

squamous cell carcinoma may occur, so close follow-up is recommended. In recalcitrant cases, biopsies should be obtained. Intraepithelial or invasive carcinoma associated with HPV may also present as hyperkeratotic plaques (*Fig. 12.13*). Spread of the infection can result in an increase in the number of warts and/or in the size of individual warts. In some cases, large plaques or masses may reach several centimeters in size, and condylomata may become so large as to cause the deformity of normal structures. These large lesions are sometimes called giant condylomata of Buschke and

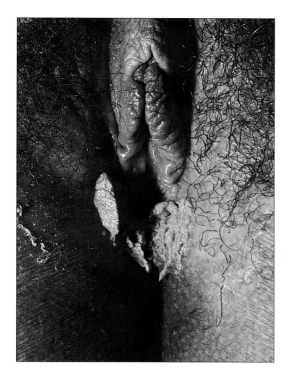

Fig. 12.8 Condylomata acuminata — vulvar. The rough, corrugated surface is characteristic and papillary projections may form as seen here.

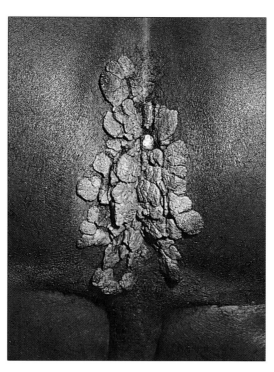

Fig. 12.9 Condylomata acuminata — perianal. Treatment of these large, recurrent warts was made more difficult by the patient's poor compliance with office follow-ups.

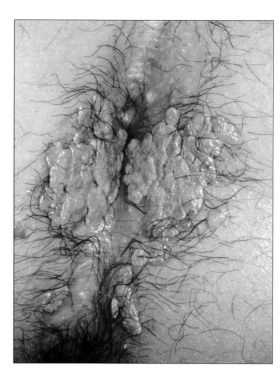

Fig. 12.10 Condylomata acuminata — perianal. Both discrete and confluent masses of condylomata are present. The large size may result in irritation or other secondary symptoms.

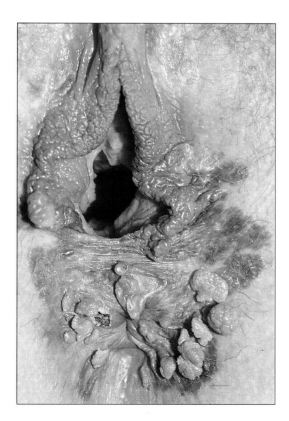

Fig. 12.12 Bowenoid papulosis — vulvar and perineal. Although these lesions resemble condylomata clinically, the presence of multiple pigmented papular lesions in a young woman should raise the possibility of bowenoid papulosis or carcinoma in situ and biopsies should be obtained.

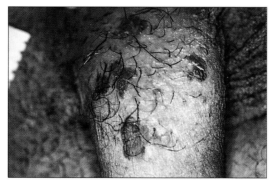

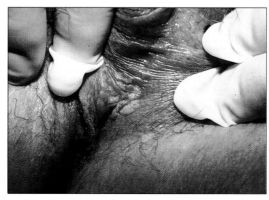

Fig. 12.13 Vulvar Bowen's disease (squamous carcinoma *in situ*). This white plaque has well-defined borders and slight ulceration. Biopsy was diagnostic of Bowen's disease.

Fig. 12.11 Bowenoid papulosis — penis. These large, hyperpigmented, flat papules on the shaft of the penis were asymptomatic. A biopsy to rule out carcinoma *in situ* is essential in such cases.

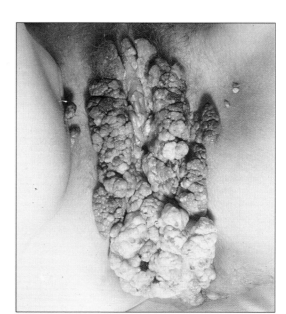

Fig. 12.14 Condylomata acuminata — vulva and perineum. The clinical diagnosis was giant condylomata of Buschke and Löwenstein. Such large and confluent lesions should be carefully examined and multiple biopsies obtained to rule out underlying malignancy.

Löwenstein (*Fig. 12.14*). Obstruction by condylomata of the urethral meatus is not infrequent in males. In males, condylomata occur earliest near the frenulum of the penis and are most frequent on the coronal sulcus, the shaft (*Fig. 12.15*) and the preputial borders (*Figs. 12.16* and *12.17*). In females, the earliest lesions are seen most often around the introitus and often on the fourchette and labia, but condylomata may be present on any part of the vulva (*Fig. 12.18*). In at least 20% of women, the perineum and perianal skin are also involved (*Fig .12.19*). The natal cleft is another frequently missed site, especially in obese patients.

Flat Warts (Condylomata Plana)

Flat warts appear on the vulva or penis as flesh-colored hyperpigmented or hypopigmented papules of about 1–4 mm diameter (*Fig. 12.20*). The application of 3–5% acetic acid enhances visualization of this form of infection (*Figs. 12.21–12.26*). Examination of the acetowhite areas with a colposcope or hand lens improves diagnostic accuracy, but the specificity is unknown. *Acetowhitening* may occur in other conditions, such as lichen planus, seborrheic dermatitis (*Figs. 12.25 and 12.26*), nonspecific inflammation, and intraepithelial neoplasia, as well as in histologically unremarkable tissue (*Fig. 10.27*). When the vulva is extensively involved, large confluent whitened areas appear after the acetic acid-soaked gauze is removed from the area. Vaginal warts are not seen as commonly as cervical or vulvar warts. They may have a spiked appearance, but may also be flat or invisible to the naked eye.

Cervical HPV Infections

Similarly, cervical HPV infections may have various presentations. These range from invisible 'flat condylomata' (subclinical infection) to 'spiked', exophytic, or florid papillomata. All are associated with the presence of HPV particles (*Fig. 12.28*). Exophytic condylomata with a rough acuminate appearance are white, gray or red, and may be hyperkeratotic or secondarily infected and ulcerated. Flat condylomata are the most common and often occur in great numbers, but they may be invisible without colposcopy and application of 3–5% acetic acid. Although colposcopic criteria have not been standardized, certain morphologic features, such as color, margin contour, vascular pattern, and iodine staining, appear to be useful in distinguishing cervical HPV infection from dysplasia or other cervical abnormalities. Cervicography is a recently developed screening tool that involves taking a photograph of the cervix through a special lens for subsequent interpretation (*Figs. 12.29* and *12.30*). Preliminary evaluation suggests that cervicography has a higher sensitivity than the Papanicolaou smear in detecting HPV and CIN.

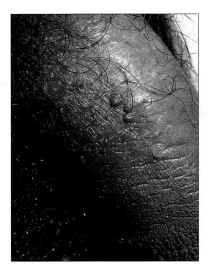

Fig. 12.15 Condylomata acuminata — penile shaft. Very early lesions may be difficult to see.

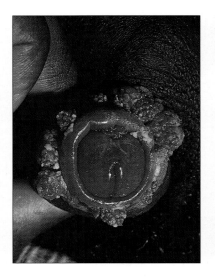

Fig. 12.16 Condylomata acuminata — preputial borders. These lesions had become secondarily infected due to occlusion of the foreskin.

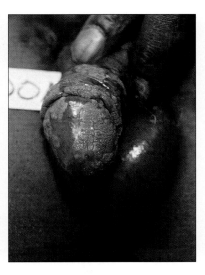

Fig. 12.17 Condylomata acuminata in a 53-year-old HIV-seropositive male. Lesions may be particularly florid in HIV-infected patients.

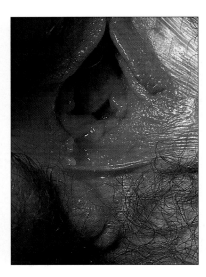

Fig. 12.18 Condylomata acuminata — vulvar introitus. These small papules seen at the fourchette are nearly invisible to the examiner and asymptomatic to the patient.

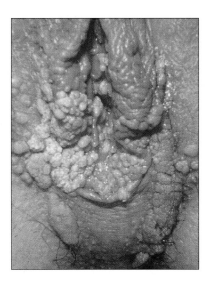

Fig. 12.19 Condylomata acuminata — vulvar and perineal. This patient has extensive involvement around the introitus and the labia with extension onto the perineum and perianal region.

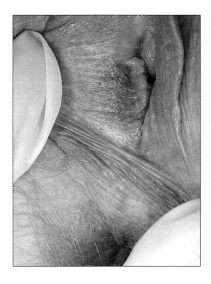

Fig. 12.20 Condylomata plana — vulva. The use of 3% acetic acid enhances visualization of these difficult-to-see flat vulvar warts on the labia minora.

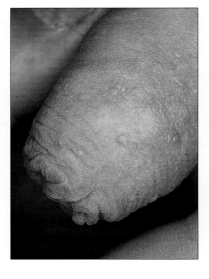

Figs. 12.21 and 12.22 Condylomata plana — penile. Acetowhite penile lesions. Penile skin showing areas of 'acetowhitening' after the application of 3–5% acetic acid in a patient with very small and recent condylomata positive for HPV 6/11. Without the use of acetic acid and a magnifying lens, these lesions were not clinically apparent. Note the area of nonspecific acetowhitening adjacent to the separate acetowhite condylomatous papules.

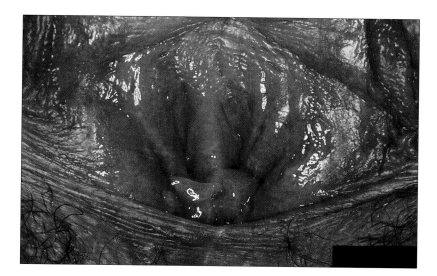
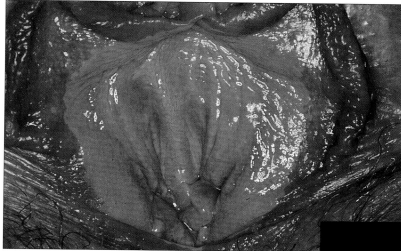

Figs. 12.23 and 12.24 Acetowhitened vulva. (**12.23**) External vulvar skin appearing normal before application of 3–5% acetic acid. (**12.24**) This is the same vulvar skin after application of acetic acid. The entire area proximal to Hart's line (demarcation of keratinized and unkeratinized stratified squamous epithelium) appears 'acetowhite'. Acetowhitening is one sign of subclinical HPV infection; however, its specificity is not known.

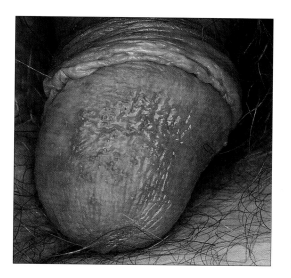
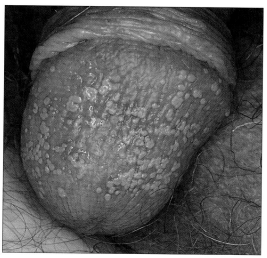
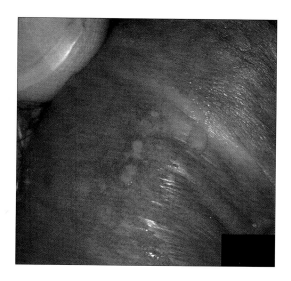

Figs. 12.25 and 12.26 Seborrheic dermatitis also acetowhitens. Pre- (**12.25**) and post-3% acetic acid (**12.26**) of a biopsy-proven HPV-negative penile seborrheic dermatitis.

Fig. 12.27 Carcinoma *in situ* — penis. These flat penile papules appeared white after acetic acid application and biopsy showed carcinoma *in situ*. All lesions that are suspicious, clinically atypical, or unresponsive to initial treatment should be biopsied to rule out premalignant and malignant changes.

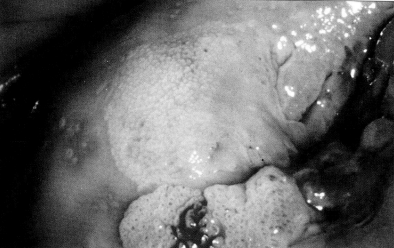

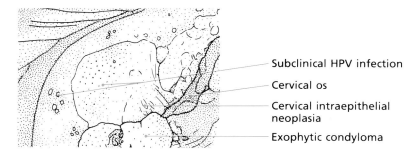

Subclinical HPV infection

Cervical os

Cervical intraepithelial neoplasia

Exophytic condyloma

Fig. 12.28 Colpophotograph of cervix showing an exophytic condyloma, an area of subclinical HPV infection, and an area of high-grade CIN. Differentiation of these lesions is difficult and should be attempted only by experienced colposcopists.

Differential Diagnosis

Condylomata acuminata ordinarily present a distinct and easily recognized clinical picture. However, the clinician should be familiar with some other common entities in the differential diagnosis. The most common of these are discussed briefly here, but for a more detailed discussion the reader is referred to *Chapter 1*.

Verruca vulgaris

Verruca vulgaris (usually caused by HPV types 2, 3, and 4) may occur in or near the genital region, especially on the skin of the lower abdomen, upper thigh, or buttocks (*Fig. 12.31*). A thickened, dry, hyperkeratotic appearance is more typical of verruca vulgaris, but differentation of the two entities may require histopathologic examination or other diagnostic tests to differentiate viral type (*see Fig. 12.34*). Treatment is similar to that for condylomata acuminata.

Molluscum contagiosum

The umbilicated papules of molluscum contagiosum infection often resemble condylomata acuminata and appear in the genital region in sexually active patients (*Fig. 12.32*). The umbilication of the papules helps to distinguish them from condylomata acuminata, but crusting or other secondary changes may obscure this helpful feature. This pox virus infection is transmitted by both sexual and nonsexual routes. It is usually self-limited but may be

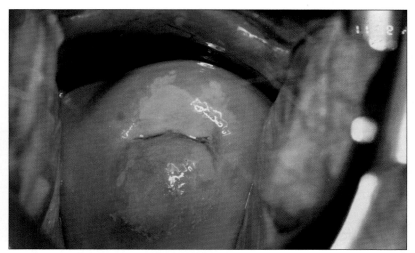

Figs. 12.29 and 12.30 Cervicography. This technique may be a useful adjunct to the Papanicolaou smear for cervical cancer screening. (**12.29**) Cervicogram showing normal cervix, including the transformation zone. (**12.30**) Cervicogram showing an area of acetowhitening with irregular borders, which is typical of subclinical HPV infection of the cervix.

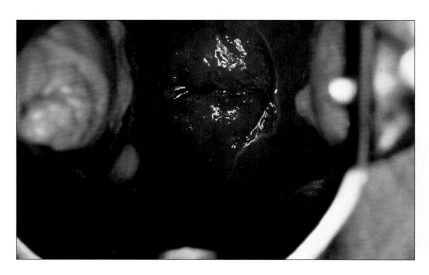

Transformation zone

Vaginal walls

Acetowhitening

Vaginal wall

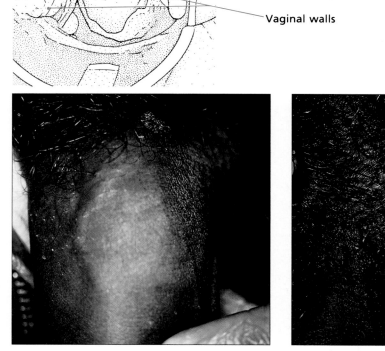

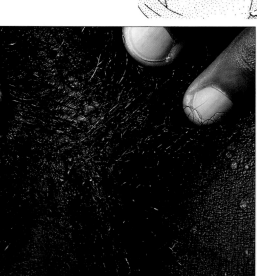

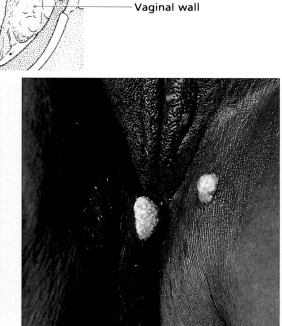

Fig. 12.31 Verruca vulgaris — penis. This raised, rough papule at the base of the penis appeared similar to condylomata acuminata but proved to be a verruca vulgaris on biopsy.

Fig. 12.32 Molluscum contagiosum — inguinal. The characteristic umbilicated papules are typically asymptomatic, but may become secondarily infected, crusted, or pruritic.

Fig. 12.33 Condylomata lata — perianal and upper thigh. The rough texture of these papules mimics condylomata acuminata. Dark-field examination and serology were positive in this case of secondary syphilis.

progressive in immunocompromised patients. It can easily be diagnosed by its characteristic inclusions seen on cytologic or histologic examination. Treatment should be conservative.

Seborrheic keratoses

Seborrheic keratoses are rough, usually brown or black hyperpigmented, flat, broad papules. They have a waxy texture and minute puncta on the surface. These benign tumors may be multiple and are treated only for cosmetic reasons.

Condylomata lata

Condylomata lata of secondary syphilis must always be considered when condylomata acuminata are present (*Fig. 12.33*). The two entities may not only look remarkably similar but may coexist, as patients with multiple sexual partners are often exposed to and become infected with more than one STD at a time. Condylomata lata, however, are typically more moist than condylomata acuminata and may even be ulcerated. In condylomata lata, dark-field examination almost always demonstrates spirochetes and syphilis serology is invariably reactive.

Other

Skin tags (acrochordons), syringomas, and pearly penile papules may also be confused with condylomata acuminata, but they have a smooth, rather than a rough, surface. They may also bleed and be tender; these features are rare in condylomata acuminata.

LABORATORY TESTS

The diagnosis of typical condylomata acuminata is made primarily on clinical appearance, aided by the application of acetic acid and the use of a magnifying lens. Clinical diagnoses should be confirmed by histology and cytology whenever necessary. Immunohistochemical and hybridization techniques are additional tools used in detecting viral antigens and viral DNA. They are used primarily in research and are particularly useful in those cases of HPV infection not readily visible by clinical means. Successful techniques for propagating HPV have recently been reported, but in vitro cultures are not available for routine diagnostic work (*Fig. 12.34*).

Fig. 12.34 The diagnosis of HPV infections and the limitations of various methods.

DIAGNOSIS OF HPV INFECTIONS

DIAGNOSTIC TEST	ADVANTAGE	DISADVANTAGE
Inspection/magnifying lens	Inexpensive	Will not detect subclinical disease
Cytology	Inexpensive	Insensitive; sampling error
Histology	Sensitive for neoplastic and morphologic diagnosis	Invasive
Colposcopy, urethroscopy, anoscopy	Magnified visualization	Differentiation from dysplasia is difficult
Southern Blot Hybridization	Sensitive, identify HPV type, use of fresh tissue or cells	Time consuming, radioactive probes, technically demanding
Dot Blot Hybridization	Sensitive, identify HPV type use of fresh tissue or cells	Cross hybridization
In situ Hybridization	Localization of HPV infection in morphologic context, identify HPV type	Sensitivity
Immunohistochemistry	Localization of HPV infection in morphologic context	Insensitive, not HPV type specific
Commercial Filter Hybridization (Virpap/Viratype, Digene Diagnostics, Inc)	Sensitive, identify HPV type, FDA approved	Radioactive
Commercial Solution Hybridization (Hybrid Capture System, Digene Diagnostics, Inc)	Sensitive, identify HPV type, non-radioactive, quantitative	Potential for cross hybridization
Polymerase Chain Reaction	Sensitive, DNA from fresh or fixed tissue or cells, identify HPV type or generate consensus HPV product, little material required	Potential for contamination or nonspecific amplification
Serology	Identification of past infection	HPV type-specific test not yet available

Histopathology
Condylomata Acuminata

In anogenital condylomata, the most obvious histologic changes are papillomatosis and acanthosis of the Malpighian layer. The dermal papillae are usually elongated, narrow, and branching, forming a pattern of pseudoepitheliomatous hyperplasia (*Fig. 12.35*). According to Lever, the most characteristic feature is the presence of 'koilocytes' in the upper stratum malpighii, stratum granulosum, and stratum corneum. These are large, epithelial cells with small or large, dense, irregular, crumpled-looking nuclei (*Fig. 12.36*). Since cytoplasmic organelles congregate at the periphery of the cell and the

remainder of the cytoplasm is clear, a 'halo' in the perinuclear area can be seen. In addition, many mitotic figures and multinucleated and dyskeratotic cells may be present (*Fig. 12.37*). Hyperplasia of the parabasal cells may be present beneath the atypical cells. Orthokeratosis and parakeratosis are common. Chronic inflammatory cells and dilated capillaries and edema are usually present in the dermis.

Cervical Condylomata

Hyperkeratosis, acanthosis, and cellular atypia create a similar overall architectural pattern in the exophytic condylomata (*Fig. 12.38*). Papillomatosis is

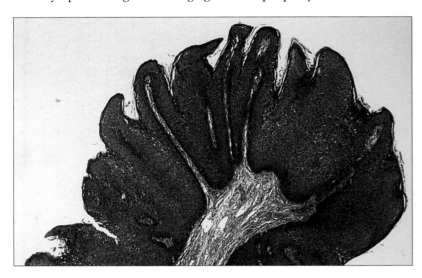

Fig. 12.35 Anogenital condyloma. Histologic preparation of condyloma showing hyperkeratotic squamous epithelium with multiple papillary fronds. The appearance of condyloma is diagnostic, irrespective of the anatomic site.

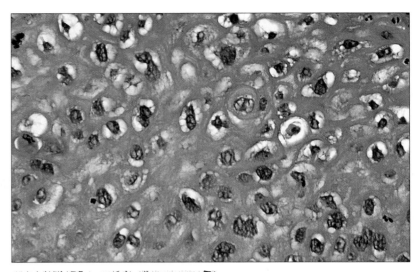

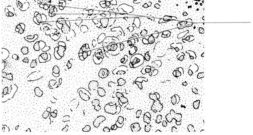

Koilocytes

Fig. 12.36 Anogenital condyloma. Histologic examination shows multiple large cells with clear cytoplasm and atypical wrinkled nuclei. These cells, called koilocytes, suggest HPV infection.

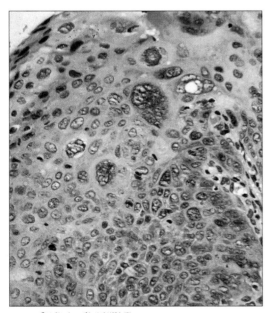

Fig. 12.37 Cervical condyloma. Histologic examination of condyloma may show large, extremely atypical, nuclei. These changes do not necessarily indicate malignancy. Condylomatous atypia and premalignant dysplastic changes are often difficult to distinguish by histologic examination alone.

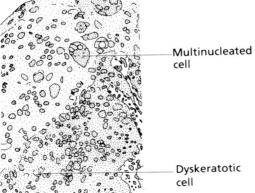

Multinucleated cell

Dyskeratotic cell

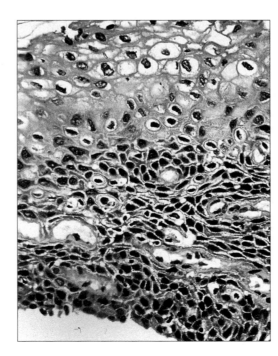

Fig. 12.38 Cervical condyloma showing large, vacuolated koilocytes in the superficial layers of the mucosa.

absent in the flat condylomata except for occasional small peaks of superficial epithelium. Koilocytosis seen in the upper layers of the cervical mucosa is a characteristic finding of flat cervical condylomata. A significant amount of cellular atypia may accompany these changes, thus mimicking CIN. It is often difficult to distinguish between condylomatous atypia and true CIN. In general, the former is seen in the superficial layers and the latter in the deeper layers of the epithelium. It is common to see both components together in a cervical biopsy. In some cases after a latent period, invasive carcinoma occurs (*Figs. 12.39* and *12.40*).

Bowenoid Papulosis, Carcinoma in situ, Intraepitheloid Neoplasia

Hyperkeratosis, parakeratosis, and psoriasiform epidermal hyperplasia with a focally prominent granular zone are accompanied by crowding of epidermal nuclei, increased mitotic figures of the upper half of the epidermis, and atypical mitotic figures (*Figs. 12.41* and *12.42*). Necrotic and large multinucleated keratinocytes may be present. Keratinocytes with hyperchromatic and pleomorphic nuclei are also characteristic and produce a pattern of squamous cell carcinoma *in situ* (*Fig. 12.43*). Koilocytosis may be present, but is less prominent than in classic forms of condylomata. Skin adnexa are gen-

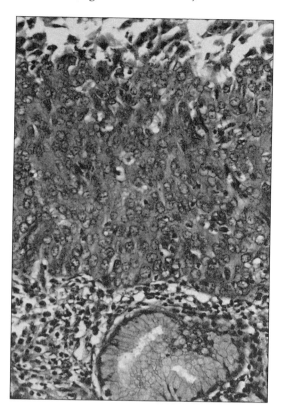

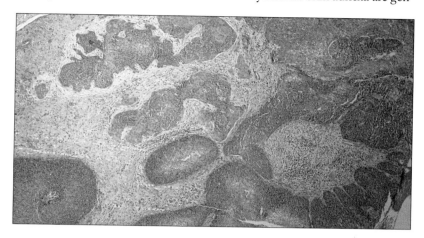

Fig. 12.39 Carcinoma of the cervix. The cervical epithelial cells have lost their regular stratified pattern, have high nucleus–cytoplasm ratios and show increased mitotic activity. As the basement membrane between the epithelium and underlying stroma is intact, this is carcinoma-in-situ or cervical intraepithelial neoplasia (CIN).

Fig. 12.40 Some of the abnormal epithelial cells have breached the basement membrane and invaded the cervical stroma; this is invasive carcinoma.

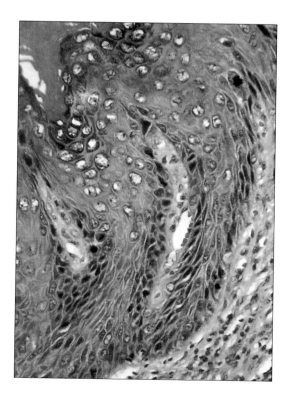

Fig. 12.42 Bowenoid papulosis of the vulva, showing the same tissue as in 12.41 at a higher magnification. Hyperkeratosis, papillomatosis, and reactive atypia of the squamous epithelium can be seen. The superficial layers of the epidermis show atypical cells with large, empty-looking nuclei suggesting a viral infection.

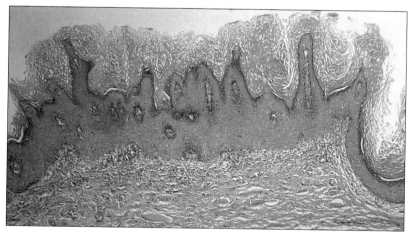

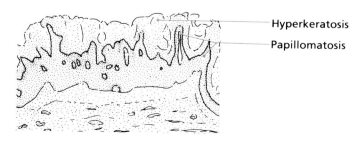

Hyperkeratosis

Papillomatosis

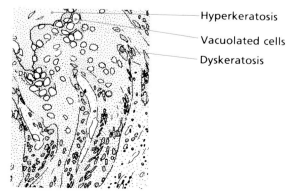

Hyperkeratosis

Vacuolated cells

Dyskeratosis

Fig. 12.41 Bowenoid papulosis of the vulva. Hyperkeratotic benign squamous epithelium with multiple papillary projections.

erally spared from the process and the confluent growth pattern of the pro-liferating epithelium is not seen. It has been recommended by the International Society for the Study of Vulvovaginal Disease that the term Bowenoid papulosis should be deleted and replaced by a report of degree of squamous dysplasia seen in a given biopsy.

Cytology

The Papanicolaou smear is the most commonly used means of detecting asymptomatic cervical HPV infections, but it is relatively insensitive and subject to sampling error. Viral atypia and koilocytosis are characteristic cytologic features of cervical HPV infection. Koilocytosis is considered fairly specific for HPV infection (*Fig. 12.44*). Koilocytes have an irregular, hyperchromatic nucleus surrounded by a clear, cytoplasmic halo, which, in turn, is surrounded by peripherally located dense cytoplasm. The diagnosis of HPV infection is further suggested by other cytologic findings, such as dyskeratocytosis, multinucleation, anucleation, and parakeratosis. The association of these changes with HPV has been confirmed by in-situ hybridization and electron microscopy studies of the same tissues.

Demonstration of Virus

Since HPV cannot be routinely propagated in tissue culture, specific viral diagnosis requires the detection of viral proteins or DNA. HPV infection can be diagnosed by a number of DNA hybridization assays. Differences in the sensitivity and specificity of the various assays has resulted in the production and FDA approval of a number of HPV DNA hybridization assays. Definitive diagnosis of HPV infection and disease requires cytology or histology and identification of the virus by at least one of the methods described below.

DNA Hybridization

Nucleic-acid hybridization identifies a specific HPV DNA type by using a DNA or RNA 'probe' made from a known type of HPV (*Fig. 12.45*). The probe is obtained by cloning the known HPV DNA in a bacterial plasmid, and labelling it either with a radioisotope, such as ^{32}P, or with a nonisotopic label,

such as biotin or digoxigenin. Cellular and viral (if present) DNA is extracted from tissue specimens and denatured before being mixed with the nucleic acid probe. In Southern blot hybridization, the homologous DNA strands combine (anneal) to form radioactive double-stranded DNA, which is visualized by autoradiography (*Fig. 12.46*). The various methods of hybridization differ mainly in the way in which DNA from the patient specimen is extracted and purified, and they therefore vary widely in sensitivity and specificity. The 'Southern blot' and 'dot blot' are popular nucleic-acid hybridization techniques that require extraction of DNA from fresh tissue or exfoliated cells. DNA is not extracted from cells for '*in situ*' methods of hybridization.

Tissue *in situ* hybridization (TISH) employs biotinylated probes to give a colorimetric reaction and may be performed on cytologic smears or formalin-fixed and paraffin-embedded tissues (*Fig. 12.47*). Automated TISH is available. The advantages of this method are cellular detail and localization of the hybridized DNA within the architecture of the tissues. Filter *in situ* hybridization (FISH) is a technique in which whole cells are collected on filter paper and then denatured; this method is quicker and more sensitive but less specific than the Southern blot technique.

Recently, a simple, nonradioactive assay has been developed by Digene Diagnostics Inc. (Springfield, Maryland) called Hybrid Capture™. This assay is designed to detect HPV DNA from exfoliated cervical cells collected with a dacron swab or by cervicovaginal lavage. It uses RNA probes to detect up to 14 different HPV DNA types. The RNA probe and HPV DNA molecule form a hybrid that is captured in a tube by an antibody that recognizes RNA/DNA hybrid molecules. The antibody–antigen complex is then recognized by an alkaline phosphatase conjugate (*Fig. 12.48*). These probes can be used in a mix to detect, for example, 'low-risk' HPV DNAs (such as HPV 6 and 11) which cause genital warts, or 'high-risk' HPV DNAs (such as HPV 16 and 18) which are associated with squamous intraepithelial lesions (SIL) (*Fig. 12.49*). The Hybrid Capture™ assay can also be used to quantitate the amount of HPV DNA in a sample. This assay is ideally suited for routine clinical use and results can be obtained from at least 25 samples in an 8-hour working day.

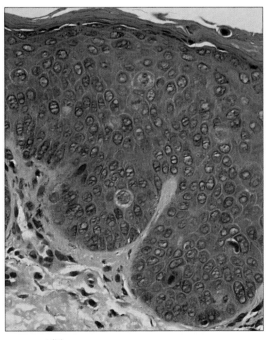

Fig. 12.43 High-grade VIN (bowenoid papulosis) of the vulva. Histologic examination shows the presence of hyperchromatic nuclei, multiple mitoses, and disruption of the maturation sequence imparting the appearance of a squamous cell carcinoma *in situ* to the epidermis.

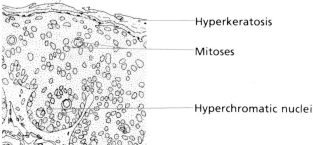

Hyperkeratosis

Mitoses

Hyperchromatic nuclei

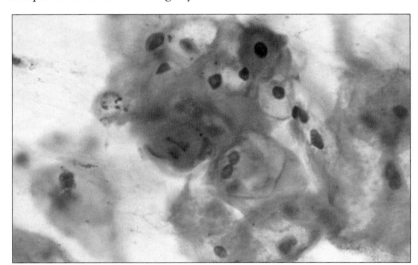

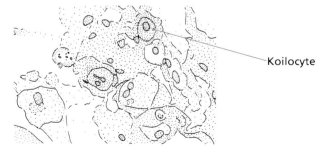

Koilocyte

Fig. 12.44 Koilocyte and superficial desquamated epithelial cells on a Papanicolaou smear. The koilocyte is the cell with the perinuclear halo. It is a relatively specific yet insensitive diagnostic indicator of HPV infection.

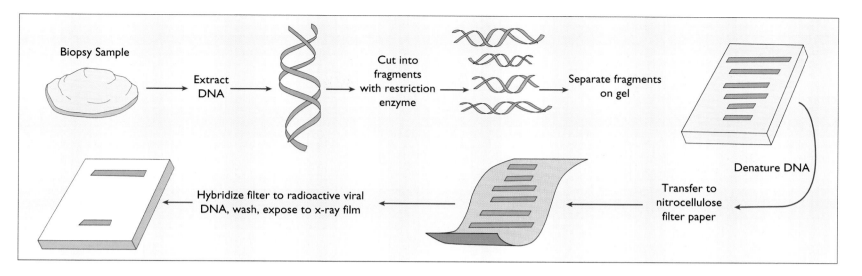

Fig. 12.45 Southern blot technique. Of all methods used to detect HPV DNA, this one is the most specific. DNA from patient specimens is cleaved into small fragments and separated by size before allowing the known DNA probe to attach.

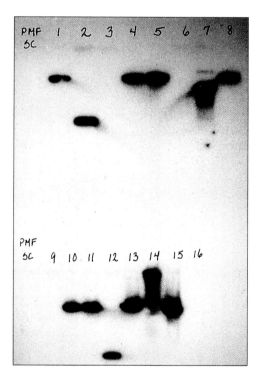

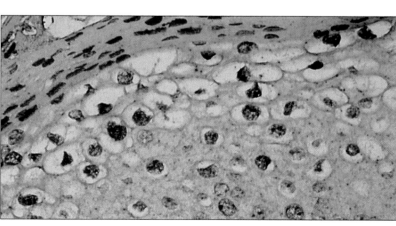

Fig. 12.46 Southern blot hybridization of DNA fragments from patient specimens on nitrocellulose filter paper. Migration patterns of DNA in the numbered lanes are compared with known standards ('fingerprints') of specific types of HPV DNA. The intensity of the black band roughly indicates the amount of DNA present.

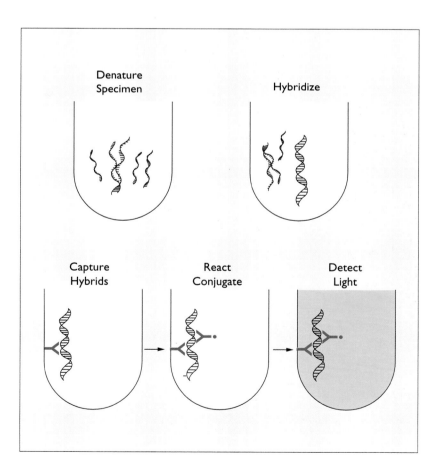

Fig. 12.47 Tissue *in situ* hybridization (TISH) of biotinylated HPV type 11 DNA to formalin-fixed, paraffin-embedded vulvar condyloma. Dark brown-black signal over nuclei indicates the presence of HPV DNA. Signal is strongest at the surface in koilocytic cells and decreases toward the basal layer. However, many nonkoilocytes also demonstrate positive hybridization indicating infection.

Fig. 12.48 Hybrid Capture™ assay. This technique employs a cocktail of unlabeled full genomic RNA probes that are hybridized in solution with denatured target DNA from a specimen. The resulting RNA–DNA hybrids are captured on the surface of a tube that is coated with an antibody that specifically binds RNA–DNA hybrids. The captured RNA–DNA hybrids are reacted with an alkaline phosphatase antibody conjugate. Detection is accomplished by addition of a chemiluminescent substrate and measurement of the light emitted, after cleavage of the substrate by the bound alkaline phosphatase conjugate, with a luminometer. The emitted light intensity is proportional to the amount of target DNA in the specimen.

IMMUNOPEROXIDASE STAIN

Immunoperoxidase staining of cells or tissues directly detects HPV capsid antigen. In this technique, commercially prepared antibodies (directed against disrupted virions) are attached to an enzyme (peroxidase) that will yield a colored reaction product. Immunoperoxidase stains may be performed on tissues (*Fig. 12.50*) or cytologic smears (*Fig. 12.51*). However, this method is even less sensitive than routine cytologic examination. Since only actively proliferating viruses produce capsid antigens, tissues that stain positively are considered infectious. The likelihood of detecting capsid antigen decreases with an increasing severity of dysplasia, and immunoperoxidase stains are invariably negative in genital cancers that contain HPV DNA.

Serology

The diagnosis of HPV infection has relied on the detection of HPV DNA; this indicates current infection but gives little information on the natural history of HPV infection in an individual. However, serology can determine whether individuals have a current or past infection by the detection of antibodies produced against a particular antigen. Within the past few years, a number of investigators have used expression systems, such as vaccinia virus or baculovirus, to produce quantities of outer capsid antigens from a number of HPV types. These antigens have been used in serologic assays to detect antibodies produced against HPV in individuals with a history of HPV infection. Currently, these assays are being optimized for sensitivity and specificity, and will be tested in large epidemiologic studies before becoming available for routine diagnostic use.

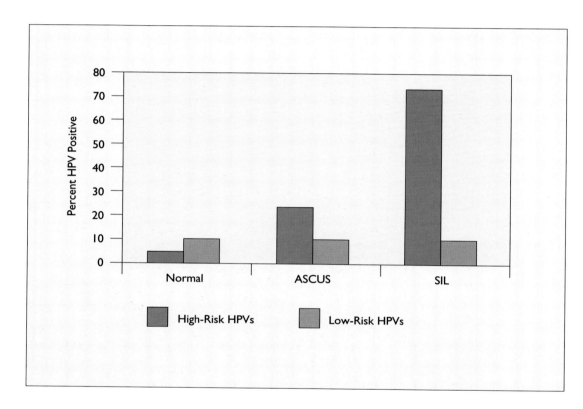

Fig. 12.49 Prevalence of high-risk HPVs and low-risk HPVs by hybrid capture in cervical specimens from normal women and women with atypical squamous cells of undetermined significance (ASCUS) or squamous intraepithelial lesion (SIL) by cytology.

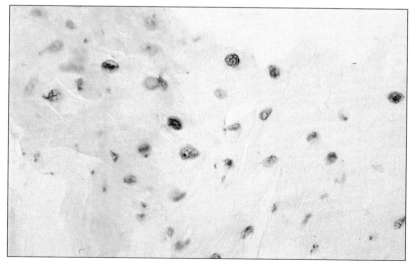

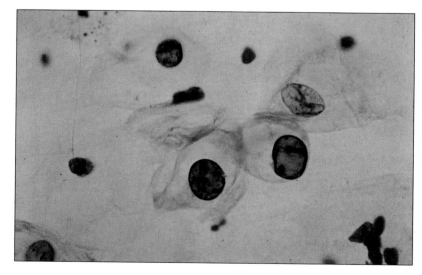

Figs. 12.50 and 12.51 Immunoperoxidase stain. Tissue (**12.50**) and cytologic smear (**12.51**) containing HPV identified by the immunoperoxidase method, which stains the intranuclear capsid antigen brown. Capsid antigen is generally found only in the superficial layers of tissue. The presence of capsid antigen indicates infectiousness.

Electron Microscopy

Electron microscopy is extremely time-consuming and insensitive compared with other diagnostic methods. Genital wart tissues contain only 1/10,000 as many virions as common skin warts, and electron microscopy is therefore not a practical diagnostic procedure.

TREATMENT

The treatment of genital warts may be frustrating since it often requires many office visits and recurrence is quite common. HPV has been recovered from seemingly uninvolved margins of surgical resection of condylomata, perhaps accounting for some clinical recurrences of the lesion. Recurrence results from a failure to eradicate completely all HPV-containing epithelial cells or from reinfection by infected sexual partners. Local treatment entails the application of antimetabolites or caustic agents (e.g. podophyllin, trichloroacetic acid, or 5-fluorouracil), cryotherapy, electrodesiccation, or surgical removal. Patients with internal (intraurethral, rectal, cervical, vaginal)

warts should be referred for appropriate specialist treatment. All women with warts should have a Papanicolaou smear to rule out coexistent CIN.

Although laser surgery is often used, its efficacy compared with that of other methods has not been established. A serious drawback of laser therapy is the destruction of the lesion without any histologic evaluation to rule out malignancy. When condylomata are large, confluent, necrotic, and rapidly growing, and the patient is old or immunoincompetent, the lesion should be properly biopsied before being treated by laser or any other locally destructive therapy. The patient should also be carefully followed. Intralesional and intramuscular injection of interferon has limited efficacy and significant adverse side-effects. The necessity for treatment of all patients with subclinical infection has not been established.

The treatment of bowenoid papulosis or other clinical forms of genital intraepithelial neoplasia should be referred to dermatologists or gynecologists familiar with these entities. Superficial destruction or excision is frequently curative. Extensive or mutilating surgical procedures are not recommended because of reports of spontaneous remission, low malignant potential, and the possibility of surrounding latent infection. However, close patient follow-up with biopsies is mandatory.

Picture credits for this chapter are as follows: Fig 12.19 courtesy of Woodruff JD, Parmley TH: Atlas of Gynecologic Pathology. New York, Gower Medical Publishing, 1988; Fig 12.20 courtesy of Marilynne McKay, MD; Fig 12.27 courtesy of Michael Campion, MD; Figs 12.23, 12.24, 12.28, and 12.29 courtesy of Richard Reid, MD; Figs 12.11 and 12.31 courtesy of Heidi Watts, PA-C; Fig 12.12 courtesy of D.R. Popkin, MD; Fig 12.30 courtesy of National Testing Laboratories Inc; Figs 12.35 to 12.37 and 12.43 courtesy of J. Michael Hall, DSS; Fig. 12.39 courtesy of Stevens A, Lowe J, Histology. London, Mosby, 1992; Fig 12.47 courtesy of Beth Unger, MD; Figs. 12.48 and 12.49 courtesy of Attila Lörincz, PhD; Fig 12.51 courtesy of Nancy Kiviat, MD.

BIBLIOGRAPHY

Beckmann AM, Myerson D, Daling JR, et al.: Detection and localisation of human papillomavirus DNA in human genital condylomas by in-situ hybridization with biotinylated probes. J Med Virol 16:265, 1985.

Beutner KR: Bridging the gap: notes of a wart watcher. Arch Derm 126:1432–1435, 1990.

Bonfiglio TA, Stoler MH: Human papillomavirus and cancer of the uterine cervis. Human Pathol 19:621, 1988.

Demeter LM, Stoler MH, Bonnez W: Penile intraepithelial neoplasia: clinical presentation and an analysis of the physical state of human papillomavirus DNA. J Infect Dis 168: 38, 1993.

Ferenczy A, Mitao M, Nagai N, et al.: Latent papillomavirus and recurring genital warts. N Engl J Med 313:784, 1985.

Ferris DG, Payne P, Frisch LE, et al.: Cervicography: adjunctive cervical cancer screening by primary care clinicians. J Family Practice 37(2):1588–164, 1993.

Gissman L, de Villiers EM, zur Hausen H: Analysis of human genital warts (condylomata acuminata) and other genital tumors for human papillomavirus type 6 DNA. Int J Cancer 29:143, 1982.

Greenberg MD, Ruttledge LH, Reid R, et al.: A double-blind randoming trial 80.5% podofilox and placebo for the treatment of genital warts. Obst Gynecol 77:735–739, 1991.

Gross G, Hagedorn M, Ikenberg H, et al.: Bowenoid papulosis. Arch Dermatol 121:858, 1985.

Grubb G: Human papillomavirus and cervical neoplasia: epidemiological considerations. Int J Epidemiol 15:1, 1986.

Guijon FB, Paraskeras M, Brunham R, et al.: The association of sexually transmitted diseases with cervical intraepithelial neoplasia: a case-control study. Am J Obstet Gynecol 151:185, 1985.

Howley PM (editorial): On human papillomaviruses. N Engl J Med 315:1089, 1986.

Jenson AB, Kurman RJ, Lancaster WD: Human papillomavirus. In: Belshe RB (ed): Textbook of Human Virology. Littleton, Mass, PSG Publishing, pp 951–968, 1984.

Kirnbauer R, Hubbert NL, Wheeler CM, Becker TM, Lowy DR, Schiller JT: A virus-like particle enzyme-linked immunosorbent assay detects serum antibodies in a majority of women infected with human papillomavirus type 16. J Natl Cancer Instit 86(7): 494–499, 1994.

Kiviat NB, Koutsky LA, Paavonen JA, et al.: Prevalence of genital papillomavirus infection among women attending a college student health clinic or a sexually transmitted disease clinic. J Infect Dis 151:293–302, 1989.

Koutsky LA, Holmes KK, Critchlow CW, et al.: A cohort study of the risk of cervical intraepithelial neoplasia grade 2 or 3 in relation to papillomavirus infection. N Engl J Med 327, 1272–1278, 1992.

Lever WF, Schaumberg-Lever G: Histopathology of the Skin. 6th edn. Philadelphia, JB Lippincott, 1983.

Mitchell H, Drake M, Medley G, et al.: Prospective evaluation of risk of cervical cancer after cytologic evidence of human papillomavirus infection. Lancet 573, 1986.

Nuovo GJ, Delvenne P, MacConnell P, et al.: Correlation of histology and detection of human papillomavirus DNA in vulvar cancers. Gynecol Oncol 43:275–280, 1991.

Oriel JD: Genital wars. In: Holmes KK, Mårdh PA, Sparling PF, Wiesner PJ (eds): Sexually Transmitted Diseases. New York, McGraw-Hill, pp 496–507, 1984.

Reid R, Greenberg M, Jenson AB, et al.: Sexually transmitted papillomaviral infections: 1. The anatomic distribution and pathologic grade of neoplastic lesions associated with different viral types. Am J Obstet Gynecol 156:212, 1987.

Reid R, Scalzi P: Genital warts and cervical cancer: VII. An improved colposcopic index for differentiating benign papillomaviral infection from high-grade cervical intraepithelial neoplasia. Am J Obstet Gynecol 153:611, 1985.

Reid R, Stanhope CR, Herschmann BR, et al.: Genital warts and cervical cancer: 1. Evidence of an association between sub-clinical papillomavirus infection and cervical malignancy. Cancer 50:377, 1982.

Reid R (ed): Obstet Gynecol Clin N Am 14(June 1987) (entire issue).

Rush-Presbyterian-St. Luke's Medical Centre, Chicago, and Sinai Hospital of Detroit: Human Papillomavirus and Squamous Carcinoma. Second International Conference. Chicago, October 27–29, pp 1–90, 1986.

Southern EM: Detection of specific sequences among DNA fragments separated by gel electrophoresis. J Mol Biol 98:503, 1975.

Spitzer M, et al.: Comparative utility of repeat Papanicolaou smears, cervicography and colposcopy in the evaluation of atypical Pap smears. Obstet Gynecol 69:731, 1987.

Von Krogh G: Genito and papillomavirus infection: diagnostic and therapeutic objectives in the light of current epidemiological observations. Int J STD AIDS 2:391–404, 1991.

Wade TR, Kopf AW, Ackerman AB, et al.: Bowenoid papulosis of the genitalia. Arch Dermatol 115:306, 1979.

CHAPTER THIRTEEN

Viral Hepatitis

C N Shapiro and M J Alter

INTRODUCTION

Five human hepatitis viruses — hepatitis viruses A through E — have been characterized to date. The corresponding clinical entities caused by each of these viruses are referred to as hepatitis A, B, C, delta, and E, respectively (*Fig. 13.1*). Hepatitis A virus (HAV) is transmitted predominantly by the fecal–oral route and can be transmitted between sexual partners. Hepatitis B virus (HBV), hepatitis C virus (HCV), and hepatitis D virus (HDV) are bloodborne viruses, and both parenteral and sexual transmission of these viruses occurs. Hepatitis E virus (HEV) is transmitted by the fecal–oral route, and sexual transmission has not been documented. Other hepatitis viruses have been recently described (e.g., "hepatitis G"), but their role in causing disease and their epidemiologic features need to be determined.

In the USA, an estimated 47% of acute viral hepatitis is due to hepatitis A; 34%, hepatitis B; 16%, hepatitis C; and 3%, other possible viral agents (*Fig. 13.2*). The clinical presentation of acute infection with each of these viruses is similar (*Fig. 13.3*), with jaundice (*Fig. 13.4*) and elevation of alanine aminotransferase (ALT) and other liver enzymes as manifestations of hepatitis. Diagnosis therefore depends on the use of specific tests for serologic markers (*Figs. 13.5–13.7*). The epidemiology of these viruses is determined by a variety of factors, including their modes of transmission, which are in turn determined by the body fluids in which each virus is found in infected persons.

Among adolescents and adults, the sexual transmission of HAV, HBV, HCV, and HDV is an important route of transmission. With the availability of vaccines to prevent HAV, HBV, and HDV transmission, specific interventions exist to protect persons who are at risk of acquiring these viruses through sexual activity.

HEPATITIS A

EPIDEMIOLOGY

Hepatitis A is caused by infection with HAV, a nonenveloped RNA agent, which is classified as a picornavirus. HAV replicates in the liver, is shed in the feces, and peak titers occur during the 2 weeks before and 1 week after the onset of illness. Virus is also present in serum and saliva during this period, though in concentrations several orders of magnitude less than in feces. Thus, the most common mode of HAV transmission is fecal–oral, with the virus being transmitted from person-to-person between household contacts or sex partners, or via contaminated food or water (*Fig. 13.8*). The transmission between sex partners occurs through oral–anal contact, and can occur both between heterosexuals and same-sex contacts. Since viremia occurs in acute infection, bloodborne HAV transmission can occur, but it has been infrequently reported. Although HAV is present in low concentrations in the saliva of infected persons, it has not been shown that saliva plays a role in transmission.

HAV infection is distributed globally, and geographic areas can be characterized by the prevalence of antibodies to HAV (anti-HAV), indicating prior HAV infection in the general population (*Fig. 13.9*). Disease patterns differ in areas of differing endemicity, and correlate with the hygienic and sanitary conditions of a given geographic region. In countries with very poor sanitary and hygienic conditions, most persons are infected as young children, at an age when HAV infection is often asymptomatic; reported disease rates in these areas are low and outbreaks are rare. In countries with variable sanitary conditions, transmission can predominate in children, adolescents, or adults, depending on the geographic region. Paradoxically, because transmission in these areas often occurs in age groups when infection is symptomatic, but conditions which promote transmission are common, disease rates can be higher than in countries with very poor sanitary conditions. Community-wide epidemics contribute significantly to the burden of disease in regions with variable sanitation. In countries with very good sanitation and hygienic conditions, infection rates in children are generally low. In these countries, disease tends to occur in circumscribed groups, such as travelers to hepatitis A endemic areas, or as outbreaks among specific risk groups, such as intravenous drug users or homosexually active men.

In the USA, hepatitis A has occurred in large nationwide epidemics approximately every 10 years, with the last increase in cases in 1989 (*Fig. 13.10*). The highest disease rates are in children aged 5–14 years old (*Fig. 13.11*). Community-wide outbreaks, with children often playing an

BASIC FEATURES OF VIRAL HEPATITIS

	HEPATITIS A	HEPATITIS B	PARENTERALLY TRANSMITTED NON-A, NON-B HEPATITIS (PT-NANB)	DELTA HEPATITIS	ENTERICALLY TRANSMITTED NON-A, NON-B HEPATITIS (ET-NANB)
INCUBATION PERIOD	15–50 days (mean 28)	60–180 days (mean 120)	15–180 days (mean 42)	15–60 days	15–60 days (mean 42)
TRANSMISSION	Fecal–oral	Bloodborne Sexual	Bloodborne Sexual	Bloodborne Sexual	Fecal–oral
PROGRESSION TO CHRONICITY	No	Occasionally	Occasionally	Occasionally	No
ETIOLOGIC AGENT	Hepatitis A Virus (HAV)	Hepatitis B Virus (HBV)	Hepatitis C Virus (HCV)	Hepatitis D Virus (HDV)	Hepatitis E Virus (HEV)
COMMENTS				Occurs only as coinfection with HBV or as superinfection of HBV carrier	Does not occur in USA

Fig. 13.1 Basic features of viral hepatitis.

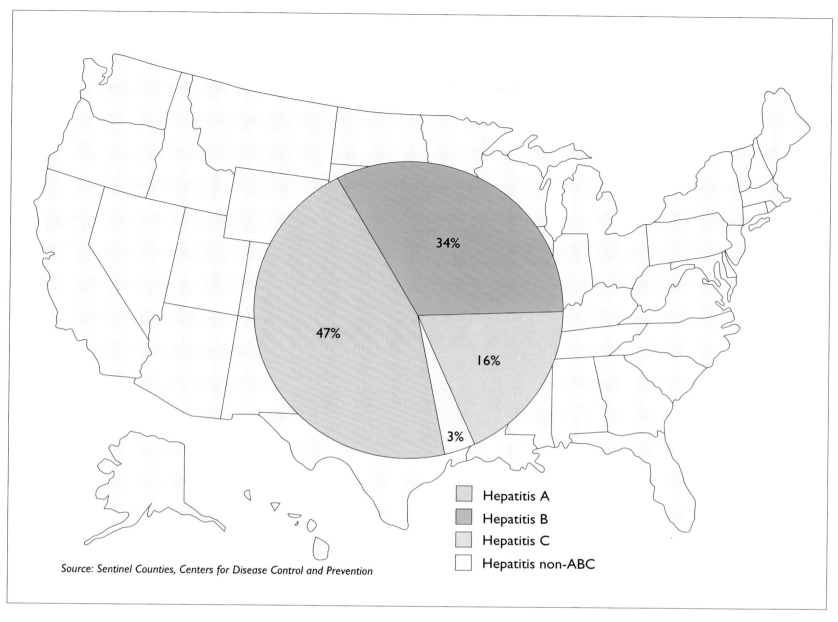

Source: Sentinel Counties, Centers for Disease Control and Prevention

34%

47%

16%

3%

Hepatitis A

Hepatitis B

Hepatitis C

Hepatitis non-ABC

Fig. 13.2 Relative proportions of acute viral hepatitis by type, in the USA, 1982–1993.

SYMPTOMS OF ACUTE VIRAL HEPATITIS

- Malaise
- Anorexia
- Nausea
- Abdominal pain
- Jaundice
- Dark urine
- Fever, rash, arthralgias
- Pruritus

Fig. 13.3 Symptoms of acute viral hepatitis. The clinical symptoms of acute viral hepatitis caused by the various hepatitis viruses are similar. Serologic tests are necessary to establish a diagnosis.

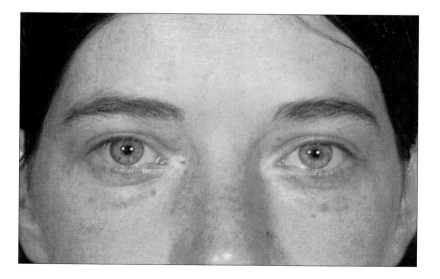

Fig. 13.4 Jaundice. This is characterized by yellowing of the skin and sclerae. Other findings in patients with hepatitis may include abdominal pain under the right costal margin, hepatomegaly, dark urine, and pale stools.

SEROLOGIC MARKERS OF HEPATITIS VIRUSES

Hepatitis A

HAV	Hepatitis A virus; etiologic agent of hepatitis A, also known as infectious hepatitis; a picornavirus with a single serotype.
anti-HAV	Total antibody to HAV; detectable at onset of symptoms; lifetime persistence.
IgM anti-HAV	IgM-class antibody indicating recent infection with HAV.

Hepatitis B

HBV	Hepatitis B virus; etiologic agent of hepatitis B, also known as serum hepatitis; agent also known as Dane particle.
HBsAg	Hepatitis B surface antigen; produced in large quantities in serum both as whole virus and as smaller surface antigen particles; originally known as Australian antigen; several subtypes.
HBeAg	Hepatitis B e antigen; soluble antigen that correlates with HBV replication and infectivity; conformational antigen of HBcAg.
HBcAg	Hepatitis B core antigen; found within the core of the virus; no commercial test available.
anti-HBs	Antibody to hepatitis B surface antigen; indicates immune response to HBV infection, due either to passive acquisition, immune response to infection, or vaccination
anti-HBc	Antibody to hepatitis B core antigen; indicates past or present infection with HBV; not present in vaccine-induced immunity.
IgM anti-HBc	IgM-class antibody to HBcAg; indicates recent infection with HBV.

Delta hepatitis

HDV	Delta virus; etiologic agent of delta hepatitis; only causes infection in the presence of HBV.
HDAg	Delta antigen; detectable in early acute infection.
anti-HD	Antibody to delta antigen; indicates past or present infection.

Hepatitis C

HCV	Hepatitis C virus; etiologic agent of most parenterally transmitted non-A, non-B hepatitis; single stranded RNA virus classified in the family Flaviviridae.
anti-HCV	Antibody to hepatitis C virus; does not distinguish between acute and chronic infection. Detectable in 90 percent of patients with hepatitis C; interval between onset of disease and seroconversion may be prolonged.

Source: *Adapted from Centers for Disease Control and Prevention. Hepatitis B virus infection. A comprehensive strategy for eliminating transmission in the United States through immunization. MMWR, in press*

Fig. 13.5 Serologic markers of hepatitis viruses.

USE OF SEROLOGIC MARKERS IN THE DIAGNOSIS OF ACUTE HEPATITIS

HBsAg	IgM anti-HBc	IgM anti-HAV	Anti-HCV	DIAGNOSIS
+	+	–	+/–	Early acute hepatitis B
–	+	–	+/–	Late acute hepatitis B (window period)
–	–	+	+/–	Acute hepatitis A
+	–	+	+/–	Acute hepatitis A in HBV carrier
–	–	–	+	Compatible with acute hepatitis C
+	–	–	+	Compatible with acute hepatitis C in HBV carrier

Fig. 13.6 Use of serologic markers in the diagnosis of acute hepatitis. Antibody to hepatitis C virus (HCV) may be present in any of these conditions, or may be present in persons without serologic markers of hepatitis A and hepatitis B. Antibody to HCV indicates HCV infection, but does not distinguish between acute infection, chronic infection, or recovery.

ADDITIONAL DIAGNOSTIC PATTERNS AND INTERPRETATIONS OF HEPATITIS B TEST RESULTS

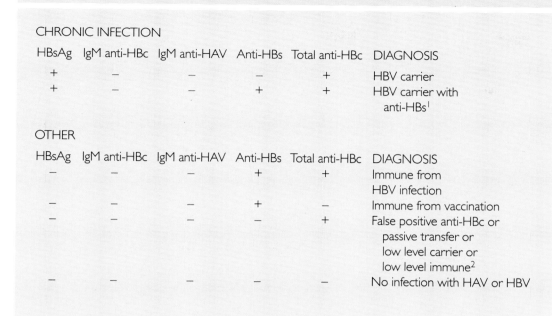

CHRONIC INFECTION

HBsAg	IgM anti-HBc	IgM anti-HAV	Anti-HBs	Total anti-HBc	DIAGNOSIS
+	−	−	−	+	HBV carrier
+	−	−	+	+	HBV carrier with anti-HBs[1]

OTHER

HBsAg	IgM anti-HBc	IgM anti-HAV	Anti-HBs	Total anti-HBc	DIAGNOSIS
−	−	−	+	+	Immune from HBV infection
−	−	−	+	−	Immune from vaccination
−	−	−	−	+	False positive anti-HBc or passive transfer or low level carrier or low level immune[2]
−	−	−	−	−	No infection with HAV or HBV

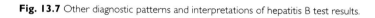

[1] <1% of carriers can have HBsAg and anti-HBs present simultaneously.

[2] Some persons with anti-HBc alone are low level carriers with subdetectable HBsAg, or low level immune with subdetectable anti-HBs.

Fig. 13.7 Other diagnostic patterns and interpretations of hepatitis B test results.

MODES OF TRANSMISSION OF HEPATITIS A VIRUS

CLOSE PERSONAL CONTACT

    Household contact
    Sexual contact
    Day care centers

CONTAMINATED FOOD/WATER

    Infected foodhandlers
    Shellfish

BLOOD EXPOSURES (RARE)

    Injecting drug users
    Blood transfusion

Fig. 13.8 Modes of transmission of hepatitis A virus (HAV).

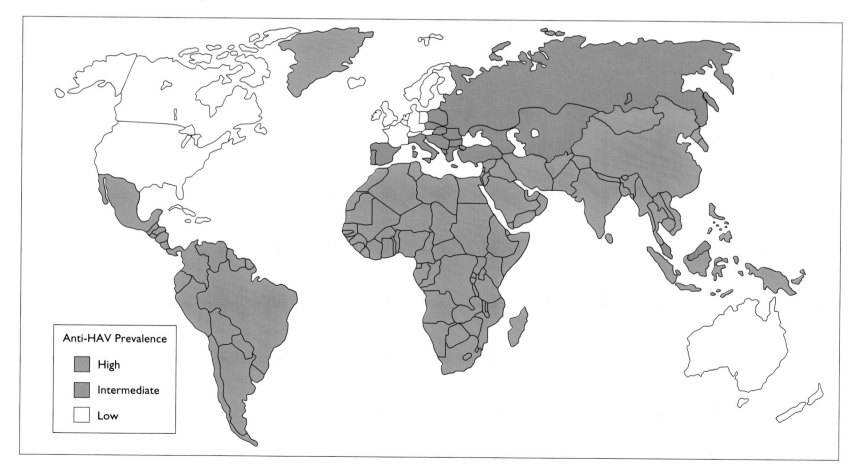

Anti-HAV Prevalence

- High
- Intermediate
- Low

Fig. 13.9 Global prevalence of antibody to HAV.

important role in disease transmission, account for a large number of cases. In 1993, approximately 24,000 persons were reported in the USA with hepatitis A. Among cases reported to the CDC, the most frequently reported risk factor was household or sexual contact with a person with hepatitis, followed by day-care attendance or employment, recent international travel, and association with a suspected food or waterborne outbreak (*Fig. 13.12*). Many persons with hepatitis A do not identify risk factors; their source of infection may be other infected persons who are asymptomatic. Based on testing from the Third National Health and Nutrition Examination Survey (NHANES III)

survey, conducted in 1989–1991, the prevalence of total anti-HAV is 33% among the general population in the USA (CDC, unpublished data).

Although, in the USA, the percentage of males with hepatitis A who report a history of male homosexual activity is generally less than 10%, hepatitis A outbreaks among homosexual men have occasionally been reported in urban areas, both in the USA and abroad. For example, in 1991–1992, outbreaks among homosexual and bisexual men occurred in New York City, Denver, and San Francisco, USA; in Toronto and Montreal, Canada; and in Melbourne, Australia. A case-control study in New York City found cases

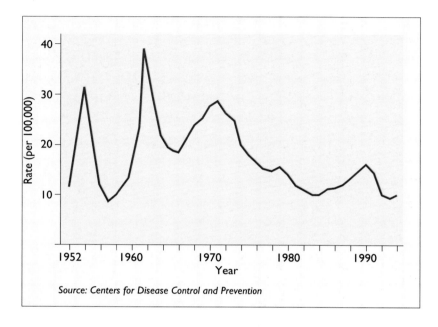

Source: Centers for Disease Control and Prevention

Fig. 13.10 Reported hepatitis A cases (per 100,000 population) USA, 1952–1993.

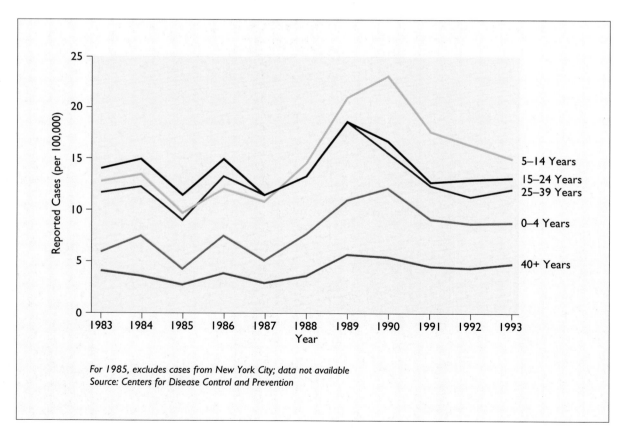

For 1985, excludes cases from New York City; data not available
Source: Centers for Disease Control and Prevention

Fig. 13.11 Reported hepatitis A cases (per 100,000 population) by age, USA, 1983–1993.

to have more anonymous sex partners and to be more likely to have engaged in group sex than controls; oral–anal intercourse (oral role) and digital–rectal intercourse (digital role) were associated with illness. Seroprevalence studies and prospective studies conducted in the late 1970s and early 1980s have found varying results for the risk of hepatitis A associated with homosexual activity (*Fig. 13.13*).

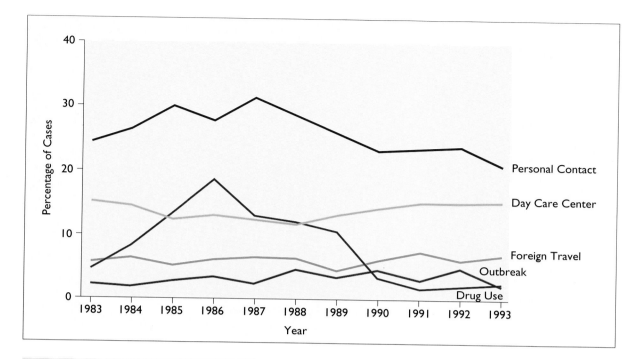

Fig. 13.12 Risk factors reported for hepatitis A by mutually exclusive groups, USA, 1983–1993. (Source: Centers for Disease Control and Prevention.)

CROSS-SECTIONAL AND PROSPECTIVE STUDIES EVALUATING THE RISK OF HEPATITIS A AMONG HOMOSEXUAL MEN

Fig. 13.13 Cross-sectional and prospective studies evaluating the risk of hepatitis A among homosexual men.

CROSS-SECTIONAL STUDIES

LOCATION	GROUP	ANTI-HAV PREVALENCE
Amsterdam, Netherlands (Couthino *et al.*)	Homosexual men Heterosexual men	30% 12%
Seattle, Washington (Corey *et al.*)	Homosexual men Heterosexual men	42% 16%
Nova Scotia, Canada (McFarlane *et al.*)	Homosexual men Heterosexual men	42% 39%

PROSPECTIVE STUDIES

LOCATION	GROUP	LENGTH OF FOLLOW-UP	ANTI-HAV SEROCONVERSION (%)
Amsterdam, Netherlands (Couthino *et al.*)	Homosexual men Heterosexual men	1.9 years 0.5 years	14%* 0%
Seattle, Washington (Corey *et al.*)	Homosexual men Heterosexual men	1 year 1 year	22% 0%

* Attack rate calculated by the product limit method

CLINICAL MANIFESTATIONS

The incubation period of hepatitis A is 15–50 days, with an average of 28 days. The illness caused by HAV infection typically has an abrupt onset of signs and symptoms that include fever, malaise, anorexia, nausea, abdominal discomfort, dark urine and jaundice (*Fig. 13.3*). Hepatitis A usually does not last longer than 2 months, though some individuals may have prolonged or relapsing signs and symptoms for up to 6 months. The likelihood of having symptoms with HAV infection is directly related to age. In children younger than 6 years of age, most infections are asymptomatic; among older children and adults, infection is usually symptomatic (*Fig. 13.14*).

HAV infection occasionally produces fulminant hepatitis A. The case-fatality rate among reported cases of all ages is approximately 0.3%, but can be higher among older persons (approximately 2% among patients of more than 40 years of age). HAV infection does not result in chronic infection or chronic liver disease.

Diagnosis

Virtually all patients with acute hepatitis A have detectable IgM antibodies to hepatitis A virus (IgM anti-HAV). The diagnosis of acute HAV infection is therefore confirmed during the acute or early convalescent phase of infection by the presence of IgM anti-HAV (*Fig. 13.15*). IgM anti-HAV generally disappears within 6 months after the onset of symptoms. IgG anti-HAV, which appears in the convalescent phase of infection, remains detectable in serum for the lifetime of the individual and confers enduring protection against disease. Commercial diagnostic tests are available for the detection of IgM and total anti-HAV in serum.

Treatment

As HAV infection is self-limited and does not result in chronic infection or chronic liver disease, treatment is generally supportive. Hospitalization may be necessary in patients who are dehydrated from nausea and vomiting, or who have fulminant hepatitis A. Medications that might cause liver damage, or that are metabolized by the liver, should be used with caution. No specific restrictions on diet or activity are necessary. In patients with fulminant hepatitis A, agents such as prostaglandin E and interferon have been studied with inconclusive results; liver transplantation is successful in some patients.

Prevention

General measures for the prevention of hepatitis A include the maintenance of good personal hygiene, with attention to handwashing before preparing food; provision of safe drinking water; and adequate disposal of sanitary waste (*Fig. 13.16*). To help control and prevent hepatitis A in communities experiencing hepatitis A outbreaks among homosexual and bisexual men, health education messages should stress the modes of HAV transmission and the measures which can be taken to reduce the risk of transmission of any STD, including enterically transmitted agents such as HAV.

Two types of products are available for the prevention of hepatitis A, immune globulin (IG) and hepatitis A vaccine. IG is a solution of antibodies prepared from human plasma. It is made with a serial ethanol precipitation procedure which has been shown to inactivate both HBV and HIV. When administered intramuscularly prior to exposure to HAV, or within 2 weeks after exposure, IG is more than 85% effective in preventing hepatitis A. IG administration is recommended for a variety of exposure situations, including persons who are sexually active or household contacts of persons with hepatitis A (*Fig. 13.17*). IG may also be used for pre-exposure

FREQUENCY OF SYMPTOMS WITH ACUTE HEPATITIS A BY AGE	
Less than 3 years of age	< 5%
4 to 6 years of age	5%–10%
6 years of age and above	75%

Fig. 13.14 Frequency of symptoms with acute hepatitis A by age.

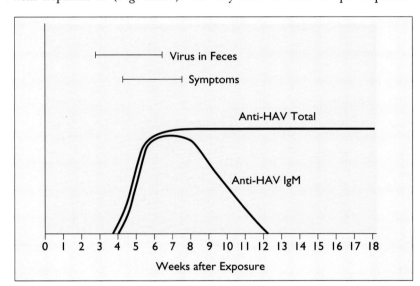

Fig. 13.15 Antibody response in hepatitis A. Symptoms, IgM anti-HAV, and total anti-HAV usually appear about 4 weeks after exposure. After several months IgM anti-HAV levels fall and only total anti-HAV is present.

PREVENTION OF HEPATITIS A
Good hygiene and sanitation
Immune globulin for postexposure prophylaxis
Hepatitis A vaccine for pre-exposure protection

Fig. 13.16 Measures for the prevention of hepatitis A.

INDICATIONS FOR IMMUNE GLOBULIN ADMINIS-TRATION FOR PROPHYLAXIS OF HEPATITIS A
POSTEXPOSURE Household and sexual contacts of hepatitis A cases Staff and children at a day care center where a child or employee is recognized to have acute hepatitis A Patrons of food establishments with an infected foodhandler with poor hygiene who handled uncooked foods or foods after cooking Selected settings where HAV transmission is occurring (hospitals, institutions)
PRE-EXPOSURE Travelers who elect not to receive hepatitis A vaccine

Fig. 13.17 Indications for immune globulin administration for prophylaxis of hepatitis A.

prophylaxis, e.g. individuals traveling to countries with endemic hepatitis A. The duration of protection is dependent on dose (*Fig. 13.18*).

Within the past several years, inactivated hepatitis A vaccines have been developed which have the potential to provide longterm protection against hepatitis A. These vaccines have been shown to be safe, highly immunogenic and highly efficacious. Immunogenicity studies indicate that between 99–100% of persons respond to one dose of hepatitis A vaccine, and that antibodies persist for at least several years after two doses of vaccine. Efficacy studies show that inactivated hepatitis A vaccines are 94–100% effective in preventing hepatitis A.

Fig. 13.19 lists the recommended doses and schedule for inactivated hepatitis A vaccine (HAVRIX®), manufactured by SmithKline Beecham Pharmaceuticals and licensed in the USA in 1995. Merck and Co. has applied for a license for another inactivated hepatitis A vaccine. Hepatitis A vaccine is recommended for individuals with a demonstrated risk of HAV infection, including men who have sex with men (*Fig. 13.20*). The targeted use of hepatitis A vaccine in communities experiencing hepatitis A outbreaks among homosexually active men should help protect such individuals. Prevaccination screening may be advisable, depending on the anti-HAV seroprevalence among potential vaccine recipients and the costs for screening and vaccination.

HEPATITIS B

EPIDEMIOLOGY

HBV is a DNA virus, with an outer envelope consisting of HBsAg and an inner core consisting of HBcAg, double-stranded DNA, and DNA poly-

merase. HBV is present in high titers in blood and exudates (e.g. skin lesions) of acutely and chronically infected persons. Moderate viral titers are found in semen, vaginal secretions and saliva. Other body fluids that do not contain blood or serous fluid, such as feces or urine, are not a source of HBV (*Fig. 13.21*). Thus, the three principal modes of HBV transmission are:

- Percutaneous (injecting drug use, blood or body fluid exposures among health-care workers, and blood transfusions)
- Sexual (heterosexual or male homosexual)
- Perinatal (from infected mothers to infants through blood exposure at the time of birth).

Transmission between siblings and other household contacts readily occurs, through contact with skin lesions such as eczema or impetigo; sharing of potentially blood-contaminated objects such as toothbrushes and razor blades; and occasionally through bites. Nosocomial outbreaks, although rare, have occurred because of the improper use or disinfection of medical devices (e.g. fingerstick devices, acupuncture needles), or from infected health-care workers to patients during invasive procedures. HBV infection occurs worldwide. Approximately 45% of the world population live in geographic areas with high HBV endemicity (> 8% of the general population are chronically infected); 43% in areas of moderate endemicity (2–7% are chronically infected); and 12% in areas of low endemicity (< 2% are chronically infected) (Fig. 13.22). Overall, an estimated 300 million persons worldwide are HBV carriers. Based on the NHANES III survey, the overall prevalence of chronic HBV infection among the general US population is 0.3%, with 0.1% among Whites and 1.1% among Blacks. Other seroprevalence studies conducted over the past several decades have identified a variety of groups at increased risk of HBV infection (Fig. 13.23).

The risk of sexual transmission among homosexual men and between heterosexual partners is well documented. Historically, HBV infection has been

RECOMMENDED DOSES OF IMMUNE GLOBULIN FOR HEPATITIS A PRE-EXPOSURE AND POSTEXPOSURE PROPHYLAXIS

SETTING	DURATION OF COVERAGE	IMMUNE GLOBULIN DOSE*
Pre-exposure	Short term (1–3 months)	0.02 ml/kg
	Long term (3–5 months)	0.06 ml/kg Repeat every 5 months if continued exposure
Postexposure		0.02 ml/kg

* IG is to be given by intramuscular injection in the deltoid muscle or the buttocks. For children < 24 months of age, it can be given in the anterolateral thigh muscle.

Adapted from: Centers for Disease Control and Prevention. Prevention of hepatitis A through active or passive immunization: Recommendations of the Advisory Committee on Immunization Practices (ACIP), MMWR (In press).

Fig. 13.18 Recommended doses of immune globulin for hepatitis A pre-exposure and postexposure prophylaxis.

RECOMMENDED DOSES OF HAVRIX® (HEPATITIS A VACCINE, INACTIVATED, SMITHKLINE BEECHAM PHARMACEUTICALS)

GROUP	AGE	DOSE (EL.U.*)	VOLUME	No. DOSES	SCHEDULE (MONTHS)**
Children and adolescents	2–18 years	360 EL.U.	0.5 ml	3	0, 1, 6–12
Adults	> 18 years	1440 EL.U.	1.0 ml	2	0, 6–12

* EL.U.–ELISA units

** 0 months represents timing of the initial dose; subsequent numbers represent months after the initial dose.

Adapted from: Centers for Disease Control and Prevention. Prevention of hepatitis A through active or passive immunization: Recommendations of the Advisory Committee on Immunization Practices (ACIP), MMWR (In press)

Fig. 13.19 Recommended doses of HAVRIX® (inactivated hepatitis A vaccine) (use of trade names is for identification purposes only and does not imply endorsement by the US Public Health Service).

GROUPS RECOMMENDED TO RECEIVE HEPATITIS A VACCINE

Persons traveling or working in countries with high or intermediate endemicity of infection

Person living in communities with high rates of HAV infection and periodic hepatitis A outbreaks

Men who have sex with men

Drug users

Persons who work with experimentally HAV-infected non-human primates or with HAV in a laboratory setting

Persons with chronic liver disease

Fig. 13.20 Groups recommended for hepatitis A vaccination.

CONCENTRATION OF HEPATITIS B VIRUS IN VARIOUS BODY FLUIDS

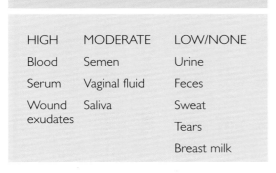

HIGH	MODERATE	LOW/NONE
Blood	Semen	Urine
Serum	Vaginal fluid	Feces
Wound exudates	Saliva	Sweat
		Tears
		Breast milk

Fig. 13.21 Concentration of hepatitis B virus (HBV) in various body fluids.

endemic among homosexual men. Studies among patients attending STD clinics have shown the prevalence of HBV infection among homosexual men to be 3 to 20 times higher compared with heterosexual patients or blood donor controls (*Fig. 13.24*). From these studies, factors associated with a higher prevalence of HBV infection include a history of multiple episodes of STDs; large numbers of sexual partners; long duration of homosexual activity; and receptive anal intercourse. The presumed mechanisms of transmission include transfer of HBV in semen or in exudates from genital lesions to open mucous membrane and skin lesions from infections or trauma.

Heterosexual partners of persons with acute or chronic HBV infection are also at substantial risk of HBV infection. Susceptible heterosexual partners of persons with acute hepatitis B followed for 3–12 months had a risk of infection of 20–27% (*Fig. 13.25*). The prevalence of serologic markers indicating past or present HBV infection (hepatitis B surface antigen [HBsAg] or antibody to HBsAg [anti-HBs]) among household (including sexual) contacts of persons with chronic HBV infection was two to 10 times higher compared with household contacts of noninfected persons. Spouses had higher rates than other household members (*Fig. 13.26*).

As with homosexual men, a history of multiple episodes of STDs, duration of sexual activity, and large numbers of sexual partners, are associated with an increased risk of HBV infection among heterosexual men and women (*Fig. 13.27*). For example, in a US study of an STD clinic's patients and a university student population, after controlling for age, gender and race, the number of lifetime sexual partners in both populations was directly associated with the prevalence of HBV infection (*Fig. 13.28*). Population-based serosurveys have also found an association between sexual activity and HBV infection. In the NHANES II serosurvey, conducted between 1976 and 1980, the prevalence of HBV infection among persons who were positive in the fluorescent treponemal antibody (FTA) test was 49%, compared with 5% among persons who were FTA-negative.

Changes in sexual practices and other risk behaviors in response to the AIDS epidemic have resulted in substantial changes in the distribution of hepatitis B cases during the past decade. Nevertheless, sexual transmission currently accounts for more reported cases than any other mode of transmission. After correcting for under-reporting and asymptomatic infections, an estimated 200,000–300,000 new HBV infections have occurred annually in the USA

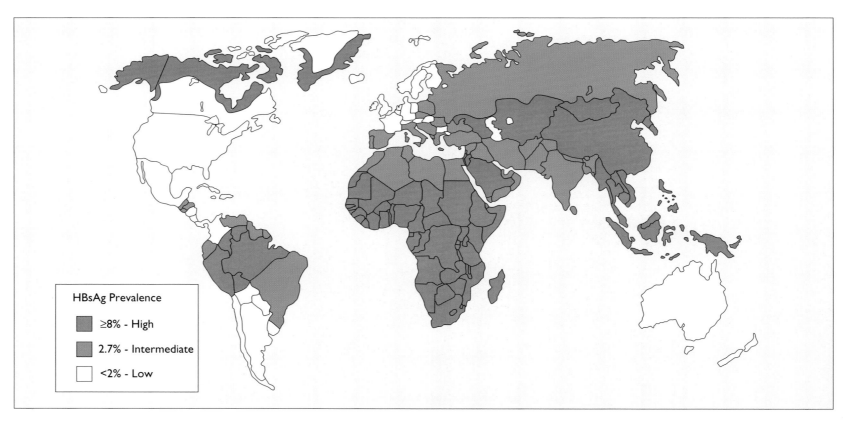

HBsAg Prevalence

≥8% - High

2.7% - Intermediate

<2% - Low

Fig. 13.22 Global prevalence of chronic HBV infection (determined by the percentage of the population positive for hepatitis B surface antigen or HBsAg).

PREVALENCE OF HEPATITIS B VIRUS SEROLOGIC MARKERS IN VARIOUS POPULATION GROUPS

POPULATION GROUP	PREVALENCE OF SEROLOGIC MARKERS OF HBV INFECTION	
	HBsAg (%)	ANY MARKER (%)
Immigrants/refugees from areas of high HBV endemicity	13	70–85
Alaska Natives/Pacific Islanders	5–15	40–70
Clients in institutions for the developmentally disabled	10–20	35–80
Users of illicit injection drugs	7	60–80
Sexually active homosexual men	6	35–80
Household contacts of HBV carriers	3–6	30–60
Hemodialysis patients	3–10	20–80
Health care workers — frequent blood contact	1–2	15–30
Prisoners (male)	1–8	10–80
Staff of institutions for the developmentally disabled	1	10–25
Heterosexuals with multiple partners	0.5	5–20
Health care workers — no or infrequent blood contact	0.3	3–10
Blood donors (per donation)	0.3	2
General population (NHANES III)*		
Blacks	1.1	11.6
Whites	0.1	3.2

* NHANES: National Health and Nutrition Examination Survey
Adapted from McQuillan et al.

Fig. 13.23 Prevalence of HBV serologic markers in various population groups.

PREVALENCE OF HEPATITIS B VIRUS INFECTION AMONG GROUPS OF MEN WITH DIFFERENT SEXUAL BEHAVIORS

GROUP	REFERENCE	PERCENT POSITIVE	
		HBsAg	ANTI-HBs
Homosexual STD Clinic Men	Jeffries	3.9	ND*
Heterosexual STD Clinic Men	et al.	0.2	ND
Blood Donors		0.1	ND
Homosexual STD Clinic Men	Fulford	3.2	21.7
Heterosexual STD Clinic Men	and	2.6	5.1
Blood Donors	Dane	0.2	0.6
Homosexual STD Clinic Men	Szmuness	4.3	48.1
Heterosexual STD Clinic Men	et al.	1.3	17.9
Blood Donors		0.3	7.3
Homosexual Men	Dietzman	5.6	39.6
Heterosexual STD Clinic Men		0.9	4.5
Controls (routine phys. exam)		0.9	4.5
Homosexual STD Clinic Men	Schreder et al.	6.1	61.5

* ND = not done.

Fig. 13.24 Prevalence of HBV infection among groups of men with different sexual behaviors.

INCIDENCE OF HEPATITIS B VIRUS INFECTION IN CONTACTS OF PERSONS WITH ACUTE HEPATITIS B

AUTHORS	TYPE OF CONTACT	OBSERVATION PERIOD	NO. INFECTED/ NO. FOLLOWED (%)
Redeker *et al.*	Heterosexual partners	5 months	9/33 (27.3)
Koff *et al.*	Heterosexual partners	12 months	3/13 (23.1)
	Other household contacts		0/68 (0.0)
Peters *et al.*	Heterosexual partners	3–12 months	2/10 (20.0)
	Household children		4/41 (9.8)
	Adults		3/60 (5.0)

Fig. 13.25 Incidence of HBV infection in contacts of persons with acute hepatitis B.

PREVALENCE OF HEPATITIS B VIRUS INFECTION IN HOUSEHOLD CONTACTS OF HBsAg CARRIERS COMPARED WITH NONCARRIERS

AUTHORS	TYPES OF CONTACT	CONTACTS OF HBsAg CARRIERS (%)		CONTROLS (%)	
		HBsAg +	ANTI-HBs +	HBsAg +	ANTI-HBs +
Irwin *et al.*	Spouses	0	58.8	0	18.2
	Children	5.7	11.4	0	4.5
Heathcote *et al.*	Sexual partners	9.1	36.4		
	Others	3.1	18.7	0	1.6
Szmuness *et al.*	Spouses	3.4	36.4		
	Children	3.6	8.9		
	Parents	8.2	34.2		
	Siblings	19.7	22.9		
	Total	6.7	23.4	0.8	7.3

Fig. 13.26 Prevalence of HBV infection in household contacts of HBsAg carriers compared with noncarriers.

PREVALENCE OF HBsAg OR ANTI-HBs IN STUDY GROUPS WHICH DIFFER ACCORDING TO SEXUAL BEHAVIOR

Fig. 13.27 Prevalence of HBsAg or anti-HBs in study groups which differ according to sexual behavior.

AUTHORS	STUDY	NUMBER OF SUBJECTS	POSITIVE (%) HBsAg+	ANTI-HBs+
Fulford *et al.*	Heterosexual women			
	0–2 sex partners within 6 mos.	339	ND*	1.4
	> 3 sex partners within 6 mos.	22	ND	18.2
Szmuness *et al.*	Heterosexual STD clinic patients	597	1.3	16.6
	Healthy adult blood donors	700	0.3	7.0
Papevangelou *et al.*	Female prostitutes	293	4.4	56.7
	Pregnant women	397	3.4	24.5
Adam *et al.*	Female prostitutes	272	5	20
	Nuns	30	10	23

* ND = not done or reported

during the past 10 years (*Fig. 13.29*). Since the mid1980s, however, the number of annual cases of acute hepatitis B reported to the CDC has decreased by approximately 50% (*Fig. 13.30*). Based upon risk-factor data collected by CDC, this decrease is believed to be due to behavior changes among homosexual men and drug users (*Fig. 13.31*). In more recent years, hepatitis B vaccination may also have had an impact in lowering disease rates. Among cases reported during

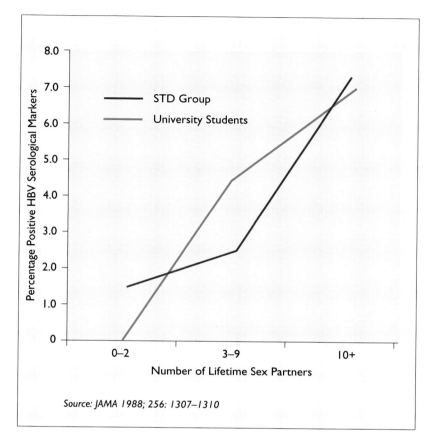

Fig. 13.28 Prevalence of HBV infection by sexual activity for white heterosexuals 18–25 years of age, with more than 12 years of education.

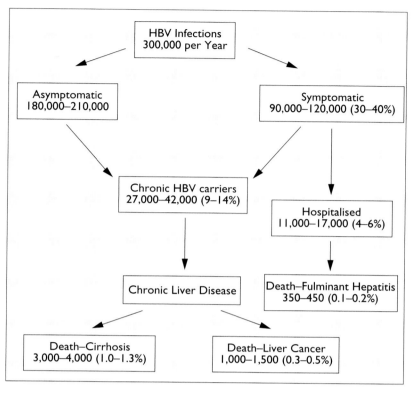

Fig. 13.29 Disease burden of acute and chronic HBV infection, showing the average annual number in all age groups, USA, 1980–1989 estimates. Overall, about 30–40% of HBV infections are symptomatic. In children and adults, about 9–14% of acute HBV infection will progress to chronic infection, and of these, 15–25% may result in premature deaths from either cirrhosis or liver cancer.

Fig. 13.30 Estimated incidence of acute hepatitis B, USA, 1978–1993. Although the incidence of acute hepatitis B has declined since the mid-1980s, the incidence in 1992–1993 is similar to that before the availability of hepatitis B vaccine.

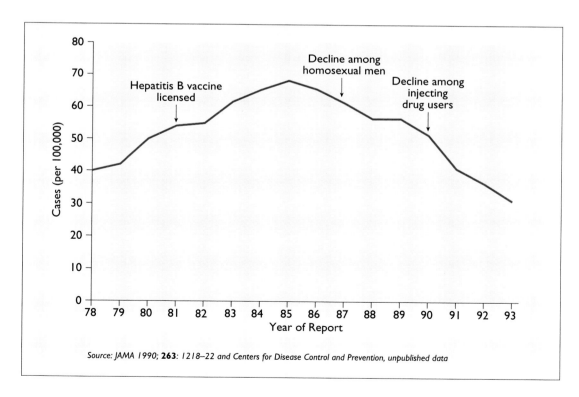

1992–1993 in the Sentinel Counties Study, a surveillance system operated by CDC in four US counties, the most frequently identified risk factor was heterosexual exposure to a contact with hepatitis or to multiple partners (41%), followed by injecting drug use (15%), homosexual activity (9%), household contact (2%), and health-care employment (1%) (*Fig. 13.32*).

CLINICAL MANIFESTATIONS

The incubation period of hepatitis B ranges from 2 months to 6 months (average 4 months). The onset of symptoms is gradual, and may include skin rashes and arthralgias, in addition to the usual symptoms of viral hepatitis (*Fig. 13.3*). Symptoms of acute hepatitis generally last 2–4 weeks, but fatigue and other symptoms may persist for several months. The clinical manifestations of hepatitis B are highly age-dependent. Infection rarely produces symptoms in infants; produces typical illness in only 5–15% of young children; and is symptomatic in 33–50% of adolescents and adults (*Fig. 13.33*). The number of deaths from acute infection is low (case fatality < 1%).

Acute HBV infection usually resolves with the development of protective antibodies, but may develop into chronic infection (the carrier state). Among the most serious consequences of hepatitis B are the sequelae associated with chronic HBV infection, including chronic hepatitis, cirrhosis, and liver cancer (*Fig. 13.34*). The risk of developing chronic HBV infection is inversely

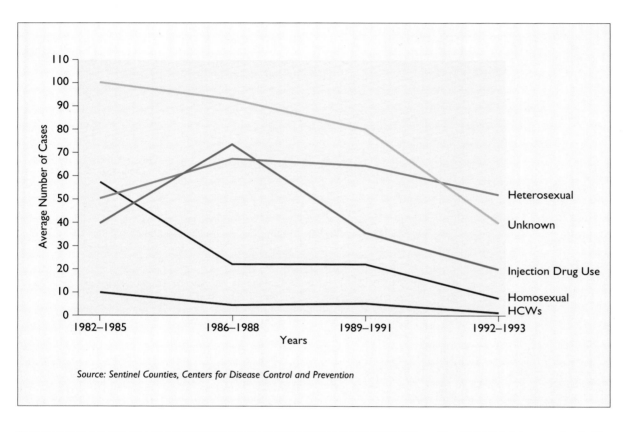

Source: Sentinel Counties, Centers for Disease Control and Prevention

Fig. 13.31 Number of reported cases of acute hepatitis B by selected risk factors, Sentinel Counties, USA, 1982–1993.

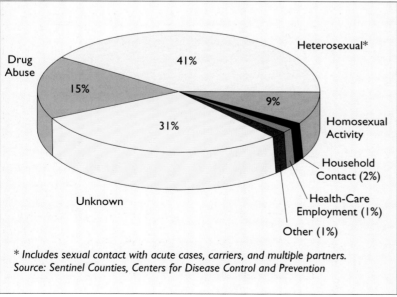

* Includes sexual contact with acute cases, carriers, and multiple partners.
Source: Sentinel Counties, Centers for Disease Control and Prevention

Fig. 13.32 Risk factors associated with reported cases of acute hepatitis B, Sentinel Counties, USA, 1992–1993. Note that heterosexual and homosexual sexual activity together account for 50% of all reported hepatitis B cases.

associated with the age at which infection is acquired (*Fig. 13.33*). Children less than 5 years old have a 20–50% risk of becoming carriers of the virus after acute infection, while older children and adults have a 5–10% risk of becoming carriers after acute infection. Persons with chronic infection have an estimated 15–25% lifetime risk of dying prematurely from cirrhosis or liver cancer.

A number of other clinical entities are associated with chronic hepatitis B. These include polyarteritis nodosa and glomerulonephritis. The pathogenesis of these diseases is thought to be due to the deposition of circulating HBsAg-antibody complexes in affected organs.

Diagnosis

As the clinical manifestations of acute hepatitis B are similar to other types of viral hepatitis, serologic testing is necessary to establish the diagnosis (*see Fig. 13.6*). Commercial assays to distinguish acute HBV infection, chronic HBV infection, susceptibility, and vaccine response are widely available. In

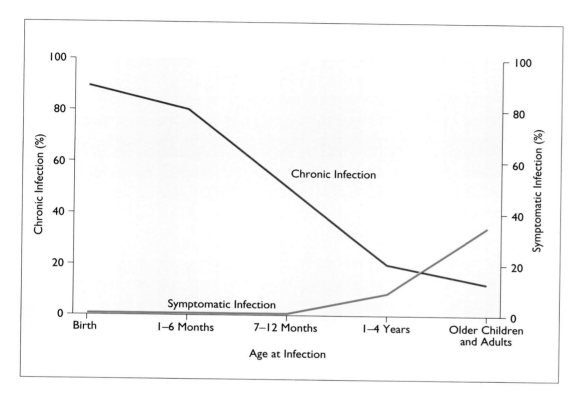

Fig. 13.33 Outcome of HBV infection by age. The frequency of symptoms with acute HBV infection is directly related to the age of acquisition. The risk of acute infection developing into chronic infection is inversely associated with age.

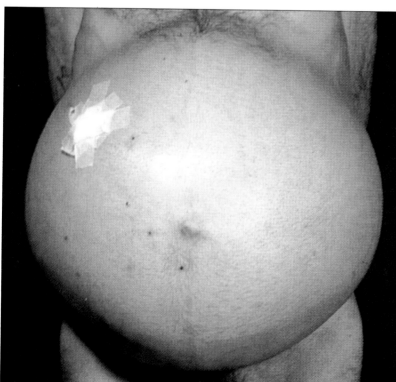

Fig. 13.34 Cirrhosis with ascites — an outcome of chronic HBV infection.

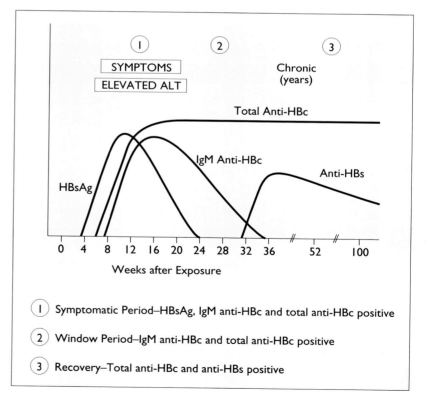

① Symptomatic Period–HBsAg, IgM anti-HBc and total anti-HBc positive

② Window Period–IgM anti-HBc and total anti-HBc positive

③ Recovery–Total anti-HBc and anti-HBs positive

Fig. 13.35 Acute HBV infection with recovery. HBsAg usually appears 1–3 months after exposure. In acute HBV infection with recovery, HBsAg disappears within 6 months, while anti-HBs and total anti-HBc persists for lifetime.

acute hepatitis B, HBsAg is the first serologic marker to become detectable, usually between 2–11 weeks after exposure. IgM antibody to hepatitis B core antigen (IgM anti-HBc) and IgG anti-HBc (measured as total anti-HBc) appear shortly after HBsAg, as does hepatitis B e antigen (HBeAg). In persons who recover from infection, HBsAg and HBeAg persist for up to several months, and then gradually become undetectable (*Fig. 13.35*). Subsequently, IgM anti-HBc gradually disappears, after which antibody to HBsAg (anti-HBs) develops, indicating recovery with lifelong immunity to reinfection. IgG anti-HBc persists for life. In some persons with acute HBV infection, there is a period referred to as 'the window', between the disappearance of HBsAg and the appearance of anti-HBs, when only IgM and total anti-HBc are detectable.

In patients with chronic HBV infection, HBsAg remains detectable, and can persist for life (*Fig. 13.36*). The diagnosis of chronic HBV infection is made by detecting HBsAg on two serum specimens at least 6 months apart, or by the presence of HBsAg and IgG anti-HBc in the absence of IgM. In chronic HBV infection, total anti-HBc is detectable, but IgM anti-HBc and anti-HBs are generally not detectable. HBeAg may be present, and is associated with active viral replication and higher circulating viral titers. The presence of HBsAg in persons with acute infection and with chronic infection indicates that the person is infectious, regardless of the HBeAg status. Since anti-HBs, but not anti-HBc, is elicited in persons who receive hepatitis B vaccine, immunity from hepatitis B vaccine can be distinguished from immunity due to natural infection by the presence of anti-HBs in the absence of total anti-HBc.

Treatment

As with hepatitis A, symptoms of acute hepatitis B are generally self-limited, and initial treatment of acutely infected patients is supportive. Liver transplantation has been used to treat patients who have fulminant acute hepatitis B, with favorable survival rates (>50%).

For chronically infected persons, treatment resulting in clearance of HBV is expected to reduce the risk of developing cirrhosis and liver cancer and of transmitting HBV to others. Numerous agents, including prednisone, interleukin-2, thymosin, ribavirin, and azidothymidine have been studied in the treatment of chronic HBV infection. To date, alpha interferon is the agent shown to be most effective, and it is the only treatment for chronic HBV infection licensed in the USA.

The most important factors associated with a favorable response to alpha interferon include high pretreatment serum ALT levels, low pretreatment serum HBV DNA levels, and adult-acquired HBV infection. The treatment course for alpha interferon is 5 million units (MU) daily or 10 MU three times a week, for 12–24 weeks, with monitoring of HBsAg, HBeAg, HBV DNA, and ALT before and after therapy to assess response. With this regimen, approximately 40% of persons have loss of viral replication (as measured by disappearance of HBeAg and/or HBV DNA), and 10–20% lose HBsAg. The response is sustained after treatment, with a relapse of hepatitis occurring in less than 10% of patients within a year of treatment. Among those in whom HBeAg has disappeared, nearly 70% lose HBsAg after 4 years of follow-up.

Prevention

The prevention of sexually transmitted HBV infection relies upon three general measures:

- Behavior modification to reduce the risk of infection, including using condoms and decreasing the number of sexual partners
- Pre-exposure immunization with hepatitis B vaccine
- Postexposure prophylaxis of contacts of acutely infected persons with hepatitis B vaccine and hepatitis B immune globulin (HBIG).

The most effective measure for preventing HBV infection is hepatitis B vaccine. Hepatitis B vaccine is safe and highly effective. Three doses of vaccine induce protective levels of antibody in 90% or greater of vaccine recipients, and studies of long-term protection indicate that protective efficacy lasts at least 12 years. The Advisory Committee on Immunization Practices (ACIP) of the US Public Health Service recommends hepatitis B vaccination of adolescents and adults at risk of sexually acquired HBV infection (*Fig. 13.37*). As some of these groups have high prevalence rates of HBV infection, prevaccination screening of some groups for prior immunity may be cost-effective. If this is done, then the proper screening test is the total anti-HBc. The recommended doses and schedules for hepatitis B vaccine are given in *Figures. 13.38* and *13.39*.

Despite these recommendations, programs targeting sexually active persons have had limited success. For example, in STD clinic vaccination programs in Birmingham, Alabama, and San Francisco, California, only 14% of the susceptible target population received two doses of vaccine, and only

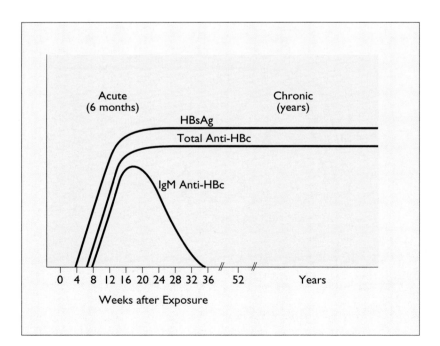

Fig. 13.36 Acute HBV infection with progression to chronic infection. HBsAg persists indefinitely and anti-HBs does not develop.

US PUBLIC HEALTH SERVICE ADVISORY COMMITTEE ON IMMUNIZATION PRACTICES RECOMMENDATIONS FOR HEPATITIS B VACCINATION OF ADOLESCENTS OR ADULTS AT RISK OF SEXUALLY ACQUIRED HBV INFECTION

Persons with a recently acquired STD

Persons identified as prostitutes

Homosexual and bisexual men

Persons with more than one sex partner in the previous 6 months

Sexual partners of HBsAg-positive persons

Fig. 13.37 US Public Health Service Advisory Committee on Immunization Practices. Recommendations for hepatitis B vaccination of adolescents or adults at risk of sexually acquired HBV infection.

4% completed the three-dose series (*Fig. 13.40*). The limited success in attempting to vaccinate individuals attending STD clinics and other persons in high-risk groups has led to a change in recommendations for hepatitis B prevention (*Fig. 13.41*). When the hepatitis B vaccine became available in 1982, initial recommendations involved targeting adult groups at high risk of infection (e.g. health-care workers, injecting drug users, homosexually active men). In 1988, recommendations were issued for HBsAg screening of pregnant women and vaccination and hepatitis B immune globulin (HBIG) administration to infants born to infected mothers. With

the realization of the limited effectiveness of a targeted vaccination approach, vaccine advisory groups in 1991–1992 recommended routine infant immunization with hepatitis B vaccine. In 1994, the ACIP recommended that all children aged 11–12 years should be given hepatitis B vaccine if they had not previously received the vaccine. Routine vaccination of infants and adolescents prevents HBV infection at an older age, when they may engage in behaviors which put them at risk for HBV infection. The implementation of infant and adolescent immunization has the potential to eventually eliminate HBV transmission in the USA. In specific exposure situations to HBV,

RECOMMENDED DOSES OF CURRENTLY LICENSED HEPATITIS B VACCINES

GROUP	RECOMBIVAX HB DOSE (µg)	ENERGIX-B DOSE (µg)
Infants of HBsAg-negative mothers	2.5	10
Infants of HBsAg-positive mothers	5	10
Children (1–< 11 years)	2.5	10
Adolescents (11–19 years)	5	10
Adults ≥ 20 years	10	20
Dialysis patients and other immunocompromised persons	40*	40**

* Special formulation in 1.0 ml
** Two 1.0 ml doses given at one site, in a 4-dose schedule at 0, 1, 2, 6 months.

Adapted from Centers for Disease Control and Prevention, Hepatitis B virus infection: A comprehensive strategy for eliminating transmission in the United States through immunization. Recommendations of the Advisory Committee on Immunization Practices MMWR (in press).

Fig. 13.38 Recommended doses of currently licensed hepatitis B vaccines. Both vaccines are routinely administered in a three-dose series. Engerix-B has also been licensed for a four-dose series administered at 0, 1, 2 and 12 months.

RECOMMENDED SCHEDULES OF HEPATITIS B VACCINATION FOR ADOLESCENTS (11–19 YEARS) AND ADULTS

0, 1, 6 months or

0, 2, 4 months or

0, 1, 4 months

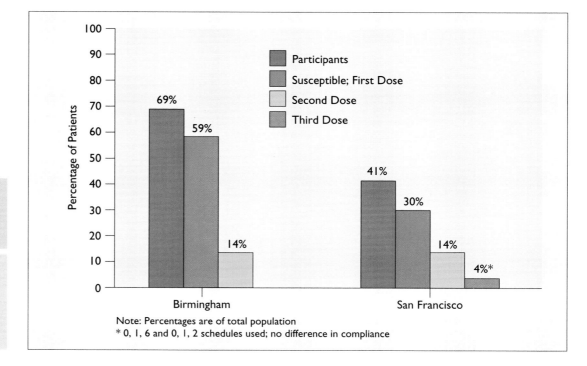

Fig. 13.39 Recommended schedules of hepatitis B vaccination for adolescents (11–19 years) and adults. The choice of schedule should be used to facilitate the highest compliance likely.

Fig. 13.40 Results of hepatitis B vaccination program: coverage among first-time patients attending STD clinics in Birmingham, Alabama, and San Francisco, California, 1990–1991. Among attendees, 41–69% enrolled, and only 4–14% received a full vaccine series (three doses).

because of the high risk of transmission, unvaccinated sexual partners of persons with acute HBV infection should receive a single dose of HBIG (0. 06 ml/kg) followed by the hepatitis B vaccine series, if prophylaxis can be started within 14 days of the last sexual contact. Sexual partners of persons found to be HBV carriers should be vaccinated.

HEPATITIS C

EPIDEMIOLOGY

Hepatitis C is caused by HCV, which is the etiologic agent of most non-A, non-B hepatitis in the USA and parenterally transmitted non-A, non-B hepatitis worldwide. As chronic infection with HCV can ultimately result in cirrhosis and liver cancer, HCV is also an important cause of chronic liver disease in the USA and worldwide.

HCV was discovered in 1989. It is an RNA virus, and has been classified as a separate genus in the family Flaviviridae. The virus circulates in low titers in the blood of infected persons, and is detected inconsistently in other body fluids. Although transmission via parenteral, sexual, and perinatal exposures has been identified (*Fig. 13.42*), many patients with hepatitis C do not report such exposures. The most efficient mode of HCV transmission is direct percutaneous blood exposure, such as via transfusion of blood or blood products or through needle-sharing among drug users. The risk of HCV transmission following a needlestick exposure to blood from a source positive for antibody to HCV (anti-HCV) is 6–10%. Studies of infants born to HCV-infected HIV-negative women have found the risk of transmission, determined by persistent anti-HCV positivity, to be from 0–13%. Two recent studies have suggested that viral titer is related to the risk of transmission. In one study, transmission occurred only from mothers with titers of greater than 10^6 genome copies per ml; in another study, transmission only occurred from one woman with a titer of 10^{10} genome copies per ml.

Although HCV can be transmitted sexually, studies examining the risk of sexual HCV transmission have been limited by small sample size, variable types of serologic testing, and methodologic problems (e.g. a lack of proper control groups). As a result, the studies have provided conflicting results (*Figs. 13.43* and *13.44*). Among contacts of patients with HCV infection, studies from Asia

---

STRATEGY FOR ELIMINATION OF HEPATITIS B VIRUS TRANSMISSION IN THE USA

OBJECTIVES

Prevent childhood hepatitis B virus infections
Prevent adult hepatitis B virus infections

ACTION PLAN

Universal screening of pregnant women for HBsAg
Universal immunization of infants
Universal immunization of adolescents (11–12 years of age)
Immunization of high risk adults

Fig. 13.41 Strategy for elimination of HBV transmission in the USA.

RISK FACTORS ASSOCIATED WITH TRANSMISSION OF HEPATITIS C VIRUS

Tranfusion or transplant from infectious donor

Injecting drug use

Hemodialysis (years of treatment)

Accidental injuries with needlestick/sharps

Sexual or household exposure to anti-HCV positive contact

Multiple sexual partners

Infants born to HCV-infected women

Fig. 13.42 Risk factors associated with the transmission of HCV.

EVIDENCE IN SUPPORT OF SEXUAL/HOUSEHOLD TRANSMISSION OF HEPATITIS C VIRUS

CASE CONTROL STUDIES

HCV infection or non-A, non-B hepatitis associated with exposure to sexual or household contacts who previously had hepatitis

Multiple sexual partners associated with HCV infection or non-A, non-B hepatitis

ANTI-HCV SEROPREVALENCE STUDIES

Higher anti-HCV rates in persons with greater number of sexual partners

Some studies have found high rates of anti-HCV in sexual partners and family members of anti-HCV positive persons

Fig. 13.43 Evidence in support of sexual/household transmission of HCV.

EVIDENCE AGAINST SEXUAL/HOUSEHOLD TRANSMISSION OF HEPATITIS C VIRUS

CASE CONTROL STUDIES

Lack of association between clinical disease and male homosexual activity

ANTI-HCV SEROPREVALENCE STUDIES

Anti-HCV rates in sexually active persons 5 to 15 fold lower than rates in injecting drug users

Anti-HCV rates in sexually active persons considerably lower than rates for HBV and HIV in same populations

Some studies have found little or no evidence of HCV infection in sexual partners and family members of anti-HCV positive persons

Fig. 13.44 Evidence against sexual/household transmission of HCV.

of spouses, who were reported to have no other risk factors for infection, found an average anti-HCV prevalence of 25% (*Fig. 13.45*). In contrast, studies of spouses and sexual partners from Western countries and Australia found an average anti-HCV prevalence of 5%. Studies of HIV-infected partners have found similar rates of anti-HCV, though in some studies anti-HCV was found in both partners only when the male was coinfected with HIV and HCV. Worldwide, studies of nonsexual household contacts have found an average anti-HCV prevalence of 3–4%; however, one study from Asia that used PCR to detect HCV RNA found an HCV RNA positivity rate of 21% among children. The substantially higher rates of HCV infection found among contacts in studies from Asia are not well explained, and common exposures occurring in the community rather than from within the household cannot be excluded. Anti-HCV seroprevalence rates of 1–19% have been found among groups with different sexual behaviors, including homosexual men, heterosexuals attending STD clinics, and female prostitutes (*Fig. 13.46*). Only a few of these studies were able to identify specific factors associated with anti-HCV positivity, which included the number of partners, a history of other STDs, and failure to use a condom. In summary, while sexual transmission can occur, the magnitude of the risk and specific factors contributing to transmission are not well defined.

An estimated 16% of acute viral hepatitis in the USA is caused by HCV (*Fig. 13.2*). Based on surveillance data for community-acquired hepatitis C, an estimated 150,000 acute HCV infections occurred annually in the USA during the past decade. The number of new cases of hepatitis C has decreased substantially since 1989, largely due to a decrease in cases associated with injecting drug use (*Fig. 13.47*). However, injecting drug use is still the risk factor most commonly identified by individuals with acute hepatitis C in surveillance studies (*Fig. 13.48*). The sexual transmission of HCV may be more important than reflected in surveillance data, because more than 40% of persons with acute hepatitis C do not report a source of infection; these persons may have denied risk factors, or have unrecognized exposures (e.g., sexual contact with a person who is asymptomatically infected).

Results from the NHANES III serosurvey indicate that the prevalence of anti-HCV among the general US population is 1.4%, which corresponds to 3.5 million anti-HCV positive individuals nationwide. These persons are at risk of developing cirrhosis and hepatocellular carcinoma. An estimated 8,000–10,000 persons die annually in the USA from the chronic consequences of HCV infection (*Fig. 13.49*).

PREVALENCE OF ANTI-HCV IN CONTACTS OF ANTI-HCV POSITIVE PERSONS BY GEOGRAPHIC REGION, SUMMARY OF SELECTED STUDIES*

TYPE OF CONTACT BY GEOGRAPHIC AREA	NO. STUDIES (NO. TESTED/STUDY)	TOTAL TESTED	AVERAGE (RANGE) % ANTI-HCV POSITIVE
ASIA			
Spouse	4 (37–154)	304	25 (18–27)
Children	3 (67–110)	284	3 (1–4)
Other	2 (34–41)	75	4 (0–9)
W. EUROPE/USA/AUSTRALIA			
Spouse/Partner	12 (18–63)	419	5 (0–15)
HIV-Pos. Partner	4 (7–164)	263	3 (0–8)
Other Household	6 (17–80)	335	4 (0–11)

* Includes only studies which determined anti-HCV positivity by enzyme immunoassay and supplemental testing, and which excluded contacts with other risk factors.

Fig. 13.45 Prevalence of anti-HCV in contacts of anti-HCV-positive persons by geographic region: summary of selected studies.

HEPATITIS C VIRUS INFECTION IN POPULATIONS WITH DIFFERENT SEXUAL BEHAVIORS

GROUP	ANTI-HCV PREVALENCE	RISK FACTORS
Homosexual men	1% to 4%	No. of partners
Heterosexual STD patients	1% to 10%	No. of partners Non-use of condoms
Prostitutes	4% to 19%	No. of partners Other STDs Non-use of condoms Sex with trauma

Fig. 13.46 HCV infection in populations with different sexual behaviors.

CLINICAL MANIFESTATIONS

Acute HCV infection is generally mild, with 25% or fewer of infected persons having a recognized illness. When symptoms do occur with acute HCV infection, the incubation period is on average 6–7 weeks (ranging from 2 weeks to 24 weeks), and the symptoms are indistinguishable from those of other types of viral hepatitis.

The most important feature of hepatitis C is the high frequency with which acute disease progresses to chronic infection. Follow-up studies of patients with acute hepatitis C show that an average of 67% (ranging from 58% to 81%) have persistently elevated ALT levels more than 6 months after illness, indicating chronic hepatitis. The risk of developing chronic hepatitis appears to be independent of the source for infection. Among patients who underwent liver biopsy within several years after acute hepatitis C, chronic active hepatitis or cirrhosis was found in 29–76%. Seroprevalence studies showing high anti-HCV rates among patients with hepatocellular carcinoma, and case-control studies finding a strong association of anti-HCV positivity with hepatocellular carcinoma, suggest that HCV infection may also be a contributory factor for this disease.

Several extrahepatic manifestations have been reported with HCV infection (*Fig. 13.50*). In several studies, approximately 50% of patients with mixed cryoglobulinema were anti-HCV positive. HCV infection has also been reported to be associated with membranous glomerulonephritis.

Diagnosis

HCV RNA is the earliest marker of HCV infection, and is detectable by PCR as early as 2 weeks after exposure. However, PCR testing for HCV RNA is not licensed for use in the USA, and the diagnosis of HCV infection is dependent on the detection of anti-HCV. The currently available second-generation EIAs for anti-HCV detect antibody to three recombinant proteins — two expressed from the nonstructural region of the HCV genome and one from the structural (core) region. On the basis of these assays, anti-HCV has been detected in an average of 70–90% of patients with parenterally transmitted non-A, non-B hepatitis. Anti-HCV is detectable within 5–6 weeks after the onset of hepatitis in 80% of patients and by 12 weeks in 90% (*Figs. 13.51* and *13.52*). As with any screening test, the proportion of repeatedly reactive EIA results that are falsely positive varies depending on the prevalence of infection in the population screened. Although no true confirmatory test has been developed, supplemental tests for specificity, such as the recombinant immunoblot assay

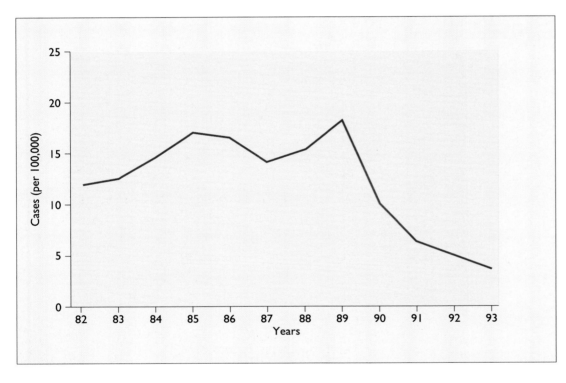

Fig. 13.47 Estimated incidence of acute hepatitis C, USA, 1982–1993.

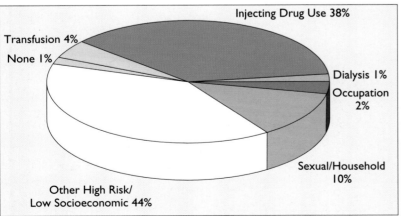

Fig. 13.48 Risk factors associated with reported cases of acute hepatitis C, USA, 1990–1993. (Source: Sentinel Counties, Centers for Disease Control and Prevention.)

(RIBA), are available and should be used to verify the results of specimens found to be positive by EIA. Other limitations of the currently available assays for anti-HCV are listed in *Figure. 13.53*. As the appearance of anti-HCV may be delayed in patients with acute HCV infection, if acute hepatitis C is suspected in a patient and initial testing is negative for anti-HCV, repeat testing should be done after at least 1 month, and possibly later. The diagnosis of chronic

1990 ESTIMATES OF ACUTE AND CHRONIC DISEASE BURDEN FOR HEPATITIS TYPES B, C, AND D, UNITED STATES

	HEPATITIS B	HEPATITIS C	HEPATITIS D
Acute	250,000	150,000	7,500
Fulminant	150	?	35
Chronic carriers	1–1.25 million	3.5 million	70,000
Deaths, chronic liver disease	5,000	8–10,000	1,000

Source: Centers for Disease Control and Prevention

Fig. 13.49 1990 estimates of acute and chronic disease burden for hepatitis types B, C, and D, USA.

HEPATIC AND EXTRAHEPATIC MANIFESTATIONS ASSOCIATED WITH HEPATITIS C VIRUS INFECTION

HEPATIC

    Acute hepatitis

    Fulminant hepatitis

    Chronic persistent hepatitis

    Chronic active hepatitis

    Cirrhosis

    Hepatocellular Carcinoma

EXTRAHEPATIC

    Mixed cryoglobulinema

    Membranous glomerulonephritis

    Leukocytoclastic vasculitis

    Aplastic anemia (?)

Fig. 13.50 Hepatic and extrahepatic manifestations associated with HCV infection.

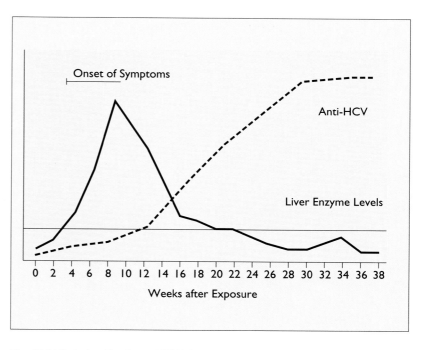

Fig. 13.51 Typical profile of acute HCV infection. With resolving infection, alanine aminotransferase (ALT) levels normalize and HCV RNA is not detectable.

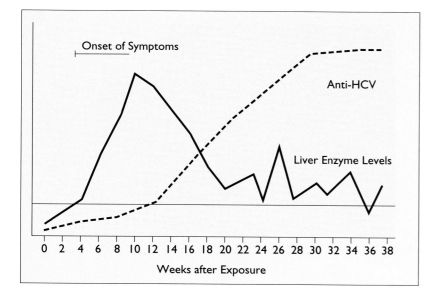

Fig. 13.52 Typical profile of acute HCV infection progressing to chronic HCV infection. In chronic HCV infection, alanine aminotransferase (ALT) levels continue to fluctuate, and HCV RNA can be detected intermittently. Approximately two-thirds of individuals with acute HCV infection develop chronic hepatitis.

LIMITATIONS OF ASSAYS FOR ANTIBODY TO HEPATITIS C VIRUS (ANTI-HCV)

Do not detect anti-HCV in approximately 10% of persons infected with HCV.

Do not distinguish between acute, chronic, or past infection.

Do not measure the presence of circulating virus.

In the acute phase of hepatitis C, there may be a prolonged interval between onset of illness and seroconversion.

In populations with a low prevalence of infection, the false positive rate of the screening enzyme immunoassay for anti-HCV is high.

Fig. 13.53 Limitations of assays for antibody to HCV (anti-HCV).

hepatitis C is made by the presence of anti-HCV and persistence of elevated liver enzymes for more than 6 months (*Fig. 13.54*). To evaluate the severity and extent of liver damage and whether specific treatment is indicated, a liver biopsy is usually necessary.

Treatment

Evaluation of therapy in patients with hepatitis C has generally focused on persons with chronic HCV infection. The only agent found to be effective is alpha interferon, but it generally suppresses infection and is rarely curative. Standard therapy is recombinant alpha-2b interferon administered at a dose of 3×10^6 units subcutaneously 3 times a week for 6 months. With this regimen, approximately 50% of persons will respond with normalization of ALT levels. However, 50–70% of these patients will relapse with elevated ALT levels and detection of HCV RNA in serum. For patients who do not respond initially, therapeutic options are limited. For patients who relapse after therapy, most will respond with repeated interferon treatment, but long term treatment is not well tolerated due to the side-effects of interferon, including bone marrow suppression, emotional lability, and depression. Studies are underway to determine the best way to maintain remission in patients who respond initially to interferon.

Since the long term response is limited, most clinicians treat HCV-infected patients who have persistently elevated liver enzymes and/or have moderate-to-severe inflammation on liver biopsy, because such patients are most likely to benefit from therapy. Since hepatitis C is slowly progressive and prolonged therapy is difficult and costly, the treatment of HCV-infected patients without symptoms and with minimal disease on liver biopsy is controversial.

Prevention

No effective vaccine exists to prevent HCV infection. Furthermore, recent studies indicate that postexposure administration of intramuscular IG does not protect against HCV infection. Thus, prevention of HCV infection must rely upon routine anti-HCV screening of blood donors to prevent transfusion-related hepatitis C, and the modification of high-risk behavior. Safer sex practices, including the use of condoms and reducing the number of sexual partners, and safer needle-using practices, may lower the risk of acquiring HCV infection.

Persons who are anti-HCV positive should be counseled to prevent transmission to others (*Fig. 13.55*). They should be informed of the potential for sexual transmission. For persons in a stable monogamous relationship, there are insufficient data to recommend changes in current sexual practices. For persons with multiple sexual partners, the number of partners should be reduced, and measures should be used to reduce the risk of acquiring STDs in general, including the use of condoms. Consideration should be given to testing exposed sexual partners for hepatitis C, and if positive, evaluating them for the presence of chronic liver disease.

HEPATITIS DELTA

EPIDEMIOLOGY

The virus HDV was discovered in 1977. It is molecularly distinct from other hepatitis viruses, but is a defective virus in that it can only infect persons who are HBV-infected, either as a coinfection with HBV or as a superinfection of someone who has chronic HBV infection. The delta viral particle has a core of delta-specific proteins (HDAg) and RNA, with an envelope of HBsAg that is contributed by the host HBV infection. Since

---

US PUBLIC HEALTH SERVICE GUIDELINES FOR MEDICAL EVALUATION OF ANTI-HCV POSITIVE PERSONS

INITIAL EVALUATION

Supplemental testing should be performed, if not already done, to verify anti-HCV screening test result

The patient should be asked about risk factors for hepatitis C as part of a medical history to support the specificity of an anti-HCV positive result

Laboratory tests to examine for evidence of liver disease may include ALT, AST, bilirubin, albumin, prothrombin time

SEQUENTIAL ALT TESTS SHOULD BE DONE TO DISTINGUISH BETWEEN ACUTE AND CHRONIC HEPATITIS C

If ALT levels remain elevated for ≥ 6 months, chronic hepatitis C is likely

If initially elevated ALT levels fall to within normal range and remain there for > 6 months, acute HCV infection was likely

Source: Centers for Disease Control. Public health service inter-agency guidelines for screening donors of blood plasma, organs, tissues and semen for evidence of hepatitis B and hepatitis C. MMWR 1991; 40 (RR–4): 1–17.

Fig. 13.54 US Public Health Service guidelines for medical evaluation of anti-HCV-positive persons.

US PUBLIC HEALTH SERVICE GUIDELINES FOR COUSELING ANTI-HCV POSITIVE PERSONS

Anti-HCV positive persons should not donate blood, body organs, other tissue, or semen

Household articles such as toothbrushes and razors that could become contaminated with blood should not be shared

Anti-HCV positive persons should be informed of the potential for sexual transmission

For persons with steady sexual partner, there are insufficient data to recommend changes in current sexual practices

For person with multiple sexual partners, safer sex practices should be used

Consideration may be given to testing exposed sexual partners for anti-HCV, and if positive, evaluating for chronic liver disease

No evidence to support advising against pregnancy based on anti-HCV status alone, or to advise any special treatment or precautions for pregnant women or their offspring

Source: Centers for Disease Control. Public health service inter-agency guidelines for screening donors of blood, plasma, organs, tissues and semen for evidence of hepatitis B and hepatitis C. MMWR 1991; 40 (RR–4): 1–17.

Fig. 13.55 US Public Health Service guidelines for counseling anti-HCV-positive persons.

HDV infection is dependent on HBV infection, the epidemiology of HDV infection is similar to that of HBV infection. The most efficient route of transmission is parenteral; sexual transmission is less efficient, and perinatal transmission rarely occurs (*Fig. 13.56*). Worldwide, the endemicity of HDV infection varies, with areas of high endemicity including southern Italy, several countries in Africa, and the Amazon basin in South America (*Fig. 13.57*). In areas of high endemicity, transmission occurs predominantly from person-to-person contact, whereas in areas of low endemicity, transmission is more common among persons with percutaneous exposures (e.g., injecting drug users).

An estimated 4% of acute viral hepatitis in the USA is HDV coinfection with HBV, corresponding to 7,500 infections annually. An estimated 1,000 persons die from chronic or fulminant HDV infection annually (*Fig. 13.49*). Studies of HDV infection among persons who are HBsAg positive show the highest prevalence among persons with frequent blood or percutaneous exposures, intermediate prevalence among persons with sexual risk-behaviors, and relatively low prevalence among immigrant and other populations in which HBV transmission occurs predominantly during early childhood (e.g. Pacific Islanders) (*Fig. 13.58*).

Both homosexual and heterosexual transmission of HDV has been described, though the efficiency of transmission appears to be less than that of HBV. Among homosexual men, the prevalence of HDV infection among HBsAg-positive persons ranges from 15% to 23%, and the risk of infection increases with an increasing number of sexual partners and the frequency of rectal intercourse. In addition, the prevalence of anti-HDV is significantly higher among homosexual men who are anti-HIV-positive compared with anti-HIV-negative men. In one study among HBV-infected female prostitutes who denied injecting drugs, the prevalence of delta infection was 6%.

MODES OF TRANSMISSION OF HEPATITIS DELTA VIRUS

MODE	GROUPS AT RISK
Parenteral	Injecting drug users Persons with mutiple blood transfusions
Indirect parenteral	Persons living in communities with endemic infection Developmentally disabled
Sexual	Heterosexual and homosexual contacts of persons with HBV–HDV coinfection or chronic HBV–HDV carriers

Fig. 13.56 Modes of transmission of hepatitis delta virus (HDV).

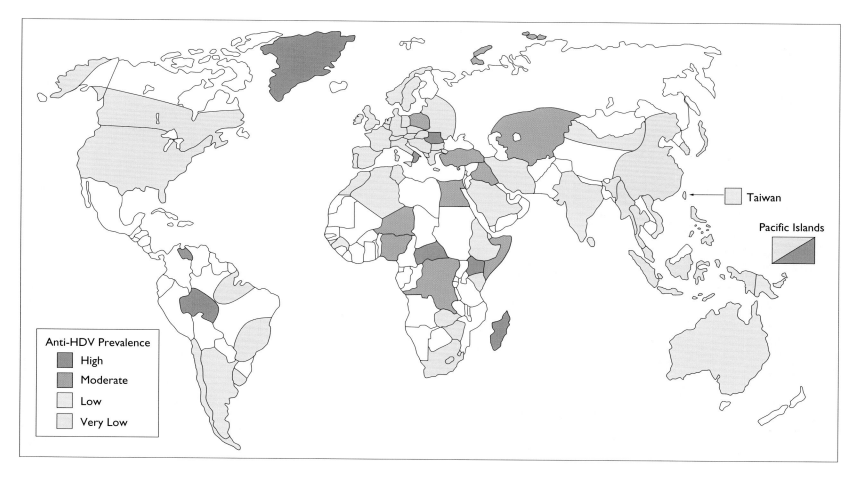

Fig. 13.57 Prevalence of HDV infection worldwide. Very low: 0–2% HDV prevalence in HBV carriers. Low: 3–9% HDV prevalence in HBV carriers. Moderate: 10–19% HDV prevalence in HBV carriers. High: >20% HDV prevalence in HBV carriers. White: no data available.

CLINICAL MANIFESTATIONS

In general, the symptoms of acute delta hepatitis (either coinfection or super-infection) are similar to those of acute hepatitis due to other viruses. However, the liver injury which occurs with acute delta hepatitis tends to be more severe. The incubation period for coinfection ranges from 6-12 weeks and for superinfection from 3-4 weeks. Coinfection with HBV and HDV does not usually result in chronic HBV or HDV infection, but is associated with a higher risk of fulminant hepatitis compared with HBV infection alone (*Fig. 13.59*). In contrast, HDV superinfection almost always results in chronic HDV infection, and the risk of development of chronic hepatitis and the rate

at which cirrhosis develops with chronic HDV infection are greater than with HBV infection alone (*Fig. 13.60*).

The clinical features of delta superinfection differ by geographic region. Large outbreaks of fulminant delta virus infection have occurred in several countries in South America, but have not been described elsewhere. In Europe, patients have been described with long term delta infection, but without liver enzyme abnormalities or histopathologic changes on liver biopsy; it has not been determined whether this is due to viral or host factors.

Diagnosis

Patients with current or resolved HDV infection have antibody to the hepatitis delta antigen (anti-HD). Patients with chronic delta hepatitis and active

PREVALENCE OF HDV INFECTION AMONG HBsAg CARRIERS IN CERTAIN GROUPS IN NORTH AMERICA

GROUP	% PREVALENCE	
	HBsAg	ANTI-HD
Blood donors	0.1–0.5	1.4–8.0
Injecting drug users	5–10	20–53
Hemophiliacs	3–5	48–80
Homosexual men	5–10	15
Prostitutes	3	15
Hemodialysis patients	2–5	8–20
Mentally retarded	5–15	4–30
Southeast Asian refugees	5–15	2–8
Alaskan Eskimos	5–15	0.6
Pacific Islanders	5–15	0–9

HBsAg: hepatitis B surface antigen
Anti-HD: antibody to hepatitis delta antigen

Fig. 13.58 Prevalence of HDV infection among HBsAg carriers in certain groups in North America.

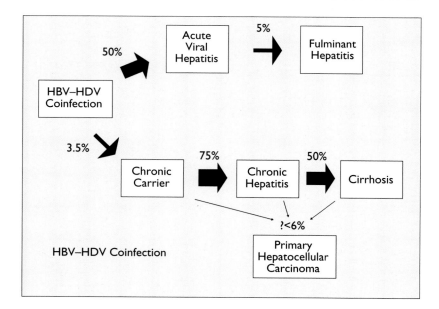

Fig. 13.59 Clinical outcome of HBV–HDV coinfection. The frequency of symptoms and of fulminant hepatitis with HBV–HDV coinfection is higher than with HBV infection alone, but infrequently progresses to chronic HBV–HDV infection.

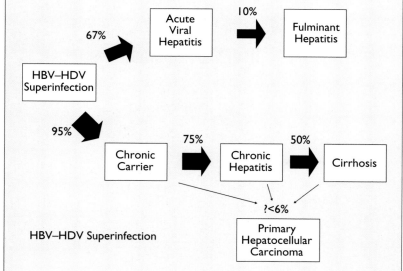

Fig. 13.60 Clinical outcome of HBV–HDV superinfection. HDV superinfection of an HBV-infected person usually results in chronic HBV–HDV infection, with a higher subsequent risk of chronic liver disease and cirrhosis.

HDV replication have very high levels of anti-HD. Patients with HBV–HDV coinfection may have only low levels of anti-HDV and IgM anti-HD (*Figs. 13.61* and *13.62*). In acute hepatitis, HDV–HBV coinfection can usually be distinguished from HDV superinfection by the presence or absence, respectively, of IgM anti-HBc (*Figs. 13.61* and *13.63*). HDV infection can also be diagnosed by the presence in serum of HDAg or HDV RNA (by either hybridization or PCR). In addition, specialized assays exist to detect HDAg or HDV RNA in liver biopsies. In general, serologic and liver assays for infection are not widely available or used, and therefore HDV infection may be underdiagnosed.

Testing for HDV infection should be considered in patients with acute and chronic hepatitis B, particularly in patients with fulminant hepatitis.

Knowledge of a patient's HDV infection status may help in counseling about prognosis and the prevention of transmission to others.

Treatment

Only α interferon has been shown to have any benefit in the treatment of chronic HDV infection. In general, 25–60% of patients respond with normalized ALT values after 3–4 months of treatment, although most will relapse with elevated ALT values and detectable HDV RNA when treatment is stopped. Prolonged treatment with α interferon (6–12 months) may result in the long term resolution of biochemical abnormalities and clearance of HDV RNA. Successful clearance of HDV RNA is associated with clearance of HBsAg.

CLINICAL DIAGNOSIS OF HEPATITIS DELTA INFECTION

CLINICAL ILLNESS	HBV		HDV			INTERPRETATION
	HBsAg	IgM ANTI-HBc	HDAg	IgM ANTI-HD	TOTAL ANTI-HD	
Acute hepatitis	+ or −	+	+ or	+ or	+	HBV–HDV coinfection
	+	−	+ or	+ or	+	HDV superinfection
Chronic hepatitis	+	−	−	+	+	Chronic HBV–HDV
None (asymptomatic)	+	−	−	+	+	Occult chronic HBV–HDV
	+	−	−	−	+	Chronic HBV with quiescent HDV

Fig. 13.61 Clinical diagnosis of HDV infection.

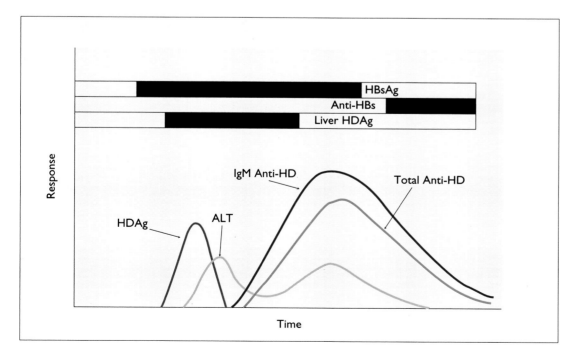

Fig. 13.62 Schematic diagram of serologic course of HBV–HDV coinfection.

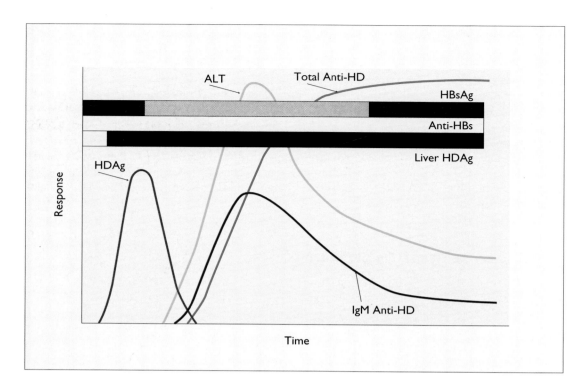

Fig. 13.63 Schematic diagram of serologic course of HBV–HDV superinfection, anti-HBs, antibodies to HBsAg.

Prevention

Pre-exposure hepatitis B vaccine, and postexposure prophylaxis with both HBIG and hepatitis B vaccine can prevent HBV–HDV coinfection (ACIP). Primary prevention of HDV infection therefore relies upon hepatitis B vaccination.

No effective vaccine exists to prevent HDV infection in persons who are chronically HBV-infected. Persons who are HBV-infected should be educated regarding measures to reduce their risk of acquiring HDV infection, including unprotected sexual intercourse and not sharing needles.

Picture credits are as follows: Figs. 13.2, 13.31, 13.48 courtesy of Sentinel Counties Study, Centers for Disease Control and Prevention; Figss. 13.5 and 13.38 adapted with permission from Centers for Disease Control and Prevention: Hepatitis B virus infection. A comprehensive strategy for eliminating transmission in the United States through immunization. MMWR (In press); Figs. 13.10 and 13.11 courtesy of National Notifiable Disease Surveillance System, Centers for Disease Control and Prevention; Fig. 13.12 courtesy of Viral Hepatitis Surveillance Program, Centers for Disease Control and Prevention; Figs. 13.18 and 13.19 adapted from Centers for Disease Control and Prevention: Prevention of hepatitis A through active or passive immunization: recommendations of the Advisory Committee on Immunization Practices (ACIP), 1995; Fig. 13.23 adapted from McQuillan et al: NHANES: Viral hepatitis. In. Everhart JE (ed): Digestive diseases in the United States: Epidemiology and impact. NIH Publication 94–1447, 1994. Fig. 13.49 courtesy of Centers for Disease Control and Prevention; Figs. 13.54 and 13.55 adapted from Centers for Disease Control and Prevention: Public Health Service inter-agency guidelines for screening donors of blood, plasma, organs, tissues and semen for evidence of hepatitis B and hepatitis C. MMWR 40(RR-4):1–17, 1991; Fig. 13.61 adapted from Polish LB et al: Delta hepatitis. Molecular biology and clinical and epidemiological features. Clin Microbiol Rev 6:211–229, 1993.

BIBLIOGRAPHY

Aach RD, Stevens CE, Hollinger FB, *et al.*: Hepatitis C virus infection in post-transfusion hepatitis. An analysis with first- and second-generation assays. *N Engl J Med* **325**:1325–1329, 1991.

Adam E, Hollinger B, Melnick JL, *et al.*: Type B hepatitis antigen and antibody among prostitutes and nuns. A study of possible venereal transmission. *J Infect Dis* **129**:317–321, 1974.

Agnello V, Chung RT, Kaplan LM: A role for hepatitis C virus infection in type II cryoglobulinemia. *N Engl J Med* **327**:1490–1495, 1992.

Akahane Y, Kojima M, Sugai Y, *et al.*: Hepatitis C virus infection in spouses of patients with type C chronic liver disease. *Ann Intern Med* **120**:748–752, 1994.

Alter MJ, Ahtone J, Weisfuse I, *et al.*: Hepatitis B virus transmission between heterosexuals. *JAMA* **256**:1307–1310, 1988.

Alter MJ, Coleman PJ, Alexander WJ, *et al.*: The importance of heterosexual activity in the transmission of hepatitis B and non-A, non-B hepatitis in the United States. *JAMA* **262**:1201–1205, 1989.

Alter MJ, Hadler SC, Judson FN, *et al.*: Risk factors for acute non-A, non-B hepatitis in the United States and association of hepatitis C virus antibody. *JAMA* **264**:2231–2235, 1990.

Alter MJ, Hadler SC: Delta hepatitis and infection in North America. In: Hadziyannis SJ, Taylor JM, Bonino F (eds): *Hepatitis delta virus. Molecular biology, pathogenesis, and clinical aspects.* Wiley–Liss Inc., New York, pp 243–250, 1993.

Alter MJ, Margolis HS, Krawczynski K, *et al.*: The natural history of community-acquired hepatitis C in the United States. *N Engl J Med* **327**:1899–1905, 1992.

Alter MJ, Margolis HS: The emergence of hepatitis B as a sexually transmitted disease. *Med Clin N Am* **74**:1529–1539, 1990.

Baddour LM, Bucak VA, Somes G, *et al.*: Risk factors for hepatitis B virus infection in black female attendees of a sexually transmitted disease clinic. *Sex Transm Dis* **15**:174–176, 1988.

Buti M, Esteban R, Allende H, *et al.*: Clinical and serological outcome of acute delta infection. *J Hepatol* **5**:59–64, 1987.

Centers for Disease Control and Prevention: Hepatitis A in homosexual men — United States, Canada, Australia. *MMWR* **41**:155–164, 1992.

Centers for Disease Control and Prevention: Hepatitis B virus infection. A comprehensive strategy for eliminating transmission in the United States through immunization. *MMWR* (In press).

Centers for Disease Control and Prevention: *Hepatitis Surveillance Report No. 55.* Atlanta, CDC, p 36, 1994.

Centers for Disease Control and Prevention: Prevention of hepatitis A through active or passive immunization: recommendations of the Advisory Committee on Immunization Practices (ACIP). *MMWR* (In press).

Centers for Disease Control and Prevention: Public health service inter-agency guidelines for screening donors of blood, plasma, organs, tissues and semen for evidence of hepatitis B and hepatitis C. *MMWR* **40**(RR-4):1–17, 1991.

Choo QL, Kuo G, Weiner AJ, *et al.*: Isolation of a cDNA clone derived from a bloodborne non-A, non-B viral hepatitis genome. *Science* **244**:359–362, 1989.

Cohen JI, Feinstone S, Purcell RH: Hepatitis A virus infection in a chimpanzee: duration of viremia and detection of virus in saliva and throat swabs. *J Infect Dis* **160**:887–890, 1989.

Corey L, Holmes KK: Sexual transmission of hepatitis A in homosexual men. *New Engl J Med* **302**:435–438, 1980.

Couthino RA, Albrecht-Van Lent P, Lelie N, *et al.*: Prevalence and incidence of hepatitis A among male homoexuals. *Br Med J* **287**:1743–1745, 1983.

Davis GL, Balart LA, Schiff ER, *et al.*: Treatment of chronic hepatitis C with recombinant interferon alfa. A multicenter randomized, controlled trial. *New Engl J Med* **321**:1501, 1506, 1989.

DeCock KM, Govindarajan S, Chin KP, Redeker A: Delta hepatitis in the Los Angeles area. A report of 126 cases. *Ann Inter Med* 1986; 105:108–114.

DeCock KM, Nilan JC, Lu HP, *et al.*: Experience with human immunodeficiency virus infection in patients with hepatitis B virus and hepatitis delta virus infection in Los Angeles, 1977–1985. *Am J Epidemiol* **127**:1250–1260, 1988.

Di Bisceglie AM, Order SE, Klein JL, *et al.*: The role of chronic viral hepatitis in hepatocellular carcinoma in the United States. *Am J Gastroenterol* **86**:335–338, 1991.

Dietzman DE, Harnisch JP, Ray CG, *et al.*: Hepatitis B surface antigen (HBsAg) and antibody to HBsAg. Prevalence in homosexual and heterosexual men. *JAMA* **238**:2625–2626, 1977.

Everhart JE, Di Bisceglie AM, Murray LM, *et al.*: Risk for non-A, non-B (type C) hepatitis through sexual or household contact with chronic carriers. *Ann Intern Med* **112**:544–545, 1990.

Farci P, Mandas A, Coiana A, *et al.*: Treatment of chronic hepatitis D with interferon alfa-2a. *N Engl J Med* **330**:88–94, 1994.

Fulford KWM, Dane DS: Australia antigen and antibody among patients attending a clinic for sexually transmitted diseases. *Lancet* i:1470–1473, 1973.

Hadler SC, Alcala de Monzon M, Bensebath G *et al.*: Epidemiology and longterm consequences of hepatitis delta virus infection in the Yucpa Indians of Venezuela. *Am J Epidemiol* **136**:1507–1516, 1973.

Heathcote J, Gateau PH, Sherlock S: Role of hepatitis B antigen carrier in nonparenteral transmission of the hepatitis B virus. *Lancet* ii:370–372, 1974.

Henning KJ, Bell E, Braun J, Barker ND: A community-wide outbreak of hepatitis A. Risk factors for infection among gay and bisexual men. *Am J Med* (In press).

Innis BL, Snitbhan R, Kunasol P, *et al.*: Protection against hepatitis A by an inactivated vaccine. *JAMA* **271**:1328–1334, 1994.

Irwin GR, Allen AM, Bancroft WH, *et al.*: Hepatitis B antigen and antibody. Occurrence in families of asymptomatic HBsAg carriers. *JAMA* **227**:1012–1013, 1974.

Jeffries DJ, James WH, Jeffries FJG, *et al.*: Australia (hepatitis associated) antigen in patients attending a venereal disease clinic. *Br Med J* **2**:455–456, 1974.

Johnson RJ, Gretch DR, Yamabe H, *et al.*: Membranoproliferative glomuleronephritis associated with hepatitis C virus infection. *N Engl J Med* **328**:465–470, 1974.

Kaklamani E, Trichopoulos D, Tzonou A, *et al.*: Hepatitis B and C viruses and their interaction in the origin of hepatocellular carcinoma. *JAMA* **265**:1974–1976, 1991.

Kao JH, Chen PJ, Yang PM, *et al.*: Intrafamilial transmission of hepatitis C virus. The important role of infections between spouses. *J Infect Dis* **166**:900–903, 1992.

Kleinman S, Alter H, Busch M, *et al.*: Increased detection of hepatitis C virus (HCV)-infected blood donors by a multiple-antigen HCV enzyme immunoassay. *Transfusion* **32**:80–813, 1992.

Koff RS, Slavin MM, Connelly LJD, *et al.*: Contagiousness of acute hepatitis B: secondary attack rates in household contacts. *Gastroenterol* **72**:297–300, 1977.

Krawczynski K, Alter MJ, Tankersley DL, *et al.*: Studies on protective efficacy of hepatitis C immunoglobulins (HCIG) in experimental hepatitis C virus infection (abstract). *Hepatology* **18**:110A, 1993.

Kuo G, Choo QL, Alter HJ, *et al.*: An assay for circulating antibodies to a major etiologic virus of human non-A, non-B hepatitis. *Science* **244**:362–364, 1989.

Lednar WM, Lemon SM, Kirkpatrick JW, *et al.*: Frequency of illness associated with epidemic hepatitis A virus infection in adults. *Am J Epidemiol* **122**:226–233, 1985.

Lin HH, Kao JH, Hsu JY, *et al.*: Possible role of high-titer maternal viremia in perinatal transmission of hepatitis C virus. *J Infect Dis* **169**:638–641, 1994.

Lin HH, Liaw YF, Chen TJ, *et al.*: Natural course of patients with chronic type B hepatitis following acute delta hepatitis superinfection. *Liver* **9**:129–134, 1989.

Lindsay KL, Davis GL, Schiff EE, *et al.*: Long-term response to higher doses of interferon (IFN) alfa-2b treatment of patients with chronic hepatitis C. A randomized multicenter controlled trial. *Hepatology* **18**:106A, 1993.

McFarlane ES, Embil JA, Manuel FR, Thiebaux HJ: Antibodies to hepatitis A antigen in relation to the number of lifetime partners in patients attending an STD clinic. *Br J Vener Dis* **57**:58–61, 1994.

McMahon BJ, Alward WLM, Hall DB, *et al.*: Acute hepatitis B virus infection: relation of age to the clinical expression of disease and subsequent development of the carrier state. *J Infect Dis* **151**:599–603, 1985.

McQuillan GM, Townsend TR, Fields HA, *et al.*: The seroepidemiology of hepatitis B virus in the United States, 1976–80. *Am J Med* **87**(suppl. 3A):5–10, 1989.

Negro F, Di Bisceglie A: Diagnosis of hepatitis delta virus infection. *Hepatology* **14**:1014–1016, 1989.

Nishioka K, Watanabe J, Furuta S,*et al.*: Antibody to the hepatitis C virus in acute hepatitis and chronic liver diseases in Japan. *Liver* **11**:65–70, 1991.

Ohto H, Terazawa S, Sasaki N, *et al.*: Transmission of hepatitis C virus from mothers to infants. *N Engl J Med* **330**:744–750, 1994.

Osmond DH, Padian NS, Sheppard HW, *et al.*: Risk factors for hepatitis C virus seropositivity in heterosexual couples. *JAMA* **269**:361–365, 1993.

Papaevangelou G, Trichopoulos D, Kremastinou T, *et al.*: Prevalence of hepatitis B antigen and antibody in prostitutes. *Br Med J* **2**:256–258, 1974.

Peters CJ, Purcell RH, Lander JJ, *et al.*: Radioimmunoassay for antibody to hepatitis B surface antigen among household contacts. *J Infect Dis* **134**:218–223, 1976.

Polish LB, Gallagher M, Fields HA, Hadler SC: Delta hepatitis. Molecular biology and clinical and epidemiological features. *Clin Microbiol Rev* **6**:211–229, 1993.

Redeker AG, Mosley JW, Gocke DJ, *et al.*: Hepatitis B immune globulin as a prophylactic measure for spouses exposed to acute type B hepatitis. *N Engl J Med* **193**:1055–1059, 1975.

Rodriguez M, Riestra S, San Roman F, *et al.*: Prevalence of antibody to hepatitis C virus in prospectively followed acute non-A, non-B hepatitis, from different epidemiological categories. *Liver* **11**:129–133, 1991.

Rosenblum L, Darrow W, Witte J, *et al.*: Sexual practices in the transmission of hepatitis B virus and hepatitis delta virus infection in female prostitutes in the United States. *JAMA* **267**:2477–2481, 1992.

Schreeder MT, Thompson SE, Hadler SC, *et al.*: Hepatitis B in homosexual men: prevalence of infection and factors related to transmission. *J Infect Dis* **146**:7–15, 1982.

Shapiro CN, Coleman PJ, McQuillan GM, Alter MJ, Margolis HS: Epidemiology of hepatitis A. Seroepidemiology and risk groups. *Vaccine* **10**:S59–S62, 1992.

Shapiro CN, Margolis HS: Worldwide epidemiology of hepatitis A virus infection. *J Hepatol* **18**:S11–S14, 1993.

Solomon RE, Kaslow RA, Phair JP, *et al.*: Human immunodeficiency virus and hepatitis delta virus in homosexual men. *Ann Inter Med* **108**:51–54, 1988.

Szmuness W, Harley EJ, Prince AM: Intrafamilial spread of asymptomatic hepatitis B. *Am J Med Sci* **270**:293–304, 1975.

Tassopoulos NC, Hatzakis A, Delladetsima I, *et al.*: Role of hepatitis C virus in acute non-A, non-B hepatitis in Greece: a 5-year prospective study. *Gastroenterology* **102**:969–972, 1992.

Tremolada F, Casarin C, Tagger A, *et al.*: Antibody to hepatitis C virus in post-transfusion hepatitis. *Ann Intern Med* **114**:277–281, 1991.

Werzberger A, Mensch B, Kuter B, *et al.*: A controlled trial of a formalin-inactivated hepatitis A vaccine in healthy children. *N Engl J Med* **327**:453–457, 1992.

Yu MC, Tong MJ, Coursaget P, *et al.*: Prevalence of hepatitis B and C viral markers in Black and White patients with hepatocellular carcinoma in the United States. *J Natl Cancer Inst* **82**:1038–1041, 1990.

CHAPTER FOURTEEN

Sexually Transmitted Infections in Infants, Children, and Adolescents

C Beck-Sague, S Larsen, and R Rice

INTRODUCTION

Sexually transmitted diseases can affect children's health at three stages in their development:
- During infancy, as a result of maternal–neonatal transmission
- During childhood, as a result of sexual abuse
- During adolescence, as a result of sexual abuse or consensual sexual activity.

PERINATALLY TRANSMITTED INFECTIONS

Vertical transmission of most recognized sexually transmitted pathogens, including *Treponema pallidum*, *Neisseria gonorrhoeae*, *Chlamydia trachomatis*, HSV, HIV, and HPV, is well documented. Although clinical manifestations of perinatally acquired STDs are distinct, there are certain similarities among these diseases, and similarities to other infectious diseases, particularly other TORCH syndromes (congenital toxoplasmosis, rubella, cytomegalovirus), which should be considered (*Fig. 14.1*).

CONGENITAL SYPHILIS

EPIDEMIOLOGY

The incidence of congenital syphilis closely reflects the incidence of primary and secondary syphilis in women (*Fig. 14.2*), as well as the effectiveness of prenatal interventions to prevent vertical transmission. The surveillance definition for congenital syphilis was simplified in 1988 (*Fig. 14.3*).

Congenital syphilis is concentrated in those populations where the incidence of primary and secondary syphilis among women is high (*Fig. 14.4*). The prevalence of reactive prenatal serologic tests for syphilis varies with population characteristics and tends to be higher in underserved areas and in some developing countries (*Fig. 14.5*).

PERINATAL TRANSMISSION OF SELECTED SEXUALLY TRANSMITTED PATHOGENS

INFECTIOUS AGENT	TYPE OF TRANSMISSION	PERINATAL MORTALITY	PRE-MATURITY	INTRAUTERINE GROWTH RETARDATION	OCULAR FINDINGS	HEPATOSPLENO-MEGALY	JAUNDICE	ANEMIA	OTHER	BONE LESIONS	SEPSIS	CNS INVOLVEMENT
Bacterial												
Treponema pallidum	Transplacental	+	+	+	Chorioretinitis, glaucoma	+	+	+	Vesiculobullous rashes	Osteitis, periostitis, metaphysitis	+	+
Neisseria gonorrhoeae	Intrapartum	+	+	+	Conjunctivitis	–	–	–	–	Arthritis	+	Rare
Chlamydia trachomatis	Intrapartum	–	+	?	Conjunctivitis	–	–	–	Pneumonitis	–	–	–
Viral												
Human papillomavirus	Intrapartum	–	–	–		–		–	Laryngeal papilloma; laryngeal cancer; oral, genital warts	–		
Human immunodeficiency virus	Intrapartum (can be transplacental & postpartum)	?	+	+	–	+	–	+	Diarrhea, failure to thrive, opportunistic and other infections, parotitis, AIDS	Abnormal skull	+	+
Herpes simplex virus	Intrapartum (can be transplacental & postpartum)	+	+	–	Chorioretinitis, keratitis	+	+	–	Vesicles, erosions	–	+	+

Fig. 14.1 Findings during infancy that are associated with perinatal infection with sexually transmitted pathogens.

Vertical transmission

The risk of congenital syphilis varies with stage of untreated maternal syphilis; it is over 80% in primary and secondary syphilis, somewhat less in early latent syphilis, and is very low during late latent and tertiary syphilis.

Prevention

Congenital syphilis is almost entirely preventable, or curable before the birth of the infant provided that the mother is diagnosed and treated before the infant has been irreversibly affected. Prenatal diagnosis and treatment with

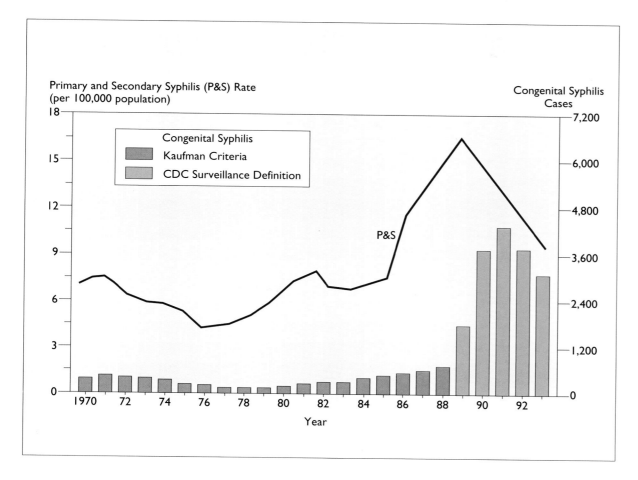

Fig. 14.2 Congenital syphilis. Reported cases in infants < 1 year of age and rates of primary and secondary (P&S) syphilis among women, USA 1970–1993.

CONGENITAL SYPHILIS CASE DEFINITION

Confirmed case: an infant in whom *Treponema pallidum* is identified by dark-field microscopy, fluorescent antibody, or other specific stains in specimens from lesions, placenta, umbilical cord, or autopsy material.

PRESUMPTIVE CASE

A. Any infant whose mother had untreated or inadequately treated[1] syphilis at delivery, regardless of signs or symptoms in the infant; or
B. Any infant or child who has a reactive treponemal test for syphilis and any one of the following:
   a. evidence of congenital syphilis on physical examination[2]
   b. evidence of congenital syphilis on long-bone x-ray
   c. reactive cerebrospinal fluid (CSF) VDRL
   d. elevated CSF cell count or protein (without other cause)[3]
   e. reactive test for FTA-ABS-19S-IgM antibody

Syphilitic stillbirth: a fetal death, occurring after 20 weeks' gestation or weighing more than 500 g, in which the mother had untreated or inadequately treated[1] syphilis at delivery.

[1] *Inadequate treatment consists of any non-penicillin therapy or penicillin given less than 30 days before delivery.*

[2] *Clinical signs in an infant (< 2 years) may include hepatosplenomegaly, characteristic skin rash, condylomata lata, snuffles, jaundice (syphilitic hepatitis), pseudoparalysis, anemia, thrombocytopenia, or edema (nephrotic syndrome). Stigmata in an older child may include: interstitial keratitis, nerve deafness, anterior bowing of shins, frontal bossing, mulberry molars, Hutchinson's teeth, saddle nose, rhagades, or Clutton's joints.*

[3] *Abnormal values for CSF are white cells > 5/mm³ and protein > 50 mg/dl. However, CSF values in preterm newborns may be higher and still be normal; these are difficult to interpret and an expert should be consulted.*

Fig. 14.3 Modified case definition for reporting of congenital syphilis cases.

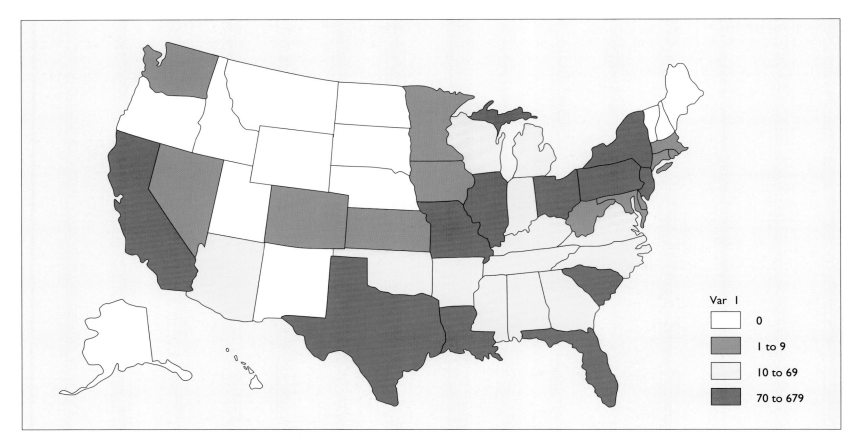

Fig. 14.4 Congenital syphilis cases, USA, 1994. Over 66% of cases are reported by seven states (New York, California, Illinois, Texas, South Carolina, Pennsylvania, and New Jersey).

Fig. 14.5 Prevalence of syphilis in selected patient populations enrolled in prenatal care and at delivery, 1980–1993.

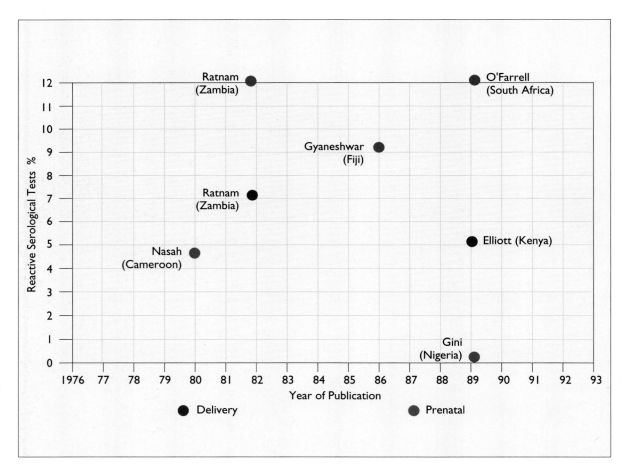

long-acting penicillin are highly effective in eradicating fetal disease. Most missed opportunities to prevent congenital syphilis occur either because a woman fails to receive prenatal care, or if she does receive it, she is not screened at her first visit and during the third trimester, or even if syphilis is detected, it is not treated (*Fig. 14.6*). Prenatal screening should be conducted in the first prenatal visit, and repeated in the third trimester in areas with a high prevalence of syphilis. Pregnant women with syphilis should be treated with a long-acting penicillin preparation (benzathine penicillin G) (*Fig. 14.7*). Alternative drugs are much more likely to fail to arrest fetal infection. It should be noted that recommended penicillin treatment regimens given during the third trimester and/or for secondary syphilis may not be as effective.

CLINICAL MANIFESTATIONS

Vasculitis and its consequences — necrosis and fibrosis — are the fundamental histologic lesions of congenital syphilis. Placental changes associated with congenital syphilis include proliferative vascular changes, chronic and sometimes acute villitis, and villous immaturity (*Figs. 14.8* and *14.9*). *T. pallidum* can also be demonstrated in the amniotic fluid and histologically normal umbilical cord or placental tissue of asymptomatic seropositive newborns, thus confirming that these infants are infected (*Fig. 14.10*). About 4% of infants reported with congenital syphilis in the USA in 1993 were still-

Fig. 14.6 Lack of prenatal screening and third trimester rescreening are the most common reasons for failure to prevent cases of congenital syphilis.

REASONS FOR OCCURRENCE OF CONGENITAL SYPHILIS (CS) AMONG US INFANTS REPORTED, 1983–1986 (N = 659)	
Failure to receive prenatal care	46%
No STS* during pregnancy	4%
STS+, mother not treated	8%
STS not repeated in third trimester	15%
Late infection, seronegative at birth	12%
Prenatal treatment failure**	15%

* STS = Serologic test for syphilis

** > 90% non-penicillin or third trimester treatments

Source: CDC CS Follow-Up Form

TREATMENT: SYPHILIS IN PREGNANCY
Benzathine penicillin G 2.4 million units im*
If patient has documented penicillin allergy, consider oral desensitization

* Consider repeating in one week if in third trimester or in secondary stage of syphilis

Source: CDC 1993 STD Treatment Guidelines

Fig. 14.7 Only parenteral long-acting penicillin regimes should be used for treatment of syphilis in pregnant women. If there is evidence of penicillin allergy, oral desensitization is indicated.

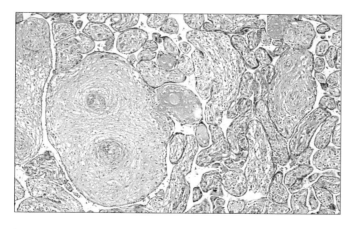

Fig. 14.8 Placental changes associated with congenital syphilis. Villi are enlarged and hypercellular, a typical finding of villous immaturity. Chronic villitis and proliferative vascular changes are also evident. Dense connective tissue almost obliterates the vessel lumen. Note villous immaturity, hypercellularity, chronic villitis, and vascular proliferation.

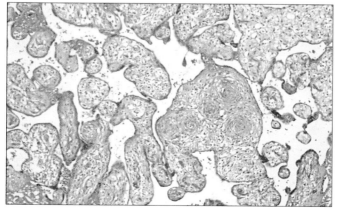

Fig. 14.9 Placental changes associated with congenital syphilis. Note villous immaturity, hypercellularity, chronic villitis, vascular proliferation, and compression of capillaries.

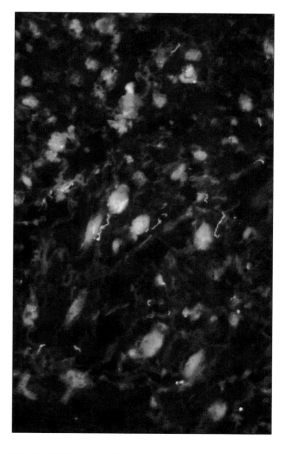

Fig. 14.10 Demonstration by direct fluorescent antibody technique of *Treponema pallidum* in histologically normal umbilical cord tissue from infant of a reactive mother diagnosed at delivery.

born (*Fig. 14.11*). Maceration is often associated with stillbirth due to congenital syphilis, but *T. pallidum* can be demonstrated even in fetuses with advanced autolysis (*Fig. 14.12*).

Most infants with early congenital syphilis are asymptomatic at birth. If infection is not diagnosed by serologic testing at birth, the first symptoms typically appear within 3–4 months, generally between 3–9 weeks of life. The earliest sign, occurring typically up to 14 days before cutaneous lesions, is a nasal discharge, which is initially watery, then becomes more mucopurulent, crusting, and sanguinous (*Figs. 14.13* and *14.14*). This discharge, 'snuffles', may be teeming with spirochetes and can result in ulceration, chondritis, septal perforation, or saddle-nose deformity typical of late congenital syphilis (*Fig. 14.15*). Mucocutaneous lesions occur

in over 50% of infants with congenital syphilis in most series, and in 17% of US cases, most of whom are diagnosed as newborns (*Fig. 14.16*). The most common mucocutaneous lesions are large round or ovoid, maculopapular or papulosquamous lesions, common on the face, arms, and legs, that resolve with a hyperpigmented patch over 1–3 months (*Figs. 14.17–14.19*). Vesicles, bullae, and scaling may occur on the palms and soles with desquamation (*Figs. 14.20* and *14.21*). Lesions on the lips, nostrils, and anus become fissured and hemorrhagic and heal into radial scars, 'rhagades' (*Fig. 14.22*).

Symptomatic bone lesions with pseudoparalysis are not common. But radiologic evidence of bone involvement is present in more than 90% of infants with confirmed congenital syphilis (*Figs. 14.23* and *14.24*).

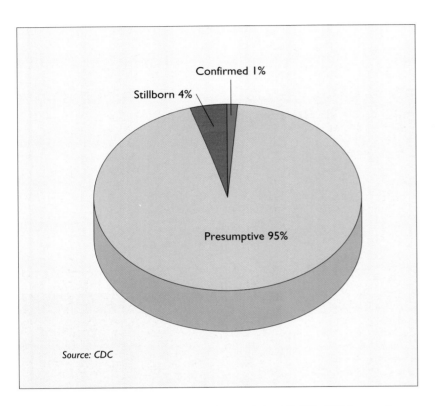

Source: CDC

Fig. 14.11 Proportion of infants reported with congenital syphilis (CS), 1993, by reporting category (N=2,920). Possible under-reporting of CS stillbirths may account for the low proportion of stillborn cases, relative to the natural history of CS.

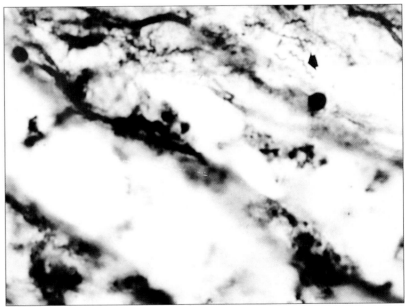

Fig. 14.12 Spirochetes (arrow) demonstrated by Warthin–Starry silver staining in autolyzed liver tissue of macerated stillbirth (× 1,000).

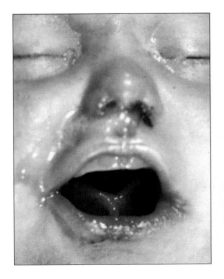
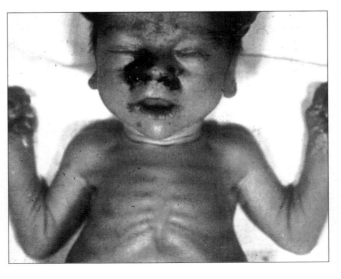

Figs. 14.13 and 14.14 Congenital syphilis. (**14.13**) Mucopurulent nasal discharge and (**14.14**) sanguinous nasal discharge in infants with snuffles.

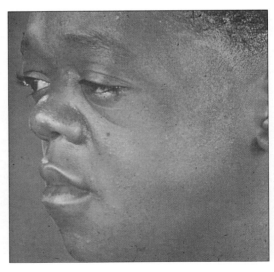

Fig. 14.15 Nasal deformity, 'saddle nose', typical of late congenital syphilis.

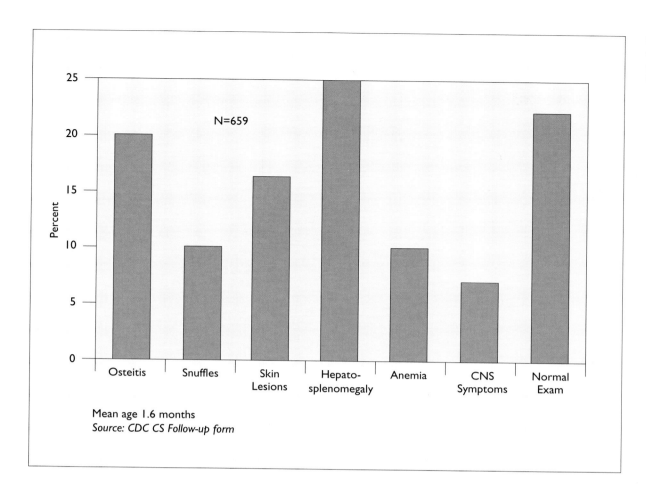

N=659

Percent

Osteitis | Snuffles | Skin Lesions | Hepato-splenomegaly | Anemia | CNS Symptoms | Normal Exam

Mean age 1.6 months
Source: CDC CS Follow-up form

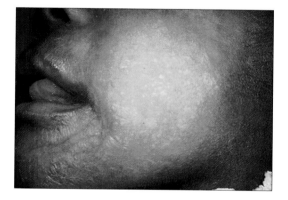
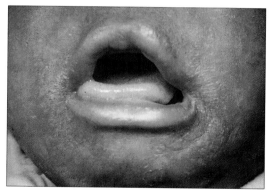
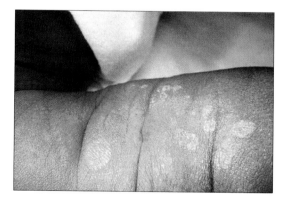

Figs. 14.17–14.19 Congenital syphilis. (**14.17**) Lesions on cheeks and (**14.18**) perioral region, and ovoid and annular lesions (**14.19**) on upper legs of 6-week-old infant with congenital syphilis, who presented with upper respiratory tract symptoms, irritability, and rash.

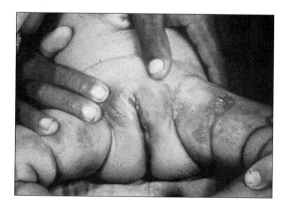
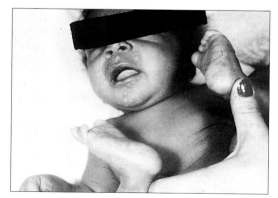
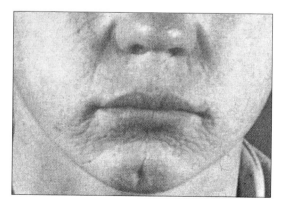

Fig. 14.20 Desquamative lesion on the thigh of an infant with dermal lesions due to congenital syphilis.

Fig. 14.21 Macular plantar rash in 2-month-old infant with congenital syphilis.

Fig. 14.22 Radiating scars (rhagades) due to healing of fissures of mucous membranes at the mucocutaneous junction around the mouth.

Pneumonia alba, so called because of the whitish appearance of the lung at autopsy, is rare and typically presents as diffuse, patchy lung densities and respiratory distress (*Figs. 14.25* and *14.26*). Hepatosplenomegaly and jaundice are very common but nonspecific findings (*Fig. 14.27*). A child with untreated late congenital syphilis may present with deafness, interstitial keratitis, and/or notched incisors (*Figs. 14.28* and *14.29*).

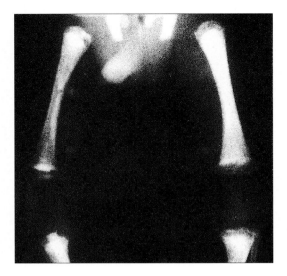

Fig. 14.23 Syphilitic metaphysitis in an infant. Note diminished density in the ends of the shaft and destruction at the proximal end of the tibia (right); this is known as the 'Wimberger sign'.

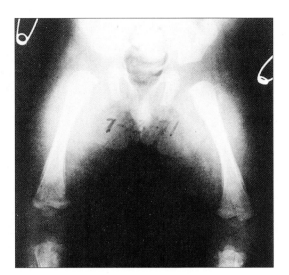

Fig. 14.24 Diaphyseal periostitis in long bones, presenting as a single-layered periosteal calcification, is the most characteristic feature of congenital syphilis in an infant.

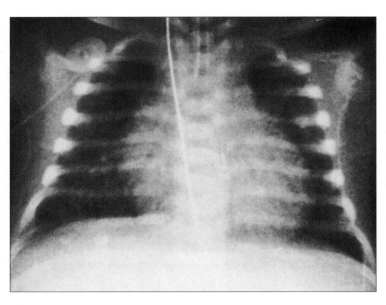

Fig. 14.25 Bilateral diffuse lung opacities in a newborn with pneumonia due to congenital syphilis.

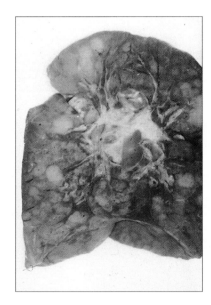

Fig. 14.26 Gross pathology of pneumonia alba in congenital syphilis. Lungs are enlarged, firm, and yellowish white in color.

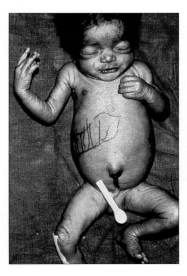

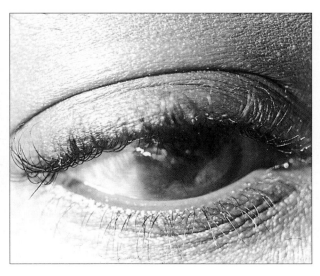

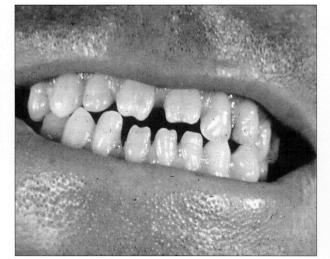

Fig. 14.27 Hepatosplenomegaly and jaundice in an infant with congenital syphilis.

Figs. 14.28 and 14.29 Hutchinson's triad of late congenital syphilis: (**14.28**) interstitial keratitis; (**14.29**) Hutchinson's notched incisors; and deafness.

The evaluation of newborns whose mothers are suspected or known to have had syphilis during pregnancy requires the careful evaluation of maternal and infant history, physical examination, and laboratory findings (*Fig. 14.30*). Currently used serologic tests for syphilis detect both IgG and IgM antibodies (*Fig. 14.31*). During the third trimester, transplacental transfer of IgG into the fetal circulation may cause an uninfected newborn to be seropositive on both nontreponemal tests, such as Venereal Disease Research Laboratory (VDRL) and rapid plasma reagin (RPR) tests, and/or treponemal tests, such as fluorescent treponemal antibody absorption test (FTA-ABS), and microhemagglutination assays for antibody to *T. pallidum* (MHA-TP). A reactive test may indicate that the infant has congenital syphilis due to failure to treat the mother adequately, but it may also indicate passively transferred antibody from a treated or untreated mother, without infant infection.

Several assays that detect only infant-produced antibody, IgM, which does not cross the placenta, have been used to help diagnose congenital syphilis. The IgM Western blot for congenital syphilis has a specificity of ≥ 90% and a sensitivity of ≥ 83%, which is greater than the sensitivity of the FTA-ABS 19S IgM test (73%). These tests may be useful confirmatory procedures to differentiate passive transfer of maternal antibody from active infection.

TREATMENT

The recommended treatment for congenital syphilis is aqueous penicillin G, 100,000–150,000 units/kg/day intravenously for 10–14 days or procaine penicillin G, 50,000 units/kg/day intramuscularly for 10–14 days (*Fig. 14.32*). Benzathine penicillin G should only be used in patients with a low likelihood of being infected, and only if follow-up can be ensured, because treatment failures with the use of this regimen for asymptomatic newborns with congenital syphilis have been reported.

NEISSERIA GONORRHOEAE INFECTIONS

EPIDEMIOLOGY

The incidence of gonorrhea among screened US pregnant women has ranged from less than 1% up to 7.5%. In some prenatal populations in

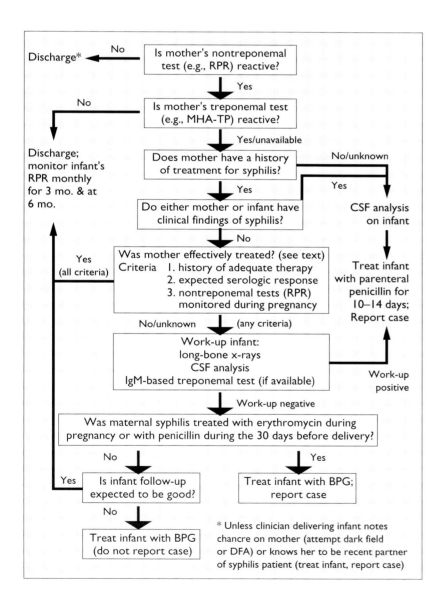

Fig.14.30 Algorithm for evaluation of seropositive newborns.

LABORATORY TESTS USED FOR THE DIAGNOSIS OF CONGENITAL SYPHILIS

NONTREPONEMAL	TREPONEMAL
Standard Tests	
Venereal Disease Research Laboratory (VDRL)	Fluorescent treponemal antibody (FTA) Fluorescent treponemal antibody-absorbed (FTA-ABS)
Rapid plasma reagin (RPR)	Microhemagglutination assay for antibody to *Treponema pallidum* (MHA-TP)
Experimental Tests	
VDRL ELISA for IgG and IgM	19S-IgM FTA-ABS* *T. pallidum* ELISA for IgG and IgM* *T. pallidum* Western blot Rabbit infectivity test (RIT) Polymerase chain reaction for *T. pallidum* (PCR) *T. pallidum* antigen-capture ELISA

* These tests are available through the Centers for Disease Control and Prevention

Fig.14.31 Standard and experimental serologic tests in the diagnosis of congenital syphilis.

developing countries, incidence rates have varied considerably, ranging from 2% in South Africa and Fiji to 27% in Gambia (*Fig. 14.33*).

Vertical Transmission

Gonococcal infection is probably only rarely transmitted through intact placental membranes. Contact with an infected birth canal is the most common way in which infection is transmitted from mother to child. The risk of transmission from an infected mother to her child in the absence of prophylaxis is estimated at 30–50%. The vertical transmission rate tends to be higher among mothers with concomitant chlamydial infection (68% versus 31%), endometritis, prolonged rupture of membranes, well-established infection at the time of birth, and possibly, delay in the application of appropriate ocular prophylaxis.

Fig. 14.32 Treatment for congenital syphilis during infancy.

RECOMMENDED TREATMENT FOR CONGENITAL SYPHILIS

Aqueous crystalline penicillin G, 100,000–150,000 units/kg/day (as 50,000 units/kg iv bid during the first 7 days of life and tid thereafter) for 10–14 days.

or

Procaine penicillin G, 50,000 units/kg im daily in a single dose for 10–14 days.

Benzathine penicillin 50,000 units in one dose should be used in an infant whose complete evaluation is normal, and whose mother was a) treated for syphilis during pregnancy with erythromycin, or b) treated for syphilis < 1 month before delivery, or c) treated with an appropriate regimen before or during pregnancy but did not yet have an adequate serologic response.

Fig. 14.33 Prevalence of *Chlamydia trachomatis* and *Neisseria gonorrhoeae* infections in selected populations enrolled in prenatal care and at delivery, 1980–1993.

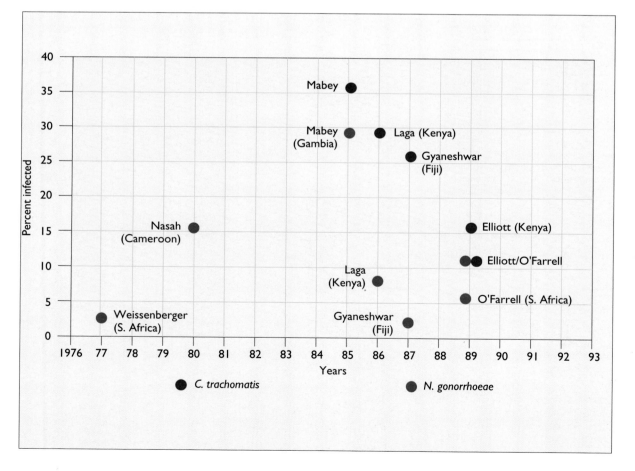

PREVENTION

Prenatal Screening

The most important strategy in the prevention of vertical transmission is the screening of pregnant women with culture at their first prenatal visit and prompt treatment. Nucleic-acid amplification tests (such as PCR or LCR) are in development and may offer increased sensitivity for detecting the presence of *N. gonorrhoeae* in anogenital specimens. Prenatal care tends to be underused due to unavailability and/or other factors in high-risk populations. For this reason, female partners of men diagnosed with gonorrhea should be sought and treated.

Treatment of Pregnant Women with Gonorrhea

Pregnant women who are diagnosed with uncomplicated gonococcal infections, or who are the sexual partners of men with gonorrhea, should be treated with ceftriaxone, 125 or 250 mg im in a single dose, or with cefixime, 400 mg orally in a single dose (*Fig. 14.34*). Both are generally effective against pharyngeal gonorrhea, which is important because pharyngeal infection appears to be higher in prenatal populations than in similar nonpregnant female populations.

Ocular Prophylaxis at Birth

The use of neonatal silver nitrate ocular prophylaxis has resulted in a dramatic reduction in neonatal disease. Ocular prophylaxis should be performed as soon after birth as possible in the delivery room, ideally before the infant opens her/his eyes (*Fig. 14.35*). Tetracycline should not be used for ocular prophylaxis in areas where high-level tetracycline-resistant strains have been reported.

CLINICAL MANIFESTATIONS

Gonococcal Ophthalmia

The most common manifestation of infant (gonococcal) infection is ophthalmia neonatorum. Arthritis, sepsis and meningitis are much less common. Before the introduction of silver nitrate prophylaxis in 1880, the incidence of gonococcal ophthalmia neonatorum varied from 1–4%, and up to 79% of children in institutions for the blind had a history of gonococcal ophthalmia. A seasonal incidence has been reported in the incidence of gonococcal ophthalmia during the year (*Fig. 14.36*).

Fig.14.34 Recommended treatment for gonorrhea during pregnancy and the neonatal period.

RECOMMENDED TREATMENTS FOR PERINATAL *NEISSERIA GONORRHOEAE* INFECTION[1]

	PREGNANT WOMEN	INFANTS
Uncomplicated gonorrhea	Ceftriaxone 125 mg im in a single dose or Cefixime 400 mg po in a single dose	*****
Pelvic inflammatory disease	Cefoxitin 2 g iv qid[2] or Cefotetan 2 g bid	*****
Maternal untreated gonorrhea	*****	Ceftriaxone 25–50 mg/kg iv or im in a single dose, not to exceed 125 mg
Gonococcal ophthalmia	Ceftriaxone 1 g im in a single dose	Ceftriaxone 25–50 mg/kg iv or im in a single dose, not to exceed 125 mg[3]
Disseminated gonococcal infection	Ceftriaxone 1 g im or iv daily continued for 24–48 hours after improvement begins	Ceftriaxone 25–50 mg/kg/day iv or im daily for 7 days
Meningitis or endocarditis	Ceftriaxone 1–2 g iv daily for 10–14 days (meningitis) or 4 weeks (endocarditis)	Ceftriaxone 25–50 mg/kg/day for 10–14 days (meningitis)

[1] Treatment for N. gonorrhoeae infections should be accompanied by effective treatment for Chlamydia trachomatis.

[2] Treatment for pelvic inflammatory disease should include a minimum of two antimicrobials, to ensure coverage for facultative bacteria, anaerobes, and streptococci.

[3] Many pediatricians continue treatment until cultures are negative at 48–72 hours; ceftriaxone should be administered with caution among infants with elevated bilirubin levels, particularly premature infants.

The severity of gonococcal ophthalmia ranges from a mild conjunctivitis similar to chemical conjunctivitis, to a process which if untreated results in corneal ulceration and perforation and blindness. Gonococcal ophthalmia is most often seen in infants, generally within 4–6.5 days after birth (range 1–28 days) (*Fig. 14.37*). Typically, gonococcal ophthalmia is bilateral and the discharge is purulent (*Figs. 14.38* and *14.39*). Gonococcal ophthalmia tends to be more severe in terms of palpebral edema, conjunctival injection, and purulent discharge than ophthalmia caused by *C. trachomatis* and ophthalmia not attributable to either pathogen.

Severe inflammation of the conjunctivae is associated with a serosanguinous exudate and may produce inflammatory membranes; these membranes are replaced by scar tissue in the conjunctivae as the disease resolves (*Fig. 14.40*). Corneal involvement presents initially as diffuse epithelial edema, giving the cornea a hazy, smoky-gray appearance, and often results in blindness due to involvement of the central cornea (*Fig. 14.41*). Prevalence of corneal involvement with residual scarring in neonates has been reported to be as high as 16%, but in numerous series and case reports, no evidence of corneal involvement has been noted.

Disseminated Gonococcal Infection

In most cases, gonococcal infection in newborns is localized, though cough, irritability or poor feeding may accompany gonococcal conjunctivitis. Nonspecific symptoms commencing within 1–2 weeks of birth, including fever, irritability, and poor feeding, however, often herald the onset of dissemination. When dissemination occurs, it usually presents as polyarthritis, though a single joint may be most prominently involved.

TREATMENT

Infants born to mothers with untreated gonorrhea are at substantial risk of infection, even if ocular prophylaxis is applied, and should be carefully evaluated with orogastric, rectal, and blood cultures if they have signs suggestive of sepsis. If there is no evidence of gonococcal infection, such infants should be treated with ceftriaxone, 25–50 mg/kg intravenously or intramuscularly in a single dose (*Fig. 14.34*).

Fig. 14.35 Ocular prophylaxis for the prevention of ophthalmia neonatorum.

RECOMMENDED OCULAR PROPHYLAXIS FOR THE PREVENTION OF OPHTHALMIA NEONATORUM

Silver nitrate	1%	Aqueous solution	Single application
Erythromycin	0.5%	Ophthalmic ointment	Single application
Tetracycline	1%	Ophthalmic ointment	Single application

Source: Centers for Disease Control. 1993 STD Treatment Guidelines. MMWR 1993;42 (No. RR–14): 1–102.

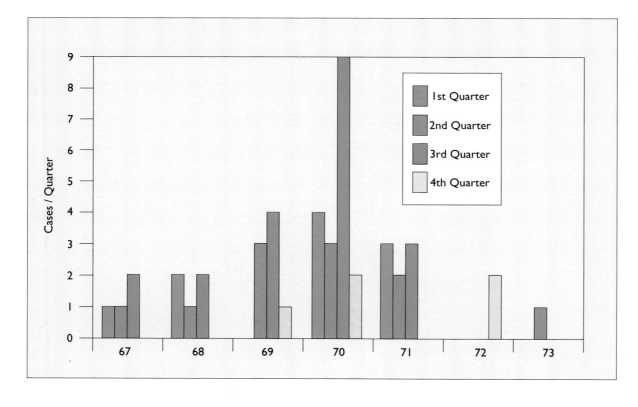

Fig. 14.36 Seasonal incidence of gonococcal ophthalmia neonatorum, showing peak occurrence in the third quarter of the year, Grady Memorial Hospital, Atlanta, GA, 1967–1973. Control measures were instituted in 1971.

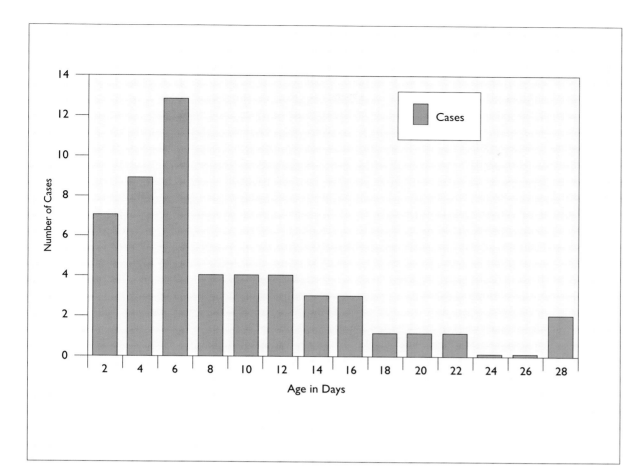

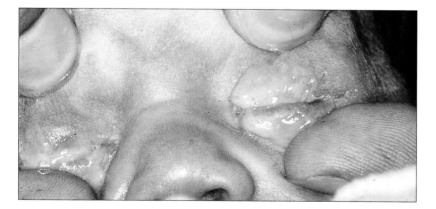

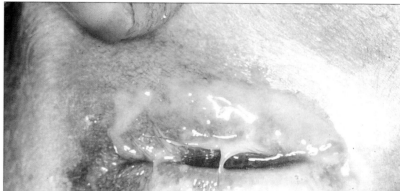

Figs. 14.38 and 14.39 Gonococcal ophthalmia. (**14.38**) Bilateral gonococcal ophthalmia in a 5-day-old infant. (**14.39**) Note purulent discharge.

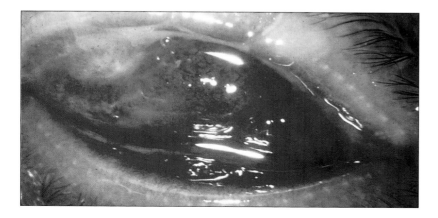

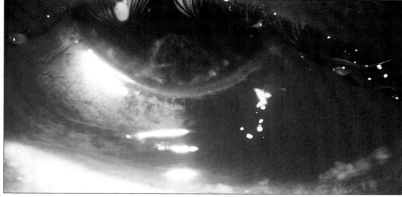

Fig.14.40 Inflammation of the conjunctivae, with sanguinous exudate and inflammatory membrane which bleeds in response to attempts to remove it.

Fig.14.41 Corneal involvement in gonococcal ophthalmia presenting as smoky, grey haziness in the peripheral cornea, resulting in partial blindness.

Infants who present with conjunctivitis should have specimens taken from conjunctivae, including exudate, for Gram stain, culture on chocolate agar for *N. gonorrhoeae* and for detection of *C. trachomatis* (*see Chlamydia trachomatis below*). Culture is essential to confirm *in vitro* susceptibility to antimicrobials used, and the laboratory should be required to perform confirmatory testing to differentiate *N. gonorrhoeae* from *Branhamella* (*Moraxella*) *catarrhalis* and other *Neisseria* species that can mimic *N. gonorrhoeae* on Gram stain (*see Chap. 6*). Patients with corneal involvement should have corneal cultures and Gram stains and be managed promptly in consultation with an ophthalmologist.

CHLAMYDIA TRACHOMATIS

EPIDEMIOLOGY

C. trachomatis appears to be the most common sexually transmitted bacterial pathogen in prenatal populations (*Fig. 14.33*). Cervical gonorrhea is a significant predictor for endocervical *C. trachomatis* infection among pregnant women. Core groups, such as have been described for gonorrhea, have not been described for chlamydial infections; these infections are broadly dispersed geographically and socioeconomically. Adolescents and young adults tend to have the highest prevalence. Studies of strains of *C. trachomatis* have resulted in their classification into 18 serotypes, or serovars, based on antigenic relationships established using a microimmunofluorescence serologic test (*see Chap. 4*). The serovars associated with sexually transmitted cervicitis, urethritis, and conjunctivitis in sexually active adults (B, D–K) are also associated with perinatally transmitted conjunctivitis, pneumonia, rhinitis and other chlamydial syndromes. Maternal chlamydial infection may be associated with adverse pregnancy outcomes, including chorioamnionitis and low birthweight, as well as infant conjunctivitis and other evidence of perinatal infection. In the USA, the incidence of neonatal infection has been estimated at 8/1,000 live births.

Vertical Transmission

Neonates often acquire *C. trachomatis* during delivery through an infected birth canal, but rare vertical transmission has occurred in spite of cesarean section. It is unclear whether symptoms in the mother tend to increase the risk of vertical transmission. Women with recent chlamydial infections are at higher risk of delivering low birthweight infants than women with chronic infections. Infant infection can persist in the conjunctivae, nasopharynx, and oropharynx for over 2 years. Conjunctivitis is seen in 20–50% and pneumonia in up to 20% of infants of mothers with *C. trachomatis* infection; up to 70% of infants have some evidence of infection, including rhinitis, pharyngitis, and possibly, otitis media. Asymptomatic anogenital infections occur in up to 15% of infants born to infected mothers.

PREVENTION

Prenatal care, particularly for those populations at highest risk (including adolescents and women from low socioeconomic groups), should include screening for cervical chlamydial infection. Screening should be performed during the third trimester, to reduce the amount of time for reinfection and to ensure treatment before delivery. An erythromycin base is recommended, though amoxicillin has been used in pregnant women who are unable to tolerate erythromycin base (*Fig. 14.42*).

Silver nitrate prophylaxis does not appear to be as effective in preventing chlamydial conjunctivitis (reduction of 68%) as it is in preventing gonococcal conjunctivitis (reduction of 83–95%) among newborns exposed to maternal infection. Tetracycline ointment has been shown to be very effective, with a reduction in incidence of gonococcal ophthalmia by 93% and a reduction in chlamydial ophthalmia by 77%, and is recommended. However, these data were collected before the presence of high-level tetracycline resistance had been described in certain strains of *N. gonorrhoeae* (*Fig. 14.35*).

Fig.14.42 Treatment of *C. trachomatis* infections during pregnancy.

RECOMMENDED TREATMENT OF CHLAMYDIA TRACHOMATIS DURING PREGNANCY

ERYTHROMYCIN BASE 500 MG PO
QID FOR 7 DAYS

Alternatives

Erythromycin base 250 mg po qid for 14 days
or
Erythromycin ethylsuccinate 800 mg po qid for 7 days
or
Erythromycin ethylsuccinate 400 mg po qid for 14 days

If erythromycin cannot be tolerated:

Amoxicillin 500 mg po tid for 7–10 days

NOTE: *Erythromycin estolate, doxycycline, and ofloxacin are contraindicated for pregnant women. The safety of azithromycin has not been established during pregnancy. Few data exist concerning efficacy of amoxicillin.*

CLINICAL MANIFESTATIONS

Conjunctivitis and Ophthalmia

C. trachomatis is the most common infectious cause of neonatal conjunctivitis, and conjunctivitis is the most common presentation of symptomatic, vertically acquired *C. trachomatis* infection in infants. Although a wide range of severity exists, chlamydial conjunctivitis tends to be milder than gonococcal conjunctivitis, and does not appear to progress to corneal scarring or blindness, or to present with preauricular adenopathy. It is more likely to be unilateral, at least initially. Chlamydial conjunctivitis generally presents in the second to third week of life, commonly with pseudomembrane formation and a diffuse matte infection of the tarsal conjunctiva (*Fig. 14.43*).

A seasonal variation has been reported, with cases peaking in the fourth quarter (*Fig. 14.44*).

All infants who present with conjunctivitis in the first 30 days of life should be evaluated for chlamydial conjunctivitis. Specimens for diagnosis should contain conjunctival cells, not exudate alone, and should be obtained from the everted eyelid using a dacron-tipped swab or the swab specified by the manufacturer's test kit. Tissue culture and nonculture tests, direct fluorescent antibody tests and immunoassays are highly sensitive, specific methods to diagnose chlamydial ophthalmia (*see Chap. 4*).

Pneumonia

Chlamydial pneumonia typically presents at 3–11 weeks of age with a history of prolonged congestion and cough. Generally, infants are afebrile and

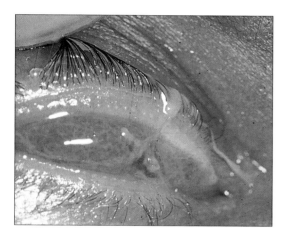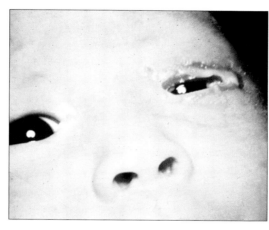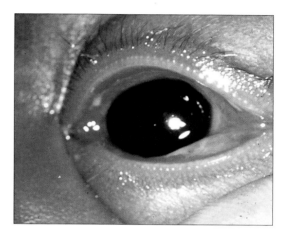

Fig.14.43 Chlamidial conjunctivitis presenting with pseudomembrane formation and diffuse matte injection of the contunctivae (left), with purulent conjunctivitis clinically indistinguishable from gonococcal conjunctivitis (center), and more typical mucopurulent ocular discharge (right).

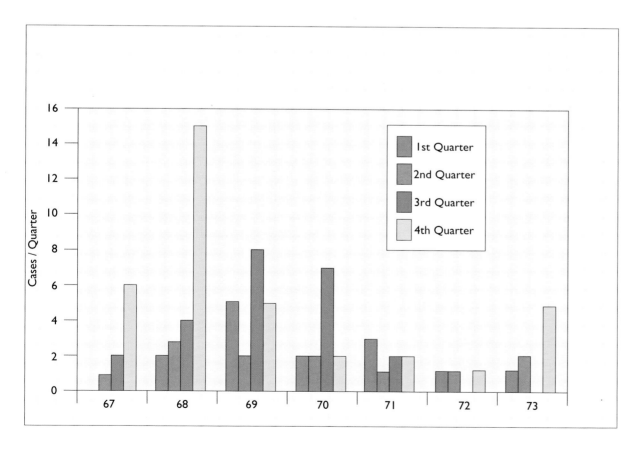

Fig. 14.44 Seasonal variation chlamydial ophthalmia neonatorum, Grady Memorial Hospital, Atlanta, GA, 1967–1973, before institution of control measures.

do not show signs of significant systemic illness. Tachypnea and rales are common physical findings. Although conjunctivitis and a pertussis-like staccato cough are not usually part of the typical presentation, these findings should alert the physician to the possibility of *C. trachomatis* pneumonia; hyperinflation with diffuse interstitial infiltrates are frequently seen (*Figs. 14.45*). Eosinophilia and elevations of serum IgG and IgM are also common.

C. trachomatis pneumonia should be considered in all cases of pneumonia in the first 3 months of life (*Fig. 14.46*). Nasopharyngeal and tracheal aspirates or lung biopsy specimens, if collected, should be tested by tissue culture. Nonculture tests of nasopharyngeal specimens may have much lower sensitivity and specificity. An acute IgM antibody titer of ≥ 1:32 is strongly suggestive.

Other Clinical Manifestations

Chronic respiratory disease characterized by chronic cough, wheezing, and abnormal functional residual capacity occurs in a small proportion of infected infants. Otitis media, rhinitis, and upper respiratory infections due to *C. trachomatis* can also occur in the first year of life.

TREATMENT

Systemic erythromycin should be used to treat chlamydial conjunctivitis and pneumonia, other infections due to *C. trachomatis* in infants, and infants born to mothers who have chlamydial infections (*Fig. 14.47*). Topical antibiotic therapy alone is inadequate to treat chlamydial infection and is unnecessary when systemic treatment is given.

HUMAN IMMUNODEFICIENCY VIRUS (HIV)

EPIDEMIOLOGY

As of December 1993, 5,228 cases of acquired immunodeficiency syndrome (AIDS) have been reported among infants and children in the USA. Well over 90% of children with HIV infection have vertically acquired infection from HIV-infected mothers. The number of cases due to perinatally acquired HIV infection has increased much more rapidly than cases due to other causes (*Fig. 14.48*). Seroprevalence rates among women delivering vary considerably by geographic area (*Fig. 14.49*).

Vertical Transmission

The prevalence of HIV infection among infants born to infected mothers generally is reported to range from 13–40%. A number of maternal factors are associated with an increased risk of HIV transmission to the infant. The highest transmission risk appears to be associated with maternal p24 antigenemia, low CD4$^+$ lymphocyte counts, maternal CD8$^+$ counts ≥ 1.80×10^9/l, and placental membrane inflammation in women without the other risk factors (*Fig. 14.50*). Infants delivered without complications, and those delivered by uncomplicated cesarean section, are less likely to be infected. Firstborn twins are more likely to be infected than secondborn twins.

It is widely believed that most vertical HIV transmission occurs during delivery. However, there is evidence that intrauterine infection does occur; HIV has been isolated from fetal and placental tissue as early as the first trimester and from the cord blood of infants at delivery. A congenital HIV syndrome has been described, but evidence of its specificity for HIV infection remains absent (*Figs. 14.51–14.53*).

PREVENTION

Strategies to prevent the perinatal transmission of HIV are just being explored. A significant reduction in vertical transmission has been associated with the use of zidovudine during pregnancy and in the perinatal period (*Fig. 14.54*). In addition, cesarean section and other strategies that reduce infant contact with maternal blood may result in reduced HIV vertical transmission. Pregnancy may accelerate the course of HIV disease in certain women, and pregnancy, oral contraception and cervical ectopy increase viral shedding in vaginal secretions. The counseling of women in high prevalence areas should include HIV serologic testing, as well as options for effective contraception or sterilization, along with barrier methods, such as condoms, to reduce the risk of sexual transmission.

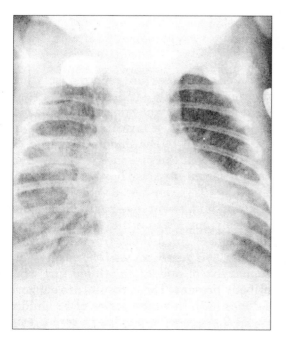

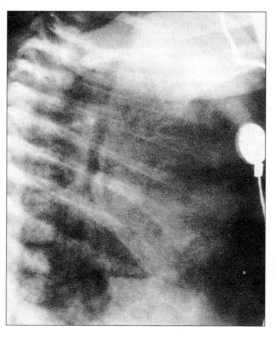

Fig. 14.45 Hyperinflation with flattening of the diaphragm and diffuse interstitial infiltrates in the anteroposterior (left) and lateral (right) views of a chest radiograph of a severely ill newborn with chlamydial pneumonia.

CLINICAL CHARACTERISTICS OF INFANT CHLAMYDIA PNEUMONIA VS. PNEUMONITIS DUE TO OTHER CAUSE

	CHLAMYDIA-POSITIVE	CHLAMYDIA-NEGATIVE
Presentation at 3–11 weeks	53/57 (93%)	19/42 (45%)
Prodrome more than 1 week	45/57 (79%)	17/42 (40%)
Conjunctivitis	26/57 (46%)	5/39 (13%)
Ear abnormalities	24/41 (59%)	0/15 (0%)
Staccato cough	24/41 (59%)	4/15 (27%)
Wheeze	9/57 (16%)	14/32 (44%)
Rales	14/16 (88%)	14/27 (52%)

Fig. 14.46 Characteristics of *C. trachomatis* including short prodrome, rales, and early presentation.

RECOMMENDED TREATMENTS FOR PERINATALLY ACQUIRED INFANT *CHLAMYDIA TRACHOMATIS* INFECTION

DIAGNOSIS	TREATMENT
Maternal untreated *C. trachomatis* genital infection	Erythromycin 50 mg/kg/day po divided in 4 doses for 10–14 days
Ophthalmia	Erythromycin 50 mg/kg/day po divided in 4 doses for 10–14 days
Pneumonia	Erythromycin 50 mg/kg/day po divided in 4 doses for 10–14 days
Others	Erythromycin 50 mg/kg/day po divided in 4 doses for 10–14 days

Fig. 14.47 Treatment of neonatal *C. trachomatis* infections.

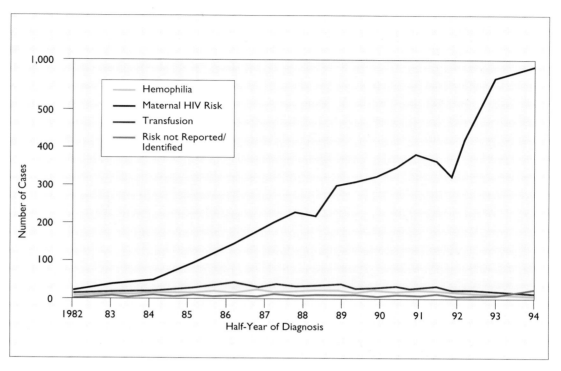

Fig. 14.48 Cases of acquired immunodeficiency syndrome (AIDS) among infants and children, USA, by mode of transmission and half-year of diagnosis through December, 1994.

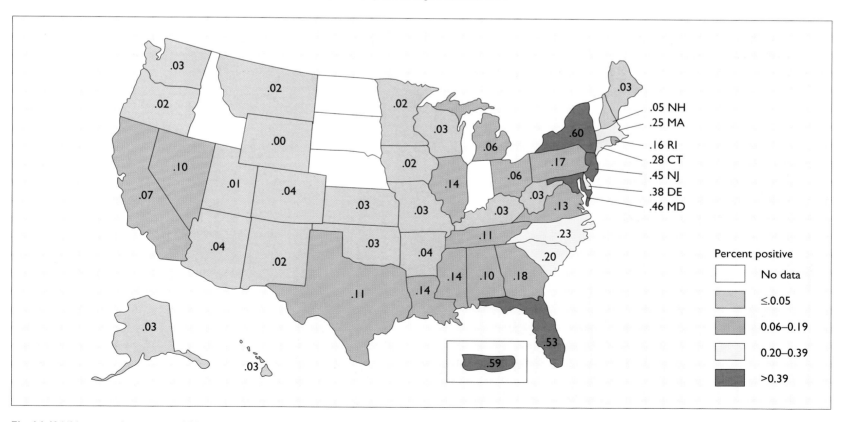

Fig. 14.49 HIV seroprevalence among childbearing women, USA, 1993. Note the variation of HIV seroprevalence in US prenatal populations.

CLINICAL MANIFESTATIONS

Preterm birth, low birthweight, premature rupture of membranes, intrauterine growth retardation and stillbirth are associated with both symptomatic and asymptomatic maternal HIV infection. These may be the result of HIV disease, or of a variety of other noxious influences on the patient, including gestational drug abuse, poor nutrition and other infections. HIV infection in children under 15 months of age is defined as: (1) the detection of virus in blood or tissues or of HIV antibody; (2) evidence of both cellular and humoral immune deficiency; and (3) one or more findings from Class P-2 or from symptoms meeting the CDC case definition for

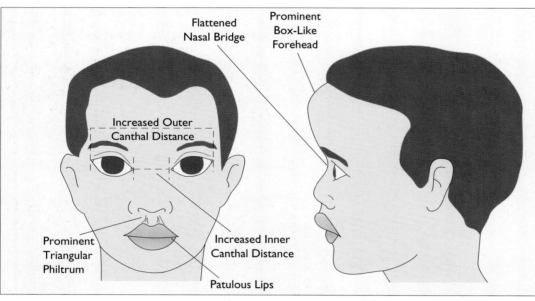

Fig. 14.50 Maternal factors associated with elevated risk of perinatal HIV-1 transmission, Zaire, October 1989–April 1990. The highest transmission risk (71%) was associated with maternal P24 antigenemia, relative risk (RR) = 3.0 and maternal CD8+ lymphocyte counts > 1.8×10^9/L (RR = 2.2). Among women with CD8+ lymphocyte counts < 1.8×10^9/L, CD4+ lymphocyte counts < 0.6×10^9/L were a risk factor (RR = 2.2). In women with neither high CD8+ nor low CD4+ lymphocyte counts, placental membrane inflammation was associated with vertical transmission.

* If CD8+ counts <0.6×10^9/L
** If neither high CD8+ count nor low CD4+ count
*Adapted from St. Louis ME, et al. JAMA 1993; **269**:2853–2859*

Figs. 14.51 Facial features in HIV embryopathy. Major facial features noted in HIV embryopathy include prominent box-like forehead, flat nasal bridge, ocular hypertelorism and obliquity, triangular philtrum, and patulous lips (frontal view).

Flattened Nasal Bridge

Prominent Box-Like Forehead

Increased Outer Canthal Distance

Prominent Triangular Philtrum

Increased Inner Canthal Distance

Patulous Lips

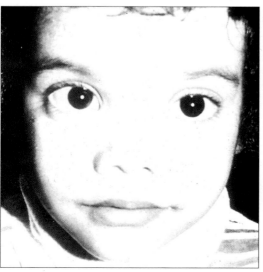
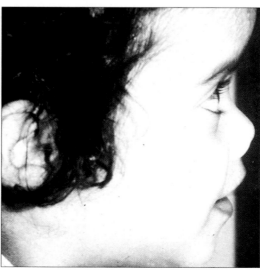

Figs 14.52 and 14.53 HIV embryopathy in a female child 37 months, with growth failure and microcephaly. Note prominent forehead, flat nasal bridge, ocular hypertelorism and obliquity, triangular philtrum and patulous lips.

AIDS (*Fig. 14.55*). The most common AIDS-defining diseases among children reported to the CDC during 1993 were *Pneumocystis carinii* pneumonia (PCP), lymphoid interstitial pneumonitis, recurrent bacterial infections, HIV-wasting syndrome, *Candida* esophagitis, and HIV encephalopathy (*Fig. 14.57*).

Pneumocystis carinii Pneumonia

Most infants diagnosed with AIDS in infancy have PCP. The median age at diagnosis is about 5–6 months. PCP presents with progressive respiratory distress, low-grade fever, and interstitial infiltrates, and rapidly advances to a diffuse bilateral airspace problem (*Fig. 14.58*).

Pulmonary Interstitial Diseases

After 1 year of age, PCP becomes less common, and diffuse interstitial processes in the lungs, due to a variety of interstitial diseases, become more common. Lymphoid lesions, including lymphocytic interstitial pneumonia (LIP) and pulmonary lymphoid hyperplasia, cause diffuse nodular or reticulonodular patterns in the lung (*Fig. 14.59*). Frequently, marked generalized lymphadenopathy, hypoxia, hepatosplenomegaly, bronchospasm, clubbing, and salivary gland enlargement accompany lymphoid interstitial processes (*Fig. 14.60*). Lymphoid lesions can progress to neoplastic lymphoproliferative diseases.

Recurrent Severe Infections

Severe bacterial infections occur commonly in children with HIV infection, particularly those with perinatally acquired infections. Over a third of infants with HIV infection have at least one episode of bacteremia. The organisms causing severe infections most commonly among HIV-infected children include *Streptococcus pneumoniae*, *Salmonella* species, *Staphylococcus aureus* and *Haemophilus influenzae* type b. *Mycobacterium tuberculosis*, *M. avium*, and cytomegalovirus infections occur less commonly. Chronic, severe skin infections are common (*Figs. 14.61–14.63*).

ELIGIBILITY CRITERIA AND ZIDOVUDINE REGIMEN FOR HIV-INFECTED PREGNANT WOMEN AND THEIR INFANTS PARTICIPATING IN AIDS CLINICAL TRIALS GROUP PROTOCOL 076

PATIENT ELIGIBILITY:

Has not received antiretroviral treatment during current pregnancy
Has no clinical indications for maternal antepartum antiretroviral therapy in the judgment of their health-care provider
Has a CD4+ T-lymphocyte count > 200 µl at initial assessment
Pregnancy 14–34 weeks

ZIDOVUDINE REGIMEN:

Oral administration of 100 mg zidovudine (ZDV) 5 times daily, initiated at 14–34 weeks' gestation and continued for the remainder of the pregnancy
During labor, intravenous administration of ZDV in a loading dose of 2 mg/kg body weight given over 1 hour, followed by continuous infusion of 1 mg/kg body weight per hour until delivery
Oral administration of ZDV to the newborn (ZDV syrup at 2 mg/kg body weight per dose given qid) for the first 6 weeks of life, beginning 8–12 hours after birth

Source: Centers for Disease Control MMWR 1993;43 (No. RR–11:3).

Fig. 14.54 Criteria and protocol for zidovudine use in pregnancy for prevention of vertical transmission.

SUMMARY OF THE CLASSIFICATION OF HIV INFECTION IN CHILDREN

Class P-0. Indeterminate infection
Class P-1. Asymptomatic infection
  Subclass A. Normal immune function
  Subclass B. Abnormal immune function
  Subclass C. Immune function not tested
Class P-2. Symptomatic infection
  Subclass A. Nonspecific findings
  Subclass B. Progressive neurologic disease
  Subclass C. Lymphoid interstitial pneumonitis
  Subclass D. Secondary infectious diseases
  Subclass E. Secondary cancers
  Subclass F. Other diseases possibly due to HIV

SUMMARY OF THE DEFINITION OF HIV INFECTION IN CHILDREN

INFANTS AND CHILDREN UNDER 15 MONTHS OF AGE WITH PERINATAL INFECTION

1. Virus in blood or tissues, or
2. HIV antibody and evidence of both cellular and humoral immune deficiency and one or more categories in Class P-2, or
3. Symptoms meeting CDC case definition for AIDS

OTHER CHILDREN WITH PERINATAL INFECTION AND CHILDREN WITH HIV INFECTION ACQUIRED THROUGH OTHER MODES

1. Virus in blood or tissues, or
2. HIV antibody, or
3. Symptoms meeting CDC case definition for AIDS

Source: Centers for Disease Control: Classification system for human immunodeficiency virus (HIV) infection in children under 13 years of age. MMWR 1987; 36:225.

Figs. 14.55 and 14.56 HIV infection in children. (**14.55**) Classification and (**14.56**) definition of HIV infection in children.

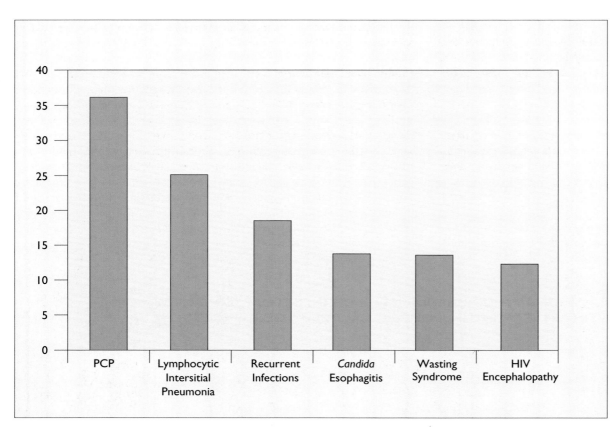

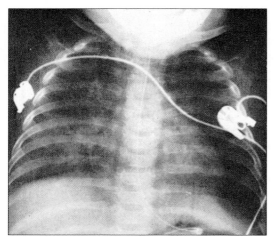

Fig. 14.58 *Pneumocystis carinii* pneumonia in a 3-month-old HIV-positive infant. Note the bilateral confluent interstitial pulmonary densities associated with hyperinflation of the lungs.

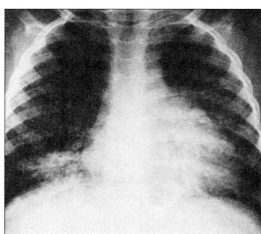

Fig. 14.59 Diffuse nodules throughout the lungs of a 20-month-old HIV-positive infant typical of lymphocytic interstitial pneumonia and pulmonary lymphoid hyperplasia.

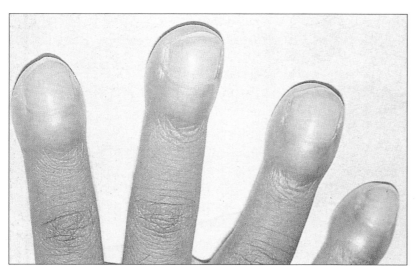

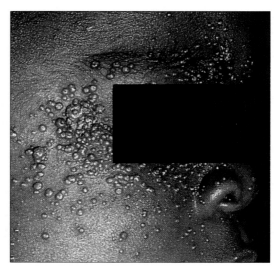

Fig. 14.61 Severe molluscum contagiosum in a child with AIDS.

Fig. 14.60 Clubbing in a child with AIDS and lymphocytic interstitial pneumonia.

HIV-Wasting Syndrome

A nonspecific syndrome characterized by chronic diarrhea, weight loss, failure to thrive, and/or refusal to feed is very common among infants and young children with HIV infection. Frequently, no causative organisms can be found. Mucosal edema and malabsorption patterns can be seen. Most radiographic changes are nonspecific (*Fig. 14.64*).

Candida Esophagitis, Oral Candidiasis and Diaper Dermatitis

Oral candidiasis, generally severe, is seen in most children with HIV infection and is associated with a more rapid progression to death (*Figs. 14.65–14.68*). *Candida* esophagitis is less common, and causes severe dysphagia. Barium esophagrams show a variety of changes including ulceration and mucosal irregularities (*Figs. 14.68* and *4.69*).

HIV Encephalopathy

Most children with HIV infection have developmental delay. Progressive HIV encephalopathy, seen less commonly, presents typically with loss of developmental milestones, spastic extremity paresis, microcephaly due to failure of brain growth and seizures. A CT scan typically shows changes consistent with cerebral atrophy and multifocal leukoencephalopathy, and less commonly, basal ganglion calcification (*Figs. 14.70* and *14.71*).

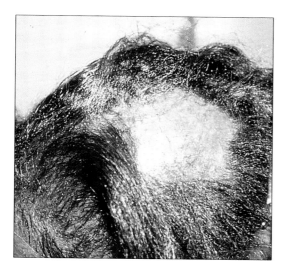

Fig. 14.62 Severe tinea capitis due to *Trichophyton tonsurans* in a child with HIV infection.

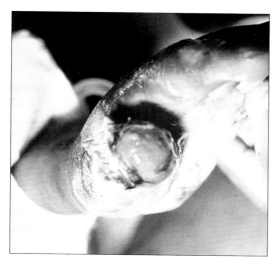

Fig. 14.63 Severe herpetic whitlow of the hand in a child with AIDS.

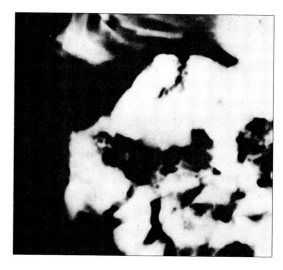

Fig. 14.64 Edema of mucosal folds in the proximal small bowel and malabsorption patterns, with nonspecific thickening of mucosal folds in the proximal small bowel of a 6-month-old HIV-positive infant hospitalized for failure to thrive. Stool was negative for pathogenic organisms.

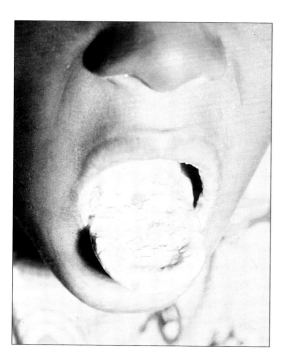

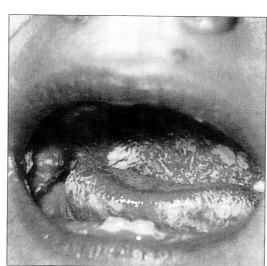

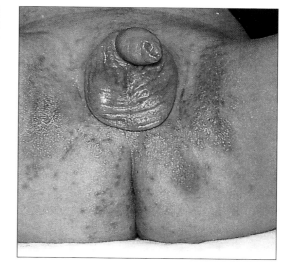

Figs. 14.65–14.67 Oral candidiasis (**14.65**, **14.66**) and *Candida* diaper dermatitis (**14.67**) in children with AIDS.

TREATMENT

In symptomatic infants and children with HIV infection, zidovudine may slow the progression of HIV disease. Prophylaxis against PCP should be given to HIV-infected children with CD4+ lymphocyte percentages of less than 20, or absolute CD4+ lymphocyte counts less than the age-defined minimum. The restricting of prophylaxis to just these infants, however, misses many infected infants, because these criteria have very low sensitivity in detecting infants at high risk of PCP. Intravenous immunoglobulin may reduce the incidence of recurrent severe bacterial infections. Management of HIV infection requires long term attention to immunizations, nutrition, and neurodevelopmental and other issues. The median survival time for children with perinatally acquired HIV infection after AIDS-defining illness develops is 2–3 years.

HERPES SIMPLEX VIRUS (HSV)

EPIDEMIOLOGY

From 1,500–2,000 cases of neonatal herpes (200–500 cases/100,000 live-births) occur yearly in the USA. Approximately 67–80% are caused by HSV type 2 (HSV-2). Most are acquired due to contact with the birth canal, but some are due to postnatal or intrauterine HSV infection (*Fig. 14.72*). The overall incidence of asymptomatic infection at delivery is 0.3%; viral shedding may be as likely in women with clinically silent genital HSV-2 infections as among women known to have genital herpes. Primary maternal infection before 20 weeks of gestation is associated with an increased incidence of abortion, stillbirth, hydroencephaly, and chorioretinitis (*Figs. 14.73* and *14.74*)

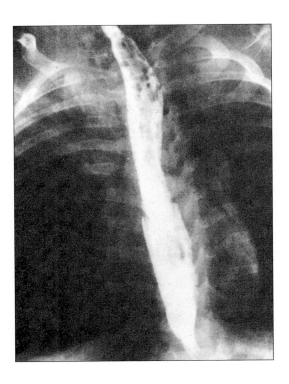

Fig. 14.68 Barium esophagram of 6-month-old infant with *Candida* esophagitis, showing mucosal irregularities and ulcerations.

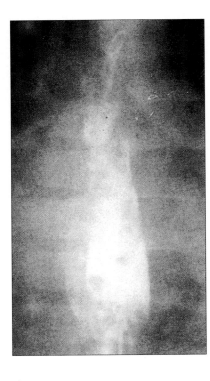

Fig. 14.69 Barium esophagram of child with AIDS, showing irregular plaques on walls of distal esophagus, and cobblestone appearance.

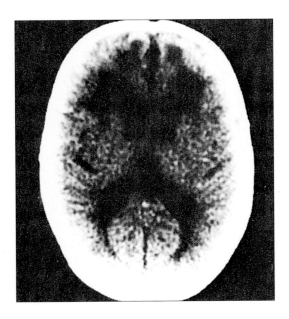

Fig. 14.70 Nonenhanced CT scan of a 3-month-old infant with HIV infection. Ventricles are dilated and interhemispheric fissure is widened, consistent with cerebral atrophy. Periventricular hypodensity, suggestive of progressive multifocal leukoencephalopathy, is present at the anterior horns.

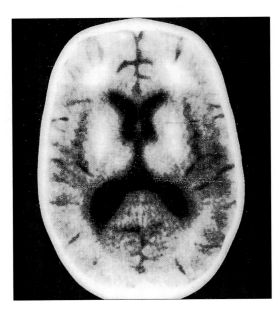

Fig. 14.71 Infant with AIDS, showing frontal lobe and basal ganglia calcification and ventricular dilation.

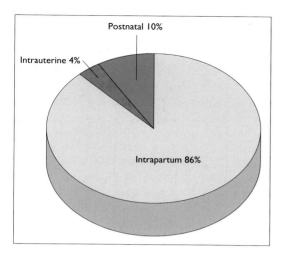

Vertical Transmission

Neonatal disease can result from primary or recurrent maternal infection. The HSV infection rate in vaginally delivered infants is influenced by the type of genital herpes in the mother (*Fig. 14.75*). Other factors, such as the use of fetal scalp electrodes or other instrumentation, may result in a greater likelihood of neonatal HSV infection.

PREVENTION

Cesarean section greatly reduces the transmission rate to infants at highest risk; of those whose mothers have active primary genital herpes at delivery, if delivered vaginally, 50% will be infected, *versus* 15–20% if delivered by cesarean section, particularly within 24 hours of membrane rupture. Maternal

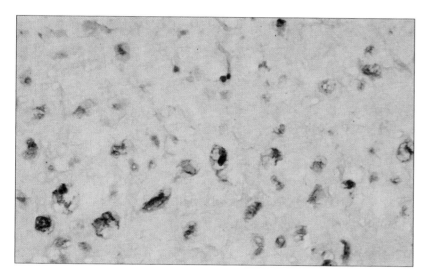

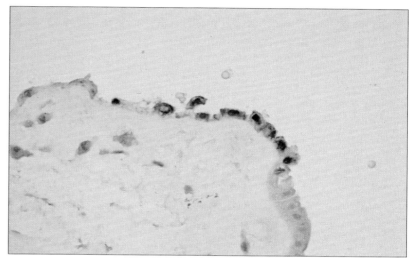

Figs. 14.73 and 14.74 Amniotic membrane from placenta of an infant with congenital HSV infection whose membranes were intact before cesarean delivery, documenting chorioamnionitis and ascending route of infection with intact membranes. (**14.73**) Section of umbilical cord (× 400) shows antigen staining pattern of inclusion consistent with HSV within mesenchymal cells. (**14.74**) Section of amniotic membrane demonstrating immunostaining pattern of cells. Cells are bordered on the right by antigen-negative cells with normal cytoarchitecture. On the left, they are bordered by debris of cells sloughed off the basement membrane.

Fig. 14.75 Risk factors for neonatal HSV infection should be considered in management of infants whose mothers are noted postpartum to have genital herpes.

RISK FACTORS FOR NEONATAL HERPES SIMPLEX VIRUS INFECTION AFTER VAGINAL DELIVERY

RISK FACTOR		POSSIBLE MECHANISM
Primary lesion	(30%–59%) vs.	Higher viral titer in primary lesions
Recurrent lesion	(3%–5%)	
Recurrent lesion, symptomatic	(3%–5%) vs.	Higher viral titer in recurrent lesions
Shedding, asymptomatic	(<3%)	
Cervical lesion* vs. lesions on vulva, buttocks, etc.		Higher viral titer in vaginal secretions
Prolonged rupture of membranes*		Longer duration of fetal exposure
Use of fetal scalp electrodes*		Provides site of entry for virus
Multiple lesions vs. single lesion		More virus from several lesions

*May be associated with higher risk

Adapted from: Overall JC. Herpes simplex virus infection of the fetus and newborn. Pediatric Annals 1994; 23:131–136.

physical examination at onset of labor, confining cesarean section to those who have evidence of genital herpes at that time, is the most cost-effective prevention strategy.

CLINICAL MANIFESTATIONS

Perinatal HSV infection tends to produce three categories of disease:
* Skin, eye, and mucous membrane involvement, generally appearing after the first 24 hours (42%)
* A nonspecific disseminated disease resembling sepsis, involving hepatic dysfunction, pneumonitis, adrenal involvement, and coagulopathy, presenting 7–10 days after birth (23%)
* Encephalitis (35%), presenting between 10 days and 1 month (*Fig. 14.76*) after birth.

The prognosis of all these categories, except localized eye, skin, and mucous membrane involvement, is poor. Without antiviral treatment, over 70% of infants with localized HSV involvement will progress to disseminated infection, and even after completing antiviral treatment, some infants with localized infection have recurrences of skin vesicles and long-term neurologic sequelae. Infants with neonatal HSV encephalitis present with fever, poor feeding, irritability, and lethargy. In approximately 67%, a skin rash develops.

Infants infected *in utero* often have skin lesions at birth, including vesicles, bullae, pustules, erosions or scarrring (*Figs. 14.77–14.79*). Chorioretinitis, microphthalmia, microcephaly, hydrocephaly, or other CNS involvement is seen in over 66% of these infants. Epidermal erosions simulating epidermolysis bullosa may occur (*Figs. 14.80–14.82*).

The diagnosis of HSV infection can be confirmed by isolating HSV from cultures of the oropharynx, CSF, and skin lesions, particularly vesicles, conjunctivae or rectum. DNA amplification methods, such as PCR, are also useful. However, these tests are not commercially available at this time. Brain biopsy may be considered in infants with suspected HSV encephalitis if there are no lesions available. The virus usually causes a cytopathic effect in tissue culture within 48–72 hours (*see Chap. 11*). Neonates with HSV infection have a variety of nonspecific laboratory abnormalities, including anemia, abnormal liver function tests, and CSF pleocytosis in the presence of CNS involvement.

CT scanning may show cerebral swelling or focal hypodensities in perinatally acquired infections, and calcifications or cystic encephalomalacia in congenital infections (*Fig. 14.83*).

TREATMENT

Vidarabine and acyclovir are about equally effective in reducing the incidence of mortality and neurologic sequelae among infants with neonatal herpes. Factors that increase the risk of mortality include dissemination, CNS involvement, coma, disseminated intravascular coagulation, prematurity, and pneumonitis. Factors associated with an increased risk of neurologic sequelae

Fig. 14.76 Categories of disease caused by perinatal herpes simplex virus infection.

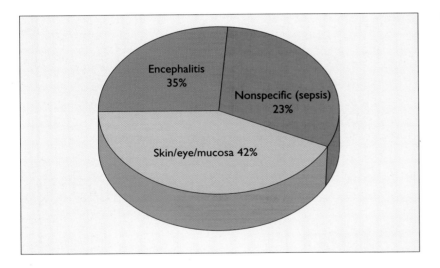

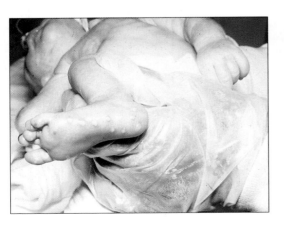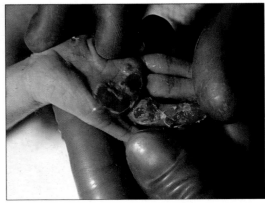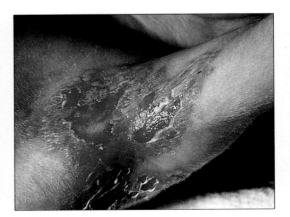

Figs. 14.77–14.79 Neonatal HSV infection. Vesicles (**14.77**) and ruptured bullae (**14.78, 14.79**) with erosion in infant with neonatal HSV infection.

include skin, eye, and mucous membrane disease with three or more recurrent skin lesions after completion of acute therapy, CNS disease, or seizures. Treatment should be initiated empirically in infants at highest risk of neonatal HSV after obtaining specimens for HSV culture (*Fig. 14.84*).

HUMAN PAPILLOMAVIRUS (HPV)

EPIDEMIOLOGY

Infections of the genital tract with HPV are among the most common STDs in adults in the USA (*see Chap. 12*). Genital warts, the most commonly recognized manifestation of these infections, appear to be very frequent, and the incidence may have increased over the last 20 years. The incidence of genital warts among women attending several STD clinics was four per 100 visits, exceeding the number of visits for genital herpes infections. Genital warts in women tend to become much larger during pregnancy or cell-mediated immunosuppression. Vaginal delivery may be complicated by large lesions.

Vertical Transmission

There is little known about the frequency of maternal-to-infant HPV transmission, the prevalence of neonatal HPV infection, what factors are associated with transmission or progression to symptomatic disease in the newborn, and whether transplacental, intrapartum, or postnatal transmission is most important. About 50% of infants born to HPV-positive mothers are found to have HPV DNA in the pharyngeal mucosa; approximately 4% of unselected infant foreskins are positive for HPV DNA. HPV transmission presumably occurs at birth due to contact with an infected birth canal. No effect of maternal HPV infection has been reported on infant birthweight or gestational age at birth. Follow-up studies of large numbers of patients delivered from mothers with anogenital warts have failed to show respiratory papillomatosis after 6 or more years of follow-up, suggesting that delivery through an infected canal alone may be insufficient to establish clinically apparent infection in the infant.

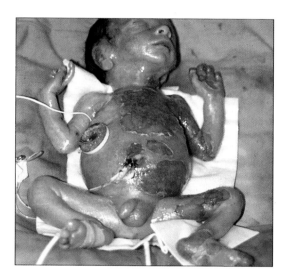

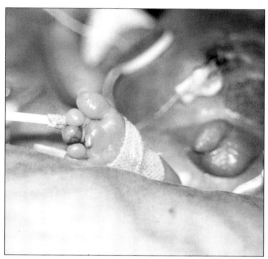

Figs. 14.80 and 14.81 Severe epidermal erosions simulating epidermolysis bullosa in infant with congenital HSV infection.

RECOMMENDED TREATMENT FOR SUSPECTED NEONATAL HERPES SIMPLEX VIRUS INFECTION

Acyclovir 30 mg/kg/day iv divided every 8 hours for 10–14 days

Source: Whitley RJ, Arvin A, Prober C, et al. N. Engl J Med 1991; 324:444–449.

Fig. 14.84 Recommended treatment for suspected neonatal HSV.

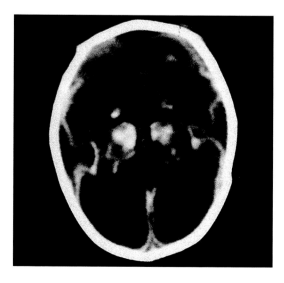

Fig. 14.82 Vesicle positive for HSV–2 on thigh of mother of infant seen in **14.80** and **14.81**.

Fig. 14.83 Unenhanced CT scan of 4-day-old infant with congenital HSV-2 infection, showing intracranial calcifications, diffuse encephalomalacia, and poorly developed gyri.

RECOMMENDED TREATMENT OF GENITAL WARTS DURING PREGNANCY

Cryotherapy with liquid nitrogen (not cryoprobes)

or

TCA 80%–90% applied only to warts; powder with talc or sodium bicarbonate to remove excess acid. Repeat weekly as needed. If warts persist after six applications, consider other method.

Use of podophyllin and podofilox are contraindicated during pregnancy.

Source: Centers for Disease Control and Prevention. 1993 STD Treatment Guidelines. MMWR 1993; 42 (No. RR–14):1–102.

Fig. 14.85 Recommended treatment for condylomata acuminata during pregnancy.

PREVENTION

Podophyllin and podofilox for the treatment of condylomata acuminata are contraindicated during pregnancy. Since lesions tend to proliferate and become friable during pregnancy, some experts advocate removal (*Fig. 14.85*). Cesarean delivery should not be performed solely to prevent transmission of HPV to the newborns, but only if the pelvic outlet is obstructed by genital warts, or if vaginal delivery would result in excessive bleeding.

CLINICAL MANIFESTATIONS

Although oral and anogenital warts in early infancy are likely to be a result of perinatal transmission (*Figs. 14.86* and *14.87*), the most important manifestation of vertical transmission is laryngeal papillomatosis, which is the most common benign laryngeal tumor of infancy. The actual incidence of the disease in the USA is unknown, but is estimated at 1 in 100,000. Laryngeal papillomatosis has a bimodal age distribution. The first peak occurs from 2–5 years of age and the second peak during adolescence.

Laryngeal papillomas appear as white or pink to red warty masses on the vocal cords (*Fig. 14.88*). Clinical symptoms generally develop prior to 4 years of age, consisting of hoarseness or abnormal cry, stridor, respiratory distress, and aphonia. Extension of disease from the larynx to the trachea occurs in up to 36% of cases; the risk increases to over 50% if the patient has undergone a tracheotomy to maintain an airway. Extension to the lung parenchyma is rare, difficult to manage, and often fatal. Malignant transformation is rare, and may be associated with radiation therapy.

Histologically, the papillomas are composed of vascular connective tissue cords covered by hyperplastic stratified squamous epithelium. HPV 11 is predominant in laryngeal papillomata, in contrast to genital condylomata, where HPV 6 predominates, suggesting that laryngeal tissues may be more susceptible to infection by HPV 11.

TREATMENT

Surgical removal is the treatment of choice. The frequent regrowth of papillomas is not due to seeding of the virus during surgery, but to the fact that clinically uninvolved sites are often infected. Even biopsies from patients in remission often contain viral DNA. Tracheostomy and radiation therapy are generally contraindicated. Interferon therapy adds little additional benefit over surgery alone.

STDs IN CHILDHOOD

Since nonsexual transmission of sexually transmitted pathogens appears to be a very unusual event, the diagnosis of an STD in a child is generally considered evidence of abuse, provided that perinatal transmission can be excluded. For this reason, diagnosis of nonvertically transmitted STDs in infants and children should be conducted using definitive techniques, preferably cultures. Follow-up tests should be performed in cases of acute assault (*Fig. 14.89*).

EPIDEMIOLOGY

Sexual abuse appears to be common in all socioeconomic groups, and may or may not coexist with other forms of maltreatment, such as physical abuse or neglect. More than 1.5 million cases of suspected child abuse or neglect are reported each year in the USA, of which about 25% are sexual abuse cases. Questionnaire surveys in the general US adult population suggest that 15–25% of adults have histories of sexual abuse before age 14. Signs of forcible coitus or overt physical trauma are generally rare, and are somewhat more common in boys than girls. In general, however, girls tend to predominate as victims.

In children in whom sexual abuse has occurred or is suspected, several studies should be routinely performed, even in asymptomatic children. Examination of the genitalia and the perianal area for warts, vaginitis, and evidence of trauma or other lesions should be undertaken. However, speculum examination should not be performed on prepubertal girls. The decision to evaluate a child by collecting specimens for STDs, when they are asymptomatic and have no physical findings suggestive of STDs, should be made on an individual basis. If specimens are collected on children without STD findings on the basis of the possibility of sexual abuse, they should be collected according to a protocol designed to maximize the predictive positive and negative values of such tests (*Fig. 14.89*). Genital examination under anesthesia is sometimes desirable for the collection of specimens. The most frequently diagnosed STD in sexually abused children is gonorrhea, but positive cultures for *C. trachomatis* are also very common among sexually abused

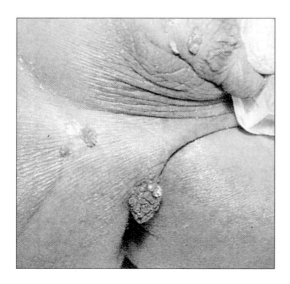

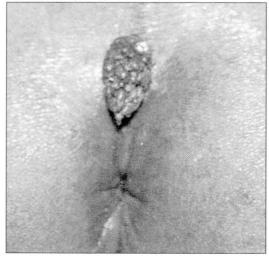

Figs. 14.86 and 14.87 Condylomata acuminata in a 9-month-old infant, probably perinatally acquired.

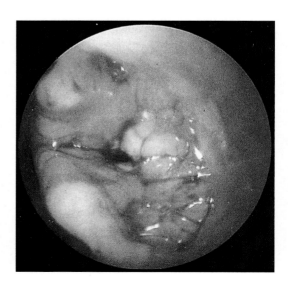

Fig. 14.88 Laryngeal papillomata presenting as warty growths almost occluding the larynx of a child with a history of chronic hoarseness.

children (*Fig. 14.90*). HIV infection is increasingly recognized as potentially acquired by children due to sexual abuse. In children with one STD, it is essential to test for a variety of others.

VULVOVAGINITIS

Vulvovaginitis is a common complaint in prepubertal girls, with an STD as the cause in only a minority of cases. Other frequent causes include *Candida*, *Streptococcus* or enteric organisms, and infestations (*Figs. 14.91* and *14.92*). However, vaginitis is the most common presentation of gonococcal infection in children. The neutral-to-alkaline pH and the thin, atrophic nature of the prepubertal vagina predispose to diffuse vaginitis and dysuria. The incubation period is brief, and while some children are asymptomatic, the child usually develops a purulent, sometimes malodorous, discharge, accompanied by labial erythema (*Figs. 14.93–14.95*). Specimens for Gram stain and culture can be obtained from the hymen or the first few millimeters of the vagina, without speculum examination, or from the discharge itself. Pelvic inflammatory disease, which presents as lower abdominal pain and tenderness, rebound, decreased bowel sounds, and vaginal discharge, occurs in about 6% of prepubertal children with gonococcal vaginitis. Suspicion of sexual abuse

among children with gonococcal infections is frequently confirmed (*Fig. 14.96*).

Chlamydial infections are generally asymptomatic, but may present with vaginitis in prepubertal children. Bacterial vaginosis and trichomoniasis can cause vaginal discharge in sexually abused children, though some children without known sexual activity have evidence of these diseases.

OTHER GONOCOCCAL INFECTIONS

Gonococcal conjunctivitis ranges from mild to extremely severe, with swelling of the conjunctivae and profuse purulent discharge. Often, the source is autoinoculation from a vaginal discharge. A presumptive diagnosis of gonococcal conjunctivitis can be made by Gram stain while awaiting culture results, but culture remains the definitive diagnostic test. Oropharyngeal infection may show exudative tonsillitis, soft-palate swelling and erythema and is seen in up to 50% of sexually abused children in some series. Gonococcal arthritis is a common cause of bacterial arthritis in children; evaluation of children with arthritis should include cultures of synovial fluid, blood, oropharynx, rectum, vagina, and urethra for *N. gonorrhoeae* prior to antimicrobial therapy.

GUIDELINES FOR SCREENING FOR STDS IN CHILDREN SUSPECTED OF BEING SEXUALLY ABUSED

INDICATIONS INCLUDE

The child has symptoms or signs of an STD, or suggestive of an STD
A suspected offender is known to have an STD or to be at high risk for STDs (e.g., multiple partners, or past history of STD)
High prevalence of STD in the community

EXAMINATIONS, INITIAL AND AT 2 WEEKS

Culture for *N. gonorrhoeae*:
  Pharynx and anus, both sexes
    Vagina, girls
    Urethral, boys (meatal specimen adequate if discharge is present)
    All presumptive isolates of *N. gonorrhoeae* should be confirmed by at least two tests that involve different principles, and should be preserved
Culture for *C. trachomatis*:
  Anus, both sexes
  Urethral specimen, only if discharge is present
  Vagina, girls
Culture and wet mount for *T. vaginalis* infection
  Significance of clue cells or other indicators of bacterial vaginosis in the absence of vaginal discharge is unclear, as is their significance as indicators of sexual exposure.
Serum sample to be preserved for subsequent analysis, if follow-up serologic tests are positive
  If last sexual exposure occurred > 8 weeks before initial examination, serum specimens should be tested immediately.
  Serum should be tested for antibodies to HIV and HBV, and with non-treponemal serologic tests for syphilis

EXAMINATION 12 WEEKS AFTER LAST SUSPECTED SEXUAL EXPOSURE

  Serologic tests for HIV, HBV, syphilis

Note: prevalence varies considerably for these conditions; HBV can be transmitted non-sexually

Fig. 14.89 Guidelines for screening for STDs in children suspected of being sexually abused.

STDS IN CHILDREN WITH HISTORY OF SEXUAL ABUSE

| | | | AGENT AND % OF PATIENTS INFECTED | | | | | |
REFERENCE	TOTAL NUMBER	POPULATION CHARACTERISTICS	NEISSERIA GONORRHOEAE	CHLAMYDIA TRACHOMATIS	CONDYLOMA ACUMINATA	HERPES SIMPLEX VIRUS	TRICHOMONAS VAGINALIS	SYPHILIS
Tilelli[1]	103	Sexually abused children aged 2–16 years, Minneapolis, Minnesota	3	–	–	–	–	0
Ingram[2]	50	Sexually abused children aged 1–12 years, North Carolina	20	6	–	–	4	–
Hammerschlag[3]	51	Sexually abused children aged 2–14.5 years, Brooklyn, New York	10	4	–	–	–	–
Grant[4]	157	Sexually abused children aged 8 months–17 years, Manitoba, Canada	9.5	–	1.5	0.5	–	0
Kahn[5]	113	Sexually abused children aged less than 13 years, Baltimore, Maryland	20*	–	–	–	–	–
White[6]	409	Sexually abused children aged less than 13 years, North Carolina	11	–	0.7	–	1	1.5
Ingram[7]	1538	Sexually abused children aged 1–12 years, North Carolina	2.8	1.2	1.8	0.1	–	0.1

*of 71 patients screened.

[1] N Engl J Med 1980; 302:319
[2] Ped Infect Dis 1984; 3:97
[3] Ped Infect Dis 1984; 3:100
[4] Am J Obstet Gynecol 1984; 148:617
[5] Clin Pediatr 1983; 22:369
[6] Pediatrics 1983; 72:16
[7] Ped Infect Dis J 1992; 11:945

Fig. 14.90 Prevalence of STDs among sexually abused children. Note that gonococcal infections tend to be most common.

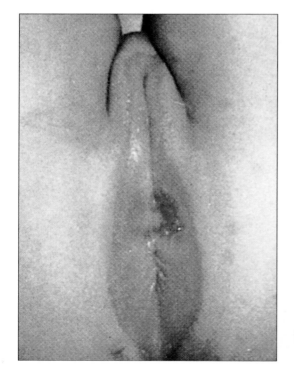

Fig. 14.91 Streptococcal vulvovaginitis presenting as sharply circumscribed erythema from the vulva to the perianal area.

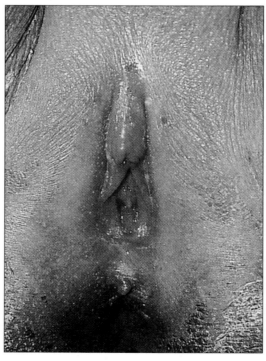

Fig. 14.92 Vulvar erythema and evident desquamation in a child with scarlet fever. Serosanguinous discharge is often seen in streptococcal vulvovaginitis. Streptococcal infections and other common nonsexually transmitted infection should be ruled out as part of the evaluation of vulvovaginitis.

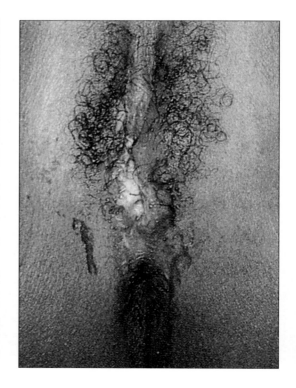

Fig. 14.93 Gonococcal vulvar erythema, edema, purulent vaginal discharge and Bartholin's cyst in a premenarchal sexually abused child.

ANOGENITAL LESIONS

Anogenital lesions are less common complaints in prepubertal children, and are more likely to be sexually acquired than vulvovaginitis. Warts, chancres, ulcers and vesicular or pustular rashes should be evaluated for the diagnosis of HPV, HSV infection, or syphilis.

CONDYLOMATA ACUMINATA

HPV anogenital infection in prepubertal children typically presents as verrucous, flesh-colored or reddish papules; the most common location is perianal in either sex (*Fig. 14.97*). The lesions may extend into the anal canal, the urethra, or hymen (*Figs. 14.98* and *14.99*). The lesions are often asymptomatic,

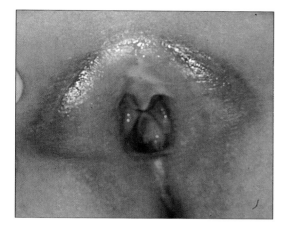

Fig. 14.94 Purulent discharge and vulvar erythema and edema due to gonococcal infection in a sexually abused child.

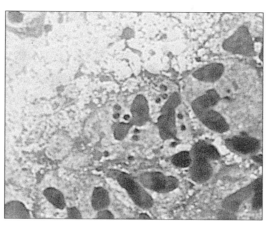

Fig. 14.95 Gram stain of vaginal discharge from patient in **14.93**, with sheets of polymorphonuclear leukocytes, several with intracellular Gram-negative diplococci. This finding, highly specific in a prepubertal child, should be confirmed by culture.

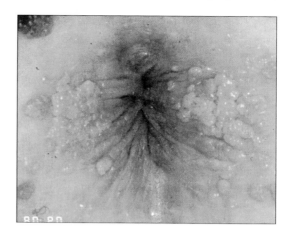

Fig. 14.97 Common presentation of perianal condylomata acuminata in a 6-year-old child.

INCIDENCE OF SEXUAL ABUSE IN CHILDREN WITH STDs OR SYMPTOMS SUGGESTIVE OF STDs

REFERENCE	TOTAL NUMBER	POPULATION CHARACTERISTICS	DISEASE	NO. (%) IN WHOM SEXUAL ABUSE CONFIRMED	
Kaplan[1]	6	Children aged 21 months – 13 years	Genital herpes	4	(67)
Jones[2]	4	Girls aged 10–12 years	Trichomoniasis	4	(100)
Samuels[3]	25	Girls ages 13 months – 11 years	Candidiasis (21%) Gonococcal vulvovaginitis (8%) Group A streptococcus (4%) Bacterial vaginosis (33%)	6	(24)
Rock[4]	5	Children aged 3–8 years	Genital warts	3	(60)
Branch[5]	45	Children aged 1–9 years	Gonococcal infection	42	(93)

[1] Am J Dis Child 1984; 138:872
[2] Am J Dis Child 1985; 139:846
[3] ICAAC, 1985, Abstract #27
[4] Arch Dermatol 1986; 122:1120
[5] Pub Health Rep 1985; 80:347

Fig. 14.96 Evidence of child abuse is established in a substantial proportion of children with STDs.

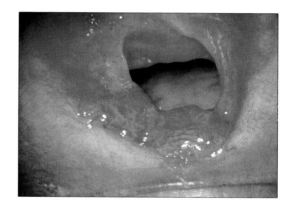

Fig. 14.98 Unusual presentation of condylomata acuminata in a 10-year-old sexually abused girl, with lesion appearing to extend from the vagina and erode the hymen.

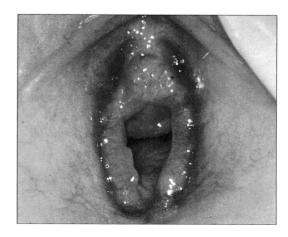

Fig. 14.99 Single condyloma in a 20-month-old girl, located on the posterior fourchette, with transection of the hymen consistent with sexual abuse.

or may become infected, causing pain, bleeding, dysuria, pruritus, or vaginitis. Molluscum contagiosum, chronic benign pemphigus, histiocytosis X, neurofibromatosis, pseudoverrucous papules, nodules and skin tags are among the conditions that must be considered in the differential diagnosis of anogenital condylomata (*Figs. 14.100* and *14.101*). HPV DNA typing of anogenital warts may help in determining the mode of transmission of anogenital warts in children. Warts due to HPV types common in genital infection, including 6 and 11, are more likely to be associated with proven sexual or vertical transmission than those types commonly seen in common skin warts, such as HPV-2. The presence of types typical of skin warts suggests the possibility of autoinoculation in patients who also have skin warts, or possibly, nonsexual transmission from caretakers. Nevertheless, the frequent association of condylomata acumi-

nata with sexual abuse, and the fact that the type of virus often does not provide proof of the presence or absence of sexual transmission, make it imperative that sexual abuse is considered in all cases of condylomata acuminata in children. HPV type information should be interpreted together with other relevant information.

SYPHILIS

Syphilis is rare among sexually abused children. When it occurs, it may present as condylomata lata, as isolated chancres, exanthems, or alopecia. Extragenital chancres are frequent in children, including chancres of the lips,

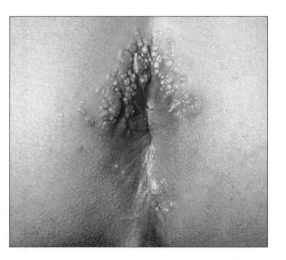

Fig. 14.100 Perianal molluscum contagiosum simulating condylomata acuminata in a 6-year-old male, necessitating biopsy confirmation.

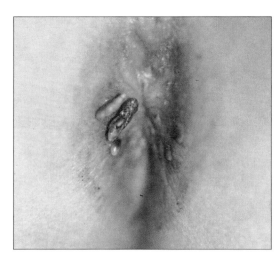

Fig. 14.101 Perianal condylomata acuminata in an 8-year-old boy. Hyperpigmented lesions were proven to be bowenoid papulosis by biopsy. Although the child had a rectal culture positive for *Chlamydia trachomatis*, confirming sexual abuse, he denied sexual activity.

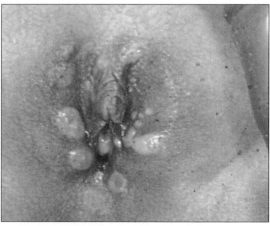

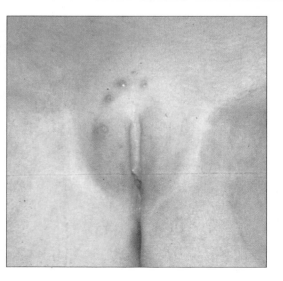

Figs. 14.102 and 14.103 Childhood sexual abuse. Perineal flat condylomata lata in sexually abused girls.

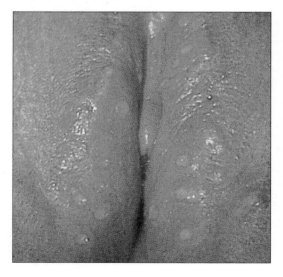

Fig. 14.104 Herpes simplex in a prepubertal child with dysuria and perineal pain.

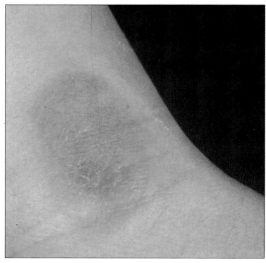

Fig. 14.105 Dermatitis due to nickel allergy from a bed-wetting alarm, simulating genital herpes.

Fig. 14.106 Confirmation of nickel allergy in **14.105** given by patch-test on wrist.

mouth, tongue, and thigh. Condylomata lata in children are generally perianal but may be perineal (*Figs. 14.102* and *14.103*). They may be indistinguishable from condylomata acuminata on physical examination. Serologic tests for syphilis may be negative during primary syphilis or immediately after an isolated assault. For these reasons, serologic tests for syphilis should be repeated 1 month after an assault if the assailant is unavailable for serologic testing.

HSV INFECTIONS

Genital HSV infection presents in children generally as painful perineal lesions, dysuria, vulvovaginitis and/or 'sores' (*Figs. 14.104–14.106*). A history of sexual contact is common among children with genital herpes. However, there is some evidence that autoinoculation from oral lesions may result in genital herpes in children who may not have been abused. This is particularly likely in children in whom the eruption of genital tract vesicles was immediately preceded by oral

lesions, generally caused by HSV-1. Since even in genital herpes due to HSV-1, evidence of sexual abuse is common, evidence of abuse should be sought in all cases of genital herpes in children, regardless of type.

STDS IN ADOLESCENTS

EPIDEMIOLOGY

Reported sexual activity has increased considerably in adolescents in the last two decades. Many behavioral and physiologic characteristics place adolescents at high risk for the many adverse consequences of STDs. When controlled for sexual activity, age-specific rates of many STDs (including gonorrhea and chlamydial infections) are highest among sexually experienced adolescents. Moreover, while the incidence of many STDs is declining in the US population, the incidence of primary and secondary syphilis and gonorrhea appears to

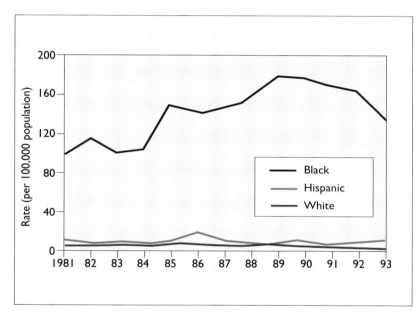

14.107

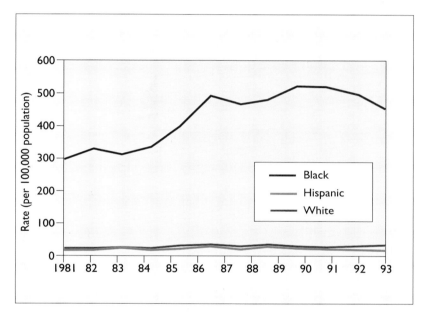

14.108

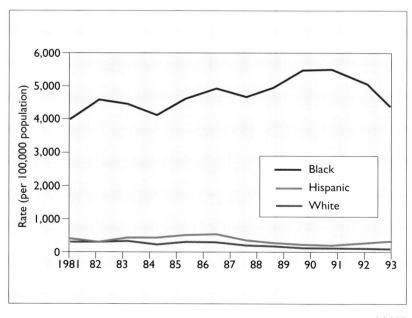

14.109

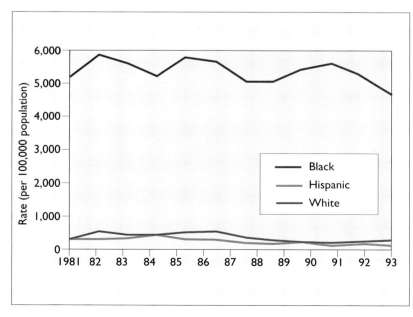

14.110

Figs. 14.107–14.110 Striking increases and high incidence of gonorrhea in selected adolescent populations by race/ethnicity, USA, 1981–1993: (**14.107**) 10- to 14-year-old males; (**14.108**) 10- to 14-year-old females; (**14.109**) 15- to 19-year-old males; (**14.110**) 15- to 19-year-old females.

be increasing among some adolescent populations (*Figs. 14.107–14.110*). In general, *C. trachomatis* infection tends to be the most frequently diagnosed STD in female adolescents (*Fig. 14.111*), but other STDs, particularly gonorrhea, are extremely common among adolescents as well. PID due to *N. gonorrhoeae* (36.4%) or *C. trachomatis* (44.7%) is one of the most serious outcomes of STDs in adolescents. It is estimated that 16–20% of women hospitalized with PID per annum are adolescents, and that a sexually active 15-year-old has 10 times the risk of developing PID than has a 24-year-old. HSV infection also appears to be common among adolescents; while less than 1% of participants in a US survey were infected before 15 years of age, between 5% and 28% had antibodies to HSV-2 at 20 years of age. Likewise, HPV infection and cervical dysplasia are becoming increasingly common among adolescent women. Finally, HIV infection due to both homosexual and heterosexual activity is also increasing rapidly among adolescents.

PREVALENCE OF STD PATHOGENS IN SELECTED ADOLESCENT POPULATIONS

REFERENCE	YEAR	POPULATION	TOTAL NUMBER	LOCATION	N. GONORRHOEAE	C. TRACHOMATIS	SYPHILIS	TRICHOMONAS VAGINALIS	OTHER
McCormack	1974–75	Female college students	431	unspecified	–	4.9	–	14.3	M. hominis U. urealyticum
Munford	1977	Indigent pregnant girls	740	Houston, TX	2.4	–	0.7	–	–
Saltz	1979–80	Low and middle income sexually active girls	100	Cincinnati, OH	3	22	–	16	–
Bell	1981	Female detainees in juvenile detention center	100	Seattle, WA	18	20	–	48	Bacterial vaginosis
Anglin	1981	Sexually active adolescent girls	75	Cleveland, OH	11	23	–	13	3
Chacko	1981–82	Urban sexually active boys and girls	280	Baltimore, MD	3	22	–	16	–
Hardy	1983	Pregnant girls in prenatal care	115	Balitmore, MD	10.4	37	–	34	M. hominis 70 U. urealyticum 90
Adger	1983–84	Working class, sexually active boys	50	San Francisco, CA	10	32	–	–	–
Eager	1983–84	Indigent & middle income sexually active girls	396	Denver, CO	7	21	–	6	–
Shafer	1985	Sexually active girls (13–21 years)	148	San Francisco, CA	–	15.5	–	–	Cytologic inflammation 44
Bump	1986	Sexually active (and virginal) middle class adolescent girls	120	Columbus, OH	6(0)	19(2)	–	9(0)	M. hominis 27 (10) U. urealyticum 75 (33)
Hughes	1989	Sexually active girls	446	Ottawa, Canada	1.5	14.7	–	–	–
Blythe	1992	Public health clinic patients	1308	Indianapolis, IN	15	31.1	–	–	–
Matson	1993	Low income pregnant girls	168	Milwaukee, WI	13	25	–	–	–

Fig. 14.111 Prevalence of selected STDs in various adolescent populations.

Both ectopy, which is common in adolescents, and the use of oral contraceptives, which are preferred by adolescents enrolled in family planning, tend to be associated with an increased risk of *C. trachomatis* infection (*Fig. 14.112*). In most studies, young age has been associated with an increased risk of cervical infection with *C. trachomatis*.

PREVENTION

STDs in adolescents, particularly in women, tend to be detected primarily by screening. Screening for STDs that are common and often asymptomatic should be part of routine care for sexually active adolescents. Screening services should be particularly geared to adolescents at highest risk (pregnant, or low socioeconomic status, drug-users), preferably by offering them at easily accessible, welcoming settings. Since specimen collection for *C. trachomatis* and *N. gonorrhoeae* involve uncomfortable procedures, such as urethral swabbing (in males) or speculum examinations (in females), adolescents may be deterred from screening, so urine-based screening strategies should be explored in high prevalence populations (*see Chap. 4*). Papanicolaou smears, and serologic tests for syphilis, in areas with a high prevalence of syphilis should be performed on sexually active adolescents at least at intake. Adolescents diagnosed with syphilis should be encouraged to seek HIV testing.

CLINICAL MANIFESTATIONS

The most commonly seen manifestations of symptomatic STDs in adolescent girls are PID (presenting as lower abdominal pain), vaginitis, vaginal discharge or cervicitis (*Fig. 14.113*). Urethritis and acute epididymitis, presenting as scrotal swelling and pain in men under 45 years of age, are commonly associated with STDs, with *C. trachomatis* established as the cause in 30–50% of cases of epididymitis. Genital warts, ulcers or vesicles are also frequently due to STDs; genital ulcers should be evaluated with dark-field microscopy and cultured for HSV regardless of appearance. Diagnosis of *C. trachomatis* in cases of epididymitis can be improved by use of a DNA amplification test such as PCR or LCR (*see Chap. 4*).

STDs are also part of the differential diagnosis in arthritis, exanthems, lymphadenopathy, and alopecia in sexually active adolescents. Most cases of

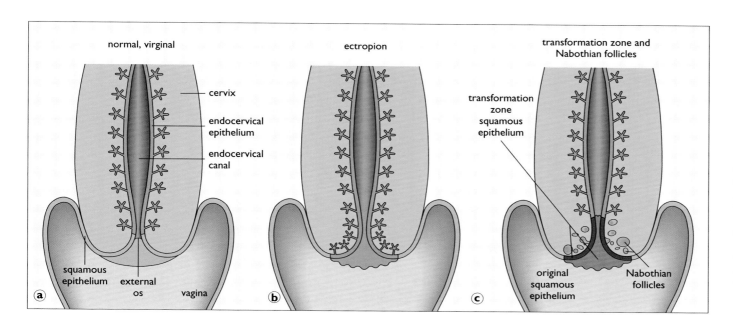

Fig. 14.112 Junction between columnar endocervical epithelium and vaginal squamous epithelium moves from the external os to the vagina during adolescence (ectopy or ectropion). Ectopy is seen commonly in adolescents and oral contraceptive users. This tissue is more susceptible to *C. trachomatis* infection. A transformation zone forms as squamous epithelium regrows over the endocervical epithelium. Openings of the crypts may be obliterated in the process, forming mucus-filled Nabothian follicles.

STD SYNDROMES (I) AND SYNDROMES SUGGESTIVE OF STDS (II) AMONG SEXUALLY ACTIVE ADOLESCENTS

I STD SYNDROMES
  Urethritis
  Vaginitis
  Cervicitis
  Genital Lesions

II SYNDROMES SUGGESTIVE OF STDs
  Lower Abdominal Pain (Female)
  Scrotal Swelling and Pain
  Arthritis
  Exanthems
  Alopecia

Fig. 14.113 Common STD syndromes (I) and syndromes with STDs in the differential diagnosis (II) among sexually active adolescents.

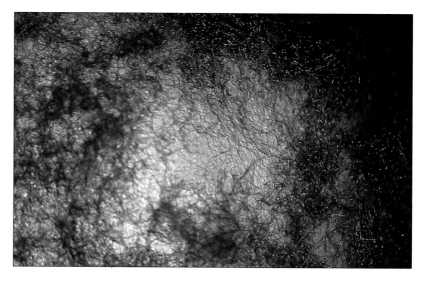

Fig. 14.114 Alopecia in a 13-year-old boy with secondary syphilis.

nontraumatic arthritis in sexually active adolescents are caused by *N. gonorrhoeae*. Generalized lymphadenopathy, papulosquamous rashes, particularly with palmar or plantar distribution, and alopecia are frequently signs of secondary syphilis in high prevalence populations (*Fig. 14.114*).

TREATMENT

In general, the treatment of STDs in adolescents is identical to that recommended for adults. Given the pressures under which sexually active adolescents generally live, and the possibility of nonadherence, it is recommended that one-dose treatments administered in the clinic be used whenever possible. Effective one-dose treatments are available for infections due to *C. trachomatis*, provided the patient is not pregnant, and for *N. gonorrhoeae* and *T. pallidum* infection. Treatment of genital warts in adolescent women should be accompanied by evaluation for cervical warts by colposcopic examination, and careful follow-up with Papanicolaou smears. Because of the high rate of reinfection among adolescents — up to 38% of those with *C. trachomatis* infections — it is imperative to identify and treat sexual partners and incorporate frequent rescreening for women previously diagnosed with STDs.

Picture credits for this chapter are as follows: Figs. 14.2, 14.90, 14.96 courtesy of Beck-Sague CM, Alexander ER: Infect Dis Clin North Am 1987;1:277–304; Fig. 14.2 courtesy of CDC: DSTD/HIVP, 1994; Fig. 14.3 courtesy of Zenker P: Sex Transm Dis 18:44–45, 1991; Fig. 14.4 courtesy of CDC: DSTD/HIVP, 1995; Fig. 14.5 compiled from Brunham RC, Embree JE: Sexually transmitted diseases: current and future dimensions of the problem in the Third World. In: Germain A, et al. (eds): Reproductive Tract Infections. Plenum Press, New York, p 44, 1992; Br J Vener Dis 58:355–358,1982; Genitourin Med 65:276–280, 1989; J Infect Dis 161:531–536, 1990; Aust NZ J Obstet Gynecol 27:213–215, 1987; Int J Gynecol Obstet 29:321–324, 1989; and Chhabra RS, Brion LP, Castro M, Feundlich L, Glaser JH: Pediatrics 91:88–91, 1993; Fig. 14.6 courtesy of CDC: DSTD, 1987; Fig. 14.7 courtesy of MMWR 42:1–102, 1993; Figs. 14.8 and 14.9 courtesy F Qureshi, MD and S Jacques, MD; Fig. 14.10 courtesy of D Schwartz, MD; Fig. 14.11 courtesy of CDC: DSTD/HIVP; Fig. 14.12 courtesy of Young SA, Crocker DW: Arch Pathol Lab Med 118:44–47, 1994; Fig. 14.16 courtesy of DSTD, CDC,1987; Fig. 14.17–14.19 courtesy of Tunnessen WW: AJDC 146:115–116, 1992; Fig. 14.20 courtesy of Wood VD: J Fam Pract 35:327–329, 1992; Fig. 14.23 courtesy of Ilagan NB, Weyhing B, Liang KC, Womack SJ, Shankaran S: Clin Pediatr 312–313, 1993; Fig. 14.25 courtesy of Edell DS, Davidson JJ, Mulvilhill DM, Majure M: Ped Pulmon 15:376–379, 1993; Fig. 14.24 courtesy of Ikeda MK, Jenson HB: J Peds 117:843–852, 1990; Fig. 14.27 courtesy of Jennifer Flood, MD; Fig. 14.30 courtesy of Zenker PN, Berman SM: Ped Infect Dis J 516–522, 1991; Fig. 14.31 courtesy of Lewis LL: Inf Dis Clin North Am 6:31–39, 1992; Fig. 14.43 courtesy of Schachter JE, Figs.

14.32, 14.35, 14.36, 14.42, 14.85, 14.89 courtesy of CDC: MMWR 42:1–102, 1993; Fig. 14.33 compiled from Brunham RC, Embree JE: Sexually transmitted diseases: current and future dimensions of the problem in the Third World. In: Germain A, et al. (eds): Reproductive Tract Infections. Plenum Press, New York, p. 44, 1992; S Afr Med J 52:119, 1977; Bull WHO 63:1107–1113, 1985; Lancet ii:1145–1148, 1986; J Infect Dis 161:531–536, 1990; Br J Vener Dis 58:355–358, 1982; Int J Gynecol Obstet 18:48–52, 1980; Aust NZ J Obstet Gynecol 27:213–215, 1987; Figs. 14.36, 14.44 courtesy of Armstrong JH, Zacarias F, Rein MF: Pediatrics 57:884–892, 1976; Fig. 14.37 courtesy of Desenclos JCA, Garrity D, Scaggs M, Wroten JE: Sex Transm Dis 19:10539–110, 1992; Figs. 14.45 and 14.46 courtesy of Harrison HR, Alexander ER: In: Holmes KK, Mardh PA, Sparling PF, Wiesner PJ (eds): Sexually Transmitted Diseases. McGraw Hill Book Co., New York, pp 270–280, 1984; Fig. 14.47 courtesy of CDC: MMWR 42:56–67, 1993; Figs. 14.48 and 14.57 courtesy of Lindegren ML, Caldwell MB, Oxtoby M. Pediatric HIV infection in the USA. In: Mok J, Newell M-L (eds). Practical Management of HIV infection in Children. Cambridge University Press, 1994; Fig. 14.49 courtesy of CDC. National HIV serosurveillance summary results through 1992. Vol 3. Atlanta, GA, US DHHS, 1994; Fig. 14.50 adapted from St Louis M, Kamenga M, Brown C, et al.: JAMA 269:2853–2859, 1993; Fig. 14.53 courtesy of CDC: MMWR 43(RR-11):1–20, 1994; Figs. 14.51–14.52 courtesy of Marion RW, Wiznia AA, Hutcheon RG, Rubinstein A: AJDC 140:636–640, 1986; Figs. 14.55, 14.56 adapted from CDC: MMWR 36:225–228, 1987; Figs. 14.58, 14.59, 14.64, 14.68, 14.70 courtesy of Marquis JR, Bardeguez AD: Clin Perinatol 1:125–147, 1994; Figs. 14.60, 14.61, 14.66, 14.67, 14.71 courtesy of Gwendolyn B. Scott, University of Miami School of Medicine, and Skoner DP, Urbach AH, Fireman P. Pediatric Allergy and Immunology. In: Zitelli BJ, Davis HW (eds). Atlas of Pediatric Physical Diagnosis. 2nd edn. Gower Medical Publishing, 1992; Figs. 14.62, 14.63, 14.65 courtesy of Prose NS: Dermatol Clin 9:543–550, 1991; Fig. 14.69 courtesy of Haller JO, Cohen HL: AJR 1994;162:387–393; Figs. 14.72, 14.76 courtesy of Whitley R, Arvin A, Prober C, et al.: N Engl J Med 324:450–454, 1991; Fig. 14.75 courtesy of Overall JC: Ped Ann 23:131–136, 1994; Figs. 14.73 and 14.74 courtesy of Hyde SR, Giacoia GP: Obstet Gynecol 81:852–855, 1993; Figs. 14.80–14.82 courtesy of Sarkell B, Blaylock WK, Vernon H: J Am Acad Dermatol 27:817–821, 1992; Fig. 14.83 courtesy of Bale JF, Murphy JR: Ped Clin North Am 39:669–690, 1992; Fig. 14.84 courtesy of Whitley RJ, Arvin A, Prober C, et al.: N Engl J Med 324:444–449, 1991; Fig. 14.88 courtesy of McBride TP, Davis HW, Reilly JS: Pediatric otolaryngology. In: Zitelli BJ, Davis HW (eds). Atlas of Pediatric Physical Diagnosis. 2nd edn. Gower Medical Publishing, 1992; Figs. 14.86 and 14.87 courtesy of Boyd AS: AJDC 144:817–824, 1990; Figs. 14.91, 14.92, 14.95, 14.104 courtesy of Murray P, Davis HW, Hamp M: Pediatric and adolescent gynecology. In: Zitelli BJ, Davis HW (eds). Atlas of Pediatric Physical Diagnosis. 2nd edn. Gower Medical Publishing, 1992; Fig. 14.94 Rimaza B, Feingold M: Picture of the month. AJDC 1989;143:381–382; Figs. 14.97–14.101 courtesy of Frasier LD: Ped Ann 23:354–360, 1994; Fig. 14.103 courtesy of Dr. Angela Robinson, University College London Hospital; Figs. 14.105–14.106 courtesy of Hanks JW: Pediatrics 90:458–460, 1992; Figs. 14.107–14.110 courtesy of CDC: MMWR 42(SS-3):1–12), 1993; Fig. 14.111 compiled from Beck-Sague CM, Alexander ER: Infect Dis Clin North Am 1:277–304, 1987; McCormack: Am J Epidemiol 121:115, 1975; Mumford: Reprod Med 19:83, 1977; Saltz J: Pediatr 98:980, 1981; Bell TA: Sex Transm Dis 12:140, 1985; Fraser: Pediatr 71:333, 1983; Anglin: Pediatr Res 15:440, 1981; Chacko: Pediatr 74:636, 1984; Shafer J: Pediatr 74:104, 1984; Hardy: Lancet ii:333, 1984; Adger: Lancet ii:944, 1984; Eager: West J Med 37:143, 1985; Shafer J: Am J Obstet Gynecol 151:765, 1985; Bump Pediatrics 77:488, 1986; Figs. 14.13, 14.15, 14.21, 14.22, 14.25, 14.26, 14.28, 14.29, 14.38–14.41, 14.51, 14.52, 14.77–14.79, 14.102, 14.114 courtesy of CDC Still Pictures Archives. Fig. 14.112 courtesy of Stevens A, Lowe J, from Histology, Mosby, 1993.

BIBLIOGRAPHY

Armstrong JH, Zacarias F, Rein MF: Ophthalmia neonatorum: a chart review. *Pediatrics* **57**:884–92, 1976.

Bale JR, Murph JR: Congenital infections and the nervous system. *Ped Clin North Am* **39**:669–690, 1992.

Batteiger BE, Jones RB: Chlamydial infections. *Infect Dis Clin of North Am* 1:55–81, 1987.

Beck-Sague CM, Alexander ER: Sexually transmitted diseases in children and adolescents. *Infect Dis Clin of North Am* 1:277–304, 1987.

Beck-Sague CM, Alexander ER: Failure of benzathine penicillin G treatment in early congenital syphilis. *Pediatr Infect Dis J* **6**:1061–1064, 1987.

Bell TA, Stamm WE, Wang SP, et al.: Chronic *Chlamydia trachomatis* infections in infants. *JAMA* **267**:400–402, 1992.

Blythe MJ, Katz BP, Batteiger BE, et al.: Recurrent genitourinary chlamydial infections in sexually active female adolescents. *J Pediatr* **121**:487–493, 1992.

Brunham RC, Embree JE: Sexually transmitted diseases: current and future dimensions of the problem in the Third World. In: Germain A, *et al.* (eds): *Reproductive Tract Infections*. Plenum Press, New York, pp 35–58, 1992.

Butler C, Hittelman J, Hauger SB: Approach to neurodevelopmental and neurologic complications in pediatric HIV infection. *J Pediatr* **119**:S41–S43, 1991.

Centers for Disease Control and Prevention: Classification system for human immunodeficiency virus (HIV) infection in children under 13 years of age. *MMWR* **36**:225–228, 1987.

Centers for Disease Control and Prevention: Recommendations for the prevention and management of *Chlamydia trachomatis* infections, 1993. *MMWR* **42**(RR-12):1–33, 1993.

Centers for Disease Control and Prevention: Recommendations of the US Public Health Service Task Force on the use of zidovudine to reduce perinatal transmission of human immunodeficiency virus. *MMWR* **43**(RR-11):1–20, 1994.

Centers for Disease Control and Prevention: 1993 Sexually transmitted diseases treatment guidelines. *MMWR* **42**(RR-14):1–102, 1993.

Desenclos JCA, Garrity D, Scaggs M, Wroten JE: Gonococcal infection of the newborn in Florida, 1984–1989. *Sex Trans Dis* **19**:105–110, 1992.

Finkelhor D, Hotaling G, Lewis IA, Smith C: Sexual abuse in a national survey of adult men and women: prevalence, characteristics and risk factors. *Child Abuse Negl* **14**:19–28, 1990.

Frasier LD: Human papillomavirus infections in children. *Pediatr Annals* **23**:354–360,1994.

Gayle HD, D'Angelo LJ: Epidemiology of acquired immunodeficiency syndrome and human immunodeficiency virus infection in adolescents. *Pediatr Infect Dis J* **10**:322–328, 1991.

Golden N, Neuhoff S, Cohen H: Pelvic inflammatory disease in adolescents. *J Pediatr* **114**:138–143, 1989.

Gutman LT, St Claire K, Herman-Giddnes M, McKinney RE: Child sexual abuse and human immunodeficiency virus transmission. *AJDC* **145**:847–848, 1991.

Gutman LT, Herman-Giddens M, Prose NS: Diagnosis of child sexual abuse in children with genital warts. *AJDC* **145**:126–127, 1991.

Gutman LT, Herman-Giddens ME, Phelps WC: Transmission of human genital papillomavirus disease: comparisons of data from adults and children. *Pediatrics* **91**:31–38, 1993.

Haller JO, Cohen HL: Gastrointestinal manifestations of AIDS in children. *AJR* **162**:387–393, 1994.

Hammerschlag MR: Chlamydial infections. *J Pediatr* **114**:727–734, 1989.

Hammerschlag MR: *Chlamydia trachomatis* in children. *Pediatr Annals* **23**:349–353, 1994.

Harrison HR, Costin M, Meder JB, *et al.*: Cervical *Chlamydia trachomatis* infection in university women: relationship to history, contraception, ectopy and cervicitis. *Am J Obstet Gynecol* **153**:244–249.

Harrison HR, English MG, Lee CK, *et al.*: *Chlamydia trachomatis* infant pneumonitis: comparison with matched controls and other infant pneumonitis. *N Engl J Med* **298**:702–708, 1978.

Hirschfield LS, Steinberg BM: Clinical spectrum of HPV infection in the neonate and child. *Clin Pract Gynecol* **2**:102–116, 1989.

Hughes EG, Mowatt J, Spence JE: Endocervical *Chlamydia trachomatis* in Canada adolescents. *Can Med Assoc J* **140**:297–301, 1989

Ikeda MK, Jenson HB: Evaluation and treatment of congenital syphilis. *J Peds* **117**:843–852, 1990.

Ingram DL: *Neisseria gonorrhoeae* in children. *Pediatr Annals* **23**:341–348, 1994.

Jones JG, Yamauchi T, Lambert B: *Trichomonas vaginalis* infestation in sexually abused girls. *AJDC* **139**:846–847, 1985.

Kaplan KM, Fleisher GR, Paradise JE, Friedman HN: Social relevance of genital herpes simplex in children. *AJDC* **138**:872–874, 1984.

Krasinski K: Retroviral therapy and clinical trials for HIV-infected children. *J Pediatr* **119**:S63–S65, 1991.

Kuhn L, Stein ZA, Thomas PA, *et al.*: Maternal–infant HIV transmission and circumstances of delivery. *Am J Public Health* **84**:1110–1115, 1994.

Laga M, Plummer FA, Nzanza H, *et al*: Epidemiology of ophthalmia neonatorum in Kenya. *Lancet* **ii**:1145–1148, 1986.

Laga M, Meheus A, Piot P: Epidemiology and control of gonococcal ophthalmia neonatorum. *Bull World Health Org* **67**:471–478, 1989.

Lewis LL: Congenital syphilis: Serologic diagnosis in the young infant. *Infect Dis Clin North Am* **6**:31–39, 1992.

Lindegren ML, Caldwell MB, Oxtoby M: Paediatric HIV infection in the United States of America. In: Mok J, Newell M-L (eds). *Practical Management of HIV Infection in Children.* Cambridge University Press, London, 1995.

Marquis JR, Bardeguez AD: Imaging of HIV infection in the prenatal and postnatal period. *Clin Perinatol* **1**:125–147, 1994.

Matson SC, Pomeranz AJ, Kamps KA: Early detection and treatment of sexually transmitted disease in pregnant adolescents of low socioeconomic status. *Clin Pediatr* **ii**:609–612, 1993.

Nahmias AJ, Josey WE, Naib ZM, *et al.*: Perinatal risk associated with maternal genital herpes simplex virus infection. *Am J Obstet Gynecol* **110**:825–836, 1971.

Overall JC: Herpes simplex virus infection of the fetus and newborn. *Ped Ann* **23**:131–136, 1994.

Pearson RC, Baumber CD, McGhie D, Thamber V: The relevance of *Chlamydia trachomatis* in acute epididymitis in young men. *Br J Urol* **62**:72–75.

Rawstron SA, Bromberg K: Failure of recommended maternal therapy to prevent congenital syphilis. *Sex Transm Dis* **18**:102–106, 1991.

Report of a concensus workshop. Maternal factors involved in mother-to-child transmission of HIV-1. *Lancet* **ii**:1007–1012, 1992.

Rothenberg R. Ophthalmia neonatorum due to *Neisseria gonorrhoeae*: prevention and treatment. *Sex Transm Dis* **6**:187–191, 1979.

Rudloff MD: Significance of *Gardnerella vaginalis* in a prepubertal female. *Ped Infect Dis J* **10**:709–710, 1991.

Schachter J, Grossman M, Sweet RL, *et al.*: Prospective study of perinatal transmission of *Chlamydia trachomatis*. *JAMA* **115**:3374–3377, 1986.

Shafer MA, Schachter, Moncada J, *et al.*: Evaluation of urine-based screening strategies to detect *Chlamydia trachomatis* among sexually active asymptomatic young males. *JAMA* **270**:2065–2075, 1993.

StLouis ME, Kamenga M, Brown C, *et al.*: Risk for perinatal HIV-1 transmission according to maternal immunologic, virologic, and placental factors. *JAMA* **269**:2853–2859, 1993.

Tipple MA, Beem MO, Saxon EM: Clinical characterisctics of afebrile pneumonia associated with Chlamydia trachomatis in infants less than 6 months of age. *Pediatrics* **63**:192–197, 1979.

Whitley RJ, Arvin A, Prober C, *et al.*: A controlled trial comparing vidarabine with acyclovir in neonatal herpes simplex virus infection. *N Engl J Med* **324**:444–449, 1991.

Whitley R, Arvin A, Prober C, *et al.*: Predictors of morbidity and mortality in newborns with herpes simplex virus infections. *N Engl J Med* **324**:450–454, 1991.

Zenker PN, Berman SM: Congenital syphilis: trends and recommendations for evaluation and management. *Pediatr Infect Dis J* **10**:516–522, 1991.

Zenker P: New case definition for congenital syphilis reporting. *Sex Transm Dis* **18**:44–45, 1991.

CHAPTER FIFTEEN

Infestations

J Long

INTRODUCTION

Scabies and pubic lice are parasitic insects that live on or within the skin. The dermatidides that they produce are generally considered to be STDs, although they are also spread by nonsexual activity involving skin-to-skin contact. Sexual acquisition can often be assumed when the patient is a young adult with multiple sexual partners. Among young children, however, most cases do not imply sexual exposure.

SCABIES

Scabies is a pruritic dermatosis caused by the mite *Sarcoptes scabiei*. This condition, recognized for centuries as the 'seven-year itch' was associated with the mite as early as 1654. The casual relationship between the mite and the rash was much debated and not generally accepted until this century.

The female mite is primarily responsible for the rash and is the form most frequently recovered from infested patients (*Figs. 15.1* and *15.2*). The adult female measures approximately 400 x 300 μm and is translucent and barely perceptible to the naked eye. Transverse grooves cover the body, and small denticles form a variable pattern on the dorsal surface. Although there is no distinct head, large, protruding jaws identify the anterior end (*Fig. 15.3*). Four pairs of legs are found in adult mites. In the female, the most posterior of these ends in long tendrils, while in the male the most posterior pair ends in suckers.

On the skin surface, the female can walk 2.5 cm/min, moving from the neck to the wrist in a few hours. Upon selecting a suitable site, the fertilized female digs into the skin down as far as the stratum granulosum, where she lays her eggs and feeds on cellular material (*Fig. 15.4*). Each day, she extends the burrow by 0.5–5 mm and lays two to three eggs. Under optimal conditions, the mite will continue to burrow and lay eggs for a month

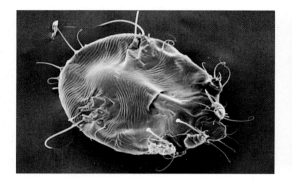

Fig. 15.1 Scanning electron micrograph of the ventral surface of a female *Sarcoptes scabiei* (× 300). A central bulge overlies the ovary, which contains a large egg.

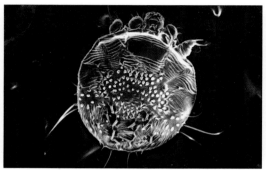

Fig. 15.2 Scanning electron micrograph of *Sarcoptes scabiei* showing the dorsal surface (× 200). Multiple small denticles are present except in a central bare area. Attempts to correlate the size of this bare area with biologic variants of the mite have had limited success.

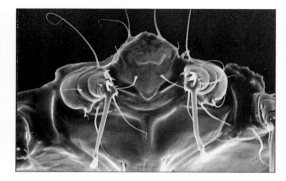

Fig. 15.3 Scanning electron micrograph of the jaw parts of *Sarcoptes scabiei* (× 1,000). These powerful jaws penetrate the skin and disrupt cells, producing a nutrient fluid on which the mite feeds.

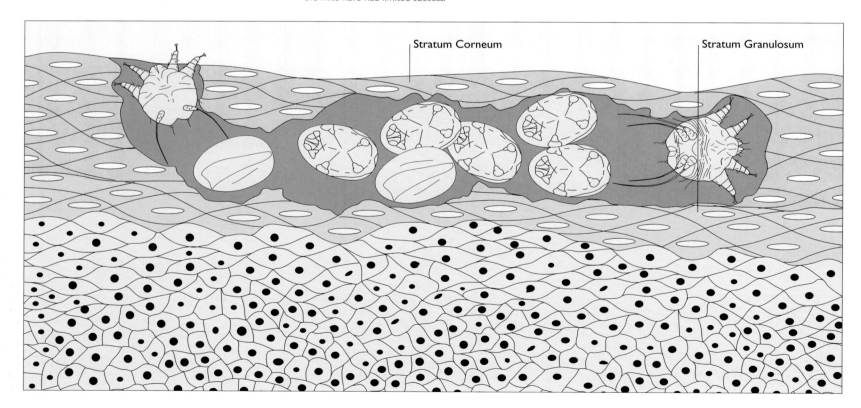

Fig. 15.4 The burrow of *Sarcoptes scabiei*. As the female mite advances through the stratum corneum, she leaves a trail of eggs and scybala behind. When the eggs hatch, the larval forms emerge onto the skin surface.

or more, never returning to the skin surface. After 3–4 days, the eggs hatch into larvae, which resemble the adults but have only three pairs of legs. The larvae leave the burrow but may penetrate the skin to feed. After 3 days, the larvae molt to produce nymphs. After a further 3 days, the larvae molt again to produce either a second nymphal stage or an adult (*Fig. 15.5*).

If all eggs survived into adulthood, an infestation could produce one million mites within 2 months. In fact, less than 10% of eggs survive to reach adulthood. Scratching, bathing, and immunologic reaction all contribute to their poor survival. The average patient with scabies is infested with 11 mites, but about 50% of patients have no more than five (*Fig. 15.6*).

The clinical manifestations of scabies primarily reflect the host's immunologic response to the invading parasite. Under experimental conditions, mites placed on volunteers initially produce only minor erythema and no symptoms, even though burrows containing mites are present. It is not until a month after infestation that the characteristic pruritus and rash appear. However, volunteers who have been previously infested with the mite will develop symptoms within a day of exposure. The number of mites infesting a patient reaches a peak at about 3 months and then begins to decline. It is not known whether the immune system can eventually clear the infestation if treatment is withheld. Under experimental conditions, it is more difficult to establish infestation in individuals with prior exposure to scabies. This suggests that there is an immunologic defense against reinfestation.

Several types of immunologic responses to the scabies mite have been studied, but investigations have been hampered by an inability to cultivate the mite in sufficient quantities to extract and purify specific antigens. The predominant response involves the cellular branch of the host's immune system. Histopathologic examination of the skin lesion shows a perivascular infiltrate, predominantly lymphocytes, histiocytes, and eosinophils (*Fig. 15.7*). Patients with impaired cellular immunity have fewer symptoms, but can develop a more severe infestation known as crusted scabies. Circulating immune complexes, vasculitis, and IgE-mediated reaction have also been associated with scabies.

Specific physical characteristics and local immunologic properties of skin at different sites may explain the mite's predilection for certain areas. The mite remains somewhat insulated from the full force of the host's immunologic response by burrowing only to the stratum granulosum, well away from the dermis.

EPIDEMIOLOGY

Scabies is known throughout the world. In underdeveloped countries, it is most prevalent among young children and adolescents, while in developed nations it is more uniformly distributed across age groups. The attack rate appears to be the same for males and females. Decreased susceptibility among various ethnic populations has been suggested; however, the idea of genetic immunity has not been proven. Although scabies is an STD, it is transmitted by skin-to-skin

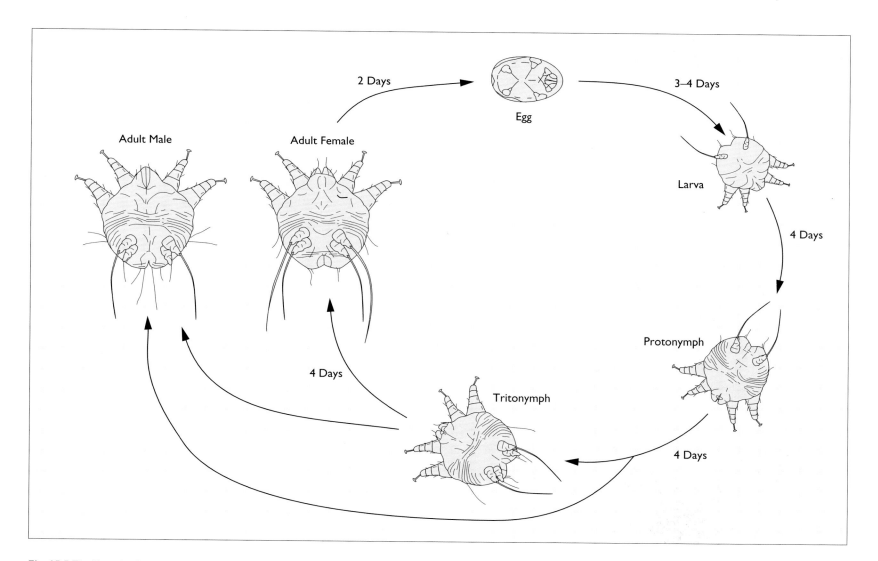

Fig. 15.5 The life cycle of *Sarcoptes scabiei*. Females complete the cycle from egg to egg in 19 days, with fertilization occuring on day 15. Males are mature after only 10 days.

contact rather than specific sexual activity. Scabies differs from other STDs in that it is not especially prevalent among young adults or homosexual men. The occurrence of scabies in infants and children further supports the view that non-sexual skin contact is an important mode of transmission. Most transmission occurs within families, although outbreaks have been observed in hospitals and nursing homes. Schools and fomites have not been shown to play an important role in the spread of scabies. Mites are immobilized by cold and killed by brief exposure to heat, so they seldom survive long away from the host. However, in a warm, moist environment they can survive for 2–3 days, suggesting at least the potential for indirect transmission. Fomites may be more important in institutional outbreaks, particularly when cases with large mite burdens occur.

It has been widely accepted that epidemics of scabies occur in 30-year cycles consisting of 15 years of high prevalence followed by 15 years of relatively few cases. Neither changes in population immunity nor a cyclical change in the mite has been found to explain this cycle. Recently, this phenomenon has been re-evaluated, and the apparent cycles may be more properly attributed to the great social upheavals caused by World Wars I and II. The scabies mite infests 40 different mammalian hosts, the largest number for any permanent parasite. Although the mites that infest different hosts are morphologically indistinguishable, there appear to be biologic differences that limit interspecies spread. Transmission to humans from domestic animals is recognized, especially from dogs.

CLINICAL MANIFESTATIONS

A patient's clinical history may offer important clues to the diagnosis of scabies. The typical patient seeks medical advice about 2–4 weeks after the onset of itching. The pruritus is usually most intense at night, especially upon first undressing and going to bed. Some patients itch only at night. Warmth intensifies the discomfort, and antipruritics may offer little relief. The rash typically begins on the hands and then spreads to the wrists, elbows, and other parts of the body. The presence of a pruritic rash on the hands and trunk is very suggestive of scabies, as is a report that other family members are also itching.

A variety of skin lesions may result from scabies infestation (*Fig 15.8*). Typical lesions of scabies are usually found on the flexor surfaces of wrists, elbows, anterior axillary folds, areolae in women, belt line, lower portion of buttocks and upper thighs, and the male genitalia (*Fig. 15.9*). The back is conspicuously free of lesions except in infants and the debilitated.

In contrast to adults, infants often show heavy infestation of the palms, soles, head, neck, face, and back (*Fig. 15.10*). The individual papules and burrows maintain their characteristic appearances. Infants may refuse food and fail to grow because of scabies infestation. Secondary bacterial infection is common.

Several specific types of skin lesions may be present in a single patient. The classically described burrow, although pathognomonic for the disease, is increasingly difficult to find. The burrow consists of a gray, dirty-appearing, 2-to-15 mm wavy line, usually seen on the wrist, interdigital web, or the side of a finger (*Fig. 15.11*). A tiny vesicle containing the mite may occasionally be seen at one end of the burrow (*Fig. 15.12*). The more typical lesion is a small, erythematous papule with surrounding erythema (*Fig. 15.13*). Lesions are usually sparse, but in some areas may become nearly confluent. These lesions are caused by larvae and nymphs that do not burrow.

In patients who bathe frequently, the manifestations of scabies may be subtle, with only a few lesions and rare burrows (*Fig. 15.14*). Bathing undoubtedly destroys many developing mites, thus limiting the number that reach maturity. Despite the paucity of characteristic lesions, the distribution and symmetry of the dermatitis provide a clue to diagnosis. In cases in which

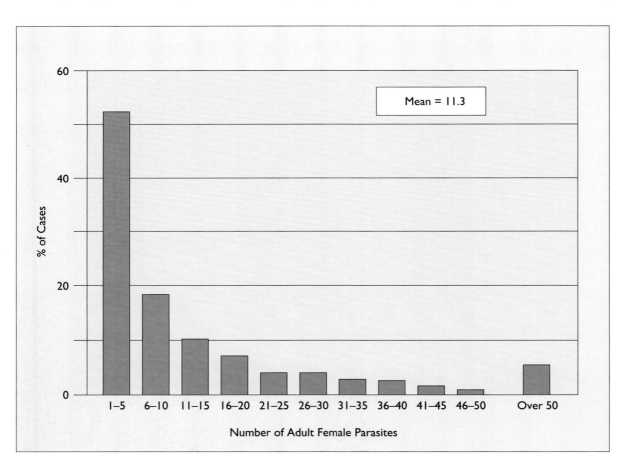

Fig. 15.6 The number of adult female mites recovered from a large series of carefully examined patients.

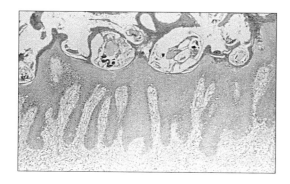

Fig. 15.7 Histology of a burrow and the inflammatory response of skin to scabies infestation. Typically, a superficial and deep perivascular infiltrate of lymphocytes, histiocytes, and eosinophils is present. When tissue sections do not reveal the mite, the pathologic pattern may be mistaken for a drug eruption, erythema multiforme, or malignant lymphoma.

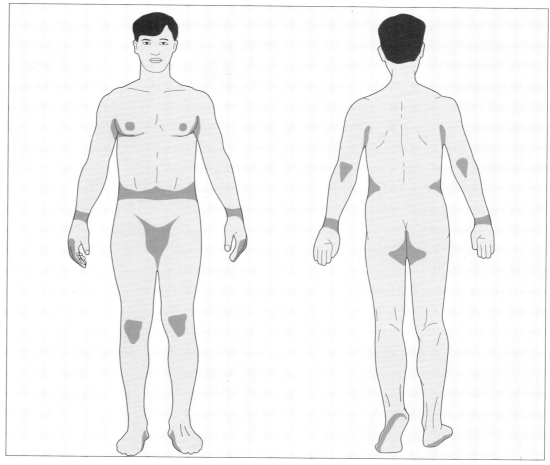

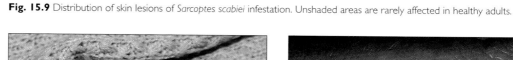

Fig. 15.9 Distribution of skin lesions of *Sarcoptes scabiei* infestation. Unshaded areas are rarely affected in healthy adults.

SKIN MANIFESTATIONS OF SCABIES

Common	Unusual
Papules	Scaling crusts
Burrows	Urticaria
Excoriations	Vasculitis
Nodules	Attenuated or exaggerated lesions
Vesicles	
Pyoderma	
Eczema	

Fig. 15.8 Skin manifestations of scabies.

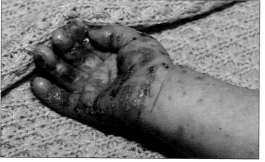

Fig. 15.10 Scabies of the palm with secondary pyoderma in an infant. Lesions on the palms, soles, head, neck and back are rare, except in infants and debilitated patients.

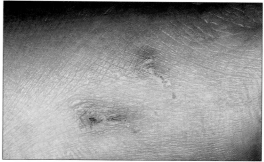

Fig. 15.11 Burrow of *Sarcoptes scabiei* on the side of a finger. Upper lesion shows the pathognomonic dirty-appearing wavy line extending out from an erythematous papule. In the lower lesion, the burrow has been nearly obliterated by excoriation.

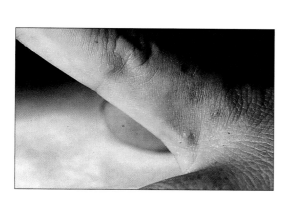

Fig. 15.12 Vesicular scabietic lesions on the lateral surface of a finger and interdigital web.

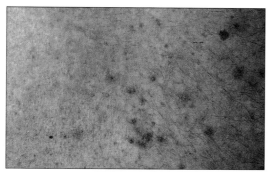

Fig. 15.13 Multiple larval papules on the abdomen. Such papules, which may be clustered or widely scattered, occur when immature mites penetrate the skin. These papules greatly outnumber burrows, which are formed only by the adult female mites.

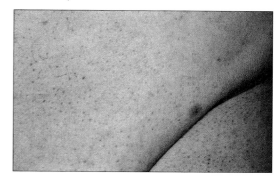

Fig. 15.14 Scabies in the clean patient. Frequent bathing kills immature mites and limits the severity of the infestation. This man had only a few pruritic papules such as this isolated lesion on the lower abdomen.

only a single body site is involved, the recognition of any infested contact may be the key to diagnosis.

Excoriation, denudation, eczematization, and subsequent infection may alter the appearance of scabies lesions so that they resemble chronic eczema or pyoderma (*Fig. 15.15*). Infection, ususally caused by *Staphylococcus aureus* or *Streptococcus pyogenes*, can produce local complications, including impetigo, ecthyma, furunculosis, and cellulitis, or more serious systemic disease such as bacteremia and internal abscesses. Eczematous changes induced by scratching may be exacerbated by the irritant or drying effect of topical antipruritic and antiscabietic medications. Scratching may also cause trauma to superficial blood vessels, resulting in petechial or ecchymotic lesions (*Fig. 15.16*).

Manifestations of scabies may be altered by the presence of any other chronic or acute dermatosis. Scabies is frequently associated with other STDs. The diagnosis of scabies in sexually active individuals indicates a need to examine for other STDs.

Nodular Scabies

Firm, reddish-brown nodules may appear on covered parts of the body (*Figs. 15.17* and *15.18*). Most commonly found on the male genitalia, including the glans penis, shaft, and scrotum, they are also frequently seen on elbows and

in the anterior axillary folds. These nodules may persist long after treatment and probably represent an immunologic reaction to the dead mite. Viable organisms are seldom found in nodules. Both clinically and histologically, nodular scabies may be confused with lymphoma and histiocytosis X.

Urticarial Reactions

A systemic allergic reaction to mite antigens may result in urticaria (*Fig. 15.19*). Such a response is not common, but when it occurs, it may completely overshadow the small number of scabies lesions. The urticaria resolves within a few days of antiscabietic therapy.

Vasculitis

Although vasculitis is often present histologically, vasculitic lesions are not common. It is possible that some lesions that appear to be ulcerated due to excoriation or superinfection may actually be the result of a localized vasculitis (*Fig. 15.20*).

Crusted Scabies

Crusted scabies is characterized by lesions, resembling psoriasis, whose thick scales contain large numbers of mites (*Figs. 15.21* and *15.22*).

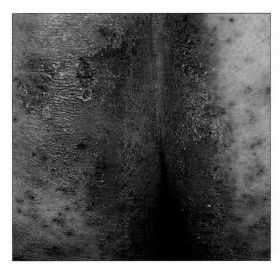 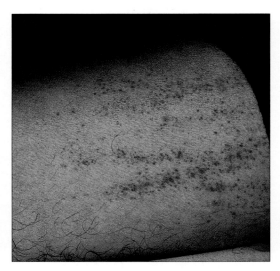 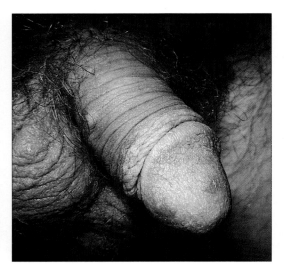

Figs. 15.15 and 15.16 Excoriated lesions. (**15.15**) Eczematization may result from repeated excoriation or from the irritating effect of topical medications. A scaling, pruritic rash on the buttocks is a common manifestation of scabies. (**15.16**) Petechiae and ecchymoses may also be caused by excoriation. These rows of petechiae resulted from capillary breakage during vigorous scratching.

Fig. 15.17 Nodular lesions of scabies on the male genitalia. Nodules generally occur on covered parts of the body. In this patient, erythematous, indurated lesions are present on the glans, penile shaft, and scrotum.

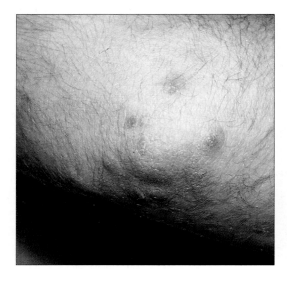 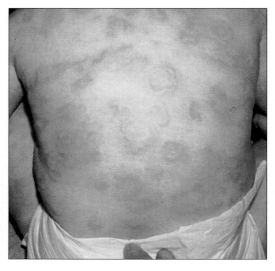 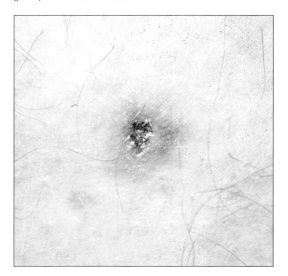

Fig. 15.18 Nodular scabies on the extensor surface of the elbow. Such lesions may persist long after antiscabietic therapy. Their clinical and histologic appearances have caused them to be mistaken for neoplasms.

Fig. 15.19 Urticaria associated with scabies. This child had multiple wheals over the face, trunk, and extremities. Typical scabietic burrows on the palms and soles were initially overlooked. The urticaria disappeared 48 hours after treatment with lindane lotion

Fig. 15.20 Lesion with necrotic center suggestive of vasculitis. Histologic evidence of localized vascular inflammation is frequently present on biopsy, but a generalized vasculitic reaction is rare.

Pruritus is minimal. The disease is usually seen in immunologically incompetent or physically debilitated patients. It has also been associated with the use of topical fluorinated steroids. Months are required for the generalized lesions of crusted scabies to develop. An impaired immune response or inability to scratch allows the mite to multiply unchecked. The shedding of tremendous numbers of mites causes this form of scabies to be extremely contagious.

Scabies Incognito
Topical application of steroids may markedly attenuate symptoms as well as reduce the number of lesions and alter their distribution. Such a presentation has been labeled scabies incognito (*Fig. 15.23*). Potent fluorinated steroids have also been associated with crusted scabies.

SCABIES AND AIDS
Patients with AIDS may have an atypical or exaggerated cutaneous response to many infections, including scabies infestation (*Fig. 15.24*). The absence of burrows, an unusual distribution of lesions, and the scaling or crusted character of the dermatitis often delay diagnosis. Repeated treatments are required to eradicate the infestation, probably because of the large mite burden.

LABORATORY TESTS

An attempt should be made to confirm the diagnosis of scabies in all suspected cases. A number of techniques have been used to demonstrate the mite, its burrow, eggs or scybala (feces), any one of which is diagnostic. Although a positive diagnosis can probably be made in all cases if one searches with sufficient diligence, the success rates of various techniques are reported to range from 30–90%. Success with any technique increases with the skill and experience of the examiner.

Skin Scraping
Preparation of a skin scraping is probably the most frequently used test for the scabies mite (*Figs. 15.25–15.27*). First, the patient should be examined carefully in good light using a magnifying lens to select a burrow or papule that has not been excoriated. Lesions on the finger webs, wrists, or elbows are most likely to yield a positive diagnosis. Place a drop of mineral oil on the lesion and use a small disposable scalpel to scrape gently across the surface until the topmost layer of skin is removed. No bleeding should occur. Gently collect the mineral oil containing the flecks of skin onto the scalpel

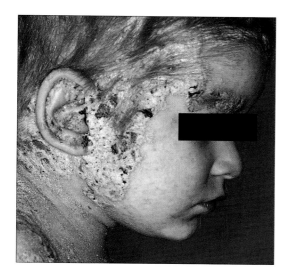

15.21 Extensive crusted lesions of the face, neck, and scalp.

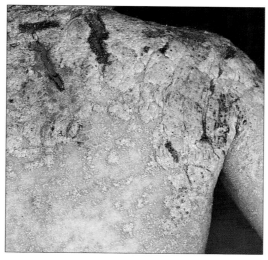

15.22 Lesions on the back, an area usually spared in typical scabies.

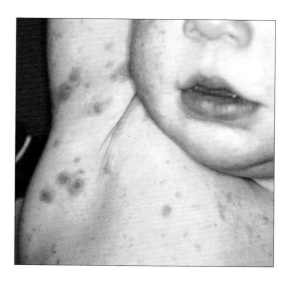

Fig. 15.23 Scabies incognito. Atypical lesions in a child treated with topical steroids. Steroids may either exacerbate or reduce the cutaneous response to infestation.

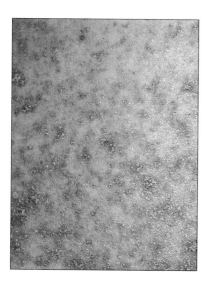

Fig. 15.24 Cutaneous lesions of scabies in a patient with AIDS. Lesions may be either diminished or exaggerated. In this patient, lesions on the back remained nearly confluent, even after multiple applications of scabicide.

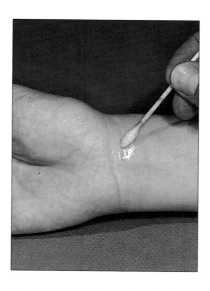
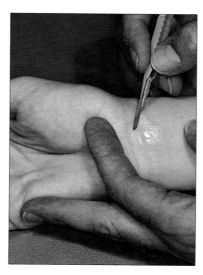
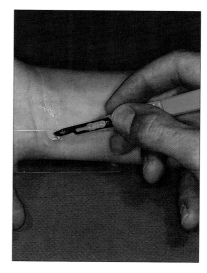

Figs. 15.25–15.27 Preparation of a skin scraping. (**15.25**) Select an unexcoriated burrow or papule, preferably on the hand or wrist. Cover the lesion with a thin layer of mineral oil. (**15.26**) Hold a sterile scalpel perpendicular to the skin. Gently scrape the lesion until the superficial skin is removed. Collect the mineral oil containing skin particles and mites onto the scalpel blade. (**15.27**) Transfer the mineral oil to a microscope slide and cover with a glass cover slip. Add another drop of oil if necessary to eliminate any air bubbles. Examine under a microscope with a low-power objective.

blade and transfer it to a glass microscope slide. Add a cover slip and examine under low magnification.

Visualization of any adult or larval mite forms, eggs, or scybala is diagnostic of scabies (*Figs. 15.28–15.31*). Some clinicians prefer to omit the mineral oil and transfer the dry skin scrapings to a slide containing a drop of 10% KOH. Although this may help to disperse the cellular material for easier examination, it will destroy the fecal pellets that in some specimens are the only clues to the diagnosis.

Epidermal Shave Biopsy
This technique offers improved sensitivity and may be less likely to cause injury in an uncooperative patient (*Figs. 15.32–15.34*). Lift the selected lesion between the thumb and index finger. Gently shave off the outer layer of skin with a sterile scalpel. Use a fine sawing movement while holding the scalpel blade tangential to the skin surface. Transfer the shaving to a microscope slide, add a drop of mineral oil, apply a cover slip, and then examine under the microscope for mites, eggs, or scybala (*Figs. 15.35* and *15.36*).

Curettage
Use a small cutting curette to scrape the epidermal layer off a selected papule or burrow. This technique is particularly useful for infants or other uncooperative patients for whom the use of a scalpel might be hazardous. Place the scrapings on a slide with oil or KOH and examine.

Burrow Ink Test
Use a fountain pen to cover a papule with ink, then clean off the ink with alcohol (*Figs. 15.37* and *15.38*). A positive result is seen when the ink penetrates the papule, revealing a dark, zigzag line running across and away from the papule (*Figs. 15.39* and *15.40*). A positive ink test is specific for scabies; however, a shave biopsy on a positive lesion will demonstrate the actual mite. Topical tetracycline may be used instead of ink and washed off with alcohol after 5 minutes. A Wood's light will reveal burrows as areas of linear yellow-green fluorescence.

Sewing Needle
An intact burrow must be present with the mite visible as either a dark point in Caucasian skin or a white point in Blacks. Using a needle or pin, perforate the burrow at this point and move the needle from side to side, holding it parallel to the skin. The mite will attach itself to the needle and can be transferred to a slide for examination.

Glue Stripping
Place a drop of methacrylate glue on a glass slide and push down firmly over an intact lesion. Allow the glue to set, then strip the slide of the lesion briskly. Repeat the process two more times to obtain deeper organisms, then examine microscopically.

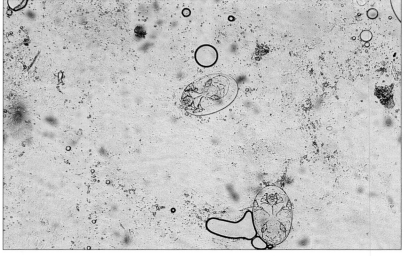

Fig. 15.28

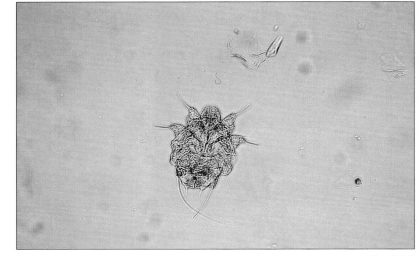

Fig. 15.29

Fig. 15.30

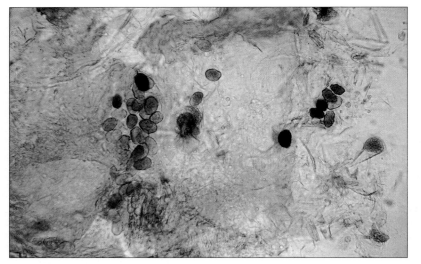

Fig. 15.31

Figs. 15.28–5.31 Positive skin scrapings. Any of the following are diagnostic of scabies infestation. (**15.28**) Adult female scabies mite. (**15.29**) Larval stage of scabies mite, which has only two hind legs. (**15.30**) *S. scabiei* eggs. (**15.31**) Feces of scabies are also called scybala.

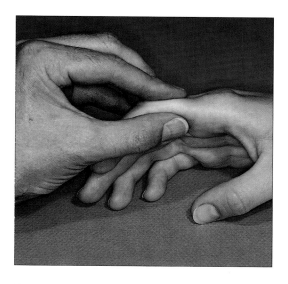
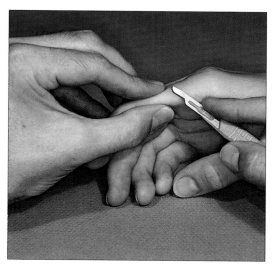
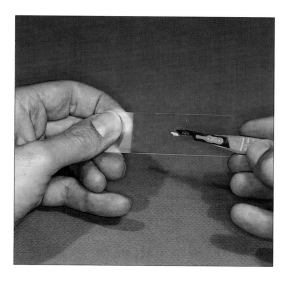

Figs. 15.32–15.34 Preparation of a shave biopsy. (**15.32**) Select a lesion and hold it firmly between the thumb and index finger, so that it is slightly elevated above the surrounding skin. (**15.33**) Hold a sterile scalpel with its blade parallel to the skin surface. Use a fine sawing motion to carefully shave off the outer layer of skin. (**15.34**) Use the scalpel blade to transfer the shaving to a microscope slide. Place a drop of oil over the specimen, then add a cover slip. Examine under a microscope using a scanning objective.

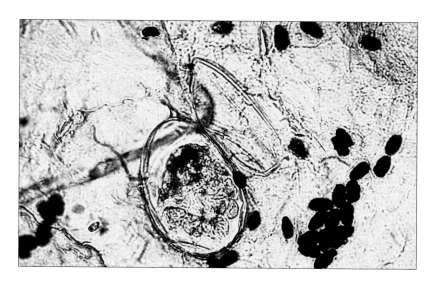
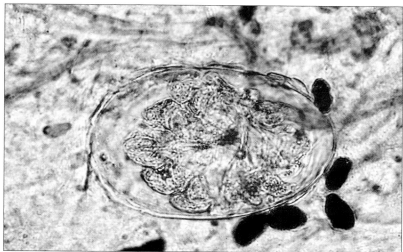

Figs. 15.35 and 15.36 Positive shave biopsies. (**15.35**) Two eggs, one hatched and one containing a developing nymph, are visible within the skin shaving. Multiple small, dark fecal particles surround the eggs (× 50). (**15.36**) Egg and scybala under higher magnification. The egg contains a larva that is nearly ready to emerge (× 100).

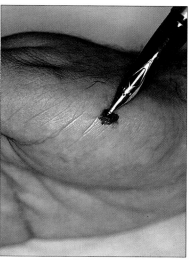
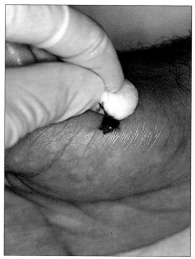
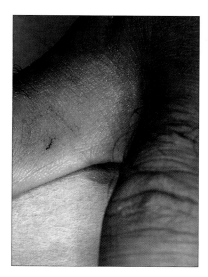
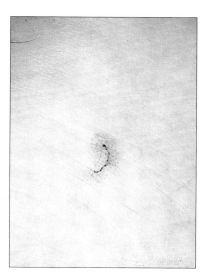

Figs. 15.37 and 15.38 Burrow ink test technique. (**15.37**) Select an unexcoriated burrow or papule for the test. Cover the lesion with water-soluble ink from a fountain pen. (**15.38**) After 5 minutes, use an alcohol-soaked cotton ball to wash all the ink off the skin surface. Examine the lesion for evidence of ink remaining within the scabies burrow.

Figs. 15.39 and 15.40 Positive burrow ink test. (**15.39**) An ink-filled burrow on the side of a finger is clearly visible after washing ink from the surface of the lesion. (**15.40**) A close-up view demonstrates the scabies burrow tracking across skin lines. The ink helps to define the morphology and limits of the burrow.

Cellophane Tape

Prepare the lesion by cleaning with ether, then apply a short length of clear cellophane tape. Briskly strip the tape from the skin and affix to a microscope slide. Repeat this several times for each lesion, using a new piece of tape each time.

Punch Biopsy

If none of the above techniques is successful, a small 2-mm punch biopsy from an unexcoriated lesion may reveal the mite. Instruct the laboratory to make serial sections, all of which should be closely studied for evidence of the mite (*see Fig. 15.7*).

TREATMENT

Decisions in scabies therapy center on the choice of drug and on selection of contacts for prophylaxis. Because scabies may not become symptomatic until 1 month following infestation, it is essential to treat contacts prophylactically in order to prevent re-exposure. In general, all household and sexual contacts should be treated. Decisions on whether to treat other contacts should be based on the degree of skin-to-skin contact they have with the patient. Four drugs are available to treat scabies: lindane, permethrin, crotamiton, and sulfur (*Fig. 15.41*).

Lindane

Lindane (gamma benzene hexachloride) in a 1% lotion is the most frequently used scabicide. After the patient bathes, lindane is applied to the entire body from the neck down. Twelve hours later, it is washed off. A second treatment is not necessary unless there is evidence of treatment failure or reinfestation. Since lindane is toxic to the CNS and approximately 10% of the drug is absorbed through the skin, it should be used cautiously. To avoid overdose, only the amount actually needed (about 1 oz for an adult) should be prescribed. Lindane should not be used by young children, pregnant women, lactating women, or patients with neurologic disorders because of the potential for toxicity.

Permethrin

Permethrin, a pyrethroid, is available in a 5% cream and is effective with a single application. Permethrin should be applied from the neck to the feet, and then washed off 8–14 hours later. Adverse reactions are infrequent and generally consist only of local burning or stinging. Permethrin is a preferred treatment for young children and pregnant women because it is not associated with CNS toxicity.

Crotamiton

Crotamiton, an effective scabicide with minimal toxicity, is suitable for use in small children and pregnant women. It is applied nightly for 2 nights, then washed off 48 hours after the last application. Crotamiton is more likely than lindane to require a second course of therapy.

Sulfur

Sulfur as 6% precipitated sulfur in petrolatum is an ancient therapy that remains effective, although it is seldom used because of its disagreeable odor and staining. It is applied nightly for 3 nights then washed off 24 hours after the last application. Upon completing the regimen of topical therapy, the patient should wash all clothes and bed linen used within the preceding 2–3 days.

Usually, pruritus begins to resolve within 2 days of therapy, but may not be completely resolved for several weeks. It is important that the patient knows what to expect because overuse of scabicides or other topical medications may lead to an irritant dermatitis that can be confused with treatment failure. Cases of apparent resistance to lindane and crotamiton are rare and may be due to improper use or reinfestation. Patients with crusted scabies may require multiple applications of scabicides over many weeks to eradicate infestation.

PHTHIRUS PUBIS

Phthirus pubis, the crab louse, is one of the three members of the order Anoplura that infests man. The other two are *Pediculus humanus capitis*, the head louse, and *Pediculus humanus corporis*, the body louse (*Fig. 15.42*). Only *P. pubis* is primarily sexually transmitted. The insect's short, broad body and large, clawlike legs bear a remarkable resemblance to a crab, thus accounting for its common name (*Fig. 15.43*). The head, conical and pointed anteriorly, contains stylets that can pierce human skin, enabling the louse to suck blood from its host. Three pairs of legs extend from the anterior abdomen. The first pair is long and thin, while the second and

---

Fig. 15.41 Treatment of scabies.

TREATMENT OF SCABIES
LINDANE 1% LOTION OR CREAM
Apply a thin layer to entire body from the neck down and allow to dry. Wash off completely after 8–12 hours. One application is usually curative.
CROTAMITON 10% CREAM
After bathing, massage cream into skin from neck down. Apply again after 24 hours. Wash off medication 48 hours after second application.
PRECIPITABLE SULFUR 6% IN PETROLATUM
Apply nightly from neck down for three nights. Wash off medication thoroughly 24 hours after final application. (May stain clothing.)
PERMETHRIN 5% CREAM
Apply from neck down and massage into skin. Wash off medication after 8–14 hours. One application is usually curative.

third have thick claws specially suited for grasping hairs (*Fig. 15.44*). Four sets of small, conical appendages ending in bristles arise from the posterior abdomen.

The life cycle of *P. pubis* includes five stages from egg to adult. The eggs, called nits, are encased in a cement substance and firmly affixed to the hair shaft. Each nit has a convex cap containing air pores through which the first nymphal stage emerges after 6–9 days (*Fig. 15.45*). Nymphs resemble adults except for their smaller size and sexual immaturity. A tough, chitinous exoskeleton restricts the nymph's growth, and a series of three molts is necessary to reach adulthood, a process requiring 2–3 weeks. Adults mate frequently, and the female begins to lay eggs shortly after fertilization, producing 20–30 eggs during her 3-week adult life.

Crab lice are found mainly in the pubic area, but may spread to the buttocks, legs, axillae, beard, scalp, and eyebrow. Their preference for certain sites is probably related to hair spacing: the 2-mm spaces between pubic hairs match the span of the louse's hind legs, with which it grasps hairs. Pubic lice are usually sedentary, moving only a few millimeters per day. They seldom travel far from the initial area of infestation unless transferred to a new site by the host. To feed, the crab louse grasps hairs with its clawlike legs and pierces the skin to obtain blood from a capillary. It often remains attached and feeds intermittently for hours before moving to a new site. *P. pubis* feeds exclusively on human blood and can survive less than 24 hours away from a human host.

EPIDEMIOLOGY

P. pubis spreads predominantly through intimate sexual contact. Transmission via nonsexual contact or fomites may occur occasionally, but it is unusual. Since *P. pubis* infestation is not reportable in the USA, limited epidemiologic information is available. Many believe that the incidence of infestation has increased markedly during the past two decades, paralleling increases in other STDs during a period of changing sexual behavior. Most available epidemiologic information comes from STD clinics. However, such data certainly underestimate cases because the availability of effective nonprescription therapy makes it unnecessary to consult a physician for this disease.

Among new patients seen in one clinic in England, the prevalence of infestation with crab lice increased from 0.8% in 1954 to 3.2% in 1968.

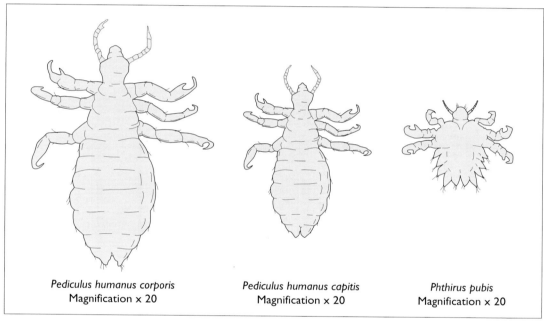

Pediculus humanus corporis
Magnification x 20

Pediculus humanus capitis
Magnification x 20

Phthirus pubis
Magnification x 20

Fig. 15.42 Lice that infest humans. The crablike appearance of *Phthirus pubis* makes it easy to distinguish from the head louse (*Pediculus humanus capitis*) and the body louse (*Pediculus humanus corporis*). *P. pubis* may be found outside the pubic area, so diagnosis must be based upon the appearance of the louse rather than its site of infestation.

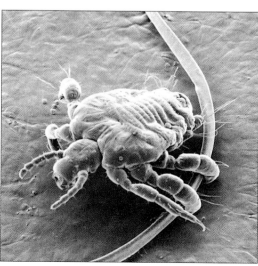

Fig. 15.43 Scanning electron micrograph of *Phthirus pubis* (× 50).

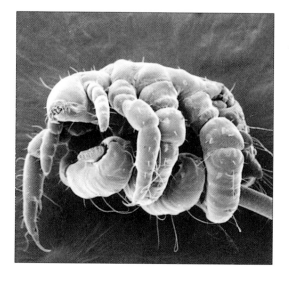

Fig. 15.44 Scanning electron micrograph of *Phthirus pubis* (× 100). Clawlike legs encircling a pubic hair produce a firm grip that can be difficult to dislodge.

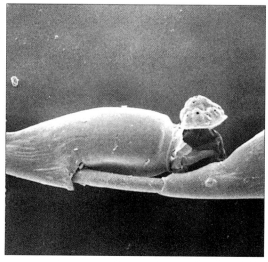

Fig. 15.45 Scanning electron micrograph of an egg, or nit, with nymphal stage of *Phthirus pubis* preparing to emerge. The cap containing air pores is pushed off during this process (× 100).

Patients with crab lice were generally similar to those with other STDs. Males were more likely to be infested than females except among 15–19 year olds. Nearly half of the patients with crab lice also had another STD. In 1986 in DeKalb County (Atlanta), Georgia, 3% of patients attending a public STD clinic were infested with *Phthirus pubis*.

CLINICAL MANIFESTATIONS

Patients who present to a physician with *P. pubis* infestation have usually seen lice or complain of severe pruritus in the pubic area. Excoriations and secondary infection are common findings in symptomatic patients. Ten or fewer adult lice are usually present at diagnosis.

In an STD clinic, half of infested patients are asymptomatic. The diagnosis is often made during examination for an unrelated problem. Occasionally the only complaint is the presence of multiple rust-colored spots on the patient's underclothes, resulting from bleeding at the sites of bites, or from excrement from the louse after a blood meal (*Fig. 15.46*). Most patients do not notice

pruritus until 1 month after exposure to an infested partner. This incubation period is probably related to development of the host's immunologic response and growth of the lice population to a size sufficient to cause discomfort.

An uncommon manifestation of *P. pubis* infestation is the macula caerulea, an asymptomatic bluish-gray macule that does not blanch under pressure. This lesion represents the bite of the louse and a resultant small hemorrhage into the skin. More commonly seen are small punctate, red lesions near hair follicles that mark the sites of recent bites (*Fig. 15.47*). These lesions, when inflamed and excoriated, resemble folliculitis.

LABORATORY TESTS

A diagnosis of *P. pubis* infestation is usually straightforward and requires finding only one of the crablike insects on the patient. The search is aided by good lighting and a magnifying lens. Their yellow-gray color makes the lice difficult to see on Caucasian skin, but after a blood meal they have a more visible rust color (*Fig. 15.48*). Occasionally, the lice are found only in extrapubic areas,

Fig. 15.46 Rust-colored spots on underclothing may result from bleeding at bite sites or from excrement from the louse after a blood meal. In patients without symptoms, these spots may be the first clue to the presence of infestation.

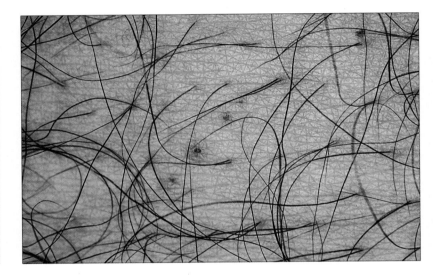

Fig. 15.47 Bite marks of *Phthirus pubis*. These punctate lesions with surrounding erythema are typical of the tiny papules that arise at sites of crab louse bites.

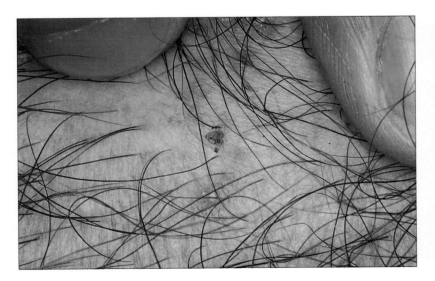

Fig. 15.48 *Phthirus pubis* feeding on its host. To obtain a meal of human blood, the crab louse uses its clawlike legs to grasp a hair on either side, then penetrates the host's skin with its mouth. Firmly anchored in this position, the louse may feed for hours. During feeding, the body takes on a red-brown color more easily seen against Caucasian skin.

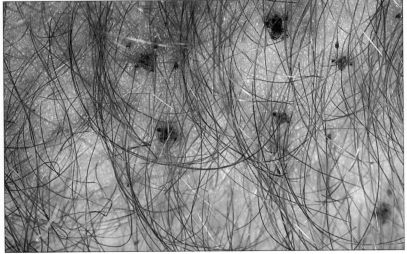

Fig. 15.49 Extrapubic infestation. *Phthirus pubis* may infest almost any area in hirsute individuals. This cluster of lice was present on the buttock of a patient whose pubic hair was not infested.

such as the axillae, extremities, buttocks, scalp, and eyelashes (*Fig. 15.49*). Demonstration of adults, nymphs, or nits is sufficient for diagnosis. Nits are usually easiest to find, but may be confused with hair casts or scales of skin from seborrhea (*Fig. 15.50*). Nits may be distinguished from the latter by microscopy and by their firm adherence to the hair shaft. Unless removed with a special fine-tooth comb, nits will remain attached to the hair after therapy and move outward as the hair grows. If treatment failure or reinfestation is suspected, only those eggs close to the base of the hair shaft should be considered significant. Empty egg casings do not indicate active infestation, but can be distinguished from viable eggs only by microscopic examination (*Fig. 15.51*).

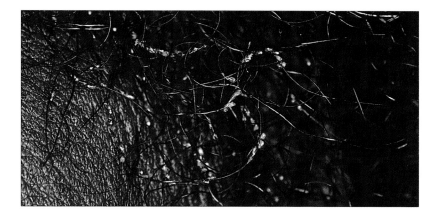

Fig. 15.50 Pubic hair with multiple nits. Hairs such as these with numerous nits are easily recognized as a sign of *Phthirus pubis* infestation. When only a few nits are present, a careful search with a magnifying lens may be necessary to establish the diagnosis.

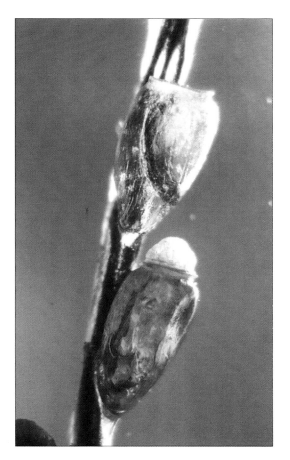

Fig. 15.51
Photomicrograph of two nits on a hair shaft. The upper egg is empty, but the lower one still contains a developing nymph. Empty nits may be a sign of past rather than current infestation. After therapy, unhatched nits at the base of hairs indicate treatment failure or reinfestation.

TREATMENT

Lindane and synergized pyrethrins are the drugs of choice for treatment of *P. pubis* infestations and are equally effective (*Fig. 15.52*). Lindane is available as a lotion, cream, or shampoo. The cream and lotion require a 12-hour application for complete killing of lice and ova, but the shampoo is effective in only 4 minutes. The use of lindane in small children, pregnant women, and patients with extensive dermatologic or neurologic disorders should be avoided. However, if used correctly, the brief exposure to the shampoo presents a very limited opportunity for absorption of the drug. Pyrethrins synergized with piperonyl butoxide are available without prescription in lotion and shampoo forms. The infested hair must be covered with the lotion or lathered with the shampoo for 10 minutes, then washed with water. Toxicity is not a problem with this drug, which may be used safely during pregnancy.

Permethrin, a synthetic pyrethrin, is available without prescription as a 1% cream rinse. It should be applied to clean hair for 10 minutes, then rinsed out immediately. Effectiveness is comparable to lindane and synergized pyrethrins and less than 1% of patients require retreatment.

It is important to instruct the patient in the proper use of these medications. In most cases, treatment of the pubic and perianal hair is sufficient, although other sites should be inspected and treated if necessary. In individuals with much body hair, medication should be applied to the lower abdomen, thighs, and buttocks, regardless of whether or not lice are found in these areas.

After treatment, any clothing and bed linen used during the preceding 24 hours should be washed. Since the louse survives for less than a day away from the host, it is not necessary to treat furniture and other potential fomites with insecticide. In cases in which the eyelashes are involved, petrolatum applied to the lashes twice a day for 8 days is safe and effective. If nits remain after this treatment, they may be removed with forceps.

Sexual contacts should be examined and treated prophylactically; household contacts should be treated only if actually infested. Patients infested with *P. pubis* should be examined for other STDs.

TREATMENT OF *PHTHIRUS PUBIS* INFESTATION

LINDANE 1% SHAMPOO

Apply shampoo to pubic hair and any other infested areas (except eyelashes). Add water to produce a thick lather, then wash off after four minutes. If the 1% cream or lotion is used, it should be washed off after 12 hours

PERMETHRIN 1% CREAM RINSE

Cream rinse should be applied after washing hair, then rinsed out after 10 minutes.

PYRETHRIN WITH PIPERONYL BUTOXIDE

Lotion, gel, and shampoo preparations are available without prescription. Apply medication to thoroughly cover infested hair (except eyelashes). Wash off after 10 minutes.

PETROLATUM

Use only for infestation of the eyelashes. Apply twice daily for eight days. Any nits remaining after treatment can be physically removed.

Fig. 15.52 Treatment of *Phthirus pubis* infestation.

Resistance of *P. pubis* to insecticides has not yet been reported. Most cases of treatment failure can be attributed to incorrect use of medication, failure to medicate all infested body sites, or re-exposure to an untreated partner. Persistent pruritus does not warrant additional therapy in the absence of active infestation. Repeated treatment with lindane may exacerbate the itching by causing a skin irritation. Delusions of parasitosis are not uncommon after successful therapy and frequently result in the overuse of medications.

Picture credits for this chapter are as follows: Figs. 15.1 to 15.3 and 15.43 to 15.45 courtesy of Patricianne Hurd, PhD, John Pietrahita, and Danny Blankenship, Fernbank Science Centre, DeKalb County Board of Education; Fig. 15.5 adapted from Orkin M, Maibach HI (eds): Cutaneous Infestations and Insect Bites. New York, Marcel Dekker, 1985. Fig. 15.6 adapted from Johnson CG, Mellanby K: The parasitology of human scabies. Parasitology 34:286, 1942, courtesy of Cambridge University Press; Fig. 15.7 courtesy of S.D. Glazer, MD; Figs. 15.18 courtesy of du Vivier A, McKee PH: Atlas of Clinical Dermatology. London, Gower Medical Publishing Ltd., 1986; Fig. 15.19 courtesy of Chapel TA: Scabies presenting as urticaria. JAMA 246:1441, 1981 with permission, © 1981 American Medical Association; Fig. 15.23 courtesy of Heidi Watts; Figs. 15.28 and 15.30 courtesy of Adele Moreland, MD; Fig. 15.40 courtesy of David Woodley, MD.

BIBLIOGRAPHY

Ackerman AB: Crabs. The resurgence of *Phthirus pubis*. N Engl J Med **278**:950, 1968.

Burkhart CG: Scabies: an epidemiologic reassessment. *Ann Intern Med* **98**:498, 1983.

Burns DA: The treatment of human ectoparasite infection. *Br J Dermatol* **125**:89, 1991.

Chapel TA, Krugel L, Chapel J, Segal A: Scabies presenting as urticaria. *JAMA* **246**:1440, 1981.

Dahl MV: The immunology of scabies. *Ann Allergy* **51**:560, 1983.

Donabedian H, Khazan U: Norwegian scabies in a patient with AIDS. *Clin Infect Dis* **14**:162, 1992.

Estes SA, Kummel B, Arlian L: Experimental canine scabies in humans. *J Am Acad Dermatol* **9**:397, 1983.

Fernandez N, Torres A, Ackerman B: Pathologic findings in human scabies. *Arch Dermatol* **113**:320, 1977.

Fisher I, Morton RS: *Phthirus pubis* infestation. *Br J Vener Dis* **46**:326, 1970.

Funkhouser ME, Ross A: Management of scabies in patients with human immunodeficiency virus disease. *Arch Dermatol* **129**:911, 1993.

Janniger CK, Kuflik AS: Pediculosis capitis. *Ped Dermatology* **51**:407, 1993.

Johnson CG, Mellanby K: The parasitology of human scabies. *Parasitology* **34**:285, 1942.

Martin WE, Wheeler CE Jr: Diagnosis of human scabies by epidermal shave biopsy. *J Am Acad Dermatol* **1**:335, 1979.

Orkin M, Maibach HI: Modern aspects of scabies. *Curr Probl Dermatol* **13**:109, 1985.

Orkin M, Maibach HI (eds): *Cutaneous Infestations and Insect Bites.* New York, Marcel Dekker, 1985.

Parish LC, Nuttig WB, Schwartzman RM (eds): *Cutaneous Infestations of Man and Animal.* New York, Praeger, 1983.

Sadick N, Kaplan MH, Pahwa SG, Sarngadharan MG: Unusual features of scabies complicating human T-lymphotropic virus type III infection. *J Am Acad Dermatol* **15**:482, 1986.

Woodley D, Saurat JH: The burrow ink test and the scabies mite. *J Am Acad Dermatol* **4**:715, 1981.

Selection and Evaluation of Test and Quality Control

JS Lewis

PURPOSE AND SELECTION OF DIAGNOSTIC TESTS

DIAGNOSIS OF DISEASE

The process of diagnosis requires two essential steps. The first is the establishment of a differential diagnosis (i.e., diagnostic hypotheses) followed by attempts to arrive at a single diagnosis by progressively ruling out specific diseases. This process requires very *sensitive* tests. Such tests, when normal, permit the physician to confidently exclude the disease. The next step is the pursuit of a strong clinical suspicion for a specific disease. This process requires a very *specific* test. Such a test, when abnormal, should essentially confirm the presence of the disease.

The use of a test to exclude or confirm a diagnosis should indicate that the physician's best estimate, after a careful evaluation of the patient's problem, is that the diagnosis in question is either unlikely or probable, respectively.

SCREENING

The primary use of screening tests in asymptomatic patients is to detect diseases whose morbidity can be reduced by early detection and treatment and to reassure patients found to be free of disease. There are several important principles in applying screening tests. First, the disease in question should be common enough to justify the effort to detect it. Next, it should be accompanied by significant morbidity if not treated, and effective therapy should exist to alter its natural history. Finally, detection and treatment of the presymptomatic state should result in benefits beyond those obtained through treatment of the early symptomatic patient. Once these criteria are met, the issue can be examined from the standpoint of laboratory tests. An acceptable test is one that will be abnormal in almost all individuals with the disease and provide the physician with confidence that the patient is free of disease when the test is normal.

PATIENT MANAGEMENT

Tests are commonly repeated for one or more of the following purposes:
1. To monitor the status of a disease process
2. To identify and reverse complications of treatment
3. To ensure therapeutic levels of one or more drugs
4. To aid in prognosis
5. To check an unexpected test result

For these purposes, the *reproducibility* of the test is the most important characteristic.

DETERMINATION OF DISEASE DISTRIBUTION

The purpose of a diagnostic test is to discriminate between patients with a particular disease and those who do not have the disease. However, most diagnostic tests measure some disease marker or surrogate (e.g., an antibody that is variably associated with the disease) rather than the presence or absence of the disease itself. The *performance level* of a diagnostic test depends on the distribution of the marker being measured in diseased and nondiseased patients and on the technical performance characteristics of the test itself (i.e., precision and reliability).

Each disease marker has a distribution in populations of diseased and nondiseased patients. Unfortunately, these distributions frequently overlap so that measurement of the marker in question does not usually permit a complete separation of the two populations (Fig. A1.1).

EVALUATION OF DIAGNOSTIC TESTS

The first step in evaluating a diagnostic test is to determine its technical performance. Does the test measure what it claims to measure? Is the test replicable? (Replicability, or precision, reflects the variance in a test result that occurs when the test is repeated on the same specimen). A highly precise text exhibits little variance among repeated measurements; an imprecise test exhibits great variance. The greater this variation, the less faith one has in results based on a single test. However, a precise test is not necessarily a good test. A test may exhibit a high level of replicability yet be in error. Is the test reliable (i.e., unbiased)? It must exhibit agreement between the mean test result and the true value of the biologic variable being measured in the sample. Evaluations of clinical tests should consider both the replicability and the reliability of the test.

The three most commonly used measures of diagnostic test performance for STDs are sensitivity, specificity, and predictive value (Fig. A1.2). These test characteristics deal with the ability of the diagnostic test to identify correctly subjects with and without the condition of interest.

SENSITIVITY

Sensitivity, which measures the ability of a test to detect infection when it is present, is of maximum concern in patient populations having a high prevalence of disease, such as STD clinics. Sensitivity measures the proportion of patients with a positive test to all infected patients.

Fig. A1.1 Relationship of test value to diseased and nondiseased populations for a hypothetical diagnostic test.

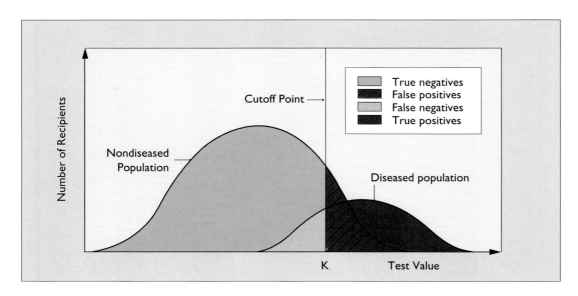

SPECIFICITY

Specificity, which measures the ability of a test to correctly exclude infection in uninfected patients, is of maximum concern when testing in patient populations having a low prevalence of disease, such as famaily planning clinics and most private practice settings. Specificity measures the proportion of uninfected patients with a negative test.

Sensitivity and specificity have been adopted widely because they are considered to be stable properties of diagnostic tests when properly derived from a broad spectrum of infected and uninfected patients. That is, their values are thought not to change significantly when applied in populations with different prevalences, presentations, or severity of disease. If diagnostic tests do not have a broad population base, their sensitivities and specificities change as the prevalence and severity of disease vary in the populations tested.

PREDICTIVE VALUE

When a test is to be used in a large, unselected population, it is important to know what its predictive value will be—that is, what is the likelihood that a person with a positive test result actually has the disease and, conversely, what is the likelihood that a person with a negative test result does not have the disease. This likelihood cannot be directly estimated from the test sensitivity and specificity value obtained in the preliminary evaluation since the predictive value is related to the actual prevalence of the disease in the total population.

Taken alone, test sensitivity and specificity do not reveal how likely it is that a given patient really has the condition in question if the test result is positive, or how likely it is that a given patient is not infected if the test result is negative. The fraction of those patients with a positive test result who actually are infected is called the predictive value positive (PVP) of a test. The fraction of patients with a negative test result who are actually free of the disease is called the predictive value negative (PVN).

The PVP and PVN of a diagnostic test measure, respectively, how likely it is that a positive or negative test result actually represents the presence or absence of disease in a given population of patients with a given prevalence of disease. The positive and negative predictive values of a diagnostic test, however, are not stable characteristics of that test. Rather, they depend strongly on the prevalence of the condition being examined in the population being tested. Where the disease prevalence (pretest likelihood of disease) decreases, the proportion of individuals with a positive test result who actually are infected falls and the proportion of uninfected patients falsely identified as being infected rises. Conversely, as the prevalence of disease increases, the proportion of patients with a positive test result who are in fact infected increases, while

the proportion of patients with a negative test result who are not suffering from the disease falls. This fact has enormous implications for all diagnostic tests, particularly when they are used in populations with a low prevalence of disease, such as in screening for the presence of an uncommon disease.

The following example will illustrate this principle: A test for gonorrhea is evaluated in 100 individuals who are known to have gonorrhea and in 100 normal control subjects with no evidence of the disease or of any factor known to result in increased risk for the disease. It is found that 95% of the infected individuals had positive test results (sensitivity, 95%), whereas only 5% of the control group had positive test results (specificity, 95%). In comparison with other tests, this test is considered highly accurate. What is the accuracy of a positive test in predicting gonorrhea in an unselected sample of 10,000 subjects in whom the actual prevalence of gonorrhea is 2%?

By simple arithmetic, there are 200 infected individuals in a population with a 2% prevalence of gonorrhea, 190 of whom will have a positive test and 10 a negative test. There are 9,800 uninfected persons in this population, 9,310 of whom will have a negative test and 490 a positive test. Therefore, the predictive value of a positive test in detecting gonorrhea in the total population will be:

$$\frac{190}{(190 + 490)} = 27.9\%$$

The predictive value of a negative test will be:

$$\frac{9,310}{(9,310 + 10)} = 99.9\%$$

Figure A1.3 shows the effect of disease prevalence on the predictive values of positive and negative test results when the sensitivity and specificity of the test are both 95%. The PVP of a test result increases with increasing disease prevalence; when the disease prevalence is 50%, PVP equals sensitivity and PVN equals specificity. Although higher disease prevalences are unlikely to occur in unselected populations, they may be obtained by preselection of the group to be tested on the basis of historical or physical data or some other test. In the example given above, the actual PVP in the positive reactor group was shown to be 27.9% under the conditions described (Fig. A1.3). The PVN of a test is not affected except at very high disease prevalences.

The value of PVP when actual disease prevalence is 2% is given for a range of sensitivities and specificities in Figure A1.4A. It is seen that the predictive value of a positive test is primarily dependent on the specificity of the test, but at this disease prevalence PVP has a maximal value of 66.9% even

---

CHARTERISTICS OF DIAGNOSTIC TESTS

Fig. A1.2 Characteristics of diagnostic tests.

MEASURE OF PERFORMANCE	CHARACTERISTIC
Sensitivity =	$\dfrac{\text{True positives}}{\text{True positives + false negatives}}$
Specificity =	$\dfrac{\text{True negatives}}{\text{True negatives + false positives}}$
Predictive value positive =	$\dfrac{\text{True positives}}{\text{True positives + false positives}}$
Predictive value negative =	$\dfrac{\text{True negatives}}{\text{True negatives + false negatives}}$

at very high sensitivity (99%) and specificity (99%). The values of PVN in a population with a 2% disease prevalence are shown in Figure A1.4B. Sensitivity and specificity have relatively little effect on this parameter.

One must be careful when applying results obtained during the preliminary evaluation of diagnostic tests using groups of known infected and uninfected individuals to unselected groups because of the magnification of false-positive errors by the generally low prevalences of disease in the general population. The concepts of sensitivity and specificity are not in themselves adequate to predict test reliability under these circumstances. This may be done, however, if the parameters of PVP and PVN are employed in unselected populations. These parameters take into account the known or assumed actual prevalence of disease in the general population.

Errors can be minimized by increasing the specificity of the test and by preselecting subjects at high risk of disease. This will produce a higher disease prevalence in the population to be tested. The preselection of the population by the first test will increase greatly the predictive value of the second test.

A good example is the screening use of the Rapid Plasma Reagin (RPR) or Venereal Disease Research Laboratory (VDRL) test to 'enrich' the group of positives, which are then subsequently tested with the Fluoroscent Treponemal Antibody Absorption (FTA-ABS) test for confirmation. A similar situation exists for the human immunodeficiency virus (HIV) enzyme-linked immunosorbent assay (ELISA) and Western blot tests. Use of the FTA-ABS or Western blot as a screening test is not indicated. These tests are no better than the screening tests for evaluation and are much more expensive and difficult to interpret.

A major problem in determining performance characteristics of many diagnostic tests is the lack of an appropriate reference standard, known as "gold standard," against which to judge the test. In practice, one is often forced to accept the best available, albeit imperfect, diagnostic test as a pseudo-reference standard. Diagnostic tests should always be evaluated in terms of their use with, and contribution to, other diagnostic tests and not merely in terms of their absolute accuracy in isolating already-known clinical information.

The effectiveness of a program to control STDs depends upon its effectiveness to detect STDs. Although most laboratories will employ a number of different tests, the range that is available is rapidly increasing.

Laboratory services are an integral part of all disease control programs, and the availability of laboratory tests considerably improves the quality of patient care. The most important characteristic and justification for the use of a laboratory test is its ability to provide information to assist patient management. The types of tests a laboratory can offer will depend on the level of its competence and its responsibilities (Fig. A1.5).

PREDICTIVE VALUES OF POSITIVE AND NEGATIVE TEST RESULTS AT VARYING DISEASE PREVALENCES WHEN SENSITIVITY AND SPECIFICITY EACH EQUAL 95%.

ACTUAL DISEASE PREVALENCE (%)	PREDICTIVE VALUES	
	POSITIVE (%)	NEGATIVE (%)
1	16.1	99.9
2	27.9	99.9
5	50.0	99.7
10	67.9	99.4
20	82.6	98.7
50	95.0	95.0
75	98.3	83.7
100	100.0	–

Fig. A1.3 Predictive values of positive and negative test results at varying disease prevalences when sensitivity and specificity each equal 95%.

PREDICTIVE VALUE OF A POSITIVE TEST (PVP) OVER A RANGE OF SENSITIVITIES AND SPECIFICITIES WHEN ACTUAL DISEASE PREVALENCE IS 2%

SPECIFICITY (%)	SENSITIVITY							
	50%	60%	70%	80%	90%	95%	98%	99%
50	2.0	2.4	2.8	3.2	3.5	3.7	3.8	3.9
60	2.5	3.0	3.4	3.9	4.4	4.6	4.8	4.8
70	3.3	3.9	4.5	5.2	5.8	6.1	6.2	6.3
80	4.8	5.8	6.7	7.6	8.4	8.8	9.1	9.2
90	9.2	10.9	12.5	14.0	15.5	16.2	16.7	16.8
95	17.0	19.7	22.2	24.6	26.9	27.9	28.6	28.8
98	33.8	38.0	41.7	44.9	47.9	49.2	50.0	50.2
99	50.5	55.0	58.8	62.0	64.7	66.0	66.7	66.9

A

Fig. A1.4 Predictive value of a positive test (PVP) (A) and a negative test (PVN) (B) over a range of sensitivities and specificities when actual disease prevalence is 2%.

PREDICTIVE VALUE OF A NEGATIVE TEST (PVN) OVER A RANGE OF SENSITIVITIES AND SPECIFICITIES WHEN ACTUAL DISEASE PREVALENCE IS 2%

SPECIFICITY (%)	SENSITIVITY							
	50%	60%	70%	80%	90%	95%	98%	99%
50	98.0	98.4	98.8	99.2	99.6	99.8	99.9	99.9
60	98.3	98.6	99.0	99.3	99.7	99.8	99.9	100.0
70	98.6	98.8	99.1	99.4	99.7	99.8	99.9	100.0
80	98.7	99.0	99.2	99.5	99.7	99.9	99.9	100.0
90	98.9	99.1	99.3	99.5	99.8	99.9	99.9	100.0
95	98.9	99.1	99.4	99.6	99.8	99.9	100.0	100.0
98	99.0	99.2	99.4	99.6	99.8	99.9	100.0	100.0
99	99.0	99.2	99.4	99.6	99.8	99.9	100.0	100.0

B

LABORATORY TESTS COMMONLY PERFORMED IN THE DIAGNOSIS OF SEXUALLY TRANSMITTED DISEASES

DISEASE	AGENT	LABORATORY TEST	SENSITIVITY	SPECIFICITY	RECOMMENDED LEVEL OF AVAILABILITY*		
					P	I	C
Syphilis	*Treponema pallidum*	Dark-field microscopy	85–95	100	+/–	+	+
		VDRL (nontreponemal) test	71–100†	79–98‡	+	+	+
		RPR card (nontreponemal) test	73–100†	79–98‡	+	+	+
		FTA-ABS (treponemal) test	85–100†	95–100‡	–	+	+
		MHA-TP (treponemal) test	70–100†	96–100	–	+	+
		Direct FA	90–95	>98	–	+/–	+
		#PCR	>95	>99	–	–	+
Gonorrhea	*Neisseria gonorrhoeae*	Gram stain					
		Urethral, symptomatic	90–95	95–99	+	+	+
		Urethral, asymptomatic	50–70	85–87	+	+	+
		Endocervix	45–65	90–99	+	+	+
		Conjunctiva	95		+	+	+
		Vagina	Not recommended		–	–	–
		Anal canal	Not recommended		–	–	–
		Pharynx	Not recommended		–	–	–
		Culture					
		Urethral discharge	94–98	>99	+/–	+	+
		Urethral, asymptomatic	80–85		+/–	+	+
		Endocervix	85–95	>99	+/–	+	+
		Conjunctiva	95		–	+	+
		Vagina	50–85		–	+	+
		Anal canal	70–85		–	+	+
		Pharynx	50–70		–	+/–	+
		Disseminated infection					
		Gram stain					
		Blood	Not recommended		–	–	–
		Joints	5–10		+	+	+
		Lesions	5–10		+	+	+
		Culture					
		Blood	25–75		–	+/–	+
		Joint	25–75		–	+	+
		Lesions	2–5		–	+	+
		Direct antigen detection					
		Urethra	90–95	81–99	–	+/–	+
		Endocervix	60–85	76–99	–	+/–	+
		Rectum	Not recommended		–	–	–
		Pharynx	Not recommended		–	–	–
		β-lactamase tests	>99		–	+/–	+
		Direct FA	90–95	95–99	–	+/–	+
		DNA probes	95–99	99	–	+/–	+
		Confirmatory tests	95–99	>95	–	+	+
		Antimicrobic susceptibility					
		Disk diffusion			+/–	+	+
		Minimum inhibitory concentration (MIC)			–	–	+
		#PCR					
		Urethra	>95	>99	–	–	+
		Endocervix	90–95	>99	–	–	+
		Urine	>95	>99	–	–	+
		#LCR					
		Endocervix	>95	>99	–	–	+
		Urine	90–95	>99	–	–	+
Genital herpes	Herpes simplex virus types 1 and 2	Tzanck test	40–50	>95	–	+/–	+
		Papanicolaou smear	30–40	>95	–	+/–	+
		Direct FA	70–80	>95	–	+/–	+
		Culture	25–90†	>99	–	+/–	+
		Neutralizing antibody	65–70	x	–	–	+
		Direct EIA	85–90	>99	–	–	+
		Direct FA	>90	>98	–	+/–	+
		#PCR	>95	>99	–	–	+
Trichomoniasis	*Trichomonas vaginalis*	Wet mount/saline	50–75	>99	+	+	+
		Culture	80–90	>99	–	+	+
		FA	85–90	>99	–	+/–	+
		EIA	90–95	>99	–	+/–	+
		#DNA probe	>95	>99	–	–	+
Candidiasis	*Candida albicans*	Wet mount/10% KOH	40–60	>99	+	+	+
		Culture	70–80	>99	–	+	+
		Latex agglutination	71–81	96–98	–	+	+
Chancroid	*Haemophillus ducreyi*	Gram stain	<50	50–70	+	+	+
		Culture	30–70	>98	–	+/–	+

continued

DISEASE	AGENT	LABORATORY TEST	SENSITIVITY	SPECIFICITY	RECOMMENDED LEVEL OF AVAILABILITY*		
					P	I	C
Chancroid	*Haemophillus ducreyi*	Serology	70–80	80–90	–	–	+
		#PCR	80–90	>99	–	–	+
Gardnerella vaginitis	*Gardnerella vaginalis*	Wet mount/saline	70–90	95–100	+	+	+
		Gram stain	60–80	95–100	+	+	+
		pH	75–80	60–70	+	+	+
		Culture	80–90	>99	–	+/–	+
		#DNA probe	>90	>99	–	–	+
Granuloma inguinale	*Calymmatobacterium granulomatis*	Direct stain/Wright–Giemsa	40–50	<50	+	+	+
		Culture	Not recommended		–	–	–
Chlamydia (also lympho-granuloma venereum)	*Chlamydia trachomatis*	Culture	60–80	>99	–	–	+
		Direct antigen EIA-confirmed					
		Urethral	70–80	>99	–	–	+
		Endocervix	80–90	>99	–	–	+
		Urine	80–90	>99	–	–	+
		Direct antigen-FA	80–92	95–98	–	+	+
		Giemsa stain	45	95	–	+	+
		Papanicolaou stain	62	96	–	+/–	+
		Conjunctiva Giemsa stain	95	90–95	–	–	+
		Conjunctiva culture	95	>99	–	–	+
		Micro-IF antibody	60–80	95	–	–	+
		Complement fixation for LGV	40–50	85	–	+/–	+
		DNA probes	90–93	96–98	–	+/–	+
		#PCR					
		Endocervix	>95	>99	–	–	+
		Urine	>90	>99	–	–	+
		#LCR					
		Endocervix	>95	>99	–	–	+
		Urine	>90	>99	–	–	+
Genital mycoplasma infections	*Mycoplasma hominis*	Culture	75–80	95–97	–	+/–	+
		Serology	Not recommended		–	–	–
	Ureaplasma urealyticum	Culture	90–95	90–92	–	+/–	+
		Serology	Not recommended		–	–	–
AIDS	Human immunodeficiency virus (HIV-1)	EIA	>99	>99	–	+/–	+
		Western Blot	>99	>99	–	+/–	+
Genital warts	Human papillomaviruses (HPV)	DNA probes	88–92	96–98	–	+/–	+

* Peripheral (P) = outpatient clinics or primary practitioner's laboratory (facilities limited); intermediate (I) = regional, state, hospital laboratory; central (C) = national research or reference laboratory.
†Varies with stage of disease
‡Varies with population being tested
For Investigational use only

Fig. A1.5 Laboratory tests commonly performed in the diagnosis of sexually transmitted diseases.

QUALITY CONTROL

Quality control of diagnostic tests depends on adherence to recommendations regarding refrigeration and/or shelf life of antibiotics, culture medium, and test reagents. More important are measures of outcome. Among these are the percentage of patients who have follow-up examinations and are found cured for each treatment regimen and, whenever possible, the level of agreement between different diagnostic tests for the same disease. For example, all intermediate and central laboratories should develop methods for comparing results of Gram-stained smears and cultures for *Neisseria gonorrhoeae*. This is the only practical way to continuously monitor the quality of gonorrhea diagnostic techniques that begins with medium production and ends with transmittal of results to patients.

BIBLIOGRAPHY

Griner PF, Mayewski RJ, Mushlin AI, Greenland P: Selection and interpretation of diagnostic tests and procedures. Ann Intern Med 94:553, 1981.

Hart G: Epidemiologic Aspects of Venereal Disease Control. US Dept of Health and Human Services publication No. 00–3633. Atlanta, Centers for Disease Control, 1980.

Hart G: The role of treponemal tests in therapeutic decision making. Am J Public Health 73:739, 1983.

Holmes KK, Mårdh P-A, Sparling PF, Wiesner PJ: Sexually Transmitted Diseases, ed I. New York, McGraw-Hill Book Co, 1984, pp 992–998.

Rothenberg RB, Simon R, Chipperfield E, Catterall RD: Efficacy of selected diagnostic tests for sexually transmitted diseases. JAMA 235:49, 1976.

Swartz JS: Assessing Medical Technologies. Washington, DC, National Academy Press, 1985, pp 70–175.

Vecchio TJ: Predictive value of a single diagnostic test in unselected populations. N Engl J Med 274:1171, 1966.

Whittington WL, Cates W Jr.: Checking out the new STD tests. Contemp Obstet Gynecol 23:135, 1984.

World Health Organization—VDT 85.437. Simplified approaches for sexually transmitted disease (STD) control at the primary health care (PHC) level. Report of a WHO working group. Geneva, Sept. 24–28, 1984.

Media, Reagents, Test Procedures, and Stains

SK Sarafian

TRANSPORT AND CULTURE MEDIA

(It should be noted that inclusion of manufacturers of media and reagents does not constitute endorsement or disapproval of any manufacturer or product).

1. A8 AGAR Growth medium for *Mycoplasma hominis* and *Ureaplasma urealyticum*.

Trypticase soy broth (BBL, Cockeysville, MD)	2.4 g
$CaCl_2.2H_2O$	0.014 g
Putrescine dihydrocholoride	0.166 g
Distilled Water	80 mL

Dissolve ingredients and adjust pH to 5.5 with 2N HCl. Add 1.05g bacteriological grade agar (Gibco Laboratories, Grand Island, NY). Autoclave at 121°C for 15 minutes, and equilibrate at 56°C. The following supplements may be combined, filter sterilized and added to the basal agar after equilibration at 56°C.

Unheated, pooled normal horse serum	20 mL
CVA enrichment (Gibco Laboratories, Grand Island, NY).	0.5 mL
Yeast extract (25% aqueous extract of pure dry yeast), pH 6.0	1.0 mL
Urea solution (10%)	1.0 mL
L-Cysteine-HCl (2% solution)	0.5 mL
GHL tripeptide (20µg/mL solution)	0.1 mL
Penicillin G, potassium (100,000 U/mL solution)	1.0 mL

Plates are incubated at 37°C in a CO_2 gassed incubator.

2. BIPHASIC BLOOD AGAR Isolation medium for *Gardnerella vaginalis* composed of a basal layer of 7mL of CNA agar base (Columbia agar, BBL, Cockeysville, MD) containing 10µg colistin, 15µg nalidixic acid, and 2µg amphotericin B per mL and a 14 mL overlayer of the same medium containing 5% (v/v) human blood.

3. BLOOD AGAR Growth medium for *Mycoplasma* spp.

Blood agar base No. 2 (Oxoid,Columbia, MD)	40 g
Dextrose	5.0 g
Thallous acetate (or thallous sulphate)	0.125 g
Distilled water	1000 mL

Boil to dissolve and autoclave at 121°C for 15 minutes. Cool to 50°C. Add 100,000 units penicillin and 200 mL horse serum; mix and pour thick plates. Inoculate and incubate separate plates at 37°C, for up to 5 or 6 days, under aerobic and anaerobic conditions simultaneously.

4. CHLAMYDIA TRANSPORT MEDIUM This medium is used for the transport of specimens for the isolation of *Chlamydia*.

Classical formula per liter distilled water:

Sucrose	74.60 g
L-Glutamic acid	0.72 g
Potassium diphosphate	0.51 g
Potassium monophosphate	1.24 g
HEPES	4.76 g
Fetal bovine serum	100.00 mL
Phenol red	3.00 mg
Gentamicin	50.00 mg
Nystatin	30.00 mg
Amphotericin B	2.50 mg

The medium is aseptically dispensed in convenient small volumes and stored at 2-8°C.

5. CHOCOLATE AGAR A complex nonselective medium used for growth of fastidious microorganisms such as *Neisseria gonorrhoeae*.

GC agar base (BBL, Cockeysville, MD)	7.2 g
Distilled water	100 mL

Mix and boil for 2 minutes. Autoclave at 121°C for 15 minutes. Cool to 50°C.

Hemoglobin	2.0 g
Distilled water	100 mL

Mix the hemoglobin with 2-3mL of the distilled water to form a smooth paste. Continue mixing and gradually add all the water. Autoclave at 121°C for 15 minutes and cool to 50°C. Aseptically combine both solutions. Add 2mL IsoVitaliX (BBL, Cockeysville, MD). Mix and pour 20-25mL per petri dish.

6. DULANEY SLANTS A medium used for growth of *Calymmatobacterium granulomatis*.

Yolks are aseptically removed from 5-8 day hen egg embryos and placed in an equal volume of sterile Locke solution containing glass beads. After vigorous mixing, the resulting homogenate is dispensed into slanted tubes and coagulated by incubating in steam at 80°C for 15 minutes.

7. GC II AGAR BASE* (BBL, Cockeysville, MD) † Basal medium used for the preparation of selective media for *N. gonorrhoeae* and *Haemophilus ducreyi*.

Pancreatic digest of casein	7.5 g
Selected meat peptone	7.5 g
Corn starch	1.0 g
Dipotassium phosphate (K_2HPO_4)	4.0 g
Monopotassium phosphate (KH_2PO_4)	1.0 g
Sodium choride	5.0 g
Agar	10.0 g
Distilled water	1000 mL

The final pH should be 7.3 ± 0.2.

* GC medium base is supplemented with 1% (v/v) IsoVitaleX enrichment.
† Similar media are also manufactured by Oxoid (Columbia, MD) and Difco (Detroit, MI) Laboratories; they differ mainly in their nitrogen sources.

8. GC-LECT ((BBL, Cockeysville, MD) A selective medium for *N. gonorrhoeae*.

This medium is prepared from a chocolate agar base supplemented with five antimicrobial agents.

9. ISOVITALEX (BBL, Cockeysville, MD) A supplement for media use for the isolation of *N. gonorrhoeae* and *H. ducreyi*.

Approximate formula per liter distilled water:

Vitamin B12	0.01 g
L-Glutamine	10.0 g
Adenine	1.0 g
Guanine HCI	0.03 g
p-Aminobenzoic acid	0.013 g
Diphosphopyridine nucleotide, oxidized (coenzyme 1)	0.25 g
Cocarboxylase	0.1 g
Ferric nitrate	0.02 g
Thiamine HCI	0.003 g
L-Cysteine HCI	25.9 g
L-Cystine	1.1 g
Dextrose	100.0 g

Each vial of IsoVitaleX enrichment is supplied with a vial of sterile rehydrating fluid diluent containing approximately 10% dextrose.
The composition of this enrichment is similar to that of Vitox (Oxoid, Columbia, MD) or CVA (Gibco Laboratories, Grand Island, NY).

10. JEMBEC This medium is used for the transport and selective growth of *N. gonorrhoeae*. The Jembec plate allows the investigator to add the CO_2 required for the growth of *N. gonorrhoeae*, after the specimen has been inoculated by placing a CO_2-generating tablet in a well provided in the plate. Jembec plates are manufactured by Flow Laboratories, Inc. (McLean, VA). Plates containing either modified Thayer-Martin or Martin-Lewis medium are available; they should be used according to the manufacturers' directions.

11. MARTIN-LEWIS MEDIUM A selective medium for *N. gonorrhoeae* identical to modified Thayer-Martin medium except for substituting anisomycin (10μg/mL) for nystatin.

12. MODIFIED DIAMOND'S MEDIUM This is a culture medium for *Trichomonas vaginalis*.

Trypticase (BBL, Cockeysville, MD)	20.0 g
Yeast extract	1.0 g
Maltose	0.5 g
L-Cystine HCl	0.5 g
L-Ascorbic acid	0.02 g
Distilled water Q.S. to	90.0 mL

Adjust pH to 6.5 and autoclave at 121°C for 15 minutes, cool to 48°C, and add the following antibiotics: sodium penicillin G (1000U/mL), streptomycin sulfate (1.5mg/mL), amphotericin B (2μg/mL). Also add 10mL horse serum that has been heat inactivated at 56°C for 30 minutes. Dispense into 5-mL aliquots in sterile tubes and store at 4°C for up to 14 days. Warm to 35°C before inoculation. This medium, without horse serum, may be stored at -20°C.

13. MODIFIED NYC MEDIUM (prepared plates may be obtained from Scott Laboratories, Inc., Fiskeville, RI).

A selective medium for *N. gonorrhoeae*.

GC agar base	36 g
Bio-enrichment	10 mL
3% lysed horse red blood cells	200 mL
Horse plasma	120 mL
Dextrose	5.0 g
Colistin	5.0 mg
Vancomycin	2.0 mg
Amphotericin B	1.2 mg
Trimethoprim lactate	3.0 mg
Distilled water	1000 mL

14. MYCOPLASMA BROTH This is a transport medium for *Mycoplasma* spp.

Mix 70mL Mycoplasma broth base with 30mL yeast extract (1 part) and horse serum (2 parts) and add the following:

0.4% Phenol red	0.5 g
Penicillin (100,000 U/mL)	0.5 mL
Polymyxin (5000μg/mL)	1.0 mL
Amphotericin (5000μg/mL)	0.1 mL

Adjust pH to 6.0 with 1N HCl and dispense into 1-mL aliquots.

15. MYCOPLASMA BROTH BASE A component of media used for transport and culture of *Mycoplasma* spp.

Beef heart infusion	50.0 g
Peptone	10.0 g
NaCl	5.0 g
Distilled water	1000 mL

Autoclave at 121°C for 15 minutes and store at 4°C.

16. NICKERSON MEDIUM (Bacto BiGGY Agar, Difco Laboratories, Detroit, MI).

A selective medium recommended for the detection, isolation, and differentiation of *Candida* spp.

Bacto yeast extract	1.0 g
Glycine	10.0 g
Bacto dextrose	10.0 g
Bismuth sulfite indicator	8.0 g
Bacto agar	20.0 g
Distilled water	1000.0 mL

Final pH should be 6.8.

Suspend 49 g Bacto BiGGY agar in 1 L distilled water. Heat to boiling to dissolve completely. Do not boil for longer than a few minutes as overheating will destroy the selective properties of the medium (do not autoclave). The medium contains a flocculent precipitate that should be evenly dispersed by swirling medium in flasks prior to dispensing in tubes or plates. Prepared medium should be stored at 4°C.

17. SABOURAUD DEXTROSE AGAR This is a culture medium for *Candida albicans* and other fungi.

Glucose	40.0 g
Neopeptone or polypeptone (BBL, Cockeysville, MD)	10.0 g
Agar	15-20.0 g
Demineralized water	1000.0 mL

Final pH should be 5.6. Heat the mixture to dissolve completely. Dispense into tubes (18-25mm in diameter) and autoclave at 121°C for 15 minutes.

18. SP-4 MEDIUM Growth medium for *M. hominis* and *M. genitalium*.

Liquid medium:

Mycoplasma broth base	1.0 g
Bacto-peptone (Difco Laboratories, Detroit, MI)	1.6 g
Bacto-tryptone (Difco)	3.0 g
Distilled water	197 mL

Dissolve ingredients and adjust pH to 7.8 (0.6mL 2N NaOH). Autoclave at 121°C for 30 minutes and cool to room temperature. Add the following sterile components:

Phenol red (0.5% solution)	1.2 mL
Penicillin G potassium (100,000 U/mL)	3.0 mL
Yeastolate (Difco) (2%)	30.0 mL
CMRL-1066 (10x) (with glutamine, without NaHCO$_3$) (Gibco Laboratories, Grand Island, NY)	15.0 mL
Fresh yeast extract (25%) (Flow Laboratories, McLean, VA)	10.5 mL
Fetal bovine serum (heat-treated, 56°C for 1 hour)	50.0 mL
Glucose (50% solution)	3.0 mL

Final pH should be 7.4.

Solid medium:
Add 2.4 to 6.8 g Difco Noble agar (depending on spiroplasma) to autoclavable fraction, before autoclaving and after adjusting pH. After autoclaving, cool to 56°C and allow nonautoclavable fraction to warm to 56°C. Combine both fractions aseptically before pouring plates.

19. 2SP MEDIUM This is a transport medium for *Chlamydia trachomatis* or *Mycoplasma* spp. consisting of 0.2M sucrose in 0.02M phosphate buffer, pH 7.2, and the following antibiotics: gentamicin (2µg/mL), amphotericin (0.5µg/mL), vancomycin (10 µg/mL).

20. SHEPARD'S 10 B BROTH Growth medium for *M. hominis* and *U. urealyticum*.

PPLO broth (without crystal violet) (Difco Laboratories, Detroit, MI)	1.47 g
Distilled water	73 mL

Dissolve powder and adjust pH to 5.5 with 2N HCI. Autoclave at 121°C for 15 minutes. The following supplements may be combined, filter sterilized, and added to the basal broth after cooling to room temperature.

Unheated normal horse serum	20 mL
Yeast extract (25%)	10 mL
L-Cysteine HCI stock solution (2%)	0.5 mL
Urea stock solution (10%)	0.4 mL
CVA supplement	0.5 mL
Sodium phenol red solution (1%)	0.1 mL
Penicillin G potassium (100,000 U/mL)	1.0 mL

The final pH of the complete 10B broth should be approximately 6.0. The medium is aseptically dispensed in convenient small volumes and stored at -20°C.

21. THAYER-MARTIN AGAR A selective medium for the isolation of *N. gonorrhoeae*.

To the complete chocolate agar (see No. 5), add 1mL of VCN inhibitor containing (per mL):

Vancomycin	300 µg
Colistin	750 µg
Nystatin	1250 U

The modified Thayer-Martin agar also contains trimethoprim lactate at a final concentration of 5µg/mL.

22. TRANSGROW This transport and selective growth medium for *N. gonorrhoeae* is similar to chocolate agar except for the addition of 2.0 g agar and 0.3 g glucose per 100mL double- strength GC agar base before autoclaving. VCN inhibitor (1mL) is added to cooled complete medium, as described for the Thayer-Martin agar. Dispense into sterile bottles, gas with 20% CO$_2$ in air, and tighten caps securely.

23. TRANSPORT MEDIUM FOR HERPES SIMPLEX VIRUS (Gibco Laboratories, Grand Island, NY)

Hanks balanced salt solution with 2% fetal calf serum (containing antibiotics to prevent bacterial overgrowth).

24. TRYPTICASE SOY BROTH + 0.5% BOVINE SERUM ALBUMIN (BSA) This is a transport medium for *Mycoplasma* spp.

Trypticase soy broth (BBL Cockeysville, MD)	3 g
BSA	0.5 g
Distilled water	100 mL

Dissolve by mixing thoroughly and warming gently until solution is complete. Dispense and autoclave at 121°C for 15 minutes.

25. TRYPTICASE SOY BROTH + 15% GLYCEROL This is a freezing solution for the storage of neisseriae at -70°C.

Trypticase soy broth (BBL, Cockeysville, MD)	30 g

Dissolve in 500mL distilled water by mixing thoroughly and warming gently until solution is complete.

Glycerol	150 mL
Distilled water Q.S. to	1000 mL

Dispense and autoclave at 121°C for 15 minutes.

26. YEAST EXTRACT, 25% [Difco Laboratories (Detroit, MI), Oxoid (Columbia, MD)] This is a component of medium used for the growth of *Mycoplasma* spp.

Sprinkle 250g active baker's yeast onto the surface of 1 L distilled water in a 2-L beaker. Heat the mixture to boiling, then clarify it by centrifuging at 1000 x g for 1 hour. Adjust the pH to 8.0 with 1N NaOH and filter sterilize.

REAGENTS AND TEST PROCEDURES

(It should be noted that inclusion or exclusion of manufacturers of reagents does not constitute endorsement or disapproval of any manufacturer or product).

1. ACETIC ACID (3%) (Acetowhitening)

Glacial acetic acid	3.0 mL
Distilled water Q.S. to	100 mL

2. Alkaline Phosphatase test

p-Nitrophenyl phosphate disodium tetrahydrate	100.0 mg
Distilled water	25.0 mL

Dissolve the substrate and add 25mL of a solution containing 0.1M glycine and 0.001M $MgCl_2$, pH 10.5.
Filter sterilize, dispense into 0.3mL aliquots, and store at -20°C. To detect alkaline phosphatase production, inoculate the substrate-containing solution with test organism and incubate at 35°C for 6 hours. Development of a yellow color is indicative of a positive test.

3. CATALASE TEST Add a drop of 3% H_2O_2 to a loopful of growth placed on a glass slide. A positive test is recorded when a brisk bubbling occurs upon addition of H_2O_2.

Hydrogen peroxide 3.0%

4. CHROMOGENIC CEPHALOSPORIN This reagent is used to detect ß-lactamase.

Cefinase is available from BBL, Cockeysville, MD.

5. CONFIRMATORY TESTS FOR *N. gonorrhoeae*

A. Coagglutination Tests. Several kits are commercially available and utilize monoclonal antibodies to epitopes on the major outer membrane protein of *N. gonorrhoeae*: Phadebact Monoclonal GC Test and Phadebact Monoclonal GC Omni Test (Pharmacia, Inc., Piscataway, NJ); Meritec-GC (Meridian Diagnostics, Inc., Cincinatti, OH); GonoGen I and GonoGen II (New Horizons Diagnostics Corp., Columbia, MD). These kits should be used for the confirmatory identification of *N. gonorrhoeae*, according to the manufacturers' directions.
B. Combined Tests. These tests are based on the enzymatic hydrolysis of chromogenic substrates, the production of acid from specific sugars, and other biochemical tests. Examples of these tests and their manufacturers are: Rapid N/H System (Innovative Diagnostic Systems, Inc., Decatur, GA); Vitek *Neisseria-Haemophilus* identification (NHI) card (Vitek Systems, Inc., Hazelwood, MO); HNID panel (American Micro Scan, Sacramento, CA).
C. Enzyme Substrate Tests. These tests are based on the enzymatic hydrolysis of chromogenic substrates by *N. gonorrhoeae*. Examples of these tests and their manufacturers are: Gonocheck II (E.I. du Pont de Nemours & Co., Inc., Wilmington, DE); Identicult-Neisseria (Scott Laboratories, Inc., Fiskville, RI).
D. NA Hybridization Tests. These tests are based on the detection of gonococcal NA using specific oligonucleotides. Examples of these tests and their manufacturers are: Orthoprobe culture confirmation test for *N. gonorrhoeae* (Ortho Diagnostic Systems, Raritan, NJ); The Gen-Probe PACE system for detection and identification of *N. gonorrhoeae* (Gen-Probe, San Diego, CA).
E. Rapid Carbohydrate Tests. These tests are based on the production of acid from specific sugars.
Examples of these tests and their manufacturers are: Minitek (BBL, Cockeysville, MD); Quadferm + (Analytab Products, Inc., Plainview, NY) (also includes β-lactamase and DNase tests); RIM-N (American Micro Scan, Campbell, CA); Niesseria-Stat (Richardson Scientific, Dallas, TX); Neisseria-Kwik (Micro Bio Logics, St Cloud, MN).

6. KOH (10%)

KOH	10.0 G
Distilled water Q.S. to	100 mL

7. KOVACS' REAGENT

p-Dimethylaminobenzaldehyde	5.0 g
Amyl alcohol	75.0 mL

Dissolve *p*-Dimethylaminobenzaldehyde by warming the solution in a 56°C water bath. Slowly add 25.0mL concentrated HCI. Dispense into a brown bottle and store at 4°C. The reagent should be a light color.

8. LOCKE SALT SOLUTION

Sodium chloride	0.900 g
Calcium chloride	0.024 g
Potassium chloride	0.042 g
Sodium carbonate	0.020 g
Glucose	0.250 g
Distilled water	100 mL

9. NITRATE REDUCTASE TEST

Heart infusion broth (Difco)	25 g
Potassium nitrate C.P.	2.0 g
Distilled water	1000 mL

Adjust pH to 7.0. Dispense into 4.0mL aliquots in 15 by 125-mm tubes containing inverted Durham fermentation tubes, autoclave at 121°C for 15 minutes, and store at 4°C. Inoculate the broth with the test organism, and incubate at 35°C for 48 hours. Add 5 drops of each of the reagents 1 and 2 (given below) consecutively and examine for the presence of a pink to red color. If negative, add a small amount of zinc dust and incubate at room temperature for 5 minutes to detect nitrate that has not been reduced.

A red color at this point indicates that the nitrate has not been reduced (a negative test for nitrate reduction); if the broth remains colorless, the nitrate has been completely reduced (a positive test for nitrate reduction).

Reagent 1:	
Sulfanilic acid	2.8 g
Glacial acetic acid	100 mL
Distilled water	250 mL
Reagent 2:	
Dimethyl-α-naphthylamine	2.1 mL
Glacial acetic acid	100 mL
Distilled water	250 mL

10. OXIDASE TEST

Tetra-methyl-p-phenylenediamine	
Dihydrochloride	1.0 g
Distilled water	100 mL

Saturate a filter paper contained in a petri dish with the reagent. Pick a portion of the colony to be tested using a platinum wire and rub it on the filter paper. A positive reaction is indicated by a deep purple color appearing in 10 seconds.

11. PHOSPHATE BUFFER, M/15, pH 6.4

KH_2PO_4	6.63 g
Na_2HPO_4	2.56 g
Distilled water Q.S. to	1000 mL

12. PORPHYRIN TEST

Delta-aminolevulinic acid	
hydrochloride (2mM)	0.034 g
$MgSO_4$. $7H_2O$ (0.8mM)	0.02 g
Phosphate buffer (0.1M) pH 6.9	100 mL

Dispense filter-sterilized solution into 0.5mL aliquots and store at −20°C. Test procedure: Add a very heavy loopful of the test organism to the substrate solution. After incubation at 35°C for 4 hours, examine under a Woods lamp for a red fluorescence. The observation of fluorescence indicates a positive reaction. If no fluorescence is observed, incubate reaction mixture overnight and re-examine. If no fluorescence is observed after overnight incubation, add an equal volume of Kovacs' reagent (see No. 7). Shake vigorously and allow the aqueous and alcohol phases to separate. The development of a red color in the lower aqueous phase indicates a positive reaction.

13. PRODUCTION OF POLYSACCHARIDE FROM SUCROSE

Strains of some *Neisseria* spp. (*N. sicca*, *N. subflava* biovar *perflava*, *N. mucosa*, *N. flavescens*, *N. polysaccharea*) produce a polysaccharide from sucrose that can be detected by the addition of iodine to the colonies. Traditionally the polysaccharide test is performed by the incorporation of 5% (w/v) sucrose into a medium, such as tryptic soy agar, which does not contain starch (which will give a positive test). Strains of *Neisseria* spp. are inoculated by the streak-plate method or spotted onto the medium and incubated at 35°C for 5 days. It was found however, that some strains were inhibited by 5% sucrose. The test may be performed on tryptic soy agar containing 1% (w/v) sucrose after incubation for 24 hours. A drop of Lugol's iodine (Gram's iodine diluted 1:4) is added to the growth. If polysaccharide has been produced, the colonies, and often the surrounding medium will immediately turn a dark blue, brown, or black.

It is important that the recommended incubation time not be exceeded. Many strains that produce polysaccharide metabolize it, and if the incubation is carried out for longer than recommended, the polysaccharide may be completely consumed and thus no longer detectable. It is also possible to detect the polysaccharide in traditional sucrose-containing media in which acid production is detected. The polysaccharide may be detected as a brown-to-black precipitate when one or two drops of Lugol's iodine are added to the sucrose-containing medium. The precipitate will range from fine brown to a course black flocculant precipitate. The reaction will fade if the test is allowed to sit at room temperature, but may be rejuvenated by the addition of a few drops of iodine. The test may be performed with fresh Gram's iodine that has been made according to the original formula; aged Gram's iodine and commercially prepared iodine will give negative results. The polysaccharide production test may not be performed using the rapid tests for the detection of acid production from sucrose.

14. SUPEROXOL TEST

The superoxol test is a variation of the catalase test, which is performed by adding a drop of 3% H_2O_2 to a loopful of growth placed on a glass slide. The superoxol test is performed by adding a drop of 30% H_2O_2 to a colony of the organism on a chocolate agar plate. A positive superoxol test is recorded when a brisk bubbling ocurrs immediately when the 30% H_2O_2 is added to the colonies. A delay of 3 seconds before a bubbling is observed is interpreted as a negative superoxol reaction. Although all human *Neisseria* spp. and *Branhamella catarrhalis* are catalase-positive, strains vary in their reactions in the superoxol test. Strains of *N. gonorrhoeae* are superoxol-positive whereas strains of other species vary in their reactions in this test. Strains of *N. meningitidis* serogroup A, *N. lactamica*, and *B. catarrhalis* may give positive superoxol tests. Thus the superoxol test must be used in combination with other tests to accurately identify strains of *N. gonorrhoeae*. It also must be noted that, similar to the catalase test, the superoxol test should not be performed on medium containing unheated blood, which will react with the H_2O_2.

15. TZANCK SMEARS In the Tzanck test the cells are smeared onto a slide, fixed, and stained with Wright or Giemsa preparations.

STAINS

(It should be noted that inclusion or exlusion of manufacturers or reagents does not constitute endorsement or disapproval of any manufacturer or product).

1. ACRIDINE ORANGE STAIN This stain is used for the detection of bacteria in clinical specimens. At pH 4.0, bateria stain red-orange while eucaryotic cells stain green-yellow. The specimen is spread onto a clean glass slide, air-dried, and fixed by immersion in absolute methanol for 2 minutes. It is then stained for 2 minutes by flooding the slide with a solution of 0.5% acridine orange in 0.15 M acetate buffer, pH 4.0. The slide is rinsed with water air-dried and examined at 400-1000x magnification under ultraviolet light.

2. FLUORESCENT ANTIBODY STAINS FOR *C. trachomatis*

Fluroescent antibody staining reagents for *C. trachomatis* elementary bodies are commercially available. Reagents utilizing anti-major outer membrane protein (MOMP) monoclonal antibodies are produced by Syva Co., Palo Alto, CA; Difco Laboratories, Detroit,MI; and Kallestad Diagnostics, Austin, TX. Reagents utlizing anti-lipopolysaccharide (LPS) monoclonal antibodies are produced by Bartels Immunodiagnostic Supplies, Inc., Bellevue, WA; Boots Celltech Diagnostics, Inc., Plainview, NY; and California Integrated Diagnostics, Inc., Berkeley, CA. In general, brighter and more consistent fluorescence is observed with those products utilizing anti-MOMP monoclonal antibodies than with those using anti-LPS antibodies. Staining with the anti-MOMP monoclonal antibodies results in the consistent appearance of elementary bodies as well defined, rough disks of a uniform size. Anti-LPS staining results in the appearance of elementary bodies of varied shapes and sizes. More cross-reactions have been observed with the reagents utilizing anti-LPS monoclonal antibodies than with those using anti-MOMP antibodies. These products should be used according to the manufacturers' directions.

3. FLUORESCENT ANTIBODY STAINS FOR *N. gonorrhoeae*

Commercially available fluorescent antibody staining reagents for the confirmatory identification of *N. gonorrhoeae* include: Syva MicroTrak *N. gonorrhoeae* Culture Confirmation Reagent (Syva Co, Palo Alto, CA), which consists of a cocktail of fluorescein-labeled antigonococcal monoclonal antibodies (This reagent also contains Evan's blue, which decreases background staining); Bacto FA *N. gonorrhoeae* (Difco Laboratories, Detroil, MI), a fluorescein-labeled rabbit polyvalent antigonococcal antibody reagent.

4. GIEMSA STAIN

Stock solution:

Giemsa powder	0.5 g
Glycerol	33.0 mL
Methyl alcohol, absolute, acetone-free	33.0 mL

Dissolve the powder in the glycerol by placing the mixture in a water bath (55°C-60°C) for 90 minutes. When crystals are dissolved, add 33ml absolute methanol. Store at room temperature.
Working solution: Prepare fresh by diluting the stock 1:23 in phosphate buffer.

Phosphate buffer:

Solution 1:
Na$_2$HPO$_4$	9.47 g
Distilled water Q.S. to	1000 mL

Solution 2:
KH$_2$PO$_4$	9.08 g
Distilled water Q.S. to	1000 mL

Mix 72.0mL of solution 1 with 28.0mL of solution 2 and 900mL distilled water. Staining procedure: The smear is air-dried, fixed with absolute methanol for at least 5 minutes, and again dried. It is then covered with the working Giemsa solution for 1 hour. The slide is then rinsed rapidly in 95% ethyl alcohol to remove excess dye, dried and examined for the presence of the typical intracytoplasmic inclusion bodies. The elementary bodies stain toward purple, whereas reticulate bodies are slightly more basophilic and tend to stain toward blue. There is some variability in commercially available prepared stock Giemsa solutions; these commercial products should be screened before being accepted for routine use. Modifications of the Giemsa stain are used to stain protozoa (parasites) and *Dermatophilus* spp. and to detect intracellular Donovan bodies in tissues.

5. GRAM STAIN

Crystal violet:
Solution 1: 10% crystal violet in 95% ethyl alcohol
Solution 2: 0.8g ammonium oxalate dissolved in 80 mL distilled water.

Mix solutions 1 and 2 together and filter after overnight storage at room temperature.

Gram's iodine:
1g iodine and 2g potassium iodine dissolved in 300mL distilled water

Decolorizers:
95% ethyl alcohol (slowest)
95% ethyl alcohol and acetone (1:1) (intermediate)
Acetone (fastest)

Counterstain:
Stock solution: 2.5% safranin O in 95% ethyl alcohol.
Working solution: 10mL stock solution in 90mL distilled water.

6. HEMATOXYLIN AND EOSIN STAIN Sections are cut at 5mm.

A. Two changes of xylol; 2 minutes each
B. Two changes of absolute alcohol; 1 minute each
C. One change of 95% alcohol; 1 minute
D. One change of 90% alcohol; 0.5 minute
E. One change of 80% alcohol; 0.5 minute
F. One change of 60% alcohol; 0.5 minute
G. Two or more changes of distilled water, until slides have cleared
H. Harris hematoxylin with glacial acetic acid (5mL acetic acid with 100mL hematoxylin); 1-2 minutes
I. Rinse in distilled water
J. Place in tap water containing 20-40 drops ammonium hydroxide; 3 seconds (section will turn blue immediately)
K. Rinse in two changes of tap water to remove the ammonia
L. Counterstain in picro-eosin solution; 30 seconds
M. Two changes of 95% alcohol; 1 minute each
N. Two changes of absolute alcohol; 1 and 2 minutes
O. Two changes of xylol; 1 minute each
P. Mount in neutral xylol-damar

7. JONES' IODINE STAIN

Potassium iodine	5.0 g
Iodine crystals	5.0 g
Absolute methanol	50.0 mL
Distilled water	50.0 mL

Combine reagents and mix until in solution. Store at room temperature in a brown bottle (to protect from direct light). Before use, filter through a #41 ashless Whatman filter paper.

8. METHYLENE BLUE STAIN

Methylene blue	0.3 g
Ethanol	30.0 mL

When the dye is dissolved, add 100 mL distilled water.
Staining procedure: Fix smear and flood slide with methylene blue stain for 1 minute. Wash the stain off the slide in tap water, blot dry, and examine.

9. MODIFIED ACID-FAST STAIN FOR *Cryptosporidium* OOCYSTS IN STOOL SPECIMENS

Basic fuchsin crystals	4.0 g
Ethanol	25 mL

After dissolving the crystals, add 12.0 mL liquefied phenol and mix well with a glass stirring rod. The following are then added:

Glycerol	25 mL
DMSO	25 mL
Distilled water	75 mL

The resulting solution is mixed well, allowed to stand for 30 minutes, and then filtered. The stain may be used immediately or kept indefinitely at room temperature in an amber glass bottle. The decolorizer–counterstain solution consists of 220 mL of a 2% aqueous solution of malachite green to which 30 mL glacial acetic acid and 50 mL glycerol are added and mixed well. Filtration is unnecessary. This solution keeps indefinitely in a closed container at room temperature.
Staining procedure: Fecal material is smeared over a 2.5 by 3.0-cm area of a clean, flamed glass slide and air-dried on a warming plate. The slide is prefixed in a Coplin jar of absolute methanol for 5–10 seconds, stained in carbol fuchsin–DMSO solution in a Coplin jar for 5 minutes, and rinsed in gently running tap water until excess solution no longer runs off. The slide is then placed in the decolorizer–counterstain for 1 minute or until a green background appears; it is then rinsed under running tap water for 10 seconds, drained, blotted, and placed on a warming plate until thoroughly dry. Slides are examined under low power ($\times$ 4). This procedure yields oocysts that are brilliant pink to fuchsia against a pale green background. Organisms seen on low-power screening are checked under oil immersion ($\times$ 100) for the typical *Cryptosporidium* internal vacuole and material clumped to one side of the 4- to 5-μm cyst.

10. MODIFIED DIENES' STAIN

Methylene blue	2.50 g
Azure II	1.25 g
Maltose	10.0 g
Na_2CO_3	0.25 g
Distilled water	100 mL

Prepare a 3% dilution of the Dienes' stain stock solution in water and filter it through a 0.22-μ filter.

Staining procedure: Cut out a small square (1 cm^2) of agar containing suspected colonies, and place it on a microscope slide with the colonies facing up. Make a petrolatum-parafin seal around the agar section, slightly higher than the agar block. Place 1 to 4 drops of the Dienes' stain working solution on the agar surface, completely covering the agar block with stain. Place a cover slip over the stained agar block, permitting it to contact the petrolatum seal. The cover slip should be as close as possible to the agar surface without touching it. Examine under oil immersion ($\times$ 1000) with a light microscope. *Mycoplasma* colonies stain blue, whereas most bacterial and fungal colonies appear colorless.

11. WRIGHT'S STAIN

Wright's stain (powder form)	3.0 g
Glycerol (C.P.)	30.0 mL
Absolute methanol (acetone-free)	970.0 mL

Place the Wright's stain in a large mortar. Add approximately 5.0 mL glycerol and 30.0 mL methanol and grind to dissolve.
Add the rest of the glycerol and methanol gradually until the dye is completely dissolved. Store in a dark, tightly stoppered bottle, and allow to mature for approximately 2 weeks. Filter before use.
Staining procedure: Cover air-dried smear with 2–3 mL Wright's stain. After staining for 2 minutes, add 2–3 mL phosphate buffer, pH 6.4, to the stain, blowing to mix stain and buffer. Rinse with buffer until all the purple stain is removed. Air dry and examine.

12. ZIEHL-NEELSEN CARBOL-FUCHSIN STAIN

Basic fuchsin	0.3 g
Ethanol (95%)	10 mL

Dissolve powder and add solution to 90 mL of a 5% aqueous solution of phenol. Store reagent in stoppered bottles to prevent evaporation. If crystals form during storage, the reagent should be filtered before use.
Staining procedure: Cover heat-fixed smear with absorbent paper. Add enough carbol-fuchsin (4–5 drops) to saturate paper. Gently heat the bottom of the slide until the stain begins to steam. Continue heating for 5 minutes but do not allow the stain to boil or dry. Add more carbol-fuchsin if necessary. Carefully lift paper from slide with forceps. Rinse smear with tap water and flood with acid alcohol (3 mL concentrated HCl to 97 mL of 95% ethanol) for 2 minutes. Rinse smear with tap water and flood slide with aqueous methylene blue (0.3 g methylene blue chloride in 100 mL distilled water) for 1–2 minutes. Rinse in tap water, drain, and dry.